Essentials of Pediatric Oncology Nursing

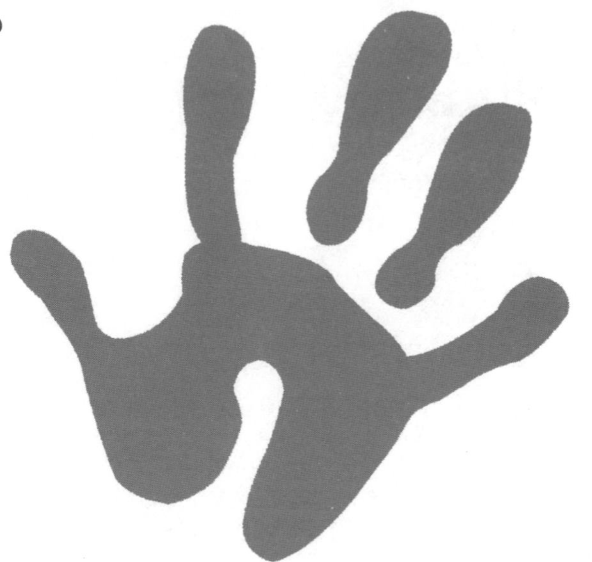

A CORE CURRICULUM, 2ND EDITION

Editor
Nancy E. Kline, PhD RN CPNP FAAN
Director of Nursing Research
Memorial Sloan-Kettering Cancer Center
New York, NY

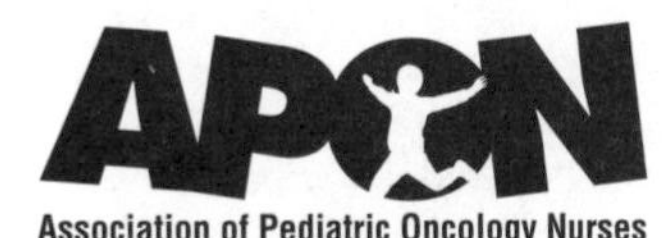

Association of Pediatric Oncology Nurses
4700 W. Lake Avenue
Glenview, IL 60025-1485

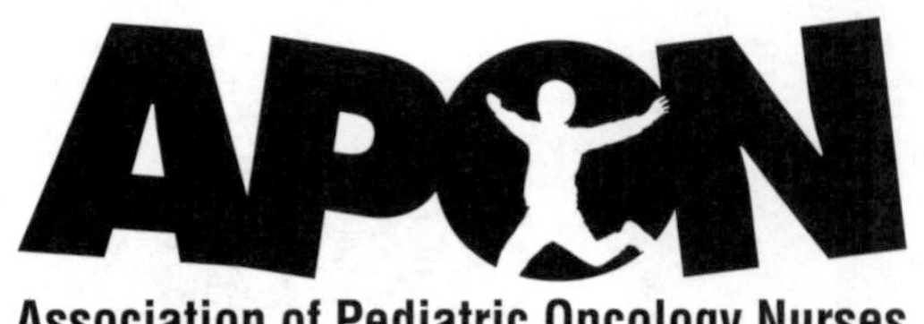

Staff

Executive Director: Louise S. Miller, MA

Managing Editor: Marilyn Ferdinand

Graphic Designer: Eric Trisilla

Editorial Assistant: Frank Broz

Printed in the United States of America

Association of Pediatric Oncology Nurses
4700 W. Lake Avenue
Glenview, IL 60025-1485

Library of Congress Catalog Number: 98-073093
ISBN 0-9666193-8-2

Note: As new scientific information becomes available through basic and clinical research, recommended treatments and drug therapies undergo changes. The authors, editors, and publisher have done everything possible to make this book accurate, up-to-date, and in accord with standards accepted at the time of publication. The recommendations contained herein reflect APON's judgment regarding the state of general knowledge and practice in the field as of the date of publication. Any practice described in this book should be applied by the healthcare practitioner in accordance with professional standards of care used in regard to the unique circumstances that may apply in each situation. The reader is advised always to check product information (package inserts) for changes and new information regarding does and contraindications before administering any drug. Caution is especially urged when using new or infrequently ordered drugs or treatments. Figures and tables in the book are used as examples only. They are not meant to be all-inclusive, nor do they represent endorsement of any particular institution by APON. Any mention of specific products and opinions related to those products do not indicate or imply endorsement by **APON. THE AUTHORS, EDITORS, AND PUBLISHER ARE NOT RESPONSIBLE FOR ERRORS OR OMISSIONS OR FOR CONSEQUENCES FROM APPLICATION OF THE BOOK, AND MAKE NO WARRANTY, EXPRESSED OR IMPLIED, IN REGARD TO THE CONTENTS OF THE BOOK.**

Editor

Nancy E. Kline, PhD RN CPNP FAAN
Director of Nursing Research
Memorial Sloan-Kettering Cancer Center
New York, NY

Section Editors

Mary C. Hooke, MSN RN APRN-BC CPON®
Clinical Nurse Specialist, Hematology-Oncology Program
Children's Hospitals and Clinics
Minneapolis/St. Paul, MN

Robbie Norville, MSN RN CPON®
Clinical Nurse Specialist
Texas Children's Cancer Center
Texas Children's Hospital
Houston, TX

Jill E. Brace O'Neill, MS RN-CS PNP
Pediatric Nurse Practitioner
Dana-Farber Cancer Institute
Boston, MA

Karla Wilson, MSN RN FNP CPON®
Family Nurse Practitioner, Department of Pediatrics
City of Hope National Medical Center
Duarte, CA

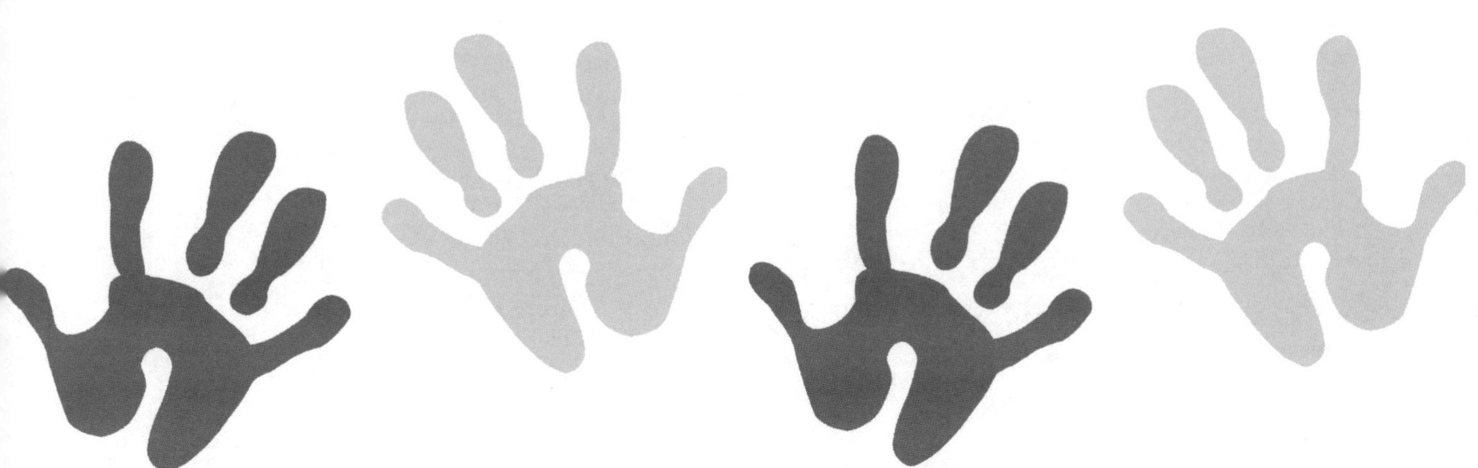

Contributors

Kathleen Adlard, MN RN CPON®
Clinical Nurse Specialist
Children's Hospital of Orange County
Orange, CA

Arlene L. Androkites, MSN RN CPNP
Pediatric Nurse Practitioner
Dana-Farber Cancer Institute
Boston, MA

Sarah J. Bottomley, MN RN CPNP
Pediatric Nurse Practitioner
Texas Children's Cancer Center
Texas Children's Hospital
Houston, TX

Brian Brooks, MDiv
Chaplain, Hematology-Oncology Program
Children's Hospitals and Clinics
Minneapolis/St. Paul, MN

Cathy J. Burks, MSN RN CPON®
Pediatric Clinical Nurse Specialist
Children's Mercy Hospital
Kansas City, MO

Sandy Call, PharmD
Clinical Pharmacist for BMT
St. Jude Children's Research Hospital
Memphis, TN

Amanda Carnes, BSN RN OCN
Clinic Nurse
Jimmy Fund Clinic
Dana Farber Cancer Institute
Boston, MA

Lorraine Cogan, LMSW
Social Worker
Texas Children's Hospital
Houston, TX

Karen A. Conley, MS RN AOCN
Program Manager, Pediatric Oncology
Dana-Farber Cancer Institute
Boston, MA

Susanne B. Conley, BSN RN CPON®
Clinical Nurse Specialist
Dana Farber Cancer Institute
Boston, MA

Virginia M. Kimball Dalton, MS RN PNP
Clinical and Research Nurse Practitioner
Pediatric Leukemia Program
Dana-Farber Cancer Institute
Boston, MA

Diane Dingley, MS CCLS
Certified Child Life Specialist
Children's Hospitals and Clinics
Minneapolis/St. Paul, MN

Shawn Elliott, MSN RNC
PC Nurse Manager
MD Anderson Cancer Center
Huffman, TX

Debra A. Eshelman, MSN RN CPNP
Pediatric Nurse Practitioner
Children's Medical Center of Dallas
Dallas, TX

Angela Ethier, MSN RN CNS CPN
Research Fellow & Clinical Instructor
Texas Children's Hospital
Houston, TX

Kathy Forte, MS RN CPNP
Advanced Practice Nurse
AFLAC Cancer Center and Blood Disorders Service
Children's Healthcare of Atlanta
Atlanta, GA

Elisa S. Frederick, MSN RN CS PNP
Pediatric Oncology Nurse Practitioner
Jimmy Fund Clinic
Dana-Farber Cancer Institute
Boston, MA 02115

Jami S. Gattuso, MSN RN CPON®
Nursing Research Specialist
St. Jude Children's Research Hospital
Memphis, TN

Marci Klein Gross, LMSW
Social Worker
Texas Children's Hospital
Houston, TX

Brittany Hardiman, BSN RN CPON®
Staff Nurse/Clinical Educator
Children's Hospital
Boston, MA

Jennifer Harley, MSN RN
Clinical Director
Riley Children's Hospital
Greenwood, IN

Contributors

Beth Hasenauer, MS RN
Clinical Research Nurse
Children's Hospital Los Angeles
Administrative Director
New Approaches to Neuroblastoma Therapy (NANT) Consortium
Monrovia, CA

Melody Hellsten, MS APRN- BC PNP
Instructor, Department of Pediatrics
Baylor College of Medicine
Houston, TX

Jane Hennessy, MPH RN CNP CPON®
Pediatric Nurse Practitioner, Hematology-Oncology Program
Children's Hospitals and Clinics
Minneapolis/St. Paul, MN

Joy Hesselgrave, MSN RNC CPON®
Clinical Nurse Specialist
Texas Children's Cancer Center
Texas Children's Hospital
Houston, TX

Barbara Anne Hieb, MSN RN CRNP
Pediatric Nurse Practitioner, Survivorship Program
Children's Hospital of Philadelphia
Philadelphia, PA

Wendy L. Hobbie, MNS RN CRNP
Coordinator, Survivorship Program and
Advanced Practice Oncology Nurses
Children's Hospital of Philadelphia
Philadelphia, PA

Mary C. Hooke, MSN RN, APRN-BC CPON®
Clinical Nurse Specialist, Hematology-Oncology Program
Children's Hospitals and Clinics
Minneapolis/St. Paul, MN

CJ Hutto, MHA RN CPON®
Division Manager
Division of Hematology/Oncology
Children's Mercy Hospital and Clinics
Kansas City, MO

Nancy E. Kline, PhD RN CPNP FAAN
Director of Nursing Research
Memorial Sloan Kettering Cancer Center
New York, NY

Asako Komiya, MSN RN PNP
Pediatric Nurse Practitioner
City of Hope National Medical Center
Duarte, CA

Ruth Landers, MSN RN CPNP CPON®
Pediatric Nurse Practitioner
Arkansas Children's Hospital
Little Rock, AR

Wendy Landier, MSN RN CPNP CPON®
Pediatric Nurse Practitioner
City of Hope National Medical Center
Duarte, CA
Assistant Clinical Professor
UCLA School of Nursing
Los Angeles, CA

Eileen Duffey Lind, MSN RN CPNP CPON®
Pediatric Oncology Nurse Practitioner
Dana-Farber Cancer Institute
Boston, MA

Kenneth J. A. Lown, MSN RN CPNP
Pediatric Nurse Practitioner
The Children's Hospital of Philadelphia
Philadelphia, PA

Catherine Fiona Macpherson, MSN RN CS CPON®
Educator of Clinical Faculty
Hematology/Oncology/HPCT Unit
Children's Hospital & Medical Center
Seattle, WA

Linda Madsen, MS RN CPON®
Certified Nurse Practitioner
Children's Hospitals and Clinics
Minneapolis, MN

Kathleen Marson MS RN PNP
Nurse Practitioner
Pediatric Hematology/Oncology
Boston Pediatric Floating Hospital at NEMCH
Boston, MA

Rebecca Monroe, MSN RN CPNP CPON®
Pediatric Nurse Practitioner, Bone Marrow Transplant
Baylor College of Medicine
Texas Children's Cancer Center
Texas Children's Hospital
Houston, TX

Revonda B. Mosher, MSN RN CPNP
Advanced Practice Clinician
Children's National Medical Center
Washington, DC

Robbie Norville, MSN RN CPON®
Clinical Nurse Specialist
Texas Children's Cancer Center
Texas Children's Hospital
Houston, TX

Contributors

Suzanne L. Nuss, MSN RN CPNP
Clinical Nurse Specialist
University of Nebraska Medical Center
Omaha, NE

Susan K. Ogle, MSN CRNP
Pediatric Nurse Practitioner, Survivorship Program
Children's Hospital of Philadelphia
Philadelphia, PA

Eileen Whyte O'Holleran, MSN RN CPNP
Bone Marrow Transplant Nurse Practitioner
Jimmy Fund Clinic
Dana Farber Cancer Institute
Boston, MA

Jill E. Brace O'Neill, MS RN-CS PNP
Pediatric Nurse Practitioner
Dana-Farber Cancer Institute
Boston, MA

Janice Post-White, PhD RN FAAN
Associate Professor
University of Minnesota School of Nursing
Minneapolis, MN

Anna Pursell, MSN RN FNP
Clinical Nurse
UCLA Medical Center
Costa Mesa, CA

Elizabeth Randall, BSN RNBC
Unit Educator–Ambulatory Care Unit
St. Jude Children's Research Hospital
Memphis, TN

Debbie Reid, BSN RN CPON®
Education Manager, Hematology/Oncology
Children's Hospital Los Angeles
Duarte, CA

Lona Roll, MSN RN
Clinical Nurse Specialist, Pediatric Hematology/Oncology
Christus Santa Rosa Children's Hospital
San Antonio, TX

Patricia M. Rubino, MSN RN CPNP
Clinical Manager
Riley Children's Hospital
Greenwood, IN

Kathy Ruccione, MPH RN FAAN
Co-Director, Health Promotion and Outcomes Program
Center Nursing Administrator
Associate Professor of Clinical Pediatrics
Keck School of Medicine
University of Southern California
Los Angeles, CA

Tamara E. Scott, MSN RN CPNP CPON®
Pediatric Nurse Practitioner
Kaiser Permanente Medical Center
Sacramento, CA

Rita Secola, MSN RN CPON®
Clinical Manager
Children's Hospital Los Angeles
Los Angeles, CA

Cynthia A. Stutzer, MS RN
Clinical Nurse Specialist-Pediatric Oncology
British Columbia Children's Hospital
Vancouver, BC, Canada

Christine Sullivan, MSN PNP RNC
Pediatric Nurse Practitioner
University of Massachusetts Medical Center
Worcester, MA

Lisa Jean Thomas, MSN RN PNP
Pediatric Nurse Practitioner
Dana-Farber Cancer Institute
Boston, MA

Debbie Toomey, MSN RN PNP CPON®
Pediatric Nurse Practitioner
City of Hope
Duarte, CA

Carolyn Walker, PhD RN
Professor, School of Nursing
San Diego State University
San Diego, CA

Joetta Deswarte Wallace, MSN RN CPON®
Clinical Nurse Specialist, Pediatric Hematology/Oncology
Miller Children's Hospital
Long Beach, CA

Melody Ann Watral, MSN RN CPNP CPON®
Pediatric Nurse Practitioner
The Brain Tumor Center at Duke University Medical Center
Durham, NC

Karla Wilson, MSN RN FNP CPON®
Family Nurse Practitioner, Department of Pediatrics
City of Hope National Medical Center
Duarte, CA

Table of Contents

Section I. Pediatric Oncology Nursing Practice

Section II. Pediatric Cancers

Section III. Overview of Hematology

Section IV. Childhood Cancer Treatment

Acknowledgments

The second edition of *Essentials of Pediatric Oncology Nursing: A Core Curriculum* is the product of many hours of hard work by numerous dedicated individuals. I am indebted to the section editors who worked tirelessly to make this the premier reference text for the core knowledge that all pediatric oncology nurses should have. I also want to acknowledge our contributors, who took time to research and update their chapters. This work was done in addition to their individual clinical responsibilities, and I certainly appreciate their expertise and dedication to this project.

Nancy E. Kline, Editor

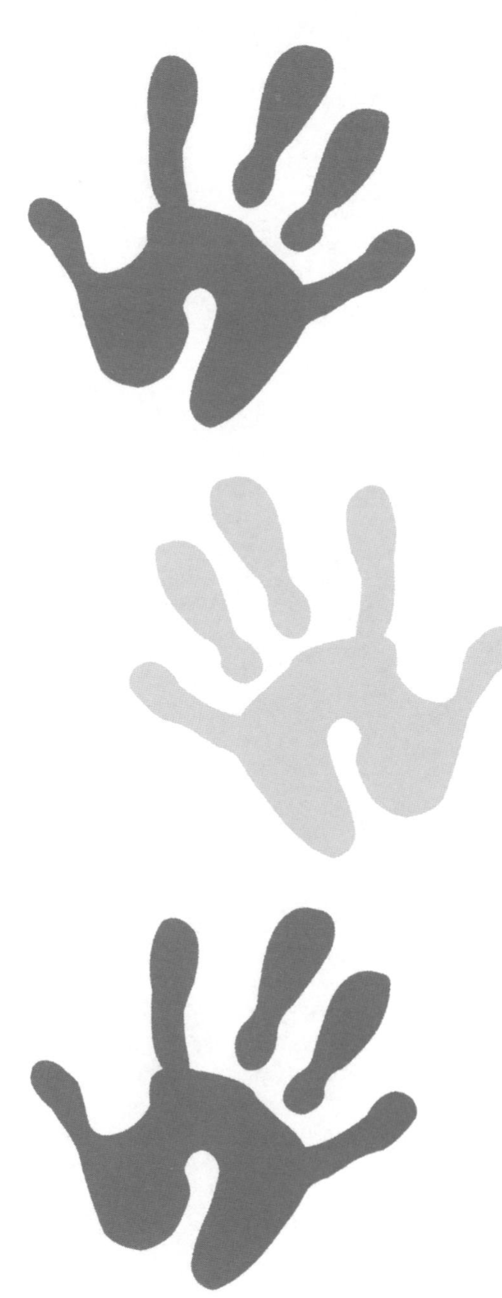

SECTION I

Pediatric Oncology Nursing Practice

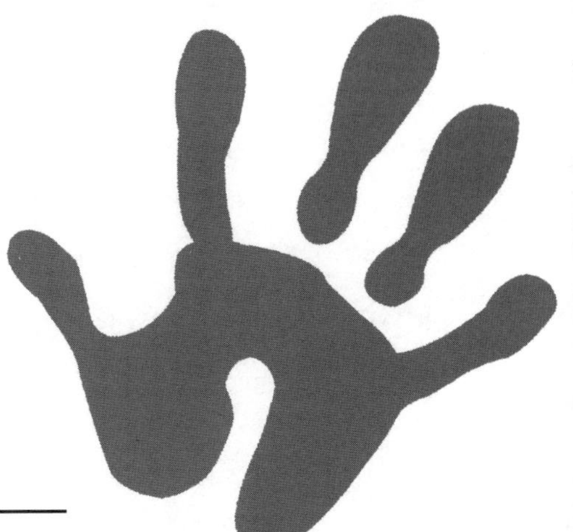

Mary C. Hooke

Section Outline

History and Philosophy of Pediatric Oncology Nursing

Carolyn L. Walker

Pediatric oncology nursing is concerned with the holistic care of children with cancer. Consequently, although some treatment necessitates hospitalization, pediatric oncology nurses support outpatient treatment whenever possible. As a pediatric specialty that includes all ages, from infancy through adolescence, pediatric oncology nursing encompasses a sound knowledge of normal growth and development and family-centered care. As an oncology discipline, pediatric oncology nursing has a knowledge base and practice that involve early detection, treatment, follow-up of late effects, as well as prevention of adult cancers through education about cancer risks during childhood.

History of Cancer

The first evidence of the existence of cancer was found among the ancient Greek and Egyptian civilizations, and it was Hippocrates, a Greek physician who lived from 460 to 370 BC, who first used the term *karbinos,* meaning crab, to describe a cancer. Hippocrates also presented one of the earliest theories of cancer's cause—an excess of black bile, or *melanchole* (Foley & Fergusson, 2003). His beliefs were virtually unchallenged for 2,000 years.

In 1792, a cancer ward containing 17 beds was opened in Middlesex, England. In 1884, Simms Hospital was opened in New York City. Simms Hospital later became Memorial Sloan-Kettering Cancer Center, the first hospital in the United States devoted to cancer care. Both of these institutions initially focused on the treatment of cancer in adults. Prior to the 20th century, rates of infant and childhood mortality were high due to infection and malnutrition, so many children died long before they would have been likely to develop cancer. In 1936, the eight leading causes of death in children were accidents, pneumonia, diarrhea, influenza, appendicitis, tuberculosis, diseases of the heart, and diphtheria—in that order. Cancer was ninth, with five deaths per 100,000 children per year (Foley & Fergusson, 2003). Health problems related to infectious diseases were so formidable that pediatric cancers were not the greatest concern.

Cancer remained a poorly understood disease until the invention of the microscope in the 18th century and X rays in the early 20th century. With these inventions, medicine had a window on the internal workings of the body. Until that time, visible tumors were the primary source of knowledge about cancer and were treated only by surgery, if at all. The discovery of radium in 1898 led to the development of radiation therapy as an important treatment modality. However, the two most dramatic events that brought the science and specialty of pediatric oncology into its own were (a) the development of antibiotic therapies that decreased infant and childhood mortality from infections and (b) the discovery during World War II that nitrogen mustard used in chemical warfare had anticancer properties. Because of the changes brought about after the discovery of antibiotics, cancer became the second leading cause of death (after accidents), as is still the case today (**Table 1-1**).

History of Childhood Cancer Treatment

The first pediatric cancer unit in the United States was established in 1939 at the Memorial Sloan-Kettering Cancer Center in New York. St. Jude Children's Research Hospital was the first facility devoted exclusively to pediatric malignancies. The first giant step in the treatment of cancer was taken in the 1940s with the discovery that folic acid antagonists produced temporary remissions in children with acute leukemia. In the 1950s and 1960s, single drugs were moderately successful until it was discovered that combinations of chemotherapy agents worked much better than single-drug therapy. This was a dramatic breakthrough. By the 1970s, childhood leukemia was responding dramatically to combination chemotherapy. Wilms' tumor is another example. Forty years ago, this most common kidney cancer in children was considered to be about 20% curable. Today, however, 90% of the children with this disease are cured. Similar success is being seen with most of the childhood cancer (Reis, 1999).

Rapid discoveries were made possible by national cooperative studies. The Children's Cancer Group and the Pediatric Oncology Group were established in 1955 under the auspices of the National Cancer Institute. Major cancer centers and most children's hospitals participated in these study groups from the very beginning, and most children with cancer were enrolled in protocol studies. As a result, information concerning cancer treatments was rapidly developed. The effect of this information reached far beyond the field of pediatric oncology, which is a relatively small field in oncology, and influenced the development of treatment for adults. The successes of national study groups in discovering the use of combination chemotherapy, developing adjunct therapies, and organizing treatment by means of cooperative studies were all pioneered in pediatrics (Hockenberry, Coody, & Falletta, 1986). In 1998, Children's Cancer Group, Pediatric Oncology Group, National Wilms' Tumor Study Group, and the International Rhabdomyosarcoma Study Group joined together in a unified group named the Children's Oncology Group (COG).

The impact of the cooperative studies in pediatrics occurred not just in the development of multidrug chemotherapy, but also in the development of individualized combinations of modalities as well. It became evident that different tumors responded differently to therapies. For example, although radiation therapy was appropriate for Ewing's sarcoma, it was not effective for osteogenic sarcoma. Protocols were adjusted accordingly. The late 1960s and the 1970s was a very exciting time of experimentation in the establishment of pediatric oncology treatment regimens.

Pediatric Oncology Nursing as a Specialty

Nursing, like medicine, was originally generic in its practice in that all nurses took care of all patients. As medicine became increasingly specialized, so did nursing. Nurse anesthetists and nurse midwives, who formed their own organizations early in the 20th century, were the first specialty

Table 1-1. Fifteen Leading Causes of Death Among Children Aged 1 to 14, United States, 2000

Rank	Cause of Death	Number of Deaths	Percent Deaths	(%) of Death Rate*
	All Causes	12,392	100.0	22.0
1	Accidents (unintentional injuries)	4,805	38.8	8.5
2	Cancer	1,434	11.6	2.5
3	Congenital anomalies	894	7.2	1.6
4	Assault (homicide)	727	5.9	1.3
5	Heart diseases	452	3.6	0.8
6	Intentional self-harm (suicide)	307	2.5	0.5
7	Chronic lower respiratory diseases	190	1.5	0.3
8	Pneumonia and influenza	190	1.5	0.3
9	Septicemia	162	1.3	0.3
10	Cerebrovascular diseases	123	0.9	0.2
11	Anemias	87	0.7	0.2
12	Meningitis	66	0.5	0.1
13	HIV disease	60	0.5	0.1
14	Complications of medical and surgical care	53	0.4	0.1
15	Nephritis, nephrotic syndrome, nephrosis	39	0.3	0.1
	All others	2,225	18.0	

* Rates are per 100,000 population and age-adjusted to the U.S. standard population.

Note: Percentages may not total 100% due to rounding.

Source: Jemal, A., Murray, T., Samuels, A., Ghafoor, A., Ward, E., & Thun, M. J., (2003). Cancer statistics, 2003. *CA: A Cancer Journal for Clinicians, 53,* 5–26.

nurses. The first recognition of oncology as a specialty was the development of the first academic course devoted exclusively to cancer nursing at Teacher's College at Columbia University in 1947 (Craytor, 1982). At that time, nurses who took care of children with cancer were pediatric nurses. Care of a child with cancer was short in duration and involved helping a family and child face certain death. For the most part, these children, who most commonly were diagnosed with leukemia, bled to death due to the unavailability of component blood therapies, such as platelets. Intravenous therapies were primitive; there were no central lines or parenteral nutrition. The nurse's role entailed encouraging fulfillment of nutritional needs (nurses themselves often cooked special foods for the child), managing infections or the constant threat of infection, and supporting the family and the child. Struggling to prevent or treat infection with first-generation antibiotics involved working in reverse isolation with patients who had fever and neutropenia.

It was not until the mid-1970s that pediatric oncology nursing began to be recognized as a distinct subspecialty. With the advent of combination therapies in the late 1960s and 1970s, patients had very specialized care needs. In addition, the increased survival of children treated for cancer demanded a very broad-based body of knowledge. A cadre of pioneers in pediatric oncology nursing started to emerge. In 1974, the Association of Pediatric Oncology Nurses (APON) was formed by a group of nurses who had attended the Association for the Care of Children's Health Conference in 1973. The incorporation of APON took place in 1976 (Greene, 1983). The roots of pediatric oncology nursing are planted securely in pediatrics for two reasons: Patients are children first and foremost, with all the special and unique needs that children have, and most of their cancers are significantly different from adult cancers because pediatric cancers, unlike those of adults, are generally systemic rather than organ-based tumors. For both of these reasons, the therapy and care of children with cancer are different from the care of adults with cancer. Today, pediatric oncology nursing is recognized as a distinct subspecialty in pediatrics as well as in oncology. This distinction was formalized with the development of specialty certification in pediatric oncology nursing in 1993.

Pediatric oncology nursing focuses on the care of children with cancer. The nurse's role has changed from one that focuses on the dying child and bereaved family to one that focuses on a broad knowledge base of childhood cancer, its treatment, side effects, and the impact on the child and the family. Because pediatric oncology nurses now work with a patient population that has an expectation of survival and probable cure, the philosophy of family-centered care is central to the practice. This philosophy is exemplified by nursing care that is mutually planned with the family from the time of diagnosis. The child is included in decisions at a developmentally appropriate level. Over the past 20 years, pediatric cancer has become, in many cases, a chronic disease that has changed the scope of practice for the pediatric oncology nurse to include the knowledge and care of long-term survivors. These children, who have the prospect of a life time ahead of them, need to receive cancer therapy with minimal long-term emotional consequences. A pediatric oncology nurse works with the child and the child's family from the day of diagnosis, helping them adjust to the probable chronicity of the illness. The goal of care is to maintain as much normalcy as possible for the child and the family throughout treatment. The philosophy of family-centered care is "recognition that the family is the constant in the child's life" (Shelton, Jeppson, & Johnson, 1992, p. 3). This philosophy permeates the entire practice of pediatric oncology nursing. Issues related to long-term survivorship require nurses to be able to recognize the effects of therapy and the necessity of educating children about adult cancer risks that start in childhood, such as skin cancer and lung cancer related to smoking. At the same time, the pediatric oncology nurse is familiar with providing care for the child and family in the event the child will die from the disease. The philosophy of family-centered care is practiced by facilitating care that will allow the child to die at home if the family wishes, as well as by organizing follow-up bereavement counseling for the child's family.

It is the philosophy of pediatric oncology nursing that the best care is provided to patients with cancer and their families when there is team collaboration. This team includes the cancer center's healthcare team, the family, community healthcare workers, and school staff. A commitment to family-centered care, strong team collaboration, and maintaining as normal a lifestyle as possible for the child with cancer are the hallmarks of the philosophy of pediatric oncology nursing. These principles allow nurses to provide individualized care in the hope of cure for the child with cancer within the child's own family and social environment.

References

Craytor, J.K. (1982). Highlights in education for cancer nursing. *Oncology Nursing Forum, 9*(4), 51–59.

Foley, G.V., & Fergusson, J.H. (2003). History, issues, and trends. In C. R. Baggott, K. P. Kelly, D. Fochtman, & G. V. Foley (Eds.), *Nursing care of children and adolescents with cancer* (pp. 2-23). Philadelphia: W.B. Saunders.

Greene, P. E. (1983). The association of pediatric oncology nurses: The first ten years. *Oncology Nursing Forum, 10*, 59–63.

Hockenberry, M. J., Coody, D. K., & Falletta, J. M. (1986). Introduction to childhood cancer. In M. J. Hockenberry and D. K. Coody (Eds.), *Pediatric oncology and hematology: Perspective of care* (pp. 3–13). St. Louis: Mosby.

Ries, L.A.G. (1999). Childhood cancer mortality. In L. A. G. Ries, M. A. Smith, J. G. Gurney, et al. (Eds.). *Cancer incidence and survival among children and adolescents: United States SEER Program 1975-1995*). National Cancer Institute, SEER Program. (NIH Pub. No. 99-4649, pp. 165–170). Bethesda, MD: National Cancer Institute.

Shelton, T. L., Jeppson, E. S., & Johnson, B. H. (1992). *Family-centered care for children with special health care needs* (2nd ed.). Bethesda, MD: Association for the Care of Children's Health.

Standards of Pediatric Oncology Nursing

Revonda B. Mosher

In 1978 the Association of Pediatric Oncology Nurses, in collaboration with the American Nurses Association, published the first pediatric oncology nursing standards, *Standards of Pediatric Oncology Nursing Practice*. In 1987 the Association of Pediatric Oncology Nurses revised the standards in the publication and published them under the title *Scope of Practice and Outcome Standard of Practice for Pediatric Oncology Nurses*. This set of standards incorporated the nursing process and outcome standards. The Association of Pediatric Oncology Nurses and the American Nurses Association published the latest edition, *Scope and Standards of Pediatric Oncology Nursing Practice,* in 2000.

Nursing standards are rules or definitions of what a nurse does to provide competent care. Standards of nursing care have three components: professional standards of care, professional performance standards, and specialty practice guidelines. *Scope and Standards of Pediatric Oncology Nursing Practice* is an example of specialty practice guidelines. Standards of care and standards of professional performance are outlined for the pediatric oncology clinical nurse and the pediatric oncology advanced practice nurse (APN). These standards are critical in guiding pediatric oncology nurses to deliver high-quality nursing care. The comprehensive standards are summarized below.

Standards of Care for the Pediatric Oncology Clinical Nurse

Standard I. Assessment: Collection and documentation of data regarding child and family. Assessment in the areas of physical care, growth and development, psychosocial care at various points in the treatment process, education, palliative care, long-term survival, and prevention and early detection are included in the data collection process.

Standard II. Diagnosis: Determination of the diagnosis by using assessment data from nursing and other disciplines. Individual problems and appropriate interventions can be identified once diagnoses are known.

Standard III. Outcome Identification: Identification of outcomes to help the nurse, child, and family work toward mutually agreed-upon goals of care. Expected outcomes may include adequate education, optimal growth and development, optimal physical and emotional health, symptom management, early detection of secondary malignancies, limited late effects, or a comfortable, dignified death.

Standard IV. Planning: Prescription of interventions that will achieve the expected outcomes. The plan of care incorporates evidence-based knowledge of oncology nursing. The child and family are active participants in achieving outcomes. The financial, social, spiritual, and cultural domains of the family are considered essential to the plan of care.

Standard V. Implementation: Implementation of the plan of care to meet the expected outcomes of the child and family. The nurse works with other healthcare professionals to implement a plan of care that will improve the child's health status and quality of life and optimize family functioning.

Standard VI. Evaluation: Measurement of the child and family's progress toward expected outcomes on an ongoing basis. The evaluation process is carried out continually. Revisions of the diagnosis, expected outcomes, and plan of care may be necessary if the evaluation reflects that the expected outcomes have not been attained.

Standards of Professional Performance of the Pediatric Oncology Clinical Nurse

Standard I. Quality of Care: Active participation in improving the quality and effectiveness of nursing care. The pediatric oncology nurse integrates new knowledge, technology, and therapeutic strategies into the care of children with cancer in order to improve outcomes and quality.

Standard II. Performance Appraisal: Self-evaluation in relation to practice standards and legal statutes and regulations. The pediatric oncology nurse acquires the required competencies needed to provide quality care. The nurse is able to identify his or her strengths and weaknesses and initiate methods to improve his or her performance.

Standard III. Education: Demonstration of competency in pediatric oncology nursing practice and maintenance of current knowledge. The pediatric oncology nurse realizes that scientific inquiry and ongoing learning are essential to one's professional development. The nurse participates in educational activities, obtains certification as appropriate, and uses skilled colleagues as resources to improve his or her knowledge base and performance.

Standard IV. Collegiality: Contribution to the professional development of peers, colleagues, and others. The pediatric oncology nurse is a leader in sharing knowledge of pediatric oncology nursing and serves as both a formal and an informal preceptor or mentor. The nurse identifies the learning needs of others and fosters their professional development, contributing to improved care for children with cancer.

Standard V. Ethics: Recognition of the rights of children and families and decision making in accordance with ethical principles. The nurse advocates for the rights of children with cancer and helps resolve the ethical crises that sometimes arise in life-and-death situations or as the result of technological advances. The nurse ensures that families have accurate information to facilitate the decision making that must be made on behalf of their children.

Standard VI. Collaboration: Collaboration with the multidisciplinary team to assess, plan, implement, and evaluate care of the child with cancer. The nurse collaborates with other team members whose unique abilities can contribute to the care of child with complex and intensive needs. This collaboration may include referrals to community and home-based resources.

Standard VII. Research: Utilization of research to deliver the best evidence-based nursing care. The nurse participates in and reviews research and utilizes research findings. The nurse ensures that protocol requirements are met for patients who are enrolled in clinical trials (most children with cancer are). The nurse identifies clinical questions for scientific inquiry.

Standard VIII. Resource Utilization: Skillful management of the care environment, ensuring that it is safe, effective, and cost-effective. The nurse uses appropriate resources so that safe, effective care can be delivered in a cost-effective way. Decisions regarding benefits and costs of care are made without compromising expected or desired outcomes.

Standards of Care for the Pediatric Oncology Advanced Practice Nurse

The pediatric oncology advanced practice nurse (APN) complies with the standards of care and professional performance of the clinical nurse while blending the roles of pediatric and oncology APN. Like the standards for the clinical nurse, the APN standards address the areas of assessment, diagnosis, outcome identification, planning, implementation, and evaluation.

Standard I. Assessment: Collection of data and use of assessment skills to determine the physical, emotional, cultural, and social needs of the child and family as well as their general well-being. The APN assesses the child in the areas of physical care, growth and development, psychosocial care, education, palliative care, long-term survival, and prevention and early detection. The data include physical assessment findings as well as diagnostic, imaging, and laboratory tests.

Standard II. Diagnosis: Analysis of assessment data to identify actual and potential diagnoses. The APN develops differential diagnoses and validates them with the child and family and with members of the healthcare team. The APN prioritizes diagnoses and resultant actions based on the child's most acute needs at the time of the assessment.

Standard III. Outcome Identification: Development of expected outcomes in collaboration with the multidisciplinary team when appropriate. Focused expected outcomes help the child return to optimal health or experience a peaceful death. The APN uses critical thinking skills, research findings, and advanced clinical knowledge to develop measurable, realistic outcomes.

Standard IV. Planning: Formulation and implementation of a prioritized plan of care, including interventions based on the diagnoses to achieve desired outcomes. The APN prescribes interventions that reflect advanced clinical knowledge and research findings. The plan should include patient and family education about potential acute side effects and late effects, as well as interventions for health promotion, restoration, and maintenance.

Standard V. Implementation: Implementation of the plan of care using the various components of the APN's role (case management, consultation, health promotion, education, prescriptive authority, referral, and research). The APN prescribes and implements plans of care that are within the scope of his or her practice.

Standard Va. Case management/coordination of care. The pediatric oncology APN provides comprehensive clinical coordination of care throughout the relationship with the child and family.

Standard Vb. Consultation. Consultation for health issues can improve the health of a particular child or a larger population or community.

Standard Vc. Health promotion, health maintenance, and health teaching. The pediatric oncology APN uses strategies and interventions to promote and maintain a return to health with minimal complications and late effects of therapy. He or she also teaches children, their families, and the community about pediatric and oncology health concerns.

Standard Vd. Prescriptive authority and treatment. In accordance with state and federal regulations, the APN prescribes and furnishes medications and treatments and performs procedures that aid in the diagnosis and treatment of children with cancer.

Standard Ve. Referral. The APN recognizes the limits of his or her knowledge base and scope of practice. The APN makes appropriate referrals to other resources or specialists, in consultation with the pediatric oncologist as needed.

Standard VI. Evaluation: Evaluation of the response to the plan and interventions, and monitoring of the progress toward achievement of expected outcomes. The APN, in conjunction with the child, family, and healthcare team, evaluates responses to interventions and revises plans and interventions as needed.

Standards of Professional Performance for the Pediatric Oncology Advanced Practice Nurse

Standard I. Quality of care: Evaluation of quality of care in terms of clinical outcomes and the effectiveness of clinical and advanced pediatric oncology nursing practice. The APN develops and monitors standards of care, analyzes outcome data, participates in quality improvement activities, and collaborates with the healthcare team to improve quality of care.

Standard II. Self-Evaluation: Accountability to oneself, the public, and the profession to provide competent care. Self-assessment includes soliciting feedback from peers, colleagues, and other healthcare members, identifying one's personal strengths, weaknesses, and learning needs, and developing performance goals.

Standard III. Education: Acquisition and maintenance of current knowledge and skills in the area of pediatric oncology nursing and related disciplines as appropriate. Certification, licensure, educational opportunities, and awareness of his or her learning needs help the APN maintain clinical expertise.

Standard IV. Leadership: Service as a leader, role model, and mentor for the professional development of peers, colleagues, staff, and students. Leadership skills are developed by contributing to the professional development and education of others and by participation in professional and specialty organizations. The APN shares knowledge by presenting or publishing in his or her area of expertise and advocating in various arenas for the needs of children with cancer and their families.

Standard V. Ethics: Respect for the rights of all children and families; conformity to ethical principles when making decisions and designing interventions. The APN ensures that the rights of children and families are respected by maintaining confidentiality, ensuring that a family is sufficiently educated to make informed care decisions, and resolving ethical conflicts. Equal care is delivered to all children regardless of race, culture, ethnicity, socioeconomic status, or ability to pay.

Standard VI. Interdisciplinary Process: Promotion of and collaboration with the multidisciplinary team to care for the child and family. Pediatric oncology care is complex and requires collaboration among healthcare team members, other medical and nursing disciplines, COG, and the child's family.

Standard VII. Research: Contribution to nursing knowledge through utilization of research findings and maintenance of an evidence-based practice. The APN promotes research by encouraging evidence-based practices, developing researchable ideas, collaborating with others to develop research proposals, participating in clinical trials research, and protecting the rights of research subjects.

Summary

Pediatric oncology nursing involves caring for children with cancer across a continuum, from diagnosis to cure or a peaceful death. The care is delivered in many settings: inpatient and outpatient settings, the home, the school, the community, and possibly, a hospice setting. Family-centered care is a consistent goal across the treatment continuum and in all settings. The core values of family-centered care include

- recognizing that the family is the constant in a child's life, while the healthcare system and personnel within that system fluctuate
- encouraging collaboration between the family and professionals in all levels and settings of care
- sharing of complete and unbiased information between families and professionals on an ongoing basis
- implementing policies and practices that recognize and honor cultural diversity, strengths, and individuality within families, including geographic, ethnic, racial, socioeconomic, educational, and spiritual diversity
- respecting different methods of coping and developing policies and programs that address the diverse needs of families
- encouraging family-to-family support and networking
- ensuring that healthcare systems are flexible, accessible, and responsive to family needs
- valuing and recognizing that families and children have multiple strengths, concerns, and aspirations beyond their specialized healthcare needs.

The facilitation of family-centered care by the pediatric oncology nurse provides the healthcare team and the family with an environment of mutual respect, quality care, and satisfactory outcomes, regardless of the outcome of the disease in the child.

Association of Pediatric Oncology Nurses

CJ Hutto

In 1973, four pediatric oncology nurses attending an Association of the Care of Children's Health (ACCH) conference envisioned the formation of an association specifically for their own specialty. At a meeting on November 3, 1974, the first members of the new group adopted a name—the Association of Pediatric Oncology Nurses (APON)—elected their first officers, began developing the bylaws, and founded the newsletter (Heiney & Wiley, 1996). Despite the significant amount of time and energy that was consumed in establishing the structure of the organization, the meeting participants also discussed educational offerings to improve the care of children with cancer (Heiney & Wiley). The association was officially incorporated on April 15, 1976, with 85 charter members. One of the premises for the development of this association was the recognition of the unique characteristics and needs of the nurse caring for the pediatric oncology patient.

In 2001, APON revised its structure. Primary objectives of encouraging membership volunteerism and promoting efficiency of operations and product development were established. The vision statement created during the developmental stages of APON was revised in 2001 to reflect changes within the organization and the healthcare industry APON's vision statement is now "Children and adolescents with cancer and blood disorders and their families will receive the highest quality of care" (APON, 2003). In support of this vision, a mission statement was also developed: "APON will provide and promote expertise in pediatric hematology/oncology nursing to its members and the public at large" (APON, 2003). APON membership has reached/surpassed 2,000, and the organization projects an annual budget of approximately $650,000. There are 36 local chapters in the United States; seven additional sites, including Toronto, Canada, are preparing for local chapter membership. The look and content of APON's newsletter, *APON Counts,* have been updated. A third edition of the pediatric oncology book, *Nursing Care of Children and Adolescents with Cancer,* was published in 2002.

Structure of APON

APON is governed by an elected board of directors, consisting of a president, president-elect or past president, secretary, treasurer, and three board members (directors-at-large). Standing APON committees include Conference, Education Provider, Local Chapter, Nominations, and Steering Committees. With the exceptions of the Nominations Committee and the Steering Committee, committee membership is voluntary, and committee chairs are appointed by the president. The Nominations Committee is elected by the general membership, and the chairperson of this committee is elected by the committee members. Steering Committee members are appointed by the board of directors; this committee directs the organization's short-term projects to ensure that volunteers' time is used effectively. APON's home office, managed by the association management firm Association Management Center, is located in Glenview, IL.

The 36 local chapters operate under policies and procedures developed at the national level and are required to offer a minimum of 4 educational offerings each year. These educational offerings, including many 1- or 2-day conferences held by local chapters, significantly increase the quality of local professionals' understanding of children with cancer and blood disorders and their families. Local chapters are the key to the continued success of APON and are the roots that keep the organization standing firm.

APON members and other interested parties can keep up-to-date on APON activities and conference highlights at APON's Web site, www.apon.org. APON members can discuss benchmarking and practice issues and concerns on the PracticeNET message boards. The Web site also contains educational materials and links to the Web sites of other organizations of interest to pediatric oncology nurses.

Conferences

APON holds a national conference each year in late September or early October. The conference is always highly rated and is an excellent opportunity for networking as well as education. In the early years, the conference was held in conjunction with other organizations, such as ACCH, the American Cancer Society, and the National Cancer Institute. Since 1979, APON has been large enough to host the conference independently. To facilitate travel arrangements, the conference is held in a different part of the country (e.g., East, Midwest, West) each year. Conference attendance ranges from 550 to 600 and consists primarily of registered nurses from a variety of practice settings (but is open to other healthcare professionals, as well).

The primary objective of the conference is to provide education to pediatric hematology/oncology nurses—an objective that is vital to APON's overall mission of pursuing excellence in the care of children and adolescents diagnosed with cancer and blood disorders. In 1996, APON was accredited by the American Nurses Credentialing Center's Commission on Accreditation as a provider of continuing nursing education. APON's national conference has become a major source of research and clinical practice information.

Publications

In 1984 the first issue of the bimonthly *Journal of the Association of Pediatric Oncology Nurses (JAPON)* was published. The journal was renamed the *Journal of Pediatric Oncology Nursing (JOPON)* in 1989, when W.B. Saunders Company in Philadelphia, PA, assumed publishing responsibilities. As of July 2003 *JOPON* has been published through Sage Publications in Thousand Oaks, CA. APON's newsletter, *APON Counts,* is published quarterly.

Publications for patient and family education include "When Your Child Has Cancer," a slide orientation program in both English and Spanish; *Pediatric Tumor Series: Handbooks for Families (Ewing's Sarcoma Family of Tumors, Germ Cell Tumors, Neuroblastoma, Osteosarcoma, Rhabdomyosarcoma,* and *Wilms' Tumor); Pain Management in Children with Cancer;* and

Cancer Treatment Fact Sheets (available in English and Spanish).

The third edition of *Nursing Care of the Children and Adolescents with Cancer,* one of APON's premier publications, was published by W.B. Saunders in 2002. APON's *Essentials of Pediatric Oncology Nursing, A Core Curriculum,* is now in its second edition. APON's *Scope and Standards of Pediatric Oncology Nursing Practice* is copublished with the American Nurses Association and considered to be the national standard for pediatric oncology nursing practice. Additionally, APON has published two position statements. Information about all of APON's publications can be found on the APON Web site.

Certification

The Oncology Nursing Certification Corporation (ONCC), in partnership with APON, provides certification for pediatric oncology nurses. Certification validates a nurse's expertise to supervisors, clients, colleagues, and the general public. Some institutions recognize certification through career ladder advancement.. Accrediting bodies such as the American College of Surgeons and Magnet Nursing Recognition assess nursing certification when recognition is given to an institution. In 1993, the first certification examination was offered to more than 500 nurses. Nurses who pass the examination may use the credential CPON® after their names to indicate they are certified pediatric oncology nurses. Recertification is required every 4 years and may be accomplished either by taking the examination or by meeting continuing education requirements.

An APON member who holds CPON certification always sits as an elected member of the ONCC board of directors. The APON board also has a liaison to ONCC, appointed by the president. ONCC conducts ongoing item-writing sessions and role-delineation surveys to ensure the examination reflects the most current practice. APON members are invited to participate in these exercises.

APON's Professional Involvement

APON supports its vision through educational endeavors and the support of professional nursing practice. With such a global vision, APON cannot operate alone and must work in cooperation with other organizations. These organizations include, but are not limited to, the Children's Oncology Group, Oncology Nursing Society, Oncology Nursing Certification Corporation, National Coalition for Cancer Research, CancerSource.com, the American Nurses Association, the American Cancer Society, the American Society of Pediatric Hematology/Oncology, the Association of Pediatric Oncology Social Workers, Candlelighters, and the Leukemia/Lymphoma Society.

APON represents experts in the care of pediatric oncology patients within the nursing profession. APON is a small organization by virtue of the relatively rare incidence of childhood cancer; however, by joining their voices with others, APON members can be a significant influence in the discipline and profession. In 2002 APON developed and published two position statements outlining specific criteria that should be met in the care of the pediatric oncology patient. APON also signed numerous letters to Congress, in partnership with other organizations that share APON's vision and mission, stating its positions on proposed or necessary legislation.

APON's founders believed that the highest standards of nursing practice are achieved through education, research, certification, advocacy, and affiliation (Heiney & Wiley, 1996). APON celebrated 27 years of service in 2003 and remains committed to this mission.

References

Association of Pediatric Oncology Nurses. (2003). *About APON.* Retrieved August 22, 2003, from http://www.apon.org.

Heiney, S. P., & Wiley, F. M. (1996). Historical beginnings of a professional nursing organization dedicated to the care of children and adolescents with cancer and their families: The Association of Pediatric Oncology Nurses from 1974-1993. *Journal of Pediatric Oncology Nursing, 13,* 196–203.

Bibliography

Standards of Pediatric Oncology Nursing

American Nurses Association & Association of Pediatric Oncology Nurses. (1978). *Standards of pediatric oncology nursing practice.* Kansas City, MO: American Nurses Association.

Association of Pediatric Oncology Nurses. (1987). *Scope of practice and outcome standards of practice for pediatric oncology nursing.* Glenview, IL: Author.

Association of Pediatric Oncology Nurses & American Nurses Association. (2000). *Scope and standards of pediatric oncology nursing practice.* Washington, DC: American Nurses Publishing.

American Nurses Association. (2000). *Recognition of a specialty, approval of scope statements and acknowledgement of nursing practice standards.* Washington, DC: Author.

Institute for Child Health Policy, http://www.ichp.edu

Association of Pediatric Oncology Nurses

Baggott, C. R., Kelly, K. P., Fochtman, D., & Foley, G. V. (2002). *Nursing care of children and adolescents with cancer* (3rd ed.). Philadelphia: W.B. Saunders.

SECTION II

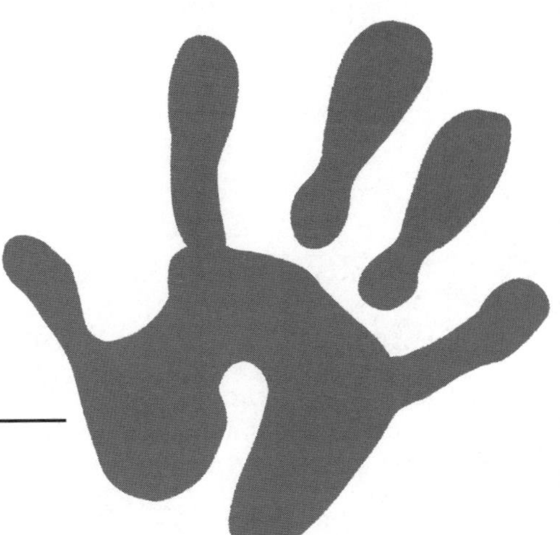

Pediatric Cancers

Jill E. Brace O'Neill

Section Outline

Overview of Childhood Cancer

Jill E. Brace O'Neill

Children comprise approximately 2% of all cancer cases. The types of malignancies in the pediatric population are totally different from those that affect adults. The most common types of cancer among adults include prostate, breast, lung, and colon cancers. Children tend to develop leukemias, brain tumors, and a variety of solid tumors. Although some adult cancers have associated risk factors that could be avoided, such as smoking and exposure to sun, very few environmental factors have been linked to pediatric malignancies.

Pediatric oncology represents only a small segment of the discipline of oncology. However, many advances in the diagnosis and treatment of cancer have resulted from treating pediatric malignancies.

Cancer is the leading cause of death from disease in children. In 2000 the death rates of children with cancer were 2.7 per 100,000 in children aged 1–4 years and 2.5 per 100,000 in children aged 5–14 years. The death rate for adults with cancer was 183 per 100,000, which made cancer the second leading cause of death from disease in adults (second to heart disease).

Most recently, cancer incidence and treatment in adolescents and young adults has become of interest and concern in pediatric oncology. In the 1990s, the annual incidence of cancer among adolescents 15–19 years of age was 203 new cases per 1 million. This rate is 50% higher than the incidence of cancer in children younger than 15 years of age. The incidence of cancer in 15–19 year olds is similar to the incidence in children 4 years old or younger. The incidence is twice that found in 5–9 year olds and is nearly twice that found in 10–14 year olds. The most common cancers among the 15–19-year-old population in the United States are Hodgkin's disease, germ cell tumors, central nervous system (CNS) tumors, non-Hodgkin's lymphoma, thyroid cancer, malignant melanoma, and acute lymphocitic leukemia (ALL). This pattern is different than in both younger and older patient populations. Many of the common malignancies in children younger than 5 years of age are virtually absent in the 15–19-year-old group. Similarly, cancers that predominate in adults are unusual among adolescents.

A partial explanation for the relative lack of progress in curing the adolescent population at the same rate as that realized in the younger pediatric population is the lack of participation in clinical trials. Of children less than 15 years of age with cancer, 90%–95% are treated at institutions that have clinical trials that are sponsored by the National Cancer Institute (NCI). By contrast, approximately 20% of 15–19-year-olds with cancer are treated at one of these institutions, and only about 10% are entered into a clinical trial. The NCI and pediatric and adult cooperative groups sponsored by the NCI have launched a national initiative to increase the numbers of adolescent and young adults in clinical trials.

Leukemia is the most common malignancy in children and the most common type of leukemia is ALL, which represents three-fourths of all pediatric leukemia cases. Although the presenting signs of the various types of leukemia may be similar, the treatment and response to treatment of childhood leukemias vary greatly.

CNS tumors are the most common types of solid tumors in children. Not all brain tumors are malignant by histology, but even a benign tumor can have devastating effects on a child. The treatment for brain tumors in children often presents difficulties because therapies such as radiation may have debilitating effects on the developing brain.

Lymphoma, including non-Hodgkin's lymphoma and Hodgkin's disease, is a malignancy common to both children and adults. However, the subtypes of lymphoma and their treatments in the two populations often differ.

Many pediatric solid tumors usually develop only in the pediatric population, but may occur in adults in rare instances.These tumors include neuroblastoma, Wilms' tumor, rhabdomyosarcoma, retinoblastoma, osteosarcoma, and Ewing's sarcoma.

Some of the factors leading to improved cure rates in pediatric oncology patients include the use of combination chemotherapy, multimodal treatment for childhood solid tumors, improvements in nursing and supportive care, development of research centers for comprehensive childhood cancer treatment, cooperation among treatment institutions and the development of cooperative study groups, recognition of the psychological effects of cancer treatment, and continued follow-up of pediatric oncology patients to track trends in the late effects of cancer treatment.

Epidemiology of Childhood Cancer

Kathy Ruccione

Incidence and Mortality

Pediatric and adolescent cancer cases make up a small proportion of overall cancer cases both in the United States and worldwide. Approximately 12,400 individuals under age 20 years are diagnosed with cancer each year in the United States, in contrast with the approximately 1.3 million adults who are diagnosed annually. Incidence is determined from reports contributed by cancer registries in several metropolitan areas and states that participate in the Surveillance, Epidemiology and End Results (SEER) Program of the National Cancer Institute (NCI). Data from the most recently published SEER monograph shaped the trends depicted in **Table 2-1**. There is considerable variation by sex, age, and race among the individual cancer types, and grouping them together masks these differences. Specific information about the epidemiology of individual types of childhood cancer is presented within the sections on these malignancies.

Patterns of Cancer in Children and Adolescents

In addition to differences in incidence and mortality, cancer in children and adolescents differs from cancer in adults in sites of origin, type of tissue involved, latency, opportunities for prevention and early detection, treatment response, and prognosis. Characteristics of childhood cancers compared with cancers in adults are listed in **Table 2-2**. Adult cancers usually are grouped by primary site, but pediatric cancers are better tabulated by their histologic type and primary site. The International Classification of Childhood Cancer (ICCC) was developed to meet this purpose. **Figure 2-1** shows the incidence rates per million children, using the ICCC groups. Highest rates are for groups I (leukemia), II (lymphoma), and III central nervous system (CNS).

Risk Factors for Cancer in Children and Adolescents

The specific stages that lead to the development of any childhood cancer are still unknown despite considerable epidemiologic research. Epidemiologists look for associations between environmental exposures or host (genetic) characteristics that increase the likelihood of developing a disease. These characteristics or exposures are risk factors. Various exposures have been investigated as risk factors for childhood cancer, but it is likely that no one factor, no single exposure or genetic trait, determines whether a person will develop cancer. Current understanding is that it is probably the interaction of many factors that produces cancer, a concept referred to as multiple causation or *multifactorial etiology*. In this view, cancer develops because of the predisposing characteristics of the person who is interacting with the environment. The concept of multiple causation is useful when the results of epidemiologic studies are interpreted. For example, laboratory and epidemiologic studies may indicate that exposure to a certain chemical can cause leukemia, but not all children exposed to that chemical will develop leukemia. Additional studies will be needed to determine what other factors must interact with chemical exposure to cause the disease. The SEER Pediatric Monograph includes summaries of current knowledge of the causes of the various childhood cancers; they are categorized as known risk factors, factors for which evidence is suggestive but not conclusive, and factors for which evidence is inconsistent or limited. Some examples of risk factors that have been studied are shown in **Table 2-3**.

Genes and the Human Genome

Human cells have 23 pairs of chromosomes; normally, one chromosome of each pair comes from the mother and the other comes from the father. Each chromosome contains a very long (unfolded, it would be 6 feet long) twisted molecule called deoxyribonucleic acid (DNA). The DNA macromolecule contains two chains of sugar and phosphate molecules. Each sugar molecule is attached to another kind of molecule called a base. The bases are purines (adenine and guanine) or pyrimidines (cytosine and thymine) known as A, G, C, T. In a chromosome, a stretch of DNA that stores the instructions for making a protein is a gene; each chromosome has thousands of genes. The protein-production instructions are in the spelling of 4-letter codes using A, G, C, and T. The beauty of the DNA structure is not only that it can produce the proteins needed for life, but also that it is self-reproducing: it can copy itself. To do that, it unzips into two ladders that are reverse images of each other. Each half then rebuilds itself, using components stored in the cell. The finished copies are identical because A's can only bond with T's, and G's can only bond with C's. **Figure 2-2** shows the DNA structure.

The human genome, the full set of instructions to make a person, contains approximately 3 billion base pairs. In 2000 scientists working on the Human Genome Project and at Celera Genomics jointly announced that they had made a draft of the map of virtually all the base pairs on the 23 chromosomes in

Table 2-1. Recent Trends in Childhood Cancer Incidence and Mortality

- Overall incidence increased from the mid-1970s, but rates in the past decade have been relatively stable. There seemed to be a slight leveling off or a slight decline during 1990–1995.
- Most experts now attribute the small increases that were seen in the incidence of CNS tumors, leukemias, and neuroblastoma in recent years to changes in diagnostic technology, reporting, and classification.
- When all sites were combined, overall cancer incidence was higher for males than for females.
- If incidence data were divided into four groups by age, the highest incidence was among the youngest and oldest, compared with the two intermediate age groups.
- If incidence data were examined year by year, the highest rates were in infants.
- The majority of cancers (57%) were leukemia, CNS tumors, or lymphoma.
- Incidence rates for African American children were lower than for European American children overall and for many of the specific disease sites. Hispanic and Asian American children had rates intermediate to those for European Americans and African Americans. The lowest incidence rates were among American Indian children.
- Surival rates have improved dramatically with newer, more effective treatment. Overall survival is now estimated at 80%, although there is variation according to tumor type. Cancer remains the leading cause of death from disease in childhood.

Note: Adapted from material in *Cancer incidence and survival among children and adolescents: United States SEER Program 1975-1995*, L.A.G. Ries, M.A. Smith, J.G. Gurney., M. Linet, T. Tamra, J.L. Young, et al. (Eds.) Bethesda, MD: National Cancer Institued (NIH Pub. No. 99-4649).

Table 2-2. Characteristics of Childhood Cancers Versus Cancers in Adults

Characteristic	Childhood Cancers	Adult Cancers
Frequency	Rare: < 1% of all cancers	Common: >99% of all cancers
Primary sites	Involves tissues of reticuloendothelial system, central nervous system, muscle, bone	Involves organs such as breast, colon, lung, prostate
Histology	Most common type: nonepithelial (leukemia, lymphoma, central nervous system, sarcomas)	Most common type: epithelial (carcinomas)
Latency (from initation to diagnosis)	Relatively brief latency	May be long (i.e., 20+ years); incidence increases with increasing age
Pathogenesis	Genetic alterations play a major role	Strong relationship to environmental and lifestyle factors; genetic factors have minor role
Preventable?	Minimal opportunity at present	80% estimated to be preventable
Opportunity for screening/early detection	Small percentage known to be at high risk can be monitored closely for early detection; screening tests generally not applicable	Many can be detected early by adherence to screening guidelines
Manifestations at diagnosis	Metastatic or system disease in ~80%	Local or regional disease
Pharmacokinetics (drug disposition, phar macodynamics (tissue and organ sensitivity)	• Markedly different in children because of rapid developmental changes; many common tumor types have been responsive to chemotherapy • May tolerate higher doses and have less difficulty with acute toxicity • Vulnerable to long-term consequences (e.g., impaired growth and development, cognitive deficits, endocrine dysfunction, cardiotoxicity)	• Common tumor types have been less responsive to available chemotherapeutic agents • May have more difficulty with acute toxicity, but fewer long-term consequences
Presymptomatic genetic testing offered	Only under specific circumstances, following established guidelines for testing in children	Yes, for malignancies where genetic mutation has been identified (e.g., *BRCA1, BRCA2*)
Treatment per research protocols in cooperative groups as standard of care	Yes	No
Prognosis	70%–90% cure (depending on tumor type, stage)	<60% cure (depending on tumor type, stage)

Note: From *Clinical pediatric oncology* (p. 2) D.J. Fernbach and T.J. Vienti (Eds.). (1991). St. Louis: Mosby–Year Book. Adapted with permission.

the human genome. Now scientists are working to understand the function of genes and their protein, to determine how a change in the spelling of the codes can lead to disease. These new discoveries will transform medicine through new treatment strategies and new possibilities for disease prevention.

Genes Associated with Cancer Susceptibility

Recent discoveries in molecular biology are helping to solve the cancer puzzle, showing how normal cellular control mechanisms malfunction to cause cancer and laying the groundwork for genetic testing and new approaches to treatment. For some time, it has been known that when a parent transmits a cancer-associated gene mutation, there is an increased susceptibility to familial cancer. Inherited cancer susceptibility syndromes (some of which are listed in **Tables 2-4** and **2-5**) account for only about 5% of newly diagnosed cancer cases in the United States each year. For the majority of childhood cancer cases, there is no evidence of familial cancer susceptibility.

Current understanding is that cancer is a genetic disease in the sense that something in the genes must go awry for cancer to develop. Three classes of genes play major roles in triggering cancer: oncogenes, tumor suppressor genes, and DNA damage response (repair) genes. When these genes are functioning correctly, they choreograph the life cycle of the cell and the intricate steps by which the cell enlarges and divides. Today, all oncology nurses must have a working

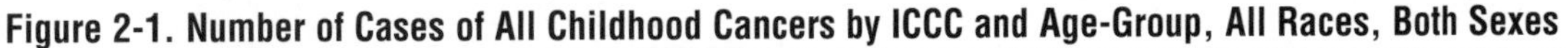

Figure 2-1. Number of Cases of All Childhood Cancers by ICCC and Age-Group, All Races, Both Sexes

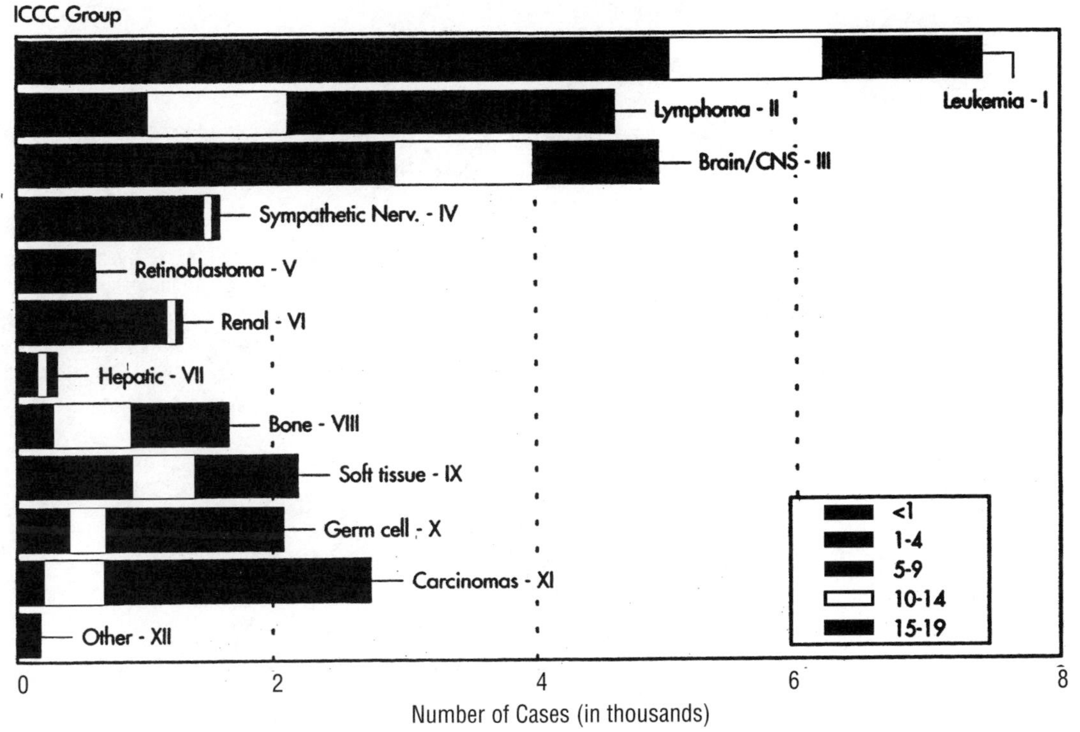

Note: From *Cancer Incidence and Survival Among Children and Adolescents: United States SEER Program 1975-1995* [p. 6], by L.A.G. Reis, M.A. Smith, J.T. Gurney, et. al., 1999, Bethesda, MD: National Cancer Institute, SEER Program. NIH pub., no. 99-4649, Reprinted with permission.

Table 2-3. Risk Factors for Cancer in Children and Adolescents

Examples of Known Risk Factors

Prenatal

- Prenatal diagnostic irradiation—modest ↑ risk of childhood leukemia
- DES exposure in utero—↑ risk of clear cell adenocarcinoma of vagina
- Transplacental transmission of certain maternal cancers (very rarely)—melanoma, lymphoma, broncogenic carcinoma

Postnatal

- Radiation (WWII atomic bomb exposure) — ↑ risk of leukemia or solid tumors in exposed children
- Radiation for thymus enlargement or ringworm (1940s and 1950s) — ↑ risk of leukemia or solid tumors of head/neck
- Chemotherapy/radiation — ↑ risk of second malignant neoplasms
- Viral—nasopharyngeal carcinoma and some lymphomas associated with Epstein-Barr virus

Examples of Possible Risk Factors

Inconclusive or inconsistent findings

- In utero exposures: antinausea medications, barbiturates, antibiotics, marijuana, frequent alcohol use, nitrosamine-containing substances.
- Exposure to pesticides, electromagnetic fields, motor vehicle exhaust

Note: Adapted from material in Ruccione, K.S. (2002). Biologic basis of cancer in children and adolescents. In Baggott, C.R., Kelly, K.P., Fochtman, D., & Foley, G.V. (Eds.), *Nursing Care of Children and Adolescents with Cancer* (3rd Edition). (pp. 24-63). Philadelphia: W.B. Saunders Company.

Figure 2-2. How DNA Works

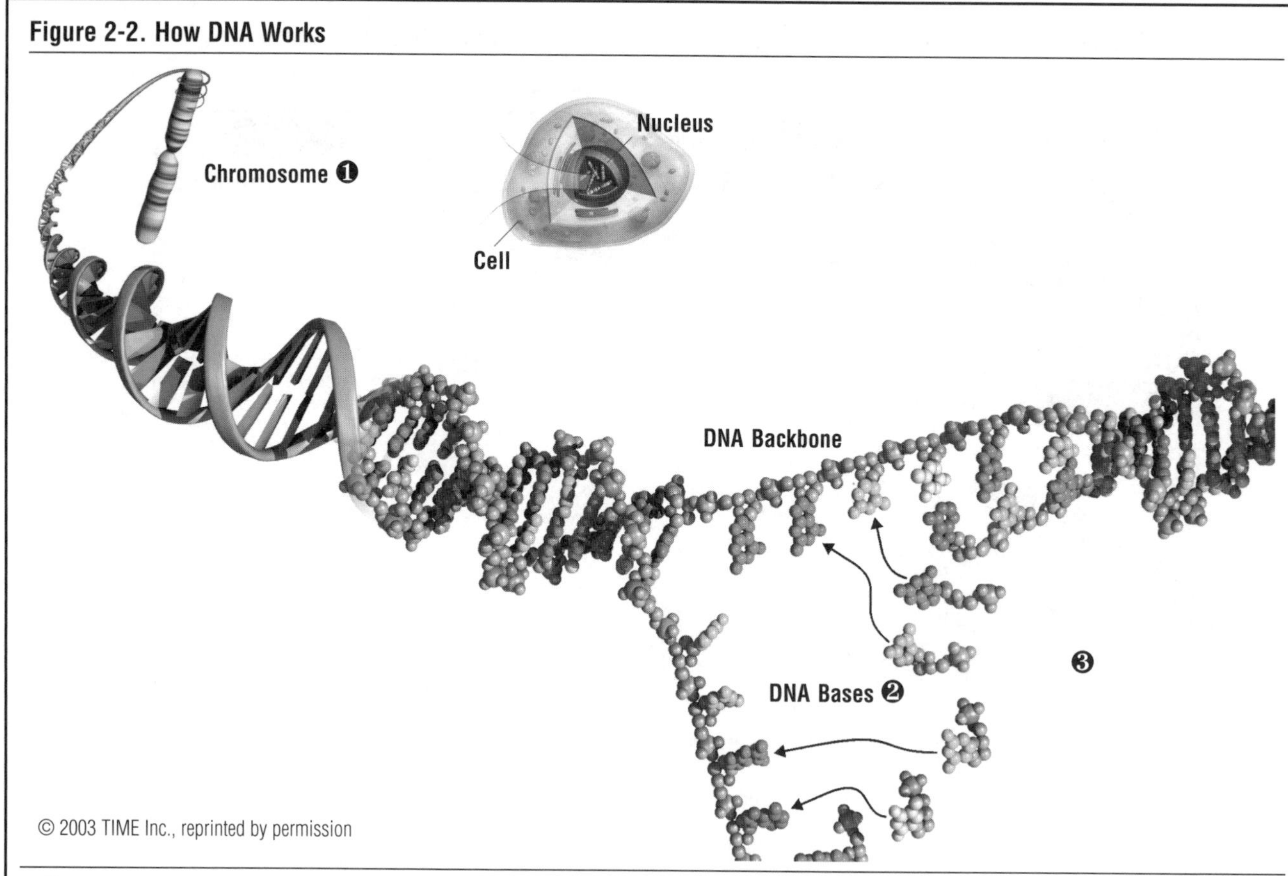

❶ Chromosomes:
DNA is twisted into packets called chromosomes and tucked into the nucleus of each cell. The blueprints for making proteins are stretched of DNA called genes; the instructions are spelled out in four letter codes: A, T, G, and C.

❷ DNA Copy:
To make a copy of itself, DNA unzips along its length, unraveling into two half-ladders that are reverse images of each other. Then each half rebuilds itself from components stored in the cell. Because As always bond with Ts and Gs with Cs, the finished copies are identical.

❸ Base Pairs:
The base pairs attach to each other with hydrogen bonds.

knowledge of genetics, including chromosomes, the DNA molecule, cell division, and protein synthesis, in order to understand new information about cancer causes and new treatment approaches.

Oncogenes. Proto-oncogenes have a role in normal cell division and growth through a signaling process that orchestrates the cell cycle. If they are mutated, proto-oncogenes become carcinogenic oncogenes. Changes produced by specific oncogenes cause the cell cycle to go out of control. An example of an oncogene in pediatric cancer is N-*myc*, which is involved in neuroblastoma and glioblastoma.

Tumor suppressor genes. Oncogenes' effects have been likened to a car's accelerator sticking in an acceleration mode. In contrast, tumor suppressor gene malfunction can be equated to the loss of a car's braking system. Normal tumor suppressor genes keep cell growth in check. When these genes are damaged or missing, the cell ignores inhibitory signals and grows out of control.

The first human tumor suppressor gene was identified in a pediatric tumor: retinoblastoma, the malignancy Dr. Knudson was studying when he proposed the "two-hit hypothesis." (Knudson, 1971). Cells have two copies (alleles) of every gene, providing a built-in safety mechanism if a normal tumor-suppressing gene is missing or inactive. Losing a functioning copy of a gene is called loss of heterozygosity (LOH). What the two-hit hypothesis proposed was that in the hereditary form of retinoblastoma, the first "hit" occurs in a germ cell. That hit predisposes cells (specifically retinal cells) to develop a tumor after another mutation occurs. In nonhereditary retinoblastoma, both hits occur later in the development of the retina, and there is no constitutional predisposition to malignancy that can passed on to future generations. The two-hit hypothesis was confirmed by laboratory experiments that showed that deletion of an *RB* gene results in LOH, which predisposes cells to tumor development. It is currently understood that the two-hit hypothesis (which

Table 2-4. Selected Autosomal Dominantly Inherited Cancer Syndromes

Syndrome	Associated Gene(s)
Familial retinoblastoma	RB1
Li-Fraumeni	*p53*
Familial adenomatous polyposis	*APC*
Hereditary nonpolyposis colorectal cancer	*MLH1, MSH2, MSH6, PMS1, PMS2*
Wilms' tumor	*WT1*
Breast and ovarian cancer	*BRCA1, BRCA2*
Von Hippel-Landau	*VHL*
Cowden	*PTEN*

Note. From American Society of Clinical Oncology, B.L. Weber (Ed.). (2000). *ONCOSEP: Genetics, an oncology self-education program curriculum text* (p. 8). Dubuque, IA: Kendall. Reprinted with permission.

Table 2-5. Selected Recessively Inherited Cancer Syndromes

Syndrome	Primary Tumor	Associated Gene(s)
Ataxia telangiectasia	Lymphoma	*ATM*
Bloom syndrome	Solid tumors	*HLM*
Xeroderma pigmentosum	Skin cancer	*XPB, XPD, XPA*
Fanconi anemia	AML	*FACC, FACA*

Note: From American Society of Clinical Oncology, B.L. Weber (Ed.). (2000). *ONCOSEP: Genetics, an oncology self-education program curriculum text* (p. 9) Dubuque, IA: Kendall.

may have more than two steps) applies to all malignancies that have both hereditable and nonhereditable forms.

More recently, several other tumor suppressor genes have been found. One of these, *p53*, is the most frequently mutated gene in human cancer. This so-called "guardian of the genome" helps monitor the health of the cell and the integrity of its DNA. Mutant inherited versions of the *p53* tumor suppressor gene are seen in Li-Fraumeni syndrome, a familial constellation of tumors that arises from various sites.

DNA repair (or damage response) genes. These caretaker genes ensure that each strand of DNA is copied correctly during cell division. If these genes are mutated, cancer can result from accumulations of mutations in critical growth-regulating genes, including proto-oncogenes and tumor suppressor genes. Some examples of disorders associated with faulty DNA repair genes and an increased risk of cancer are Bloom syndrome, ataxia-telangiectasia, Fanconi anemia, and heredity nonpolyposis colon cancer.

Hallmarks of Cancer

Understanding the dynamic interactions between tumor cells and other cells and substances in their vicinity, and how they modulate each other, has opened a new view of cancer as a disease of the cell's microenvironment. Cancer results from genetic mutations in a cell. These mutations can change the amount or the activity of proteins involved in regulating cell life. The transformation from normal cell to malignant cell is a progressive multistep process, involving a succession of genetic changes. In this process, a cancer acquires the ability to circumvent normal control mechanisms and manipulate its local environment. Recently, Hanahan and Weinberg (2000) proposed that there are six essential alterations in normal cell physiology that collectively dictate malignant growth (**Figure 2-3**).

Self-sufficiency in growth signals. In normal cells, growth-stimulating signals communicate from outside the cell to deep within its interior. This happens when one cell secretes proteins known as growth factors that move through spaces between cells and bind to specific receptors. A succession of other proteins relays the signal until it reaches the nucleus, alerting the cell to go through its growth cycle. Recent research that focused on these normal cell activities has helped explain what happens in malignant tumors. A hallmark of cancer is that cancer cells are not dependent on normal mechanisms to move from a quiescent state into an active proliferative state. The concept is that tumors are complex tissues in which cancer cells have hijacked normal endothelial cells and fibroblasts and forced them to release growth-stimulating signals. In this model, immune cells attracted to sites of malignant cells may promote rather than eliminate the cancer. Thus, cancer cells do not rely on normal growth signals.

Insensitivity to antigrowth signals. Another characteristic of cancer is an overstimulation of growth-promoting mechanisms that is combined with evading or ignoring normal braking systems. An important discovery was that there is a destination point in the cell's nucleus that promotes or inhibits growth; this has been called the cell clock. In normal cells, the cell clock programs the events of the cell cycle

Figure 2-3. Acquired Capabilities of Cancer

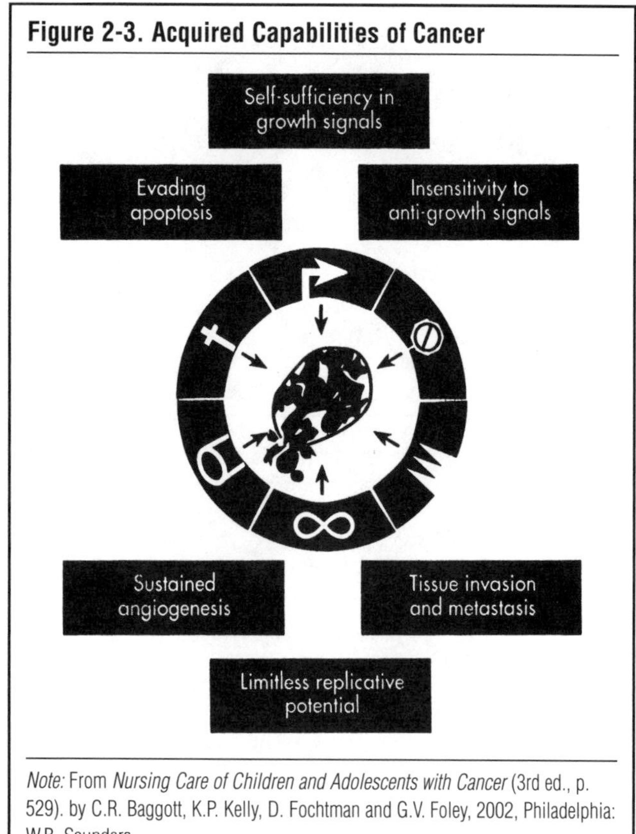

Note: From *Nursing Care of Children and Adolescents with Cancer* (3rd ed., p. 529). by C.R. Baggott, K.P. Kelly, D. Fochtman and G.V. Foley, 2002, Philadelphia: W.B. Saunders.

through various molecules. Two molecules important in this process are cyclins and cyclin-dependent kinases (CDKs). In almost every malignancy, the cell clock is malfunctioning.

Evading apoptosis. The ability to escape an important cellular defense against runaway cell growth contributes to cancer development. Apoptosis refers to a backup system that tells the cell to destroy itself if something essential is damaged or if controls are deregulated. Evading apoptosis allows tumors to grow and also may make them more resistant to treatment.

Limitless replicative potential. Counters within cells, called telomeres, keep track of how many times cells reproduce themselves as a defense against uncontrolled growth. Telomeres are located in DNA segments at the end of chromosomes. In normal cells, telomeres shorten a bit every time chromosomes are replicated. When they shrink below a certain threshold length, an alarm signals the cell to enter senescence and stop reproducing. But with cancer, the malignant cell's ability to produce an enzyme called telomerase, which replaces telomeric segments, permits the cell to reproduce endlessly.

Sustained angiogenesis. Angiogenesis is the proliferation of new capillaries. When cells are functioning normally, angiogenesis is activated during menstruation, placental nourishment of the fetus, and wound healing. Tumors also can switch on angiogenesis, which increases their blood supply and enables them to expand. Tumors can produce growth factors such as the vascular endothelial growth factor (VEGF) and basic fibroblast growth factor (bFGF). Their actions are counterbalanced by angiogenesis inhibitors such as angiostatin or endostatin. Regulatory molecules moving between cells and their microenvironment relay signals that change the balance of angiogenesis inducers and inhibitors, thereby activating an "angiogenic switch." Close proximity to capillaries is necessary for cells to survive, and tumors cannot expand beyond 1–2mm^3 unless new blood vessel growth occurs. In cancer, angiogenesis is literally the lifeblood of the malignancy.

Tissue invasion and metastasis. When cancer spreads, it is because some cells in the tumor have mutated with the characteristics for successful metastasis. Such cells disregard the normal tissue barrier of the extracellular matrix (ECM), the structure that provides support for the development and organization of tissues. These mutated cells have alterations in the proteins that are involved in tethering cells to their surroundings. The proteins include cell-cell adhesion molecules (involved in mediating cell-to-cell interactions), integrins (involved in linking cells to the ECM structure), and proteases (enzymes that can facilitate invasion of cancer cells into nearby tissue, across blood vessel walls, and through normal epithelial cell layers). Together, these substances play a role in degrading the ECM, which permits cancer cells to untether from the tumor and to establish themselves in other tissue. Local invasion starts the multistep process of metastasis, known as the metastatic cascade (**Figure 2-4**). Angiogenesis is essential in this process. If clinically significant metastases are to develop, every step of the cascade must be completed. Particular types of primary tumors metastasize preferentially to specific anatomic sites (**Table 2-6**). The capacity for tissue invasion and metastasis is deadly in cancer; metastatic disease is responsible for most deaths caused by cancer.

Common Parental Concerns

There are still no definitive, clear, cause-and-effect answers for parents who want to know exactly what caused their child's cancer. Many parents of children with cancer form

Figure 2-4. The Metastatic Cascade

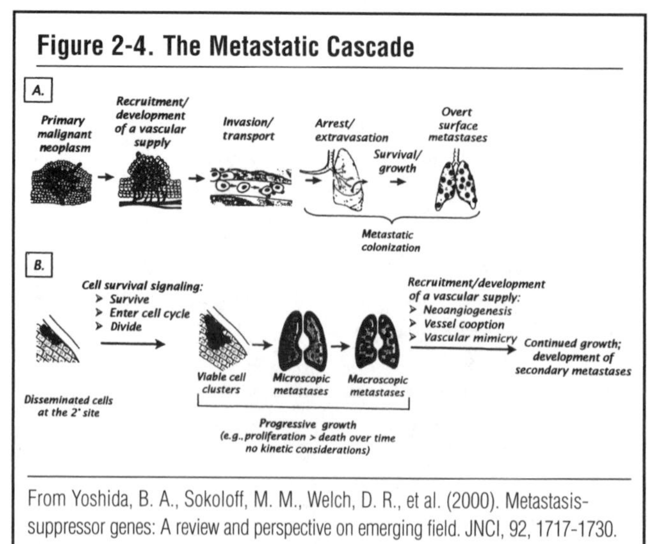

From Yoshida, B. A., Sokoloff, M. M., Welch, D. R., et al. (2000). Metastasis-suppressor genes: A review and perspective on emerging field. JNCI, 92, 1717-1730.

Table 2-6. Metastasis in Selected Childhood Cancers

Primary Tumor	Incidence at Diagnosis	Metastatic Sites
Neuroblastoma	60%	Lymph nodes, bond marrow, liver, bone
Rhabdomyosarcoma	10–30%	Lymph nodes, lung, bone, bone marrow, liver
Ewing sarcoma	14–50%	Bone, brain
Osteosarcoma	10–20%	Lung, bone
Wilms' tumor	16%	Lung, liver
Retinoblastoma	5%	Bone, brain, bone marrow
Brain	Very rare	Spine

Courtesy Yves DeClerck, MD, 2001

theories about the origin of their child's cancer as they search for its cause and meaning. It can be helpful to discuss these ideas and to reassure parents that this searching for answers is a normal part of the process of adjusting to the cancer diagnosis. Another common area of parental concern is the possibility that the child's cancer was part of a cancer cluster. Although several clusters have been investigated, such studies have taught us very little about the causes of cancer; more has been learned from epidemiologic and laboratory research. Newer epidemiologic studies are collecting direct evidence of exposure (such as carcinogenic effects on DNA) and are searching for inherited variations in genes that would predispose children to cancer. Nurses are in a key position to facilitate patient and family participation in these studies. As biologic science progresses, and especially as particular genes are implicated in specific childhood cancers, there will be different challenges: helping parents who may struggle with "genetic guilt," and understanding the ethical, legal, and social issues in predictive genetic testing. Fortunately, resources are increasingly available for nursing education, as well as patient/family education, in the rapidly evolving field of epidemiology and genetics.

Nursing Assessment and Intervention

Understanding the biologic basis of cancer and all of its implications for young people and their families is a critical challenge for pediatric oncology nurses in the 21st century. As recent discoveries become integrated in clinical practice, nurses will care for patients and families who need well-informed, sensitive, and ethical nursing assessments and interventions with regard to the epidemiology and genetics of cancer.

Goal: The patient (as appropriate for age and developmental level) and family will be adequately informed about the diagnosis and epidemiologic/genetic factors related to the cancer.

Assessment:

- Assess the learning styles of the patients and family (see Section VIII, "Patient and Family Education").
- Assess the patient's and the family's knowledge of, and prior experience with, cancer.
- Assess the patient's and the family's knowledge of risk factors (environmental exposures, genetic factors) related to the cancer.
- Update and maintain the family's medical history (this is particularly relevant for nurses who practice in ambulatory settings, especially in posttreatment clinics), with special attention given to cancers that may have developed in first-, second-, and third-degree relatives.

Interventions:

- Communicate with the patient and the family in a style that is appropriate for them. If their perspective on cancer is based on what they have seen in adult friends and relatives, it may be helpful to discuss the important differences between cancer in children and adults.
- Provide the patient and family with honest, compassionate answers to their questions and concerns. Help them formulate questions, as needed, and guide them to appropriate resources.
- Provide the patient and family with appropriate informational resources. Use the most current version of the SEER Pediatric Monograph, or the Children's Oncology Group Epidemiology Committee materials, or both, as a basis for discussing risk factors related to the cancer.
- Inform the patient and family about pertinent epidemiology studies that may be recruiting patient participants.
- Encourage families that are at increased risk for hereditary cancer syndromes to provide medical documentation of family members' cancers for confirmation purposes. Collaborate with the medical team to refer these people for genetic counseling and possible genetic predisposition testing, as appropriate.

Goal: The patient and the family will adequately cope with information that has been provided regarding the epidemiology of the disease.

Assessment:

- Assess the family's communication and coping styles in general (See Section VII, "Family Resources").
- Assess the family's response to information presented about any known risk factors related to the cancer.
- Assess the family's response to genetic aspects (if any) of the cancer.
- Assess the patient's and the family's concept of why the cancer occurred (i.e., their explanation for the cancer and its meaning in their lives).

Interventions:

- Encourage the patient and family to share their beliefs about the cause of the cancer, acknowledging and validating that forming a theory about why the cancer happened is a normal reaction to a cancer diagnosis.
- Provide emotional support.
- Ensure that the family is aware of when and how to contact members of the healthcare team.
- Anticipate the need for referral services (e.g., genetic counseling, social work, chaplain).

Expected Patient and Family Outcomes

The patient and family can

- Name the type of malignancy and describe any known risk factors related to it.
- Use informational and support resources appropriately.
- Identify available resources for genetic counseling and testing, if relevant.
- Determine whether participation in epidemiologic studies is appropriate.
- Verbalize how and when to contact the healthcare team with concerns or questions.

Reference

Hanahan, D., & Weinberg, R.A. (2000). The hallmarks of cancer. *Cell, 100,* 57–70.

Leukemia

Virginia Kimball Dalton

Definition

Leukemia is a malignant disorder of the blood and blood forming organs, including the bone marrow, lymph nodes, and spleen.

Pathophysiology

The hematopoietic system is composed of undifferentiated pluripotent stem cells. Signals from the hematopoietic microenvironment regulate the proliferation and differentiation of the stem cells into mature elements (red blood cell, granulocyte, monocyte, lymphocyte, or platelet). Malignant stem cells result in cells that lose the ability to regulate cell division and to differentiate to mature functioning cells. Immature cells (blasts) accumulate in the marrow spaces, peripheral vasculature, and organs. Then, normal cell proliferation is blocked because of the lack of space and nutrients in the marrow. Presenting symptoms, which include anemia, neutropenia, and thrombocytopenia, are a direct result of the replacement of normal cells with leukemia cells. An accumulation of leukemia cells in other organs and tissues also may cause symptoms.

Acute lymphoblastic leukemia (ALL) results from abnormalities in differentiation and proliferation in the lymphoid cell lineage. Acute myelogenous leukemia (AML) results from abnormalities in differentiation and proliferation of primitive cells of the myeloid/erythroid or megakaryocytic lineages. AML also is referred to as acute non-lymphoblastic leukemia (ANLL). Chronic myeloid leukemia (CML) results from an abnormality in proliferation of myeloid cells.

Classification

Leukemia is classified by morphology, cytochemistry, immunology, and chromosomal analysis. The three major classifications of childhood leukemia are

- acute lymphocytic leukemia (ALL), which accounts for 75%–80% of childhood leukemia
- acute nonlymphocytic leukemia (ANLL), or acute myelogeneous leukemia (AML). The two account for 20%–25% of childhood leukemia.
- chronic myelocytic leukemia (CML), which accounts for less than 5% of childhood leukemia.

French-American-British morphological classification: The French-American-British (FAB) morphological classification is a systematic and reproducible system for leukemia developed in 1976. It is based on the morphology (descriptive appearance, structure, and cytochemistry) and numbers of cells.

Morphology

Morphology is based on the descriptive appearance of the cells under the light microscope. The current classification system was developed in 1976 and revised in 1985 by the French-American-British (FAB) Cooperative Group. This classification is extremely important in the treatment of AML (**Table 2-7**). Auer rods (abnormal lysosomal granules) are one morphologic feature found only in some subtypes of AML.

Immunophenotyping

Normal hematopoietic cells undergo changes in the expression of cell surface antigens as they mature in the bone marrow. Monoclonal antibodies have been developed that react with lineage-specific and stage-specific lymphoid and myeloid activation and differentiation antigens. These antibodies help confirm the differentiation between ALL and ANLL. Each monoclonal antibody is identified with a classification number with the prefix CD (**Table 2-8**). By immunophenotyping, the malignant cell lines in ALL can be identified and described as B-cell, T-cell, or biphenotypic (both lymphoid and myeloid cell lines are present).

Biochemical Markers

Various biochemical markers have been identified; some are useful in the diagnosis and classification of leukemias.

Cytogenetics

Cytogenetic abnormalities are found in more than 90% of patients with ALL. Abnormalities exist both in the number of chromosomes (known as ploidy, also measurable as a DNA index) and structure (translocations). These abnormalities can be detected by conventional chromosome analysis methods but often are found with reverse transcriptase polymerase

Table 2-7. French-American-British Cooperative Group Classification (FAB) for Leukemia

FAB	Name	Morphology
M1	Acute myeloblastic; no maturation	Undifferentiated; >90% blasts; <10% promyelocytes/monocytes
M2	Acute myeloblastic with maturation	>30% and <89% blasts; >10% promyelocytes; <20% monocytes
M3	Acute promyelocytic: hypergranular	>20% abnormal hypergranular promyelocytes; auer rods present
M3v	Acute promyelocytic: microgranular variant	Fine granularity of cytoplasm in promyelocytes; folded nuclei
M4	Acute myelomonocytic	>30% blasts nonerythroid series; >20% but <80% monocytic
M4Eo	Acute myelomonocytic with eosinophilia	>5% abnormal eosinophils with basophilic granules
M5a	Acute monocytic	>80% monocytic cells are monoblasts; remaining promonocytes/monocytes
M5b	Acute monocytic with differentiation	<80% of monocytes are monoblasts; remaining promonocytes/monocytes
M6	Acute erythroleukemia	>30% of nonerythroid cells are blasts; 50% are erythroblasts
M7	Acute megakaryoblastic	>30% nonerythriod cells are megakaryoblasts; myelofibrosis common

Table 2-8. Immunophenotyping for Leukemia

T Cell	Myeloid	B Lineage	Miscellaneous
CD1	CD11	CD19	CD9
CD2	CD13	CD20	CD10
CD3	CD14	CD21	CD34
CD4	CD15	CD24	CD41a
CD5	CD33		CD45
CD7			
CD8			

chain reaction (RT-PCR) and fluorescence in situ hybridization (FISH), which are more sensitive techniques.

Aberrations in chromosome number (ploidy) are associated with prognosis. Leukemia cells can be described as diploid (containing 46 chromosomes), hyperdiploid (>46 chromosomes), hypodiploid (<46 chromosomes) and pseudodiploidy (46 chromosomes with structural change). Hyperdiploidy is associated with a good prognosis, whereas hypodiploidy and pseudodiploidy are associated with poor outcomes. Trisomies 4 and 10 are associated with a low risk of treatment failure.

Both ALL and ANLL are associated with common translocations that hold prognostic significance. Common translocations associated with ALL are TEL-AML1, BCR-ABL, and MLL. TEL-AML1 is the most common abnormality (occurring in 20%–25% of cases), and occurs when the TEL gene on chromosome 12p13 fuses with the AML1 gene on chromosome 21q22; it is associated with a favorable outcome. BCR-ABL, also known as the Philadelphia chromosome, is t(9;22), associated with B-cell ALL, present in approximately 4% of the cases and responds poorly to conventional chemotherapy. MLL arrangement, t(4;11), is located on chromosome 11q23. This translocation, the most common within this subtype, is found in infant ALL and is associated with a poor prognosis.

ANLL is a highly molecular heterogeneous disease with many chromosome abnormalities. Since so many changes occur, it is difficult to assign prognostic significance. Translocation may continue even when the child is considered in remission; it usually is indicative of an impending relapse. Common translocations associated with ANLL include PML/RARA, AML1-ETO, and Inv (16). PML/RARA, t(15;17)(q22;q12), is observed in M3 AML (acute promyelocytic leukemia APL) and is associated with the best prognosis of all AML subgroups. AML1-ETO, t(8;21), is observed in M2 AML and carries a better than average prognosis. Inv (16) is found in myelomonocytic leukemia and is characterized by the presence of abnormal basophilic granules.

Incidence and Etiology

Despite concerted efforts to determine the cause of leukemia, its etiology remains unknown. However, there are known factors that increase the risk for the development of leukemia.

Acute Lymphocytic Leukemia (ALL)

There are 3,000 new cases of ALL per year in the United States and ALL accounts for 75%–80% of all cases of childhood leukemia (25% of all childhood cancers). The peak age of onset is 4 years. ALL affects more Caucasians than children of African heritage, and more males than females. Male predominance is greater in T-cell disease. There also is a higher incidence of ALL in Western and industrialized nations.

Environmental exposure to ionizing radiation has been associated with ALL development. The following genetic factors are associated with disease:

- Trisomy 21, also known as Down's syndrome (15 times the risk over unaffected children)
- Fanconi's anemia
- Ataxia telangiectasia, Klinefeltzer syndrome, Shwachwan syndrome, Bloom's syndrome
- Older maternal age at birth
- Maternal history of fetal loss
- A sibling with ALL (2–4 times the risk over an only child; monozygotic twins <7 years of age have a 25% chance of developing ALL once one twin does)

Acute Nonlymphoblastic Leukemia (ANLL)

ANLL accounts for 15% of all cases of childhood leukemia in the United States, with 500 children diagnosed per year. Peak incidence is in the neonatal period. Frequency of ANLL remains stable with a slight increase during adolescence. It is more common in the Hispanic population, with a higher incidence in African Americans than in Caucasians. The subtype acute promyelocytic leukemia (APML) has a higher incidence in the Hispanic population.

Genetic Predisposition

The following genetic factors are associated with disease:

- Trisomy 21, also known as Down's syndrome (greatest occurrence <3 years of age; thereafter, incidence is the same as with ALL)
- Fanconi's anemia, aplastic anemia, Bloom's syndrome, Diamond-Blackfan anemia
- Neurofibromatosis
- Myelodysplastic syndrome (Monosomy 7)
- Sibling with ANLL (2–4 times the risk over an only child); monozygotic twins <6 years of age have a 20%–25% chance of developing ANLL once one twin does).

Environmental Exposure

The following environmental factors are associated with disease:

- Certain drugs and chemicals (e.g., alkylating agents [etoposide(VP-16)], nitro-soureas, benzenes, herbicides, pesticides)
- Ionizing radiation
- Prenatal maternal cigarette smoke exposure
- Prenatal maternal alcohol use
- Petroleum product exposure

Clinical Presentation

Patients may present with one or more of the following symptoms. **(Table 2–9):**

- Abnormal complete blood count (CBC)
- Fatigue
- Pallor
- Weight loss
- Malaise
- Lymphadenopathy
- Hepatosplenomegaly
- Bone pain
- Abdominal pain
- Signs and symptoms of infection
- Painless testicular swelling (ALL)
- Chloroma (ANLL)

Diagnostic

A diagnostic includes disease staging to determine the classification of leukemia before beginning therapy. Diagnosis is made through the use of a history, physical examination, and bone marrow aspirate.

The history should include a review of the medical history; current illnesses; duration of symptoms (pain, fatigue, infection, fever, bleeding, central nervous system symptoms, including headache, vision changes, or facial palsy); prior exposures; and familial history of malignancies. A psychosocial assessment also should be done. The physical examination should note liver/spleen size from costal margin, presence of testicular swelling, and lymphadenopathy.

A chest X ray is done to rule out anterior mediastinal mass and to evaluate airway status before sedation for bone marrow aspirate/biopsy.

CBC and differential may reveal a low, normal, or high white blood cell count and peripheral blasts that may or may not be present on differential. Platelets may be low or normal.

Bone marrow aspiration can reveal more than 25% blasts (cytogenetics, immunophenotyping, morphology, and special stains are done to differentiate the type of leukemia.) Bone marrow biopsy can reveal the cellularity of the marrow (as indicated should the aspirate be of poor quality or yield).

Lumbar puncture is done to rule out central nervous system disease for cell count, cytology (if blasts are present in the differential, it is an indication of central nervous system disease), glucose, and protein.

Evaluations prior to chemotherapy are essential. Baseline liver enzymes should be taken to evaluate the hepatic ability to metabolize chemotherapeutic agents. Blood chemistries

Table 2-9. Presenting Signs and Symptoms of Leukemia

Acute Lymphocytic Leukemia	Acute Nonlymphocytic Leukemia
Anemia: malaise, fatigue, and pallor	Lymphadenopathy
Thrombocytopenia: gingival, cutaneous, or nasal bleeding	Fever
Neutropenia: fever	Pallor
Hepatosplenomegaly	Anorexia, weight loss
CNS disease (<10% of cases at diagnosis): increased intracranial pressure, headache, vomiting, and visual disturbances	Weakness, fatigue
Bone pain (23% of cases present with bone pain)	Sore throat, recurrent infections
Lymphadenopathy	Other respiratory symptoms
	Gastrointestinal symptoms: abdominal pain, nausea, and vomiting
	Gingival hypertrophy
	Chloromas

including potassium, calcium, phosphorous, magnesium, BUN, and LDH levels should be taken. These values can reach critically abnormal values with the start of chemotherapy (tumor lysis syndrome). High uric acid and creatinine levels often are associated with renal failure. LDH provides an estimate of tumor burden.

Prognostic Considerations

Symptoms at presentation, and diagnostic methods for defining subtypes of leukemia, allow the patient to be classified according to a risk group.

With ALL, the risk group classification will determine therapy.

ALL: 70%–80% of children are cured of the disease.

ANLL: 45%–50% of children are cured of the disease (**Table 2-10**).

Treatment and Prognosis

ALL: Principles of treatment include

- Use of central nervous system (CNS) prophylaxis (either cranial irradiation or intrathecal chemotherapy)
- Use of combination chemotherapy to maintain remission
- Observation of tumor for lysis syndrome
- Understanding of prognostic features at diagnosis to determine therapy.

Induction therapy: The goal is to eliminate leukemic blasts and obtain a remission bone marrow (<5% blasts) with normal peripheral count (absolute neutrophil count >1,000/mm^3 and platelet count >100,000/mm^3). Prednisone (Deltasone) plus vincristine (Oncovin) produce remission in 90% of patients. The addition of L-asparaginase (Elspar) or doxorubicin (Adriamycin) increases the remission rate to 95%. Prevention of tumor lysis syndrome is a major concern.

Consolidation therapy: Induction chemotherapy kills much of the leukemia, but an even greater reduction of leukemia cells is needed to ensure eradication of the disease. Intravenous methotrexate (Mexate) or an anthracycline is usually added at this stage. Prophylactic treatment of the CNS is by cranial radiation in combination with intrathecal methotrexate and cytarabine or triple therapy (methotrexate/cytarabine/hydrocortisone) when radiation is not used.

Maintenance therapy: The goal is to maintain remission. This therapy usually continues for 2–3 years and includes daily mercaptopurine (Purinethol) and methotrexate, but it may include the use of other drugs. CNS prophylaxis continues throughout maintenance.

Table 2-10. Prognostic Factors in ANLL

	Good	Poor
Age	N/A	Age <2 years old
White Blood Cells	N/A	WBC >100,000
French-American-British Classification	M3	M4 or M5
Platelets	>100,000	<100,000
Chromosomes	T(8;21)	T(9;11)

ANLL: Assessment of patients receiving maintenance therapy includes the following:

- Observe or monitor for bleeding due to thrombocytopenia and disseminated intravascular coagulation.
- Observe for fever, neutropenia, and infection.
- Observe for tumor lysis syndrome (much less common than with ALL).
- Observe for leukostasis if the white blood count is more than 200,000.

Induction chemotherapy: This therapy comprises a combination of three to seven or more drugs in a highly intensive regimen, except for M3, which utilizes retinoic acid as a differentiation agent and lower doses of chemotherapy. Dosages must be high enough to achieve bone marrow aplasia. Active drugs are cytarabine, doxorubicin, thioguanine (6-TG), prednisone, and etoposide (VP-16).

Therapy is of shorter duration than for ALL—usually 6 months of intensive induction-like courses.

Allogeneic bone marrow transplantation is usually recommended if there is a matched related donor.

CNS prophylaxis: Twenty percent of patients who do not receive CNS treatment will relapse. CNS leukemia at diagnosis does not adversely affect long-term prognosis. CNS is treated with intrathecal chemotherapy before each cycle of induction therapy.

Recurrent Disease

ALL: If there is a relapse while a patient is receiving therapy, prognosis is extremely poor. Those who relapse more than 12 months after completion of therapy have a better chance at long-term survival.

Extramedullary relapse: CNS relapse occurs in 10% of patients. Testicular relapse is treated with testicular radiation and chemotherapy.

ANLL: A patient has a 25% chance of a second remission if relapse occurs while receiving chemotherapy and a 50% chance of achieving a second remission if relapse occurs after completing chemotherapy. Bone marrow transplantation (autologous or allogenic) may be considered.

Nursing Assessment and Interventions

Goal: The patient will experience minimal complications related to the diagnosis of leukemia.

Assessment:

- Assess presenting symptoms and determine the type of leukemia.
- Obtain a complete history, including the incidence and duration of symptoms (e.g., pain, fatigue, infection, bleeding, neurological changes), predisposing factors (e.g., exposure to radiation, cytotoxic drugs, genetic abnormalities), and pertinent family history.
- Perform a complete physical examination, and assess for pallor, petechiae, bleeding, signs of infection, rash, lymphadenopathy, hepatosplenomegaly, and neurological changes.
- Review laboratory findings.

- Review radiological imaging studies (e.g., chest X ray).
- Review surgical and pathology reports as indicated.
- Assess the child's degree of pain and or discomfort.

Interventions:

- Provide comfort measures.
- Provide pain medication as needed.
- Monitor for tumor lysis syndrome (i.e., maintain strict intake and output of fluids and monitor serum chemistries). (See Section V, "Side Effects of Treatment".)
- Administer irradiated, leuko-reduced blood products, and chemotherapy as indicated.
- Take measures to prevent tumor lysis syndrome; provide intravenous hydration with alkalization and allopurinol.
- Explain all tests, procedures, and results to the patient and the family.

Goal: The patient will experience minimal complications related to treatment.

Assessment:

- Assess the child for signs of toxicity related to specific chemotherapy agents (see the discussion of chemotherapy in Section IV, "Childhood Cancer Treatment").
- Assess the child for toxicity if he or she has had radiation therapy (see the discussion of radiation therapy in Section IV, "Childhood Cancer Treatment").
- Assess the child for signs of infection.
- Assess the child for evidence of fatigue, bleeding, pain, and nutritional deficits.
- Monitor fluids and electrolytes.
- Determine the type of intravenous access that is needed.
- Assess for signs and symptoms of emergency complications.
- Assess for the patient's response to therapy (i.e., a decreased number of blasts in peripheral blood, decrease in the size of enlarged nodes, or hepatosplenomegaly; decrease in blast cells in bone marrow).

Interventions:

- Refer the child for central intravenous access, as needed.
- Provide comfort measures.
- Administer pain medication, as needed.
- Provide instruction on proper mouth care, nutrition, and hygiene.
- Educate the family about neutropenia, anemia, thrombocytopenia, the signs and symptoms of infection, and fever precautions.
- Obtain cultures and radiological examinations, as ordered, when infection is suspected, and initiate antibiotics if indicated (see Section V, "Side Effects of Treatment").
- Provide alternative methods of nutrition (e.g., oral supplements, nasogastric [NG] and parenteral supplements).
- Review all findings of laboratory studies and radiological studies with the patient and the family.

Goal: The patient and the family will be adequately informed regarding diagnosis, disease, and treatment.

Assessment:

- Assess level of knowledge of the patient and family about the diagnosis and disease.
- Assess their level of knowledge about treatment (i.e., surgery, radiation therapy, chemotherapy).
- Assess their learning styles (see Section VIII, "Patient and Family Education").
- Assess how well they understand the role of the multidisciplinary team in treating children with leukemia.

Interventions:

- Communicate with the patient and the family in an appropriate style.
- Provide them with appropriate educational resources and review the material with them.
- Ensure that the family is aware of when and how to contact the healthcare team.
- Encourage the patient and the family to ask questions about the diagnosis, disease, and treatment.
- Clarify the information provided by various members of the multidisciplinary team.

Goal: The patient and family will cope adequately with the diagnosis.

Assessment:

- Assess the family's communication and coping styles in general.
- Assess the family's adjustment to the diagnosis.

Interventions:

- Give honest answers to questions from the patient and the family.
- Provide emotional support.
- Anticipate the need for referral for services (e.g., social work, chaplain, Candlelighters, American Cancer Society, Leukemia Society).
- Offer age-appropriate "hospital play."
- Offer to help the patient and the family contact another family with experience with a similar malignancy to exchange information.

Expected Patient and Family Outcomes

The child and parents are able to do the following:

- Describe the type of leukemia and the plan of care.
- List the expected and the possible toxic side effects of therapy.
- Outline methods for preventing infection.
- Describe the schedule of treatment, procedures, and follow-up care.
- Describe available community resources.
- Demonstrate the skills needed to care for the child at home.
- Verbalize how and when to contact the healthcare team if problems or questions arise.

Non-Hodgkin's Lymphoma

Eileen Whyte O'Holleran

Definition

Non-Hodgkin's lymphoma (NHL) is a malignant solid tumor of the immune system. The cells of origin are malignant, undifferentiated lymphoid cells or their precursors.

Pathophysiology

NHL differs from most cancers, which originate from an overgrowth of cancerous cells in a particular organ or tissue that then may spread by local invasion or metastasis. However, because lymphoma is a neoplasm of the immune system and cells of that system normally circulate throughout the body, lymphomas are most commonly generalized diseases at presentation. In NHL, malignant lymphoid cells spread in a random, diffuse, unpredictable, and aggressive pattern. Expedient diagnosis and prompt initiation of treatment are critical. NHL responds rapidly to chemotherapy; therefore, tumor lysis syndrome is a complication that must be anticipated and prevented.

Three Types of Histology

Histologic classification of NHL attempts to identify the malignant cell of origin that will help clinicians understand the biologic behavior of the tumor. NHL is divided into T and B cell lymphomas, with subdivisions specific to precursor characteristics. The World Health Organization classification system defines the histologic classification system for NHL as lymphoblastic lymphoma (LL), Burkitt's lymphoma (BL) or Burkitt's-like lymphoma (BLL) and large cell lymphoma (LCL).

Lymphoblastic Lymphoma

Lymphoblastic lymphoma accounts for one-third of all childhood lymphomas. More than 95% are derived from immature T cells undergoing differentiation in the thymus, and about 10%–15% express the phenotype of pre-B cells, accompanied by multiple cytogenetic abnormalities. LL typically presents in the thorax, with approximately 50%–70% involving the anterior mediastinum with pleural effusions. Neck, supraclavicular, and axillary lymphadenopathy may be present. T-cell disease commonly spreads to the bone marrow, central nervous system (CNS) and gonads. If the marrow has more than 25% blasts, the patient is considered to have acute lymphoblastic leukemia.

Burkitt's Lymphoma or Burkitt's-like Lymphoma

Burkitt's and Burkitt's-like lymphoma accounts for about 50% of all childhood NHL. The most common cytogenetic abnormality is t8:14. It is a lymphoma of mature B cell origin. Endemic BL refers to lymphomas occurring in equatorial Africa. More than 50% of children with endemic BL will have tumors involving the abdomen and approximately 50% will have tumors involving the jaw. Ninety-five percent are associated with Epstein-Barr virus (EBV) infection. Metastasis to the CNS is more common than in sporadic BL.

Sporadic BL generally refers to lymphomas found in Europe and the United States, 80%–90% of which have abdominal involvement at presentation; only 20% show evidence of EBV disease. Metastasis to the bone marrow is more common than in endemic BL.

Large Cell Lymphoma

Large cell lymphoma accounts for 15% of all childhood lymphomas, 50% of which are large B-cell lymphoma and 50% are anaplastic large cell lymphomas (ALCL). CNS involvement is rare, and most presentations involve the mediastinum or abdomen. Other common presentations for ALCL include the lymph nodes (unlike other lymphomas that often present in extranodal regions), skin, soft tissue, bone, lung, and testes. ALCL tumors arise from T cells or NK cells, which typically have a t2:5. cytogenetic abnormality and express the Ki-1 (CD30) antigen. Metastasis to the bone marrow or CNS is unusual.

Other

Adult lymphomas are seen occasionally in pediatrics, such as follicular lymphoma, marginal zone B-cell lymphomas (typically in children with acquired immunodeficiency syndrome (AIDS), and peripheral T-cell lymphomas that are not related to the ALCL subdivision. In addition, posttransplant lymphoproliferative disorder (PTLD) is a more recent diagnosis in posttransplant patients who are on immunosuppressive therapy.

Incidence and Etiology

In developed countries, lymphomas (including Hodgkin's and NHLs), rank third in incidence after acute leukemia and brain tumors, and comprise 10%–15% of all childhood cancers. NHL comprises 60% of all childhood lymphomas. The incidence is two times greater in males than females, and twice as common among European Americans as it is among other groups. The incidence of NHL increases steadily with age, however, most patients are between 5 and 15 years old. Between 1973 and 1996, the average annual incidence of lymphoma in the United States increased by approximately 35% for reasons that remain unknown.

There is an increased incidence of lymphoma in children with congenital immunodeficiency syndromes such as Wiskott-Aldrich syndrome, severe combined immunodeficiency (SCIDS), X-linked lymphoproliferative disease, and ataxia-telangiectasia, as well those with AIDS. Increased incidence of NHL also is associated with immunosuppression after solid organ and stem cell transplants, particularly T-cell-depleted stem cell transplantation.

NHL accounts for 6.3% of all childhood cancers and for 60% of all childhood lymphomas. The peak ages of onset are 5–15 years. The incidence is higher in males than in females (2.5:1). There is increased incidence in children with congenital immunodeficiency syndromes (e.g., Wiskott-Aldrich syndrome, severe combined immunodeficiency syndrome, ataxia telangiectasia). Increased incidence is associated with posttransplant immunosuppression, especially in children undergoing a T-cell-depleted bone marrow transplant.

It is likely that geographic, immunologic, viral, and genetic factors have important roles in the etiology of NHL. There is an increased incidence of NHL in patients with EBV and AIDS . There also are variations in incidence in different countries (e.g., Burkitt's lymphoma is endemic in Africa and sporadic in other parts of the world). EBV is linked to the development of endemic Burkitt's, with the jaw being the primary tumor site, though abdominal tumors also may be present.

Clinical Presentation

Clinical features typically are determined by the initial sites of disease and by the degree of tumor spread. In addition to symptomatology correlating to the primary site, a child may have systemic symptoms of fever, malaise, weight loss, anorexia, and night sweats. Patients with ALCL often have these symptoms. Almost two-thirds of patients will initially present with locally advanced or metastatic disease.

- *Abdomen* (presenting in 31% of ALCL cases): Symptoms may include abdominal pain, nausea, vomiting, change in bowel habits, abdominal distention, palpable mass, intussusception, obstructive jaundice, gastrointestinal (GI) bleed. In addition to intestinal sites, tumors may be present in the liver, spleen, kidneys, pancreas, and ovaries.
- *Mediastinum* (presenting in 26% of ALCL cases): Symptoms may include dysphagia, subtle cough, wheezing, stridor, dyspnea, orthopnea, pericardial effusion, superior vena cava (SVC) syndrome with distended neck veins, head and neck edema, inferior vena caval obstruction, pericardial tumor or effusion, or cardiac tamponade.
- *Head and neck* (presenting in 29% of ALCL cases): Symptoms may include cervical lymphadenopathy, jaw swelling, unilateral tonsillar enlargement, nasal obstruction, snoring, rhinorrhea, or cranial nerve palsies.
- *CNS* (rare): Symptoms may include headache, vomiting, irritability, or papilledema.
- *Bone marrow* (presenting in 50% of LL cases and 20% of sporadic Burkitt's lymphoma cases): Symptoms may include pallor, anemia, or thrombocytopenia.
- *Other presentation sites:* Symptoms may include breast, testicular, skin, pharyngeal, nasopharyngeal, adrenal gland, thyroid, salivary gland, orbital, bone, muscle, or lung parenchyma.

Diagnostic

Given the rapidity of tumor growth, diagnostic should be performed as promptly as possible. Burkitt's lymphoma is the fastest-growing tumor in humans, with a doubling time of 24 hours. The diagnostic evaluation includes determining the extent of disease before therapy is started. This evaluation should include the following:

- A complete history of the current illness, including the incidence and duration of symptoms, such as pain, fatigue, bleeding, neurological changes; existence of predisposing factors, such as genetic abnormalities, previous solid organ or bone marrow transplant, family history, risk factors for HIV, and/or exposure to radiation, cytotoxic drugs, and immunosuppressive medications.
- A complete physical examination, including possible detection of pallor, petechiae, signs of infection, rash, lymphadenopathy, hepatosplenomegaly, neurological changes, other masses (especially abdominal), and respiratory symptoms.
- Laboratory studies, including complete blood count with differential, reticulocyte count, liver function studies, lactate dehydrogenase, urinalysis, hepatic and renal studies, erythrocyte sedimentation rate, and electrolytes. Alterations of potassium, calcium, phosphorous, magnesium level may be seen in acute tumor lysis syndrome. Testing to rule out other diagnoses, including alpha-fetoprotein, CA 125, or urinary catecholamines, should be done.
- Bone marrow aspiration and biopsy, bilateral (patients with more than 25% blasts are diagnosed with acute leukemia).
- Surgical biopsy of the involved site. Open biopsy of a node or mass is ideal, since it permits sufficient tissue for histologic, morphologic, cytogenetic, immunophenotypic, molecular and enzymatic studies. If it is not possible to obtain open biopsy because of the patient's condition (i.e., respiratory distress from a large mediastinal mass), a fine needle aspiration or biopsy of a mass or pleural fluid or cerebrospinal fluid is recommended.
- Chest X ray.
- Chest CT scan, if chest X ray is abnormal or suspicious.
- Thoracic ultrasound for monitoring thoracic tumor.
- Abdominal ultrasound that includes, liver, spleen, kidneys, abdomen, and pelvis.
- Gallium scan.
- Head and neck CT and/or MRI, depending on the disease site.
- If indicated, bone scan, MRI for CNS disease, endoscopy, serum lactate.

Staging

The majority of childhood lymphomas are high grade, in contrast with adult NHL, which is primarily low and intermediate grade. Prompt staging of a patient's disease is paramount because of the aggressive and rapid growth rate of NHL. In addition, accurate staging is crucial since it dictates the intensity and duration of therapy, and therefore has an impact on prognosis. Staging systems describe the tumor, its primary site, and sites of spread or metastases. Pediatric NHL historically has been staged according to the Murphy Ann Arbor system. The staging system most commonly used currently is that of St. Jude Children's Research Hospital (**Table 2-11**). Patients are staged with limited-stage disease (one or two masses on one side of the diaphragm), or as patients with extensive intrathoracic or intra-abdominal disease. Histologic classification is considered for patients with advanced stage disease.

Prognostic Considerations

Age and sex are not considered prognostic factors for NHL. Factors associated with a poor prognosis include

Table 2-11. St. Jude Children's Research Hospital Staging System for Non-Hodgkin's Lymphoma

Stage I

A single tumor (extranodal) or single anatomic area (nodal) with the exclusion of mediastinum or abdomen

Stage II

A single tumor (extranodal) with regional node involvement

Two or more nodal areas on the same side of the diaphragm

Two single (extranodal) tumors with or without regional node involvement on the same side of the diaphragm

A primary gastrointestinal tract tumor, usually in the ileocecal area, with or without involvement of associated mesenteric nodes only

Stage III

Two single tumors (extranodal) on opposite sides of the diaphragm

Two or more nodal areas above and below the diaphragm

All the primary intrathoracic tumors (mediastinal, pleural, and thymic)

All extensive primary intraabdominal disease*

All paraspinal or epidural tumors, regardless of the other tumor site(s)

Stage IV

Any of the above with initial central nervous system or bone marrow involvement†

* A distinction is made between apparently localized gastroin testinal tract lymphoma and more extensive intraabdominal disease. Stage II disease typically is limited to a segment of the gut plus or minus the associated mesenteric nodes only, and the primary tumor can be completely removed grossly by segmental excision. Stage III disease typically exhibits spread to para-aortic and retroperitoneal areas by implants and plaques in mesentery or peritoneum or by direct infiltration of structures adjacent to the primary tumor. Ascites may be present, and complete resection of all gross tumor is not possible.

† If marrow involvement is present initially, the number of abnormal cells must be 25% or less in an otherwise normal marrow aspirate with normal peripheral blood picture.

Note: From Nursing Care of Children and adolescents with Cancer (3rd ed., p. 539, by C.R. Baggott, K.P. Kelly, D. Fochtman and G.V. Foley, 2002, Philadelphia: W.B. Saunders.

incomplete remission within 2 months after treatment is started, large tumor burden, lactate dehydrogenase (LDH) greater than 1,000 mg/ml, Stages III and IV with bone marrow and/or CNS involvement, delay in initiating therapy, and relapse. Factors associated with a good prognosis are Stages I and II with primary tumors of the head and neck, peripheral lymph nodes, or GI tract.

Treatment

Initial treatment may focus on managing the presenting symptoms that are associated with marrow involvement, mediastinal and intra-abdominal tumors, and biochemical disturbances (hyperuricemia and acute tumor lysis syndrome). Before a patient receives chemotherapy, his or her chemistries must be stabilized because the chemotherapy could exacerbate such abnormalities, thereby potentially placing the patient at further risk.

Surgery is necessary for staging and if a resection is needed, as with emergency situations or when a complete resection of an isolated GI tumor is possible. In the case of resection, however, surgery may delay chemotherapy, since it puts patients at risk for fistula and perforation after the surgery. A second surgery also may be indicated, particularly with patients who are not responding to chemotherapy and who are being treated as low risk.

Radiation has no "routine" role as a therapeutic modality for childhood NHL. The exception is emergency situations when airway, intestinal, or spinal obstruction mandate immediate reduction in tumor size. Cranial radiation therapy (XRT) may be used for patients with T-cell lymphoblastic lymphoma.

Multiagent Chemotherapy

The primary therapeutic modality for childhood NHL is chemotherapy, regardless of stage or site(s) of the disease. The tumor responds to many different agents. Many children with NHL receive intrathecal agents (methotrexate [Mexate] and/or cytarabine [Cytosine Arabinoside]) for CNS prophylaxis.

Histology and Staging as Determinants of Treatment Protocol

Limited-Stage Disease (Stage I and II):

Children with Stage I or II NHL have an excellent prognosis, with a 5-year disease-free survival rate of 85%–95%. Burkitt's lymphoma, Burkitt's-like lymphoma, and large B-cell lymphoma typically are treated similarly, given their similar histology as B-cell lymphomas. Such patients have overall survival rates of approximately 90% when treated with multiagent, intensive chemotherapy for 3–6 months. Regimens include these chemotherapeutic agents: cyclophosphamide [Cytoxan], vincristine [Oncovin], methotrexate, prednisone, and Adriamycin. Newer protocols include high-dose methotrexate in initial therapy and other agents, such as etoposide, ifosfamide, and high-dose Ara-C.

Lymphoblastic lymphoma.

LL is optimally treated with chemotherapeutic regimens similar to ALL protocols—three-phase multiagent therapy (8–10 agents) involving induction, consolidation, and maintenance that typically spans 15–36 months. CNS prophylaxis also is given. Patients with limited disease have an 80%–90% overall survival rate, and patients with extensive disease have an overall survival rate of 60%–80%.

Anaplastic large cell lymphoma.

ALCL is a recently identified subtype and, therefore, standard therapy has yet to be determined. Anaplastic large cell lymphoma patients also have an 80%–90% overall survival and are treated with protocols similar to those used for B-cell lymphomas. Protocols used for lymphoblastic lymphoma, Hodgkin's disease, and adult "diffuse aggressive lymphomas" also have been used for ALCL.

CNS prophylaxis.

CNS prophylaxis is used for most NHLs, except for those diseases in which CNS spread is uncommon and for patients who have minimal disease that does not involve the head, neck, or epidural regions. CNS therapy typically includes MTX alone or MTX and Ara-C. In some institutions, patients with T-cell lymphoblastic lymphoma receive cranial radiation.

Advanced-Stage Disease (Stages III and IV)

Burkitt's lymphoma.

Cyclophosphamide, high-dose methotrexate, cytarabine and, more recently, ifosfamide and etoposide are used to treat advanced stages of BL. Among patients treated for more than 6 months, 75% are cured.

Lymphblastic lymphoma.

LL is treated similarly to high-risk ALL, with 2 years of multiagent systemic chemotherapy, intrathecal therapy, and cranial XRT with a 5-year disease-free survival rate of 80%.

Large cell lymphoma and recurrent disease.

Early Pediatric Oncology Group (POG) studies of large cell lymphomas and recurrent diseases have shown that cyclophosphamide can be omitted and the cumulative dose of Adriamycin reduced, substituting methotrexate after the cumulative dose has been reached in the protocols used to treat LCL and recurrent disease. These approaches have resulted in a 2-year, disease-free survival rate of 65%–80%.

The prognosis generally is grave for children who relapse. Although "salvage" therapy may be effective, many clinicians feel that a more aggressive initial approach is warranted and that limited stages should be treated with the same intensive and prolonged regimen used to treat advanced stage disease. As a result, some chemotherapeutic agents that were initially considered to be salvage therapy now are used for initial therapy. Ifosfamide, carboplatinum, and etoposide (ICE) chemotherapy is sometimes used for palliation, but it is unlikely to benefit patients who previously received full dose ifosfamide and etoposide.

Often an attempt is made to treat chemosensitive disease using high-dose chemotherapy, ideally with agents to which the child has not been exposed previously. Patients who have responsive relapsed disease, even in the absence of complete remission, then are candidates for stem cell transplantation. Such patients have a 50% disease-free survival rate at 5 years. Conditioning therapy regimens have included both total body irradiation (TBI) containing regimens and chemotherapy-only regimens (particularly for patients who have already received XRT), but no clearcut advantage to either has been found. Anaplastic large cell lymphoma patients generally do not have favorable outcomes with autologous stem cell transplant and may benefit from repetitive chemotherapy agents, such as vincristine, cis-retinoic acid, or alpha-interferon. The role of allogeneic transplant currently is being explored with the theoretical premise that there will be a graft-versus-tumor effect.

Nursing Assessment and Interventions

Goal: The patient will experience minimal complications related to lymphoma.

Assessment:

- Know the type of lymphoma being treated and its presenting symptoms.
- Obtain a complete history, including the incidence and duration of symptoms (e.g., pain, fatigue, infection, bleeding, neurological changes), predisposing factors (e.g., exposure to radiation, cytotoxic drugs, genetic abnormalities), and pertinent family history.
- Perform a complete physical examination and assess for pallor, petechiae, bleeding, signs of infection, rash, lymphadenopathy, hepatosplenomegaly, neurological changes, and masses.
- Review the laboratory findings.
- Review radiological imaging studies, as indicated.
- Review surgical and pathology reports, as indicated.
- Assess the child's degree of pain.

Interventions:

- Provide comfort measures.
- Provide pain medication as needed.
- Monitor for tumor lysis syndrome (i.e., strict intake and output and monitoring serum chemistries) (see Section V, "Side Effects of Treatment").
- Administer blood products and chemotherapy, as needed.
- Monitor for signs of tumor lysis syndrome by providing intravenous hydration with alkalization and allopurinol.
- Explain all tests, procedures, and results to the patient and the family.

Goal: The patient will experience minimal complications related to treatment.

Assessment:

- Assess the child for toxicity related to specific chemotherapy agents (see the discussion of chemotherapy in Section IV, "Childhood Cancer Treatment").
- Assess the child for toxicity related to radiation therapy, if used (see the discussion of radiation therapy in Section IV, "Childhood Cancer Treatment").
- Assess for signs of infection.
- Assess the child for evidence of fatigue, bleeding, pain, and nutritional deficits.
- Monitor intake and output of fluids and electrolytes.
- Determine the type of intravenous access that is needed.
- Assess the child for emergent complications.
- Assess the child for response to therapy (e.g., decrease in the size of enlarged nodes or hepatosplenomegaly, absence of disease in bone marrow).

Interventions:

- Refer the child for additional intravenous access, as needed.
- Provide comfort measures.

- Give pain medication, as needed.
- Provide instruction on proper mouth care, nutrition, and hygiene.
- Educate the family about neutropenia, anemia, thrombocytopenia, the signs and symptoms of infection, and fever-related precautions.
- Obtain cultures and radiological examinations, as ordered, when infection is suspected, and initiate antibiotics, if indicated.
- Provide alternative methods of nutrition (e.g., oral supplements, NG or parenteral supplements).
- Review all laboratory findings and radiological studies with the patient.

Goal: The patient and family will be adequately informed regarding diagnosis, disease, and treatment.

Assessment:

- Assess the level of knowledge of the patient and the family about the diagnosis and disease.
- Assess their level of knowledge about treatment (i.e., surgery, radiation therapy, chemotherapy).
- Assess their learning styles (see Section VIII, "Patient and Family Education").
- Assess their understanding of the role of the multidisciplinary team in treating children with lymphoma.

Interventions:

- Communicate with the patient and the family in an appropriate style.
- Provide them with appropriate educational resources and review the materials with them.
- Confirm that the family is aware of the healthcare team, as well as when and how to contact members of the team.
- Encourage the patient and the family to ask questions about the patient's diagnosis, disease, and treatment.
- Clarify information provided by various members of the multidisciplinary team.

Goal: The patient and the family will adequately cope with the diagnosis.

Assessment:

- Assess the family's general communication and coping styles.
- Assess the family's adjustment to the diagnosis.

Interventions:

- Provide emotional support.
- Anticipate the need for referral for services (e.g., social work, chaplain, Candlelighters, American Cancer Society, Leukemia Society).
- Offer age-appropriate "hospital play."
- Offer to introduce a contact family who has dealt with a similar malignancy to talk with the patient and family.

Expected Patient and Family Outcomes

The child and the family can do the following:

- Describe the type of lymphoma and the plan of care.
- List the expected and possible toxic side effects of therapy.
- Outline methods to prevent infections.
- Describe the schedule of treatment, procedures, and follow-up care.
- Describe available community resources.
- Demonstrate the skills needed to care for the child at home.
- Explain how and when to contact the healthcare team if problems or questions arise.

Hodgkin's Disease

Arlene L. Androkites

Definition

Hodgkin's disease (HD), a type of lymphoma, is a malignancy that involves the spleen and lymphatic system. Thomas Hodgkin first described the disease in 1932.

Pathophysiology

The exact nature of HD remains controversial and speculative. It is characterized by the presence of binucleate or multinucleated giant cells, as first described by Sternberg in 1898, and again by Reed in 1902. HD is unusual because its malignant cells account for less than 1% of a tumor's total cell population. Most of the tumor is composed of inflammatory cells and fibrosis, a result of cytokine release. The presence of Reed-Sternberg cells or their variant establishes the diagnosis.

The classic Reed-Sternberg cell is large, with abundant cytoplasm and either multiple or multilobed nuclei. The nucleoli are large and prominent. The nucleolus often resembles an "owl's eye" because of its delicate chromatin network.

Histologic Subtypes

The Rye classification system has been adopted universally for diagnosis and classification of Hodgkin's disease. The system divides HD into four categories. All histologic subtypes of HD are equally responsive to treatment.

Nodular sclerosis (NS): The most common subtype of HD, NS accounts for 40% of all cases in younger children and 70% of all cases in adolescents. The disease often involves the lower cervical, supraclavicular, and mediastinal lymph nodes. The lymph node capsule appears thickened, and the lymphoid tissue appears nodular. The radiographic appearance of these nodes slowly returns to normal with treatment.

Mixed cellularity (MC): This subtype occurs in approximately 30% of all cases and is seen most commonly in children 10 years of age or younger. Frequently, the disease is advanced, with extranodal involvement. The lymph node usually is diffusely effaced, and contains an inflammatory background of lymphocytes, plasma cells, eosinophils, histiocytes, and malignant reticular cells. Reed-Sternberg cells and their variants often are numerous in tissue samples.

Lymphocyte predominance (LP): LP type is more common in males and younger children and affects 10%–15% of all patients. LP usually presents as localized disease. Cellular proliferation consists of benign-appearing lymphocytes that may be misinterpreted as reactive hyperplasia.

Lymphocyte depletion (LD): This is a rare type of HD that is associated with patients with human immunodeficiency virus (HIV). It is associated with late stage, extensive disease that is widespread in bones and bone marrow. The disease is characterized by many Reed-Sternberg cells, few lymphocytes, and diffuse fibrosis and necrosis.

Incidence and Etiology

HD accounts for 5% of all childhood cancers and 1% of all oncology-related deaths in children and adolescents. It has a unique bimodal age distribution that differs geographically and ethnically. In industrialized countries, the early age peak occurs in the mid- to late 20s, and the second peak occurs after age 50. In developing countries, the early peak occurs before adolescence. There appear to be three distinct forms of HD—a childhood form (14 years of age and younger), a young adult form (ages 15–34), and an older adult form (ages 55–74). The incidence in the childhood form reveals a slight male predominance. With adolescents, there is equal incidence among males and females. Rarely is HD seen in a child who is under 5 years of age.

HD in childhood increases with family size and lower socioeconomic status. In contrast, the young adult form of HD is associated with industrialized countries and higher socioeconomic status. Mixed cellularity type is more common in younger children, whereas nodular sclerosis is more common in adolescents and young adults.

There is increased incidence in children with immunologic disorders such as genetic (Wiskott-Aldrich Syndrome, ataxia-telangiectasia), infectious (HIV), and iatrogenic agents. Epstein-Barr virus (EBV) has been associated with HD because large numbers of HD patients have high EBV antibody titers; this finding suggests that EBV may precede the development of HD.

Clinical Presentation

The presenting sign of HD is usually painless supraclavicular or cervical adenopathy (**Figure 2-4**). The lymph nodes are characteristically firmer than inflammatory nodes, feel rubbery, and, if they have grown rapidly, are sensitive to palpation. Approximately two-thirds of HD patients present with mediastinal involvement, which may cause pressure on the trachea and bronchi and lead to coughing or symptoms of airway obstruction. Axillary or inguinal lymphadenopathy is unusual as a presenting sign. Other symptoms may include fatigue, anorexia, and weight loss. Pruritis occurs more commonly in patients with advance stage disease and may be mild to severe. The three constitutional "B"symptoms that correlate with prognosis are: unexplained fever above 38°C, orally; unexplained weight loss of 10% within 6 months of diagnosis; and drenching night sweats.

When "B" symptoms are absent, the disease is referred to as "A." Splenomegaly is observed frequently on physical examination, but it is not necessarily indicative of splenic involvement. Liver size also is not an indicator of disease involvement (**Table 2-12**).

Diagnostic

Diagnostic evaluation begins with a thorough history and physical examination. Lymph node chains are assessed for size and measured. Evaluation of a child with suspected Hodgkin's disease should include:

Table 2-12. Classification of Hodgkin's Disease

Clinical or Pathologic Stage *

Stage	Criteria
I	Involvement of a single lymph node region (I), with extension from that node to an adjacent extralymphatic region (IE)
II	Involvement of two or more lymph node regions on the same side of the diaphragm (II), with extension to an extralymphatic organ or site (IIE)
III	Involvement of lymph node regions on both sides of the diaphragm (III), which may be accompanied by extension to an extralymphatic organ (IIIE), involvement of the spleen (IIIS) or both (IIIS+E)
IV	Diffuse or disseminated (multifocal) involvement of one or more extralymphatic organs or tissues with or without associated lymph node involvement, or isolated extralymphatic organ involvement with distant nodal involvement

* *Stages:* Clinical stage is when extent of disease is determined by history, physical examination, radiologic and other imaging studies, laboratory tests, and initial biopsy results. Pathologic stage is when a staging laparotomy provides histologic confirmation of the presence or absence of involvement of specific sites.

Symptoms: The presence of unexplained fever higher than 38°C for 3 consecutive days, drenching night sweats, or unexplained loss of more than 10% of body weight in the 6 months preceding diagnosis are to be denoted by the suffix B; the absence of these symptoms is denoted by the suffix A.

Subscripts: X is bulky disease > or equal to 10 cm at maximal dimension; E is extranodal extension with involvement of extralymphatic tissues by limited direct extension from an adjacent nodal site or a single extranodal deposit consistent with extension from a regionally involved node; PS sites are indicated by a subscript: D-skin, H-liver, L-lung, M-bone marrow, O-bone, P-pleura.

Source: Data from National Cancer Institute NCI–PDQ

- A complete blood count with differential.
- Sedimentation rate.
- Renal and liver function tests, alkaline phosphatase level.
- Serum copper and ferritin.
- Lymph node biopsy.
- Chest radiograph with measurement of mediastinal ratio. It is important to determine "bulky disease," which is lymphadenopathy measuring greater than or equal to 33% of the maximum intrathoracic cavity.
- CT scan, for evaluating mediastinal, pulmonary, and upper abdominal disease. (CT scan is less effective for evaluating abdominal adenopathy).
- MRI scan, for visualizing infradiaphragmatic structures and retroperitoneal lymph nodes.
- Lymphangiogram (LAG) for children with equivocal infradiaphragmatic imaging, and if expertise is available at center.
- Bone marrow biopsy for all children except those with stages IA/IIA disease.
- Bone scan for all children with bone pain and elevated alkaline phosphatase.
- Gallium scan.
- Surgical staging, only if the findings will alter the choice of therapy.

Prognostic Considerations

Favorable prognostic indicators are generally characterized by localized nodal involvement in the absence of B symptoms and bulky disease.

Unfavorable prognostic indicators are those associated with the presence of B symptoms, bulky mediastinal or peripheral lymphadenopathy, extra nodal disease, and stages IIIB and IV disease.

Children and adolescents with HD in the favorable prognostic group have a 95% cure rate. Modern combination chemotherapy regimens yield cure rates of 60%–80% in advanced stage and bulky HD.

Treatment

The goal of treatment is to cure disease while preventing radiation-related organ dysfunction, infertility, musculoskeletal abnormalities, and secondary neoplasms or leukemias.

Treatment depends on age, stage, and clinical presentation. It may include radiation therapy alone, chemotherapy alone, or, most commonly, combined-modality treatment including low-dose involved field radiation therapy (**Table 2–13**) and combination multiagent chemotherapy regimens.

Types of chemotherapy regimens: (repeat cycle every 28 days)

MOPP: Mechlorethamine (nitrogen mustard), vincristine (Oncovin), procarbazine (Matulane), and prednisone

COPP: Cyclophosphamide (Cytoxan), vincristine, procarbazine, and prednisone

ABVD: Doxorubicin (Adriamycin), bleomycin, vinblastine, dacarbazine

VEPA: Vinblastine, etoposide, prednisone, doxorubicin, (Adriamycin)

OPPA: Vincristine, procarbazine, prednisone, doxorubicin

Recurrent Disease

Most relapses occur within 3 years of diagnosis, although relapses have been reported 10 years after diagnosis. Relapsed Stage I disease that was treated initally with radiation therapy alone, is associated with a long-term survival rate of 50%–80% when treated with salvage chemotherapy. A myeloablative treatment regimen followed by autologous transplantation, using bone marrow or peripheral stem cell rescue, is a treatment option for relapsed high-risk patients. These include patients who develop refractory disease during or within 1 year of completing therapy, who respond poorly to conventional salvage therapy, or who have had multiple relapses. Survival rates in these high-risk children and adolescents range from 30%–50%.

Nursing Assessment and Interventions

Goal: The patient will experience minimal complications related to the onset of the tumor.

Assessment:

- Review the patient's type and stage of Hodgkin's disease.
- Assess the presenting symptoms and obtain a complete history, including the incidence and duration of symptoms (e.g., lymphadenopathy, fevers, weight loss, night sweats, pain, fatigue, infection, bleeding, neurological changes), predisposing factors (e.g., exposure to radiation, cytotoxic drugs, genetic abnormalities), and family history.
- Perform a complete physical examination to determine the presence of enlarged lymph nodes, pallor, petechiae, signs of infection, rash, hepatosplenomegaly, and neurological changes.

Table 2–13. Involved-Field Radiotherapy for Hodgkin's Disease

Type	Description
Mantle	Supradiaphragmatic disease involving medistinum as well as one or more cervical, supraclavicular, infraclavicular, or axillary lymph nodes (egs. Minimantle, hemiminimantle)
Mediastinum	Disease in mediastinum, one or both hila.
Para-aortic/	Subdiaphragmatic disease hilar/spleenin spleen, splenic hilar, or para-aortic areas
Spade	Subdiaphragmatic disease in spleen, splenic hilar, para-aortic, and iliac areas
Pelvis	Disease in bilateral iliac and inguinal-femoral areas (egs. Hemipelvis)
Inverted Y	Subdiaphragmatic disease in spleen, splenic hilar, para-aortic, and pelvic areas

Source: Data from National Cancer Institute NCI–PDQ

- Review the laboratory findings.
- Review radiological imaging studies, as indicated.
- Review surgical and pathology reports, as indicated.
- Assess the child's degree of pain.

Interventions:

- Provide comfort measures.
- Provide pain medication as needed.
- Monitor serum chemistries for tumor lysis syndrome. Provide intravenous hydration with alkalinization and allopurinol and strict intake and output monitoring.
- Monitor for signs of respiratory compromise.
- Monitor for signs of superior vena cava syndrome.
- Monitor for signs of abdominal complications.
- Administer blood products and chemotherapy as needed.

Goal: The patient will experience minimal complications related to treatment.

Assessment:

- Assess for toxicity related to specific chemotherapy agents (see the discussion of chemotherapy in Section IV, "Childhood Cancer Treatment").
- Assess for toxicity related to radiation therapy, if that treatment was given (see the discussion of radiation therapy in Section IV, "Childhood Cancer Treatment").
- Assess for complications related to any surgery performed (see the discussion of surgery in Section IV, "Childhood Cancer Treatment").
- Assess for signs of infection.
- Assess for evidence of fatigue, bleeding, pain, and nutritional deficits.
- Monitor intake and output of fluid and electrolytes.
- Determine the type of intravenous access that is needed.
- Assess for the possibility of emergency complications.
- Assess for a response to therapy (i.e., decrease in the size of the mass or enlarged lymph nodes, decrease in sedimentation rate, improved weight, and resolution of pruritis).

Interventions:

- Refer the child for central intravenous treatment, as it is needed.
- Provide comfort measures.
- Provide pain medication, as needed.
- Provide medication to relieve pruritis.
- Provide instruction on proper mouth care, nutrition, and hygiene.
- Educate the family regarding neutropenia, anemia, thrombocytopenia, the signs and symptoms of infection, and fever precautions.
- Obtain cultures and radiological examinations, as ordered, when infection is suspected, and initiate antibiotics, if it is indicated.
- Provide alternative methods of nutrition (e.g., oral supplements, NG or parenteral supplements).
- Review all findings of the laboratory and radiological studies with the patient and the family.

Goal: The patient and family will be adequately informed regarding diagnosis, disease, and treatment.

Assessment:

- Assess the level of knowledge of patients and family about the diagnosis and disease.
- Assess their level of knowledge about treatment (i.e., surgery, radiation therapy, chemotherapy).
- Assess the learning styles of the patient and family (see Section VIII, "Patient and Family Education").
- Assess how well they understand the role of the multidisciplinary team in treating children with Hodgkin's disease.

Interventions:

- Communicate with the patient and the family in an appropriate style.
- Provide them with appropriate educational resources and review the material with them.
- Ensure that the family is aware of when and how to contact the healthcare team.
- Encourage the patient and the family to ask questions related to the diagnosis, disease, and treatment.
- Clarify information provided by various members of the multidisciplinary team.

Goal: The patient and the family will cope adequately with the diagnosis.

Assessment:

- Assess the family's communication and coping styles, in general.
- Assess the family's adjustment to the diagnosis.

Interventions:

- Provide the patient and the family with honest answers.
- Provide emotional support.
- Anticipate the need for referral services (e.g., social work, chaplain, Candlelighters, American Cancer Society, Leukemia Society).
- Offer the child age-appropriate "hospital play."
- Offer to introduce a contact family who has dealt with a similar malignancy to talk with the patient and the family.

Expected Patient and Family Outcomes

The child and family can do the following:

- Describe Hodgkin's disease and the plan of care.
- List the expected and possible toxic side effects of therapy.
- Outline methods to prevent infection.
- Describe the schedule of treatment, procedures, and follow-up care.

- Describe available community resources.
- Demonstrate the skills needed to care for the child at home.
- Explain how and when to contact the healthcare team if problems or questions arise.

Central Nervous System Tumors

Melody Watral

Definition

A tumor in the regions of the brain that can be malignant or benign, based upon the microscopic appearance of the mass, is defined as a brain tumor.

Pathophysiology

Astrocytomas: These tumors account for 50% of all pediatric brain tumors and are classified according to the degree of anaplasia. Per the World Health Organization (WHO) classification system for astrocytomas, Grade I tumors are pilocytic astrocytomas; Grade II tumors are low-grade fibrillary astrocytomas; Grade III tumors are anaplastic astrocytomas; and Grade IV tumors are glioblastoma multiforme. Grades II and IV tumors have higher mitotic activity, and Grade IV tumors have vascular changes and necrosis.

Thirty-five percent of astrocytomas occur in the cerebellum (the majority have a benign histology), 25% in the cerebral hemispheres (with an equal distribution of benign and malignant histology), 15% in the brainstem (the majority have a malignant histology), 11% in the optic chiasm or optic nerves (the majority with a benign histology), and 7% occur in the hypothalamus (the majority have a benign histology).

Brainstem glioma (anaplastic astrocytoma or glioblastoma of the brainstem): There is a rapid onset of symptoms in this type of tumor. It appears as a diffuse tumor on MRI. Less than 10% of patients will survive more than 18 months from the time of diagnosis. The tumor is surgically inoperable in the majority of cases (see Section IV, "Childhood Cancer Treatment," for exceptions).

Medulloblastoma: This tumor type, which accounts for 25% of all pediatric brain tumors, is the most common malignant primary central nervous system (CNS) tumor. It is a highly cellular, small, round, blue cell tumor, and usually arises in the cerebellum or in the fourth ventricle. It grows aggressively and may metastasize through the CNS and extraneurally into the bone marrow and viscera.

Ependymoma: This type of tumor accounts for 8%–10% of all pediatric brain tumors. Two-thirds of the cases occur as infratentorial lesions, often in the posterior fossa, with the remaining cases occurring supratentorially. WHO classifies Grade I tumors as sub-ependymomas (benign, slow growing), and myxopapillary ependymomas (a variant with favorable prognosis). Grade II tumors are classic epnedymomas. Grade III tumors are anaplastic ependymomas, which may develop through malignant progression from low-grade ependymomas, but typically show anaplastic features on the first biopsy.

Craniopharyngioma: Seven percent of all pediatric tumors are of this type. This tumor arises from the sella, which is adjacent to the pituitary gland, the hypothalamus, and the optic nerve.

Incidence and Etiology

An estimated 3,110 new cases of childhood primary brain tumors were expected to be diagnosed in the United States in 2002. At least 2,330 of the cases would occur in children under 15 years of age. Tumors of the CNS are the second most common neoplasm and the most common solid tumor in children. Sixty percent are in the posterior fossa (infratentorial tumors such as cerebellar astrocytomas, medulloblastomas, ependymomas) and 40% are supratentorial (astrocytomas, hypothalamic and optic pathway tumors, craniopharyngiomas). The causes are as yet unknown. Possible sites of oncogenesis include chromosome 17 in medulloblastoma and astrocytoma tumors and chromosome 10 in glioblastoma tumors.

Clinical Presentation

Diagnosis often is difficult to establish; symptoms often mimic common childhood illnesses, and vary, depending upon the location and growth rate of the tumor (**Figure 2-5**). A sudden onset of symptoms tends to occur in more aggressive (malignant) tumors. A slow, indolent course and incidental radiological finding tend to indicate slowly growing (benign) tumors.

Posterior fossa symptoms (i.e., headache, vomiting, ataxia, nystagmus, diplopia) most commonly are caused by increased intracranial pressure. Cranial nerve deficits are associated with brain stem involvement, either from tumor, infiltration, compression on the surrounding structures, or

Figure 2-5. Structures and Functions of the Brain

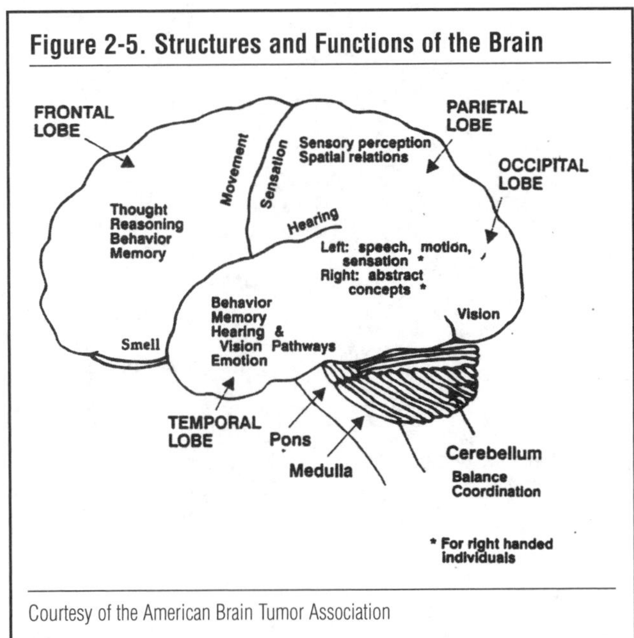

Courtesy of the American Brain Tumor Association

from hydrocephalus. Supratentorial symptoms include hemiparesis, seizures, visual changes, and intellectual problems. Midline tumors in the hypothalamus/pituitary region present with visual changes, endocrine abnormalities, and increased intracranial pressure (ICP).

ICP may result from the mass effect exerted by the tumor on the surrounding structures, or result from the obstruction of CSF flow. The "classic triad" of symptoms from elevated ICP are morning headaches, lethargy, and nausea and/or vomiting (headaches usually improve after vomiting). However, most initial signs of increasing ICP are subacute, including declining academic performance, personality changes, fatigue, and complaints of vague intermittent headaches. Signs of increased ICP in younger children include increased irritability, increased head circumference, bulging fontanel(s) and the "sun setting" sign (limited upward gaze and a forced downward deviation of the eyes), which may be seen in infants with ICP.

When possible, the mass lesion responsible for the increased ICP should be removed. An external ventricular drain may be placed for cerebral spinal fluid (CSF) diversion after surgery. A ventriculoperitoneal (VP) shunt may be required to treat persistent hydrocephaul that does not resolve after tumor resection or biopsy (**Figure 2-6**). An endoscopic anterior third ventriculostomy (establishing an opening in the floor of the third ventricle to reestablish CSF pathways) may eliminate the need for a permanent VP shunt.

Diagnostic: The diagnostic includes an evaluation of the extent of the disease before therapy is started. An evaluation should include the following:

- A complete history of the current illness, specifically, the incidence and duration of symptoms such as pain, fatigue, weakness, neurological changes (e.g., developmental delay or regression, morning vomiting, headache, seizures, visual changes, ataxia); predisposing factors (e.g., exposure to radiation, cytotoxic drugs, genetic abnormalities); and family history.
- A physical examination that includes growth and development, cranial nerve examination, gait, strength, sensory examination, coordination, deep tendon reflexes, head circumference, mental status.
- MRI of the brain—the gold standard test—which has replaced computed tomography (CT) in most cases.
- MRI of the spine, done before surgery if there is an infratentorial tumor.
- Magnetic resonance angiography is used if concerned with the vascularity of the tumor.
- Positron emission tomography (PET), which may be used to evaluate the metabolic activity of the tumor.
- Bone marrow aspirates and bone scan, which are done only in cases of medulloblastoma.

Prognostic considerations:

- The rate of cell growth of the tumor is a consideration (high-grade tumors have a poorer prognosis).
- Surgical accessibility allows for more than 95% of patients with low-grade tumors to be cured and for improved survival in patients with high-grade tumors when more than 95% of the tumor is removed.
- Deep tumors, even those that are histologically benign, have significant sequelae.
- Infants with malignant tumors have a poor prognosis.
- Younger children tend to recover deficits after surgery to a fuller extent than do older children.

Treatment and prognosis: Surgery is the primary treatment, with the goal being maximal surgical resection. Advances in surgical techniques in the past decade are responsible for maximal surgical resection with lower morbidity. MRI and stereotactic, or MRI computer-guided, surgery permit surgeons to plan an approach that minimizes injury to the adjacent brain tissue. Intraoperative electrophysiological monitoring of the motor strip and motor pathways identify the tumor's location with respect to other tissue. Surgical procedures are performed in stages, and second-look operations keep the surgeon involved throughout all stages of the illness.

Posterior fossa syndrome, which can occur after surgery, can include different signs and symptoms comprising mutism or speech disturbances, dysphagia, decreased motor movement, cranial nerve palsies, and emotional lability. Signs and symptoms occur 24–107 hours after surgery. Recovery may take weeks or months, depending upon the severity of the symptoms.

Figure 2–6. A Shunt Used to Treat Hydrocephalus

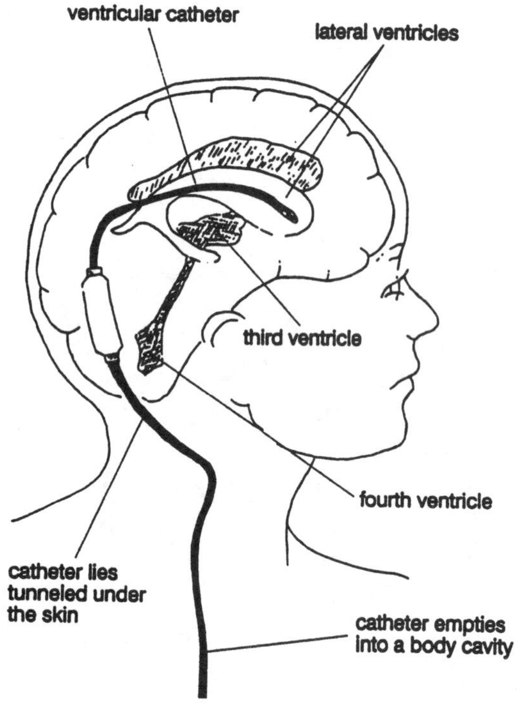

Courtesy of the American Brain Tumor Association

Radiation therapy: Radiation therapy, the oldest treatment for brain tumors, is used to treat malignant tumors or deep benign lesions with a large amount of residual disease. Radiation therapy affects the ability of cells to continue dividing by targeting the cells' DNA. Improved technology (i.e., three-dimensional imaging utilizing CT and MRI, focused irradiation) has improved accuracy while causing minimal damage to normal tissue.

Radiation therapy is delayed in children under 3 years of age because of its detrimental effects on the developing brain. Use of local field or cranial-spinal radiation therapy is dependent upon the histological findings. Standard radiation therapy, with approximately 200 cGy per treatment to a total 5,500–6,000 cGy to the local field, is given once daily. Spinal doses are usually 2,400 cGy.

Hyperfractionated radiation treatment: This treatment consists of 100 cGy given twice daily at least 6 hours apart, which permits a higher total dose (usually 7,200 cGy) and a lower ultimate morbidity.

Chemotherapy: Chemotherapy is a standard treatment for certain brain tumors and is given with, or as an adjuvant treatment to, radiation therapy. Clinical studies by the Children's Oncology Group and the Pediatric Brain Tumor Consortium have tested specific chemotherapy agents against histologically malignant and benign tumors.

Chemotherapy agents most commonly used to treat pediatric brain tumors include vincristine (Oncovin), carmustine (BCNU), lomustine (CCNU), carboplatin (CBDCA), cisplatin (Platinol), etoposide (VP-16), cyclophosphamide (Cytoxan), thiotepa (Thiotepa), temozolomide (Temodar), and irinotecan (CPT-11). High-dose chemotherapy followed by autologous bone marrow rescue has replaced radiotherapy in patients who are diagnosed with highly malignant tumors (with minimal residual disease) before 3 years of age.

Supportive care: Supportive care should focus on the risk of increased ICP. Hydration is aimed at maintaining an isovolemic state to avoid fluid and electrolyte shifts that could result in brain edema. Maintenance fluids are administered with mannitol (osmitrol) and furosemide (Lasix) to maintain diuresis and fluid balance.

Treatment for Specific Types of Brain Tumors

Low-grade astrocytoma of the cerebellum. The goal is gross total resection (greater than 95% removal). If that total is not achieved with the first surgery, another operation may be performed. Surgically accessible tumors of this type can be cured with gross total resection alone. The recurrence rate is very low. Patient progress is followed with periodic MRI scans.

Low-grade astrocytoma supratentorial area. A gross total resection, if possible, has the best prognosis and is usually obtainable in frontal, parietal and temporal tumors. Chemotherapy or local field radiation is given to midline tumors that are not completely resected.

Low-grade (exophytic) astrocytomas of the brainstem. This type of tumor, which accounts for less than 20% of all brain stem tumors, is often located in the medulla (based upon MRI appearance). Surgical debulking of exophytic brain stem tumors may be possible, but there is a significant risk of lower cranial nerve problems after surgery, which can affect swallowing and breathing. Local field radiation therapy has been used with older children with good results. Children with large residual disease are given chemotherapy.

High-grade astrocytoma of the supratentorial area. The prognosis is poor for this type of tumor. Gross total resection offers the best prognosis. Chemotherapy and focal radiation therapy are given after surgery. High-dose chemotherapy with autologous bone marrow rescue—an experimental treatment—possibly can be effective for patients with minimal residual disease.

High-grade astrocytoma of the brain stem. This tumor has a rapid onset of symptoms (i.e., increased intracranial pressure, cranial nerve deficits, hemiparesis) and a diffuse appearance on MRI involving multiple levels of the brain stem. Morbidity from surgery outweighs its advantages. Treatment consists of local standard fraction or hyperfractionated radiation therapy with or without adjunctive chemotherapy. Overall survival in patients with diffuse pontine gliomas is less than 10%; the median survival time is 18 months from diagnosis, despite radiation therapy, with or without chemotherapy.

Medulloblastoma. The presenting symptoms associated with medulloblastoma are related to increased intracranial pressure (i.e., morning headaches, with forceful or projectile vomiting). Hydrocephalus occurs secondary to mass effect and obstruction of CSF flow from the fourth ventricle. Surgical resection is the initial treatment. MRI of the spine, CSF sampling, and bone marrow studies are done to determine the extent of the disease. The best prognosis is associated with gross total resection without metastatic disease at diagnosis. Cranial-spinal radiation is used in children older than 3 years of age. Chemotherapy is given during and after radiation therapy. High-dose chemotherapy, with autologous bone marrow rescue, is administered in children under 3 years of age. The overall, average, long-term survival rate is 60%–65% and has been reported as high as 70% in patients who are considered "good-risk" cases.

Ependymoma. Approximately 60%–75% of ependymomas are found in the posterior fossa (fourth ventricle); 25%–40% of ependymomas are supratentorial. The best prognosis is associated with gross total surgical resection, which is difficult in the fourth ventricle because of its close proximity to the brain stem. Radiation (focal or cranial-spinal) with or without chemotherapy is used after surgery. Prognosis is dependent upon histology, the degree of metastatic disease, and the extent of surgical resection (the most significant prognostic indicator).

Craniopharyngioma. Surgical resection is the primary treatment for this type of tumor; however, gross total removal is difficult because of its proximity to the hypothalamus, pituitary gland, and optic chiasm. Surgical morbidity (i.e., hypothalamic or pituitary dysfunction, neurocognitive dysfunction, visual problems, and psychosocial problems) and mortality are significant. Focal radiation therapy, intracystic radioactive implants, and chemotherapy are used to treat recurrent or residual tumor. Gross total resection is associated with long-term survival but often results in significant morbidity.

Recurrent disease: Disease commonly reoccurs in infants and in patients with malignant astrocytomas and subtotally resected low-grade tumors. Late recurrence is most frequently associated with medulloblastoma. Patients should be evaluated for possible surgical debulking, radiation therapy (if it has not previously been administered), or experimental chemotherapy. Placement of a ventriculoperitoneal shunt may be required if hydrocephalus is present. High-dose chemotherapy, followed by autologous marrow rescue, is used for patients with recurrent malignant tumors and minimal residual disease. Pain management and supportive care should be given as needed and patients should be referred to a hospice.

Spinal Cord Tumors

Definition: Spinal cord tumors are intramedullary tumors within the spinal cord.

Pathophysiology: Of these tumors, 58% are astrocytomas, 28% are ependymomas, and the remainder consist of metastatic medulloblastomas, dermoid tumors, and lipomas. The majority of spinal cord tumors have low-grade histology, but exceptions are anaplastic astrocytoma and glioblastoma multiform tumors.

Incidence and etiology: Spinal cord tumors account for 6% of all pediatric CNS tumors. They occur most frequently in children who are between 10 and 16 years of age. The incidence in males and females is the same.

Clinical presentation: Symptoms, which may be present for months before a tumor is diagnosed, include scoliosis, pain, motor weakness, and sensory disturbances (e.g., paresthesias, dysesthesias, radiculopathy, and, rarely, sphincter dysfunction).

Diagnostic: An MRI will reveal an intramedullary tumor that is either extensive or focal in nature. Radiographs may detect scoliosis, along with a diffusely widened spinal canal.

Prognostic considerations: The majority (85%–90%) of spinal cord tumors in children are not fatal. High-grade astrocytomas account for only 10%–15% of all spinal cord tumors. These tumors are not responsive to current aggressive surgical, radiation, and chemotherapy regimens. Patients with deficits before surgery have a greater risk that those deficits will persist after surgery or any adjunctive treatment. Younger children tend to recover postoperative deficits more completely than do older children.

Treatment and prognosis: Surgical resection, which has the goal of achieving a radical—or even total—excision when technically possible, is desirable. Ependymomas are clearly demarcated from the adjacent normal spinal cord and are more easily resected than most tumors. Low-grade astrocytomas that have an interface between the normal spinal cord and tumor are more easily removed than most tumors. The use of intraoperative sensory and motor-evoked potentials by electrophysiological monitoring can facilitate surgical resection. Ideally, surgery should be performed by a pediatric neurosurgeon in a large tertiary care center.

Radiation therapy often is used. The use of chemotherapy to treat malignant spinal cord tumors has been limited. Physical and occupational therapy are often necessary after surgery.

Recurrent disease: Surgical resection may be possible for recurrent disease. Radiation therapy may be administered after surgery.

Nursing Assessment and Interventions

Goal: The patient will experience minimal complications related to the onset of the tumor.

Assessment:

- Know the type of brain or CNS tumor, location of the tumor, and presenting symptoms.
- Assess the presenting symptoms and obtain a complete history, including incidence and duration of symptoms (e.g., pain, fatigue, weakness, developmental delay, morning vomiting, headache, seizures, ataxia), predisposing factors (e.g., exposure to radiation, cytotoxic drugs, genetic abnormalities), and family history.
- Perform a complete physical examination that includes growth and development, cranial nerve examination, gait, strength, sensory examination, deep tendon reflexes, head circumference, and mental status.
- Review laboratory findings.
- Review radiological imaging studies as indicated.
- Review surgical and pathology reports as indicated.
- Assess the child's degree of pain.

Interventions:

- Provide comfort measures.
- Provide pain medication as needed.
- Explain all tests, procedures, and results to the patient and the family.

Goal: The patient will experience minimal complications related to treatment.

Assessment:

- Assess the child for toxicity associated with specific chemotherapy agents (see the discussion of chemotherapy in Section IV, "Childhood Cancer Treatment").
- Assess the child for toxicity associated with radiation therapy, if it was given (see the discussion of radiation therapy in Section IV, "Childhood Cancer Treatment").
- Assess the child for complications associated with surgery, if surgery has been performed (see the discussion of surgery in Section IV, "Childhood Cancer Treatment").
- Assess for signs of infection.
- Assess the child for evidence of fatigue, bleeding, pain, and nutritional deficits.
- Monitor fluid intake and electrolytes.
- Determine the type of intravenous access that is needed.
- Assess for the possibility of emergency complications.
- Assess for response to therapy (i.e., decrease in size of mass, evaluation of any metastatic disease).

Interventions:

- Refer the child for central intravenous access, as needed.
- Provide comfort measures.
- Provide pain medication, as needed.
- Provide instruction on proper mouth care, nutrition, and hygiene.
- Educate the family regarding neutropenia, anemia, thrombocytopenia, signs and symptoms of infection, and fever precautions.
- Obtain cultures and radiological examinations, as ordered, when infection is suspected, and initiate antibiotics, if indicated.
- Provide alternative methods of nutrition (e.g., oral supplements, NG and parenteral supplements).
- Review all findings of laboratory and radiological studies with the patient and the family.

Goal: The patient and family will be adequately informed regarding the diagnosis, disease work-up, and treatment.

Assessment:

- Assess the level of knowledge of patient and family about the diagnosis and disease work-up.
- Assess their level of knowledge about treatment (i.e., surgery, radiation therapy, chemotherapy).
- Assess their learning styles (see Section VIII, "Patient and Family Education").
- Assess how well they understand the role of the multidisciplinary team in treating children with CNS tumors.

Interventions:

- Communicate with the patient and the family in an appropriate style.
- Provide them with appropriate educational resources and review the material with them.
- Determine that the family is aware of when and how to contact the healthcare team.
- Encourage the patient and the family to ask questions related to the diagnosis, disease work-up, and treatment.
- Clarify the information provided by various members of the multidisciplinary team.

Goal: The patient and the family will cope adequately with the diagnosis.

Assessment:

- Assess the family's communication and coping styles in general.
- Assess the family's adjustment to the diagnosis.

Interventions:

- Give the patient and the family honest answers to their questions.
- Provide emotional support.
- Anticipate the need for referral services (e.g., social work, chaplain, Candlelighters, American Cancer Society, Leukemia Society, Brain Tumor Assocation).
- Offer the child age-appropriate "hospital play."
- Offer to introduce a contact family who has dealt with a similar malignancy to talk with the patient and the family.

Expected Patient and Family Outcomes

The child and parents can do the following:

- Describe the type of brain or CNS tumor and the plan of care.
- List the expected and possible toxic side effects of therapy.
- Outline methods for preventing infection.
- Describe the schedule of treatment, procedures, and follow-up care.
- Describe available community resources.
- Demonstrate the skills needed to care for the child at home.
- Explain how and when to contact the healthcare team if problems or questions arise.

NEUROBLASTOMA

Eileen Duffey-Lind

Definition

A neuroblastoma is a malignant tumor that develops from neural crest cells normally found in the sympathetic ganglia, adrenal medulla, and other sites, such as the chest and abdomen. The cells are primitive neuroblasts that may differentiate into neuroblastoma or ganglioneuroblastoma (malignant forms), or into ganglioneuroma, (the benign form, without metastatic potential). Neuroblastoma has diverse clinical and biological characteristics and natural history.

Pathophysiology

A neuroblastoma is a solid soft mass with microscopic nests of small tumor cells, separated by fibrovascular septa, with areas of hemorrhage, calcification, and necrosis. This type of tumor is derived from neural crest cells and is composed of small round cells with blue granules. It has a varied spectrum of maturation, including neuroblastoma, ganglioneuroblastoma, and ganglioneuroma (the most mature).

Electron microscopy and immunohistochemistry help differentiate neuroblastoma from other small, round, blue-cell tumors, such as rhabdomyosarcomas. Pseudorosettes can be seen in 15%–50% of cases. Depending upon its size and location, this tumor can cause clinical effects as it enlarges.

Having multiple copies of the oncogene *N-myc* ("*N-myc* amplification") is associated with advanced stages of disease, rapid tumor progression, and a poor prognosis. A gene called TRK-A may be associated with cell differentiation and tumor regression. High TRK-A expression is associated with a biologically and clinically favorable group; age younger than 1 year and stages 1, 2, and 4S.

In infants, tumors that are hyperdiploid (i.e., they have a DNA index [DI] greater than 1) are more likely to reflect lower-stage disease and be more responsive to chemotherapy. Tumors in infants with a DI of 1 are more likely to have advanced disease and not be responsive to these drugs. Older children with hyperdiploid tumors do not have favorable outcomes.

Incidence and Etiology

Neuroblastoma is the most common extracranial solid tumor in children, accounting for 8%–10% of all childhood cancers. The prevalence is approximately 1 case per 7,000 live births, and there are approximately 600 new cases per year in the United States. It is the most common malignancy in infants, accounting for 50% of all malignancies in newborns. Its actual incidence may be higher; the phenomenon of spontaneous tumor regression and maturation of the tumor make it difficult to know its precise incidence. Neuroblastoma is more common in boys than girls (1.1:1.0).

The most commonly diagnosed neoplasm occurs in the first year of life; the average age at diagnosis is 2 years. Most children are diagnosed with neuroblastoma by the age of 5; a diagnosis after age 10 is rare.

Known as the "silent tumor," neuroblastoma presents with widespread metastatic disease at diagnosis in 70% of patients. Increased incidence has been reported in patients with neurofibromatosis Type I, Hirschsprung disease, and central hypoventilation (Ondin's curse).

Although neuroblastoma usually occurs sporadically, 1%–2% of patients report a family history of the disease. A small subset of patients have familial transmission through an autosomal dominant gene, with an increased incidence among siblings and identical twins, following Knudson's two-mutation theory of the origin of childhood cancer. The first mutation may be germinal (present in all cells prezygotically): the second may be environmental. Mass screenings for early detection that use urine catecholamines have been attempted, but are problematic due to issues such as specimen collection, unreliability of test results, lack of access to all infants, infants lost to follow-up, consumption of healthcare resources, and the subjection of infants to cancer treatment that may not be necessary. Screening studies at 6 months of age or younger, therefore, do not reduce the incidence of late-appearing, advanced-stage disease. Although longer follow-up will be needed, it is unlikely that screening infants will reduce neuroblastoma mortality.

Clinical Presentation

Neuroblastoma most commonly includes pain, abdominal mass (which may cross the midline), mass in other anatomic sites, and malaise. Tumors can occur anywhere along the sympathetic nervous system. More than half occur in the retroperitoneal area and present as an abdominal mass that often involves the adrenal gland. Although the frequency of adrenal tumors is slightly higher in children (40%) than in infants (25%), infants have more thoracic and cervical primary tumors. Other disease sites include the head, posterior mediastinum, pelvis, and neck. Sites of metastatic spread include the lymph nodes, bone, bone marrow, liver, and subcutaneous tissue. Rarely does disease spread to the lung and brain except as a manifestation of relapsing or end-stage disease.

If metastases to bone or bone marrow, or both, are present, the patient may have malaise, or low-grade fever, or may limp. Catecholamine secretion may produce hypertension, flushing, periods of excessive sweating, and irritability. Subcutaneous tumors may appear as hardened bluish nodules that can be seen or palpated; they have been described as a "blueberry muffin" sign. Periorbital lesions with proptosis and periorbital ecchymoses have been mistaken for signs of child abuse. A tumor in the intervertebral ganglion tends to grow into intervertebral foramena that forms a dumbbell-shaped mass that produces symptoms of cord compression that include paralysis, weakness in the extremities, incontinence, and pain. This is an oncology emergency, and early recognition is imperative because cord compression can result in permanent paralysis.

High thoracic and cervical masses can be associated with Horner's syndrome, which consists of unilateral ptosis, myosis, and anhydrosis.

Several unique paraneoplastic syndromes have been associated with both localized and disseminated neuroblastoma. Opsomyoclonus (myoclonic jerking and random eye movement) and cerebellar ataxia have been observed in as many as 4% of patients.

From 7%–9% of patients with neural crest tumors have symptoms related to tumor secretion of vasoactive intestinal polypeptide (VIP) that causes intractable diarrhea that results in hypokalemia and dehydration. Most tumors secreting VIP are mature histologically (ganglioneuroblastoma or ganglioneuroma) and these patients almost always have favorable outcomes.

Diagnostic

A diagnostic includes an evaluation of the extent of disease before initiation of therapy. This evaluation should include the following:

- A complete history of the current illness, including symptoms of increased catecholamines (e.g., hypertension, flushing, periods of excessive sweating, and irritability); weight loss, anorexia, cachexia, and diarrhea; pain, limping, refusal to walk or use extremities; symptoms associated with pressure to surrounding systems such as changes in bowel or bladder function due to compression.
- A complete physical examination that includes observation for periorbital ecchymosis or proptosis or both; bluish, movable cutaneous or subcutaneous nodules (almost exclusively in infants); abdominal mass that may cross midline, hepatomegaly, or pelvic mass; lymph nodes; paralysis; extremity weakness.
- CT or MRI with gadolinium to identify the location(s) of a solid tumor.
- A bone scan to assess for metastases.
- Radiographs to reveal any lesions not noted on a bone scan.
- Laboratory studies, including a complete blood count (if the bone marrow is involved, one or more cell lines may be affected; elevated ferritin is present in 50% of the patients with advanced disease and is associated with poor prognosis).

- Urinary catecholamines (vanillymandelic acid and homovanillic acid), which are elevated in 90%–95% of cases.
- Bilateral bone marrow aspirate and biopsy (biopsies are positive in 11%–30% of samples in which aspirate yielded negative results).
- Tumor tissue, for a determination of N-myc amplification and ploidy (DNA index or DI) and possible other studies.
- Meta-iodobenzylguanidine (MIBG) scan that determines bone and tissue involvement (included in routine evaluation with suspected or proven neuroblastoma).

Prognostic Considerations

Stage: This is the process that determines the location of the disease at diagnosis. A cooperative group effort to develop a universal staging system was started in 1987 and was refined in 1991. This system is the International Neuroblastoma Staging System (**Table 2-14**). Children under 1 year of age have the best prognosis. Patients more than 1 year old with advanced disease can still have excellent cure rates; some have spontaneous regression of tumors. These tumors are classified as Stage 4S. Infants with an elevated DI have improved prognoses.

After infancy, children with advanced disease have a poor prognosis. Patients with abdominal primary tumors have a poorer survival rate than do those with chest, neck, or pelvic primary tumors. N-myc amplification in the neuroblastoma cells indicates poor prognosis.

Treatment and Prognosis

Treatment and prognosis depend on the staging of the disease and the age of the child. Therapy is multimodal (i.e., surgery, chemotherapy, radiation, and bone marrow transplant).

Surgery: Surgery has a pivotal role in the management of neuroblastoma, both for treament and diagnosis. Tumor removal consists of debulking or total removal. Surgery alone is curative in low-stage disease. Second-look surgery is performed after a tumor has been exposed to chemotherapy, radiation, or both, and has decreased in size.

Chemotherapy: Chemotherapy is the predominant modality of management in neuroblastoma patients who have intermediate or high-risk disease. Commonly used drugs include vincristine (Oncovin), etoposide (VP-16), ifosfamide (Ifex), cyclophosphamide (Cytoxan), cisplatin (Platinol), carboplatin (CBDCA), and doxorubicin (Adriamycin).

Radiation therapy: Radiation therapy is given to the primary tumor site. Neuroblastoma cells are very radioresponsive. It may be useful to decrease the tumor mass initially, and radiation therapy may be required for palliative care if it is later indicated. Radiation therapy may proceed or follow surgery and chemotherapy and may be used to alleviate an emergency situation caused by proptosis, respiratory compromise, or cord compression.

Bone marrow transplant: Children with a poor prognosis who receive conventional treatment alone may benefit from intensive short-term chemotherapy followed by single or tandem autologous bone marrow transplantation.Children under 1 year of age have the best prognosis. Topotecan, a topoisomerase I inhibitor, is a new agent that currently is in phase II studies to treat neuroblastoma. Other chemotherapeutic agents under investigation include Taxol, Irinotecan, and Rebeccamycin.

Treatment is based on risk stratification. Neuroblastoma patients are divided into three risk groups (low, intermediate, high) based upon combination of biology (N-myc and ploidy), age, stage, and histology.

Low risk: Treatment of low-risk neuroblastoma consists of surgical removal of the primary tumor. Patients with stage 1 (gross total resection) can be expected to have a relapse-free survival probability of greater than 90%, regardless of

Table 2-14. International Neuroblastoma Staging System (INSS)*

Stage	Description
1	Localized tumor with complete gross excision, with or without microscopic residual disease; representative ipsilateral lymph nodes negative for tumor microscopically (nodes attached to and removed with the primary tumor may be positive).
2A	Localized tumor with incomplete gross excision; representative ipsilateral nonadherent lymph nodes negative for tumor microscopically.
2B	Localized tumor with or without complete gross excision, with ipsilateral nonadherent lymph nodes positive for tumor. Enlarged contralateral lymph nodes must be negative microscopically.
3	Unresectable unilateral tumor infiltrating across the midline, with or without regional lymph node involvement; or localized unilateral tumor with contralateral regional lymph node involvement; or midline tumor with bilateral extension by infiltration (unresectable) or by lymph node involvement. The midline is defined as the vertebral column. Tumors originating on 1 side and crossing the midline must infiltrate to or beyond the opposite side of the vertebral column.
4	Any primary tumor with dissemination to distant lymph nodes, bone, bone marrow, liver, skin, and/or other organs (except as defined for stage 4S).
4S	Localized primary tumor (as defined for stage 1, 2A, or 2B), with dissemination limited to skin, liver, and/or bone marrow (limited to infants less than 1 year of age). Marrow involvement should be minimal (<10% of total nucleated cells identified as malignant by bone biopsy or by bone marrow aspirate). More extensive bone marrow involvement would be considered to be stage 4 disease. The results of the MIBG scan (if performed) should be negative for disease in the bone marrow.

Source: Data from National Cancer Institute NCI – PDQ

*Combines features of the previously used POG and CCG systems

age. The majority of stage 2 patients who receive surgery alone for treatment fall into the low-risk category, as do most patients with stage 4S disease.

Intermediate risk: The approach to treatment for intermediate risk is moderate-dose, intensive chemotherapy with carboplatin, cytoxan, doxorubicin, and etoposide. Radical surgery and external beam radiation is avoided in the majority of these patients. Most infants with stage 4 are treated as intermediate risk because they do not typically have N-myc amplification.

High risk: Historically, high-risk neuroblastoma patients have had long-term survival probabilities of less than 15%. Treatment with intensive induction chemotherapy, myeloablative consolidation treatment with stem cell rescue, and minimal residual disease treatment, have improved overall survival rates. Some studies that involve this intense treatment result in a 3-year event-free survival rate of approximately 40%–60%.

Recurrent Disease

The treatments for recurrent therapy are high-dose therapy with bone marrow transplant or peripheral stem cell rescue and often, palliative therapy. The rate of cure of patients who recur after treatment for high-risk disease remains low. Current innovative approaches include novel cytotoxic agents, targeted delivery of radionuclides, retinoids, and immune-mediated therapy.

Radioactive MIBG is a targeted delivery of radiation to neuroblastoma cells used in the United States for recurrent or refractory disease with or without stem cell rescue.

13-Cis-retinoic acids are effective treatments in cases of minimal residual disease. Newer retinoids, such as fenretinide, are being developed for use in neuroblastoma treatment.

Neuroblastoma also can be treated with antibodies against ganglioside GD2 for minimal residual disease. These antibodies, alone or with cytokines, have been active against neuroblastoma cells.

Nursing Assessment and Interventions

Goal: The patient will experience minimal complications related to the onset of tumor.

Assessment:

- Determine the type of malignancy and the location and extent of disease.
- Obtain a complete history, including symptoms associated with catecholamines (hypertension, flushing, periods of excessive sweating, and irritability); weight loss, anorexia, cachexia, and diarrhea; pain, refusal to walk, limping, or refusal to use extremities; symptoms associated with pressure to surrounding organs (e.g., changes in bowel or bladder function); family history of cancer.
- Perform a complete physical examination to assess for periorbital ecchymosis and/or proptosis; bluish, movable cutaneous or subcutaneous nodules; abdominal mass that may cross the midline, hepatomegaly, or pelvic mass; enlarged lymph nodes; paralysis, extremity weakness.
- Review laboratory findings.
- Review radiological imaging studies as indicated.
- Review surgical and pathology reports as indicated.
- Assess the child's degree of pain.

Interventions:

- Provide comfort measures.
- Provide pain medication, as needed.
- Explain all tests, procedures, and results to the patient and the family.

Goal: The patient will experience minimal complications related to treatment.

Assessment:

- Assess the child for toxicity related to specific chemotherapy agents (see the discussion of chemotherapy in Section IV, "Childhood Cancer Treatment").
- Assess the child for toxicity related to radiation therapy, if it is being given (see the discussion of radiation therapy in Section IV, "Childhood Cancer Treatment").
- Assess the child for complications related to surgery, if used (see the discussion of surgery in Section IV, "Childhood Cancer Treatment").
- Assess for signs of infection.
- Assess the child for evidence of fatigue, bleeding, pain, and nutritional deficits.
- Monitor fluids and electrolytes.
- Determine the type of intravenous access that is needed.
- Assess for the possibility of emergency complications.
- Assess for a response to therapy (i.e., a decrease in the size of the mass or enlarged lymph nodes, evaluation of any metastatic disease).

Interventions:

- Refer the child for central intravenous access, as needed.
- Provide comfort measures.
- Provide pain medication as needed.
- Provide instruction on proper mouth care, nutrition, and hygiene.
- Educate the family regarding neutropenia, anemia, thrombocytopenia, as well as the signs and symptoms of infection and fever precautions.
- Obtain cultures and radiological examinations, as ordered, when infection is suspected, and initiate antibiotics, if indicated.
- Provide alternative methods of nutrition (e.g., oral supplements, NG and parenteral supplements).
- Review all findings of laboratory tests and radiological studies with the patient and the family.

Goal: The patient, the family, or both will be adequately informed regarding the diagnosis, disease, and treatment.

Assessment:

- Assess the level of knowledge of the patient and family about the diagnosis and disease.

- Assess their level of knowledge about treatment (i.e., surgery, radiation therapy, chemotherapy).
- Assess their learning styles (see Section VIII, "Patient and Family Education").
- Assess their understanding of the role of the multidisciplinary team in treating children with neuroblastoma.

Interventions:

- Communicate with the patient and the family in an appropriate style.
- Provide them with appropriate educational resources and review the material with them.
- Ensure that the family is aware of when and how to contact the healthcare team.
- Encourage the patient, the family, or both to ask questions related to the diagnosis, disease, and treatment.
- Clarify the information provided by various members of the multidisciplinary team.

Goal: The patient and the family will cope adequately with diagnosis.

Assessment:

- Assess the family's communication and coping styles in general.
- Assess the family's adjustment to the diagnosis.

Interventions:

- Provide the patient and the family with honest answers to their questions.
- Provide emotional support.
- Anticipate the need for referral services (e.g., social work, chaplain, Candlelighters, American Cancer Society, Leukemia Society).
- Offer the child age-appropriate "hospital play."
- Offer to introduce a contact family who has dealt with a similar malignancy to talk with the patient and the family.

Expected Patient and Family Outcomes

The child, the parents, or both can do the following:

- Describe the type of neuroblastoma and the plan of care.
- List the expected and possible toxic side effects of therapy.
- Outline methods to prevent infection.
- Describe the schedule of treatment, procedures, and follow-up care.
- Describe available community resources.
- Demonstrate the skills needed to care for the child at home.
- Explain how and when to contact the healthcare team if problems or questions arise.

Osteosarcoma

Melody Hellsten

Definition

Osteosarcoma is a primary malignant tumor of bone.

Pathophysiology

Osteosarcoma is distinguished from other bone tumors by the production of osteoid substance. These tumors have varying degrees of osteoblastic, chondroblastic, and fibroblastic differentiation.

Incidence and Etiology

Osteosarcoma is the most common bone tumor and the sixth most common malignancy in children; in adolescents and young adults, it is the third most frequent neoplasm (after leukemias and lymphomas). There are 5.6 cases per 1 million European ancestry children under the age of 15 years, with approximately 400 children and adolescents less than 20 years old, diagnosed in the United States each year. Incidence is slightly lower in children without European ancestry. Peak incidence is in the second decade of life, during the adolescent growth spurt. Osteosarcoma often occurs earlier in girls because of their earlier growth spurt, but it is more common in boys because of their large bone volume.

Three percent of osteosarcomas result from irradiation, but this applies to the older population and occurs from 4 to 40 years (the median is 12–16 years) after receiving irradiation. Two percent of patients with Paget's disease, a premalignant condition, will develop osteosarcoma after age 50. Patients with hereditary retinoblastoma or carriers of the mutations of the p53 gene have a genetic predisposition to develop osteosarcoma, but the majority of cases are of unknown cause. Li-Fraumeni syndrome describes a condition in which mutations of the p53 gene are inherited. People have a 50% chance of developing a malignancy (usually bone or breast) by the age of 30 and a 90% chance of developing a cancer by the age of 70. (**Table 2-15.**)

Clinical Presentation

The patient may have pain that is dull, aching, and constant and is often worse at night; the average duration of the pain is 3 months before osteosarcoma is diagnosed. Pain often is attributed to trauma, which is common in active adolescents. Patients may or may not have a soft-tissue mass or swelling. This disease most commonly involves the long bones (e.g., femur, tibia, humerus). Patients may have altered gait or function of the extremity because of their reluctance to use the affected limb. Twenty percent of patients have visible metastatic disease, most commonly pulmonary, at presentation.

Diagnostic

The diagnostic includes an evaluation of the extent of disease before therapy is initiated. An evaluation should include the following:

Table 2-15. Causes of Osteosarcoma

Exposure or Characteristic	Comments
Known risk factors	
Prior treatment for childhood cancer with radiation therapy and/or chemotherapy	There is an increased risk following radiotherapy for childhood cancer.
	Independent of radiotherapy, treatment with alkylating agents increases the risk of developing osteosarcoma.
Hereditary retinoblastoma, Li-Fraumeni syndrome, and Rothmund-Thomson syndrome	Increased risk is well documented for these genetic conditions.
Radium	High doses of the radioisotope radium are known to cause osteosarcoma in adults. Whether the low levels sometimes found in drinking water confer risk to children or adults is unknown.
Factors for which evidence is limited or inconsistent	
Growth and development	There has been some suggestion that taller stature is associated with increased risk, but the results of more recent studies do not support this finding. One study showed an association with earlier age at onset of secondary sex characteristics in females and lower weight gain during pubertal growth spurt in males.
Prior trauma to tumor site	One study found a small positive association between damage to the tumor site and increased risk of osteosarcoma.
Prenatal exposure and development	Short birth length and fetal X rays were associated with an increased risk in a single study.
Parental exposures	An association with chicken farming and another with gardening fertilizer, herbicides, or pesticides have been reported in single studies
Fluoride in drinking water	The few epidemielogic studies as well as ecologic and time trend analyses suggest that fluoride is unlikely to cause osteosarcoma.

Source: National Cancer Institute SEER data 1975-1995

- A complete history of the current illness, including the location, duration, and intensity of pain; limping or refusal to bear weight; and the presence of mass.
- A complete physical examination, including observation for soft-tissue mass, abnormal gait, limited range of motion, circumference of the affected and nonaffected limb, and warmth and tenderness associated with the affected limb.
- Radiographic findings of the extremity, which often may include a sunburst pattern, mixed regions of sclerosis and lytic lesions of bone; Codman's triangle (an isolated cuff of reactive subperiosteal new bone at the boundary of any benign or malignant mass that rapidly elevates the periosteum); and chest X ray to assess for the possible presence of metastatic disease.
- An assessment for a pathological fracture, which can be present with any malignant or benign bone tumor.
- A bone scan to assess for an increased uptake of radioisotope at tumor sites or areas of healing bone.
- A CT scan of the chest to reveal the presence and extent of pulmonary lesion(s).
- An MRI scan to assess for soft tissue, nerve, and vessel involvement, tumor boundaries.
- Laboratory studies such as serum alkaline phosphate, which is increased in 40% of patients (Elevations are not uncommon in adolescents because they are undergoing normal bone growth).
- Arteriography, which may be helpful for determining the extent of blood or vascular flow to the tumor that is not noted with MRI.
- Fine-needle, core, or open incisional biopsy, which is important for determining histology. An open biopsy is preferred to allow for obtaining an ample bone specimen for testing. The initial biopsy should be done at a pediatric oncology center.

Prognostic Considerations

The most important prognostic factor is extent of disease at diagnosis. Pulmonary metastasis is present in 20% of patients and greatly decreases the survival time. The location of the tumor will direct the surgical procedure (i.e., limb salvage or surgical resection). Spinal osteosarcoma has a poor prognosis because it is not possible to completely resect the tumor. A poor prognosis is associated with patients under 10 years of age, males, and serum and tumor tissue alkaline phosphatase levels. Patients who respond to preoperative chemotherapy (more than a 98% necrosis) have more favorable outcomes.

Treatment and Prognosis

Successful treatment requires chemotherapy inasmuch as all patients are presumed to have microscopic metastases. Chemotherapy consists of high-dose methotrexate [Mexate], doxorubicin (Adriamycin), cisplatin (Platinol), and possibly ifosfamide (Ifex) and etoposide (VP-16). Initial chemotherapy is given, then surgery for tumor resection and reconstruction of the limb is performed, followed by additional chemotherapy. The overall survival rate is 65%–70%.

Although osteosarcoma is a typically radioresistant tumor, radiation may be used for metastatic disease or palliation. Treatment of a lung metastasis includes resection and possible irradiation of the areas. The event-free survival rate for metastatic osteosarcoma is approximately 20%–30% (**Figure 2-7**).

Surgery: The goal is to obtain a wide margin—a zone of 5 mm or more of normal healthy tissue—around the tumor. The type of surgery is dependent upon the tumor type and location, age of the patient, response to preoperative chemotherapy, surgeon's preference, and the decision of the patient or the family.

Patients undergoing either limb salvage or amputation often achieve similar functional outcomes. However, these two surgical groups of patients are at risk for decreased quality of life, social isolation, poor self-esteem, and limitations in employment and future health insurance coverage.

Limb salvage procedure: An endoprosthetic device, such as a total knee or hip joint, is implanted after the diseased bone is removed. The allograft, bone, or soft tissue can become infected and can result in additional surgeries and even amputation. Ten percent of patients will have mechanical failure of the endoprosthesis resulting from routine use and will need to undergo replacement procedures.

Arthodesis (fusion of the joint): This involves replacement of the joint with allograft or cadaver bone.

Amputation: This procedure is used especially for expendable bones, such as a fibula, rib, toe, finger, or ulna.

Rotationplasty: This involves an excision of the femur (and preservation of the lower leg), after which the lower

Figure 2–7. Osteosarcoma 5-year Relative Survival Rates

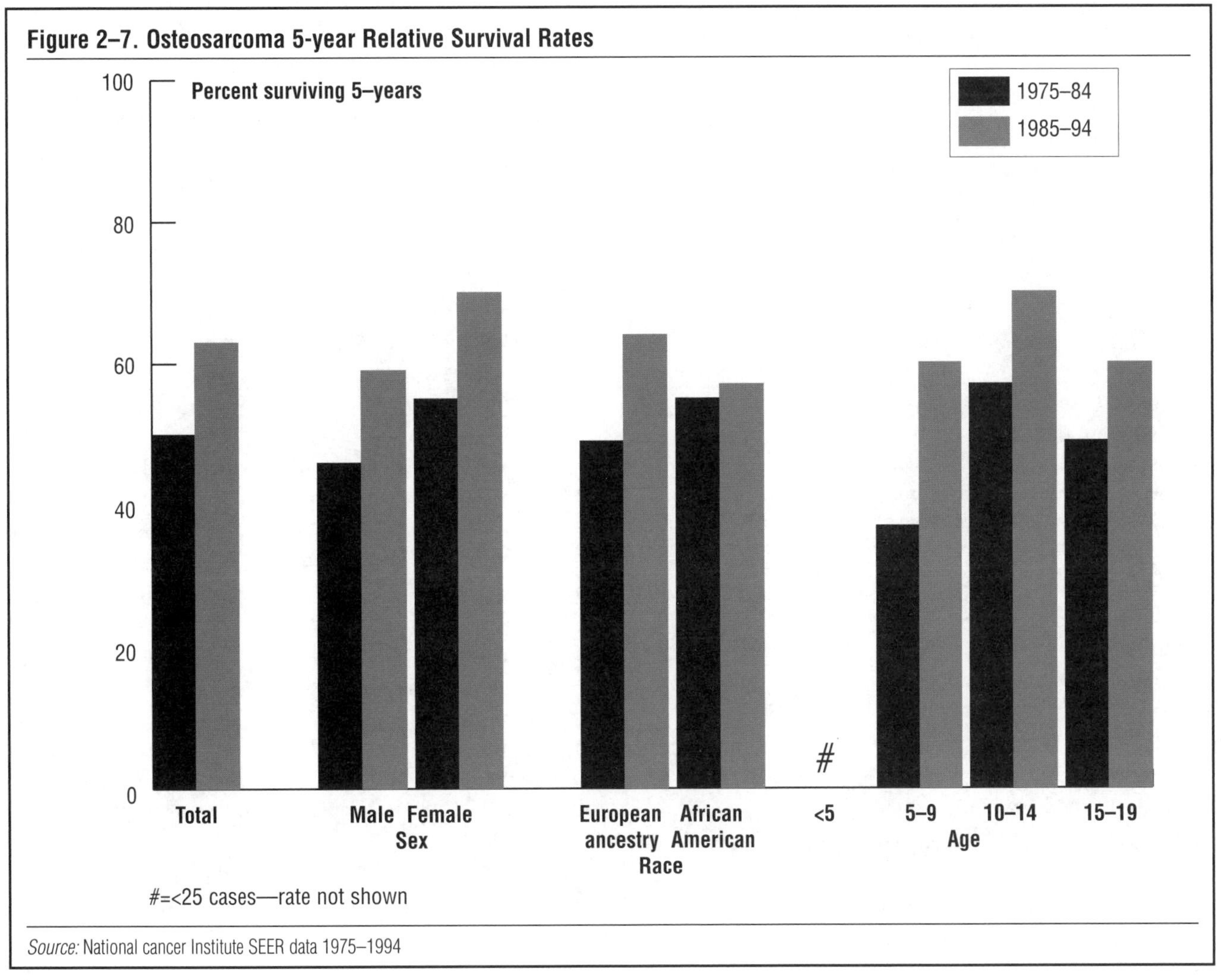

Source: National cancer Institute SEER data 1975–1994

leg is turned 180 degrees. The foot, which is now facing backward, becomes the knee. This procedure improves functional ability, as it is similar to a below-the-knee amputation and the patient can be fitted with a prosthesis.

Recurrent Disease

A routine chest radiograph and plain films of the affected limb are needed if a recurrence is to be detected early. Recurrent disease most commonly occurs within 3 years of the original diagnosis; 85% of recurrences occur in the lung. There is less possibility of a cure if a recurrence appears within 2 years after therapy is discontinued.

Nursing Assessment and Interventions

Goal: The patient will experience minimal complications related to the onset of tumor.

Assessment:
- Review the type of bone cancer and the location and extent of the disease.
- Obtain a complete history, including the incidence and duration of symptoms (e.g., limping, presence of masses), predisposing factors (e.g., exposure to radiation, cytotoxic drugs, genetic abnormalities), and family history.
- Perform a complete physical examination to assess for the presence of a mass, warmth, tenderness, and bilateral limb circumference.
- Review the laboratory findings.
- Review the radiological imaging studies, as indicated.
- Review the surgical and pathology reports, as indicated.
- Assess the child's degree of pain.

Interventions:
- Provide comfort measures.
- Provide pain medication, as needed.
- Explain all tests, procedures, and results to the patient and the family.

Goal: The patient will experience minimal complications related to the treatment.

Assessment:
- Assess the child for toxicity related to specific chemotherapy agents (see the discussion of chemotherapy in Section IV, "Childhood Cancer Treatment").
- Assess the child for toxicity related to radiation therapy, if it has been given (see the discussion of radiation therapy in Section IV, "Childhood Cancer Treatment").
- Assess the child for complications related to surgery, if it has been done (see the discussion of surgery in Section IV, "Childhood Cancer Treatment").
- Assess need for rehabilitative therapies.
- Assess the child for signs of infection.
- Assess the child for evidence of fatigue, bleeding, pain, and nutritional deficits.
- Monitor fluid intake and output and electrolytes.
- Determine the type of intravenous access that is needed.
- Assess for the possibility of emergency complications.
- Assess for response to therapy (i.e., a decrease in the size of the mass or enlarged lymph nodes, evaluation of any metastatic disease).

Interventions:
- Refer the child for central intravenous access, as needed.
- Provide comfort measures.
- Provide pain medication, as needed.
- Provide instruction on proper mouth care, nutrition, and hygiene.
- Educate the family regarding neutropenia, anemia, thrombocytopenia, as well as the signs and symptoms of infection and fever precautions.
- Obtain cultures and radiological examinations, as ordered, when infection is suspected, and initiate antibiotics if they are indicated.
- Provide alternative methods of nutrition (e.g., oral supplements, NG and parenteral supplements).
- Review all findings of laboratory tests and radiological studies with the patient and the family.

Goal: The patient or the family or both will be adequately informed regarding the patient's diagnosis, disease, and treatment.

Assessment:
- Assess the level of knowledge of the patient and the family about the diagnosis and disease.
- Assess their level of knowledge about treatment (i.e., surgery, radiation therapy, chemotherapy).
- Assess their learning styles (see Section VIII, "Patient and Family Education").
- Assess their understanding of the role of the multidisciplinary team in treating children with osteosarcoma.

Interventions:
- Communicate with the patient and the family in an appropriate style.
- Provide them with appropriate educational resources and review the material with them.
- Determine that the family is aware of when and how to contact the healthcare team.
- Encourage the patient, the family, or both to ask questions related to the diagnosis, disease, and treatment.
- Clarify information provided by various members of the multidisciplinary team.

Goal: The patient and the family will cope adequately with the diagnosis.

Assessment:
- Assess the family's communication and coping styles in general.
- Assess the family's adjustment to the diagnosis.
- Assess the patient and family for adjustment to limb salvage or amputation.

Interventions:

- Provide the patient and the family with honest answers to their questions.
- Provide emotional support.
- Provide counseling resources, as needed, for patients experiencing amputation or rotationplasty.
- Anticipate the need for referral services (e.g., social work, chaplain, Candlelighters, American Cancer Society, Leukemia Society).
- Offer the child age-appropriate "hospital play."
- Offer to introduce a contact family who has dealt with a similar malignancy to talk with the patient and the family.

Expected Patient and Family Outcomes

The child, the parents, or both can do the following:

- Describe the type of osteosarcoma and the plan of care.
- List the expected and possible toxic side effects of therapy.
- Outline methods to prevent infection.
- Describe the schedule of treatment, procedures, and follow-up care.
- Describe available community resources.
- Demonstrate the skills needed to care for the child at home.
- Explain how and when to contact the healthcare team if problems or questions arise.

Ewing's Sarcoma of Bone and Soft Tissue and Peripheral Primitive Neuroectodermal Tumors

Melody Hellsten

Definition

Ewing's sarcoma was first described by James Ewing in 1921 as a bone tumor that differs from osteosarcoma because of its radiosensitivity. It was initially thought to be of endothelial origin and was later found to be of neural origin. Ewing's sarcoma most frequently occurs in the bone. Tumors arising from the soft tissue present in a way that is similar to rhabdomyosarcoma, such as extraosseous Ewing's sarcoma (EES) or peripheral primitive neuroectodermal tumor (peripheral PNET), are now thought to be of similar pathology along the same spectrum of tumors as Ewing's sarcoma of bone. (**Authors' note:** For this text, Ewing's sarcoma family of tumors [ESFT] will refer to Ewing's sarcoma of bone, EES, and peripheral PNET.) PNET is the most highly differentiated tumor on the spectrum.

Pathophysiology

Ewing's sarcoma is a tumor composed of small, round cells with blue granules and characteristic chromosomal translocations. EWS-FLI1 [t(11,22)(q24,q12) occurs in 90%–95% of tumors within the ESFT. EWS-ERG (t(21;22 (q22;q12) occurs in 5%–10% of these types of tumors. The most commonly occurring cytogenetic alternations in this family of tumors is Trisomy 8 (55%), Trisomy 12 (33%), and 9q21 LOH (p16,INK4)(33%). Ewing's sarcoma cells require special markers or staining to differentiate them from other small round cell tumors. The ESFT stain with vimentin and express CD 99.

Incidence and Etiology

The ESFT are the second most common bone malignancies in childhood and adolescence. The annual incidence in the United States is 2.1 cases per 1 million children. They are most common in the second decade of life, with a slight predominance in males. The majority of patients are European American or Hispanic (the tumors are exceedingly rare among Asians and Africans) and they are not commonly associated with congenital diseases of childhood (**Table 2–16**).

Clinical Presentation

Nearly all patients present with pain that often is intermittent, and often has been present for 3 to 9 months prior to diagnosis. The majority of patients have a palpable mass. It may be difficult to determine if the primary tumor is bone with an associated large soft-tissue mass or soft-tissue mass that invades the bone. Pathological fractures are commonly present. Patients may present with fever.

Distribution of primary sites is split evenly between the extremities (53%) and the central axis (47%) (e.g., pelvis, chest wall, spine, or head and neck). Hemorrhage and necrosis often are seen and may be mistaken for infection. Approximately 25% of patients have metastatic disease at diagnosis (e.g., lung, bone, or bone marrow).

Diagnostic

The diagnostic includes an evaluation of the extent of disease before therapy is started. Evaluation should include the following:

- A complete history of the current illness regarding pain (i.e., location, duration, and intensity), limp or limited range of motion, presence of a mass.
- A physical examination to assess for soft tissue mass, warmth, tenderness; abnormal gait and limited range of motion; circumference of the affected and nonaffected limb.
- Radiography (including: X rays/plain films, MRI of the primary site, computed tomography (CT) of the chest, and bone scan) The ESFT often appear as a loss of the normal sharp, dense cortical bone, or has an onion-skin appearance. Pathological fractures can be present with any malignant or benign bone tumor. A chest X ray should be done to assess for metastatic disease.
- A bone scan to assess for increased uptake of radioisotope at the tumor sites or areas of healing bone.
- A CT of the chest to reveal the presence and extent of pulmonary lesion(s).

Table 2-16. Causes of Ewing's Sarcoma

Exposure or Characteristic	Comments
Known risk factors	
Race	ES is almost exclusively a disease of European ancestry children, with rates approximately 9 times those in African Americans.
Risk factors for which evidence is limited or inconsistent	
Growth	As for osteosarcoma, recent studies have not found a consistent association with increased height or weight, or age at pubertal growth.
Hernia	An association was found between hernias and increased risk in one study.
Paternal occupation	Paternal occupation in agriculture has been associated with increased risk in two studies, although only in one were the results statistically significant.
Ingestion of poison or overdose of medication	A prior poisoning episode was more common among cases than controls in a single study.
Family history of cancer	ES has been reported in several pairs of siblings. However, more than one family member with ES is rare. In a study of over 200 cases, none had a relative with ES. Unlike ostoesarcoma, ES is not part of te Li-fraumeni syndrome.

Source: National Cancer Institute SEER data 1975-1995

- MRI scan to reveal soft tissue, nerve, and vessel involvement and tumor boundaries. Scans rarely are normal after treatment.
- Laboratory studies, including complete blood count, chemistries, and erythrocyte sedimentation rate. An elevated sedimentation rate and white blood cell count can be seen with the ESFT and can be confused with osteomyelitis.
- An initial biopsy at a pediatric oncology center. Poorly planned biopsies of bone may lead to pathological fractures or contamination of other tissue.
- Bilateral bone marrow aspirations and biopsies.
- Baseline cardiovascular, pulmonary, renal, and hepatic function studies.
- Baseline assessment of neurologic, musculoskeletal, and psychological function.

Prognostic Considerations

The presence of clinically detectable metastatic disease at diagnosis is associated with poor outcomes and is the most significant prognostic indicator. Patients with ESFT with a primary lesion in the pelvis have a poor prognosis; patients with primary lesions in a distal extremity or rib fare best. Tumor size is related significantly to outcome in some studies. The serum LDH level may be a prognostic indicator (i.e., a higher level is associated with a poorer prognosis) (**Figure 2-8**).

Treatment and Prognosis

Chemotherapy: Chemotherapy for ESFT consists of a combination of several agents: ifosfamide (Ifex), cyclophosphamide (Cytoxan), vincristine (Oncovin), etoposide (VP-16), doxorubicin (Adriamycin), and dactinomycin (Actinomycin D).

Local control: Surgery or radiation therapy is dependent upon the tumor's location and its response to chemotherapy, as noted with disease restaging. ESFT responds well to radiation therapy, with total tumor dose equal to 55–60 Gy. Surgical procedures, such as limb salvage or amputation, may be necessary to achieve maximal tumor resection. Local control measures should not compromise systemic therapy. If there are lung metastases at presentation, the patient will receive lung irradiation.

Cure rates: Cure rates of localized ESFT are 50%–70%. Distal lesions are more easily cured than axial lesions. The cure rate for metastatic ESFT is less than 20%.

Recurrent Disease

Recurrent disease is indicative of a poor prognosis. The chance of survival is related to the site and extent of recurrence, biology of tumor cells, aggressiveness of previous treatment, length of time between treatment, and recurrence and age (patients younger than 11 years old have improved survival rates). Chemotherapy agents not previously used are considered when there is a recurrence. Treatment may include surgery, radiation, or both. Currently, metastatic,

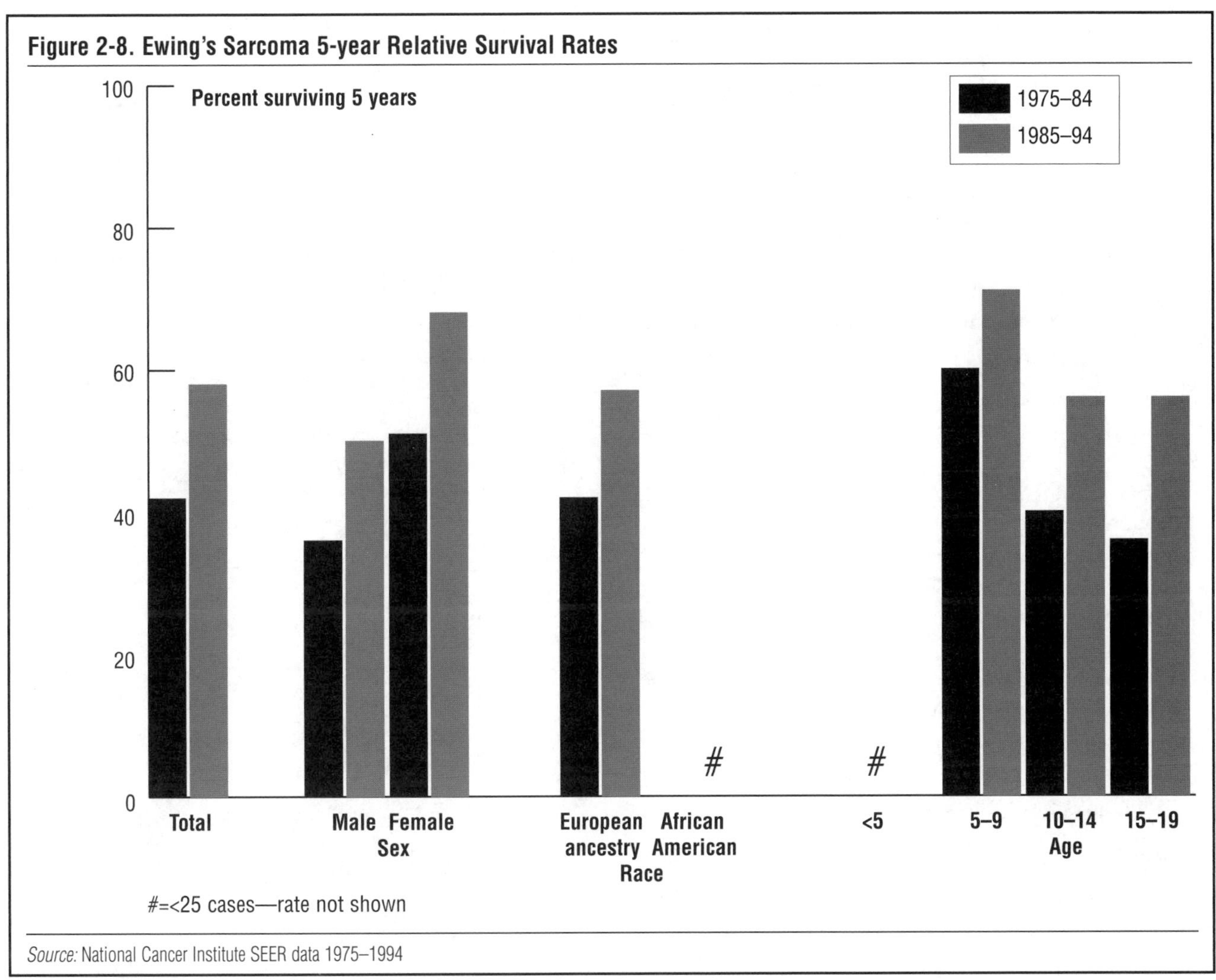

refractory or relapsed disease, or large inoperable tumors, are being treated with high dose therapy with autologous stem cell rescue. There is no conclusive evidence that this type of high-dose therapy is beneficial. The secondary malignancy rate may be as high as 30%.

Nursing Assessment and Interventions

Goal: The patient will experience minimal complications related to the onset of ESFT.

Assessment:

- Know the type of malignancy, location and extent of disease, and presenting symptoms.
- Obtain a complete history, including the incidence and duration of symptoms (e.g., the presence of mass, warmth, tenderness, limited range of motion) and family history.
- Perform a complete physical examination to determine the presence of mass, warmth, tenderness, and bilateral limb circumference.
- Review the laboratory findings.
- Review radiological imaging studies, as indicated.
- Review surgical and pathology reports, as indicated.
- Assess the child's degree of pain.

Interventions:

- Provide comfort measures.
- Provide pain medication, as needed.
- Explain all tests, procedures, and results to the patient and the family.

Goal: The patient will experience minimal complications related to treatment.

Assessment:

- Assess the child for toxicity related to specific chemotherapy agents (see the discussion of chemotherapy in Section IV, "Childhood Cancer Treatment").
- Assess the child for toxicity related to radiation therapy if it has been given (see the discussion of radiation therapy in Section IV, "Childhood Cancer Treatment").
- Assess the child for complications related to surgery, if performed (see the discussion of surgery in Section IV, "Childhood Cancer Treatment").
- Assess the need for rehabilitation therapies after surgery.
- Assess for signs of infection.

- Assess the child for evidence of fatigue, bleeding, pain, and nutritional deficits.
- Monitor fluid intake and output and electrolytes.
- Determine the type of intravenous access that is needed.
- Assess for the possibility of emergency complications.
- Assess for the child's response to therapy (i.e., decrease in size of the mass or enlarged lymph nodes, evaluation of any metastatic disease).

Interventions:

- Refer the child for central intravenous access, as needed.
- Provide comfort measures.
- Provide pain medication, as needed.
- Provide instruction on proper mouth care, nutrition, and hygiene.
- Educate the family regarding neutropenia, anemia, thrombocytopenia, as well as the signs and symptoms of infection and fever precautions.
- Obtain cultures and radiological examinations, as ordered, when infection is suspected, and initiate antibiotics, if indicated.
- Provide alternative methods of nutrition (e.g., oral supplements, NG and parenteral supplements).
- Review all findings of laboratory studies and radiological studies with the patient and the family.

Goal: The patient, the family, or both will be adequately informed regarding the diagnosis, disease, and treatment.

Assessment:

- Assess the level of knowledge of the patient and the family about the diagnosis and disease.
- Assess their level of knowledge regarding treatment (i.e., surgery, radiation therapy, chemotherapy).
- Assess their learning styles (see Section VIII, "Patient and Family Education").
- Assess their understanding of the role of the multidisciplinary team in treating children with ESFT.

Interventions:

- Communicate with the patient and the family in an appropriate style.
- Provide them with appropriate educational resources and review the material with them.
- Determine that the family is aware of when and how to contact the healthcare team.
- Encourage both the patient and the family to ask questions related to the diagnosis, disease, and treatment.
- Clarify information provided by various members of the multidisciplinary team.

Goal: The patient and the family will cope adequately with the diagnosis.

Assessment:

- Assess the family's communication and coping styles in general.
- Assess the family's adjustment to the cancer diagnosis and treatment.

Interventions:

- Provide the patient and the family with honest answers to their questions.
- Provide them emotional support.
- Anticipate their need for referral services early (e.g., social work, chaplain, Candlelighters, American Cancer Society, Leukemia Society).
- Offer the child age-appropriate "hospital play."
- Offer to introduce a contact family that has dealt with a similar malignancy to talk with the patient and the family.

Expected Patient and Family Outcomes

The child and the parents can do the following:

- Describe ESFT and the plan of care.
- List the expected and possible toxic side effects of therapy.
- Outline methods for preventing infection.
- Describe the schedule of treatment, procedures, and follow-up care.
- Describe available community resources.
- Demonstrate the skills needed to care for the child at home.
- Explain how and when to contact the healthcare team if problems or questions arise.

Tumors of the Kidney

Eileen Duffey-Lind

Definition

Tumors of the kidney are primary tumors arising from the kidney.

Pathophysiology

Description: Tumors of the kidney are most often Wilms' tumors, which are large, rapidly growing, vascular abdominal tumors. They frequently have a fragile gelatinous capsule. Wilms' tumors are divided into two categories:

Favorable histology: This tumor has an undifferentiated, primitive development. It is composed of stromal, epithelial, and blastemic tissue (precursor of stromal and epithelial cells).

Anaplastic: This type of tumor has anaplastic nuclear changes, is present in about 5% of patients with Wilms' tumor, and is more common in older children. It is rarely seen in the first 2 years of life, then increases in frequency in patients older than 5 years of age, accounting for approximately 13% of patients with Wilms' tumor. It is significantly more frequent in African American than in Caucasian children. Anaplasia in only a few cells is associated with high relapse rates, thus an adequate sample is necessary for an appropriate diagnosis.

Clear-cell sarcoma of the kidney: This tumor is the second most common pediatric renal neoplasm and is associated with a significantly higher rate of relapse and death than favorable histology Wilms' tumor. It also is associated with a wider distribution of metastases, including to the brain and bone.

Rhabdoid tumor of the kidney: This is not Wilms' tumor, but it is a rare, highly malignant, renal tumor. It may metastasize to the brain and lungs. Rhabdoid tumor of the kidney occurs more frequently in infants, with 85% of cases occurring within the first 2 years of life.

Nephrogenic rests: These are precursor cells to Wilms' tumor. Nephroblastomatosis refers to multiple nephrogenic rests, which are classified by their position within the kidney. Only a small number develop a clonal transformation into Wilms' tumor.

Renal cell carcinoma: The classic form of renal cell carcinoma is rare in children who do not have a genetic predisposition to it. It is a rare subtype that is seen in adolescence and young adulthood, with a male predominance.

Renal medullary carcinoma: This is a rare, highly lethal tumor that is virtually restricted to patients with sickle cell hemoglobinopathy, most commonly sickle cell trait. The median age at which it occurs is 13 years.

Congenital mesoblastic nephroma: This is a distinctive renal neoplasm of infancy. It occurs predominantly in infants, with a median age of 2 months. The poor response to chemotherapy and radiation highlights the importance of surgical resection.

Incidence and Etiology

Wilms' tumor represents 6% of childhood cancers, and the total incidence in the United States is estimated at 500 cases per year. From 1975 to 1995, the annual incidence was 7.6 cases per 1 million in children younger than 15 years.

Wilms' tumors are seen slightly less frequently in boys (0.92:1.00) than in girls; the median age at diagnosis is slightly younger for boys. The age at diagnosis peaks at 2 to 3 years; these tumors are rare in children more than 5 years of age.

Familial cases account for approximately 1%–2% of all Wilms' tumor cases. These are usually autosomal dominant with variable penetrance. Tumors of the kidney are associated with aniridia (congenital absence of iris), hemihypertrophy, genital or renal malformations, Beckwith-Wiedemann syndrome (including macroglossia, omphalocele, hemihypertrophy, and visceromegaly), and other overgrowth syndromes **(Table 2-17)**.

Table 2-17. Causes of Wilms' Tumor (WT)

Exposure or Characteristic	Comments
Known risk factors	
Race	Incidence in Asians is about half that in African Americans and European Americans.
Aniridia, genitourinary anomalies, WAGR syndrome (Wilms' tumor, aniridia, genitourinary abnormalities, mental retardation), Beckwith-Wiedemann syndrome, Denys-Drash syndrome, Simpson-Golabi-Behmel syndrome	Risk is increased in children with these congenital anomalies and genetic conditions. The study of children with WAGR led to the identification of one of the WT genes.
Factors for which evidence is suggestive but not conclusive	
Paternal occupation	An increased risk for fathers employed as a welder or mechanic has been reported in several studies.
Factors for which evidence is inconsistent or limited	
High birth weight	Association with birth weight over 4,000 grams has been reported in some studies.
Parental exposure to pesticides	One study found an increased risk for parental occupational exposure to pesticides. Another study found an association with household insect extermination.
Ionizing radiation (in utero)	Prenatal diagnostic X ray was associated with increased risk in one study.
Maternal consumption of coffee and tea during pregnancy	Three studies reported association with coffee and/or tea; another did not replicate this finding.
Maternal hair dye use during pregnancy	Use was associated with risk in one study, but not in others.
Maternal medication use during pregnancy	Studies reported associations with various drugs including hormones, antibiotics, dipyrone, metoclopramide, pethrane anesthesia during delivery. Most of these results were found in a single study.
Maternal occupation	One study found an association with job groupings that included hairdressers, electronic and clothing manufacturing workers, laboratory workers, dental assistants.

Source: National Cancer Institute SEER data 1975-1995

Most patients with Wilms' tumor have normal chromosomes, but a gene deletion at 11p13 is noted in the tumor cells of many patients and, frequently, in all cells of patients with aniridia. A hypothesis is that the Wilms' tumor suppressor gene (*WT1*) located at 11p13 suppresses the activity of the tumor-transforming gene located elsewhere on chromosome 11. A second Wilms' tumor gene (WT2) has been found at 11p15; the same gene deletion is seen in Beckwith-Wiedemann syndrome. Alterations on band 11p15 may predispose a person to the development of Wilms' tumor.

Clinical Presentation

Tumors of the kidney most often present with an asymptomatic abdominal mass and are frequently found by family members, or during a routine physical examination. Pain, malaise, and hematuria are present in 20%–30% of patients with kidney tumors. Twenty-five percent of patients have hypertension, which has been attributed to an increase in renin activity. Rapid abdominal enlargement, anemia, and hypertension occur in a subset of patients who have a sudden subcapsular hemorrhage; eggshell-type calcifications may be visible on plain film. The lungs, liver, and regional lymph nodes are the most common sites of metastatic disease. Seven percent involve both kidneys, either at diagnosis or subsequently; 7% of bilateral lesions are not noted on preoperative imaging studies; and 12% are unilateral with multicentric foci. Neurological signs may indicate brain metastases. The primary tumor may extend to the inferior vena cava or right atrium.

Diagnostic

The diagnostic includes an evaluation of the extent of the disease before therapy is started. An evaluation should include the following:

- A complete history of the current illness, including information about the location of the pain, its duration, and intensity (bone pain may indicate metastases, often in the long bones); presence of abdominal mass, including location and size; and hematuria.
- A complete physical examination to assess for hemihypertrophy (partial or complex), aniridia, Beckwith-Wiedemann syndrome, distended abdominal veins, cryptorchidism, hypospadius, and abdominal mass.
- A CBC, urinalysis, renal function and liver function tests, and serum chemistries.
- An abdominal ultrasound to determine tumor size and shape, vessel involvement, the presence of thrombus in the inferior vena cava and right atrium.
- An abdominal CT is recommended to further evaluate the nature and extent of disease.
- A chest radiograph to assess for metastases.
- A chest CT, which may reveal lesions not noted on a chest X ray. A biopsy might have to be obtained to determine if Stage IV disease is present.
- Bone scan and X ray skeletal survey should be obtained in children with clear cell sarcoma of the kidney.
- Brain imaging with MRI or CT should be obtained for children with clear cell sarcoma or rhabdoid of the kidney.

Other considerations: Liver, bone, and brain metastases are not routinely assessed for in the initial of Wilms' tumor unless warranted by presenting signs and symptoms.

Staging: Wilms' tumors are classified by stage (**Table 2-18**).

Prognostic Considerations

Histology (i.e., a favorable histology versus anaplastic) is the most significant prognostic consideration. Lymph node involvement is an adverse prognostic factor. Metastatic disease at the time of diagnosis remains an important prognostic indicator. Children entered in the National Wilms' Tumor Study (NWTS)-1 are younger than 24 months of age and have a significantly better prognosis than do older children. However, the prognostic significance of age and tumor size have lessened as treatment efficacy has improved.

Treatment and Prognosis

The NWTS has systematically studied Wilms' tumor since 1969. The overall cure rate, including that for Stage IV disease, is 80% to more than 90%.

Table 2-18. National Wilms' Tumor Study (NWTS) Group Staging for Renal Tumors

Stage	Description/Incidence
I	Tumor confined to the kidney and completely resected. No penetration of the renal capsule or involvement of renal sinus vessels – 43%
II	Tumor extends beyond the kidney but is completely resected (negative margins and lymph nodes). At least one of the following has occurred: penetration of the renal capsule, invasion of the renal sinus vessels, biopsy of tumor before removal, spillage of tumor locally during removal – 23%
III	Gross or microscopic residual tumor remains postoperatively, including inoperable tumor, positive surgical margins, tumor spillage involving peritoneal surfaces, regional lymph node metastatses, or transected tumor thrombus – 23%
IV	Hematogenous metastases or lymph node metastases outside the abdomen (e.g., lung, liver, bone, brain) – 10%
V	Bilateral renal Wilms' tumors at onset – 5%

Source: Data from National Cancer Institute NCI–PDQ

Surgery: Surgery, with a transperitoneal approach and nephrectomy, is most frequently used as an initial treatment. The contralateral kidney and sample lymph nodes must also be examined for tumor. Extensive lymph node dissection is not necessary, however. Small amounts of residual tumor are not associated with a major decrease in the survival rate. Preoperative chemotherapy is given to patients with an intravascular spread of disease, for very large invasive tumors, or for patients for whom there is an anesthesia-related risk. Preoperative chemotherapy prevents an adequate assessment of staging. Patients whose tumors are staged on the basis of imaging only should be considered to have a Stage III tumor.

When bilateral disease is present, an initial staging and biopsy of both kidneys are performed, followed by approximately 5 weeks of chemotherapy and by a nephrectomy of the more involved side and a partial nephrectomy of the other kidney. Seventy-five percent of patients with bilateral disease will have residual tumor in the remaining kidney after surgery, but the survival rate remains high.

Chemotherapy (based on the National Wilms' Tumor Study V)

Stage I & II, favorable histology or Stage I focal or diffuse anaplastic: Treatment includes 18 weeks of vincristine, and actinomycin-D, without radiation.

Stage III & IV, favorable histology or II-IV focal anaplastic: Treatment includes 24 weeks of vincristine, actinomycin-D, doxorubicin, abdominal radiation, and radiation to metastatic disease.

Stage I-IV clear cell sarcoma: Treatment includes 24 weeks of vincristine, doxorubicin, cytoxan, etoposide, abdominal radiation and radiation to metastatic disease.

Stage I-IV rhabdoid tumor: No satisfactory treatment has been developed. Treatment includes 24 weeks of carboplatin, etoposide, and cytoxan; abdominal radiation, and radiation to distant metastatic sites.

Radiation therapy: The port is extended to cross the midline to prevent scoliosis. With tumors that have a favorable histology, radiation therapy is needed only for Stage III and Stage IV disease. After lung irradiation, the doses of chemotherapy may have to be decreased. The whole abdomen is treated when patients have had tumor spillage during surgery or when patients have had diffuse peritoneal seeding.

Recurrent Disease

There is less chance of a cure if a recurrence appears within 12 months of diagnosis. Patients who have an abdominal recurrence after radiation or a recurrence after treatment with doxorubicin (Adriamycin) have a poor prognosis and need aggressive treatment. This treatment often consists of etoposide (VP-16) and ifosfamide (Ifex) or autologous bone marrow transplantation. The first site of disease recurrence with all stages is most frequently the lungs. Most recurrences (approximately 90%) occur within the first 2 years after diagnosis, and the remainder occur in the next 2 years. Children in a more favorable group should be treated aggressively with relapse because they generally have a good response to retrieval therapy. Longer follow-up for clear cell sarcoma patients is needed because relapses are known to occur as long as 5 years after diagnosis.

Nursing Assessment and Interventions

Goal: The patient will experience minimal complications related to the onset of tumor.

Assessment:

- Know the type of malignancy, location and extent of disease, and presenting symptoms.
- Obtain a complete history, including the incidence and duration of symptoms (e.g., presence of abdominal mass, hematuria), predisposing factors (e.g., hemihypertrophy, aniridia, Beckwith-Wiedemann syndrome), and family history.
- Perform a complete physical examination to assess for the presence of abdominal mass, hypertension, hemihypertrophy, aniridia, distended abdominal veins, genitourinary abnormalities, and neurological changes.
- Review the laboratory findings.
- Review the radiological imaging studies, as indicated.
- Review surgical and pathology reports, as indicated.
- Assess the child's degree of pain.

Interventions:

- Provide comfort measures.
- Provide pain medication, as needed.
- Explain all tests, procedures, and results to the patient and the family.

Goal: The patient will experience minimal complications related to treatment.

Assessment:

- Assess the child for toxicity related to specific chemotherapy agents (see the discussion of chemotherapy in Section IV, "Childhood Cancer Treatment").
- Assess the child for toxicity related to radiation therapy, if it has been given (see the discussion of radiation therapy in Section IV, "Childhood Cancer Treatment").
- Assess the child for complications related to surgery, if it has been performed (see the discussion of surgery in Section IV, "Childhood Cancer Treatment").
- Assess for signs of infection.
- Assess the child for evidence of fatigue, bleeding, pain, and nutritional deficits.
- Monitor fluid intake and output and electrolytes.
- Determine the type of intravenous access that is needed.
- Assess for the possibility of emergency complications.
- Assess for the child's response to therapy (i.e., a decrease in the size of mass or enlarged lymph nodes, evaluation of any metastatic disease).

Interventions:

- Refer the child for central intravenous access, as needed.
- Provide comfort measures.

- Provide pain medication, as needed.
- Provide instruction on proper mouth care, nutrition, and hygiene.
- Educate the family regarding neutropenia, anemia, thrombocytopenia, as well as about the signs and symptoms of infection.
- Obtain cultures and radiological examinations, as ordered, when infection is suspected, and initiate antibiotics, if it is indicated.
- Provide alternative methods of nutrition (e.g., oral supplements, NG and parenteral supplements).
- Review all of the findings of laboratory studies and radiological studies with the patient and the family.

Goal: The patient, the family, or both will be adequately informed regarding diagnosis, disease, and treatment.

Assessment:

- Assess the level of knowledge of the patient and the family about diagnosis and disease.
- Assess their level of knowledge regarding treatment (i.e., surgery, radiation therapy, chemotherapy).
- Assess their learning styles (see Section VIII, "Patient and Family Education").
- Assess the patient's and the family's understanding of the role of the multidisciplinary team in treating children with renal tumors.

Interventions:

- Communicate with the patient and the family in an appropriate style.
- Provide them with appropriate educational resources and review the material with them.
- Determine that the family is aware of when and how to contact the healthcare team.
- Encourage both the patient and the family to ask questions related to diagnosis, disease, and treatment.
- Clarify information provided by various members of the multidisciplinary team.

Goal: The patient and the family will cope adequately with the diagnosis.

Assessment:

- Assess the family's communication and coping styles in general.
- Assess the family's adjustment to the diagnosis.

Interventions:

- Provide the patient and the family with honest answers.
- Provide them with emotional support.
- Anticipate the need for referral services (e.g., social work, chaplain, Candlelighters, American Cancer Society, Leukemia Society).
- Offer the child age-appropriate "hospital play."
- Offer to introduce a contact family who has dealt with a similar malignancy to talk with the patient and the family.

Expected Patient and Family Outcomes

The child, the parents, or both are able to do the following:

- Describe the type of kidney tumor and the plan of care.
- List the expected and possible toxic side effects of therapy.
- Outline methods for preventing infection.
- Describe the schedule of treatment, procedures, and follow-up care.
- Describe available community resources.
- Demonstrate the skills needed to care for the child at home.
- Describe how and when to contact the healthcare team if problems or questions arise.

Rhabdomyosarcoma

Elisa Frederick

Definition

Rhabdomyosarcoma (RMS) is a malignant tumor of mesenchymal cell origin, most often arising from cells of skeletal muscle lineage. This type of tumor can develop in tissues in which striated muscle cells are not normally found.

Pathophysiology

RMS is a small round blue-cell tumor. It is classified as a RMS when muscle cell characteristics (e.g., cross striations on muscle proteins, such as actin, myosin, desmin, myoglobin, Z-band, protein and myoD) are noted on pathologic review, using both microscopic techniques and molecular genetic techniques.

The histological classifications of RMS are botryoid, spindle-cell, alveolar, and undifferentiated. The botryoid and spindle-cell types generally have the best prognosis. The undifferentiated sarcoma subtype has a poorer prognosis, as does the alveolar type. Although these tumors may develop almost anywhere in the body, there exist certain clusters of features specific to age at diagnosis, site of primary tumor, and histology that are more common. Children younger than 8 years of age are most commonly diagnosed with head and neck tumors, which are most commonly embryonal if they arise from the orbit. Adolescents are more likely to have extremity tumors of the alveolar variety. RMS is seen almost exclusively in infants, developing from the vagina or the bladder. In older children, botryoid arises from the nasopharynx.

Incidence and Etiology

There are 350 new cases of RMS in the United States each year, 4.3 cases per 1 million children. After neuroblastoma and Wilms' tumor, RMS is the most common extracranial solid tumor of childhood. The majority of RMS cases are diagnosed before age 9, with another peak incidence during early-to-mid adolescence.

African American girls have just half the incidence rate of Caucasian girls, but no demonstrated difference has been noted among boys in these two racial groups. Lower incidence rates are seen in Asia than in industrialized Western countries. This tumor is slightly more common in males than in females (a 1.3–1.4:1 ratio).

Genetics and Molecular Biology

The development of RMS occurs sporadically in the majority of cases, however, its development has also been associated with certain familial syndromes. Neurofibromatosis and the Li-Fraumeni syndrome are linked to the *p53* tumor suppressor gene, and Beckwith-Wiedeman syndrome, which is marked by abnormalities on 11p15—where the insulin-like growth factor-2 (IGF-2) gene is located—have been associated with RMS. It has been argued that children with these germline mutations should have their therapy altered because of the increased risk of developing cancer associated with the syndromes. Treatment, including radiation, epipodophyllinotoxins, and alkylating agents—which also have potential carcinogenic properties—may need to be adjusted for this patient poulation in the future.

The two major histologic subtypes of RMS, embryonal and alveolar, have been found to have different genetic alternations as well. The alveolar subtype is associated with the translocation of chromosome 2 and 13, designated as t(2;13), and the involvement of the *PAX3* gene. This gene is believed to regulate early neuromuscular development, thus interfering with normal growth and contributing to the development of RMS. The embryonal subtype is associated with loss of heterozygosity at the 11p15 corresponding position (locus). Both alveolar and embryonal RMS have been associated with the overproduction of IGF-2.

Clinical Presentation

Rhabdomyosarcoma, depending on the site, is detected by the appearance of a mass or a disturbance of normal body function. The head and neck, including the orbit and parameningeal areas, are the sites of 35% of these tumors. The signs and symptoms for orbital tumors include proptosis and ophthalmoplegia; for nonorbital parameningeal tumors, they are nasal, aural, or sinus obstruction, muco-purulent or sanguinous discharge, cranial nerve palsies, or signs of increased intracranial pressure. For nonparameningeal tumors, the symptoms include painless growth, which often is localized. The genitourinary tract is the site of 22% of RMS, which are found most often in the bladder or prostate. The signs and symptoms include hematuria, urinary obstruction, extrusion of the tumor, vaginal discharge, pelvic or testicular mass, and constipation. Eighteen percent are found in the extremities, where the signs and symptoms include swelling of the soft tissue, either with or without tenderness or erythema. Other sites (i.e., trunk, pelvis, retroperitoneal areas, perineum, biliary tract, liver, brain, trachea, heart, breast, ovary) account for 25%, and the signs and symptoms depend upon the location of the tumor. On occasion, no primary tumor is found.

Diagnostic

The diagnostic includes an evaluation of the extent of disease before therapy is initiated. An evaluation should include the following components:

- A complete history of the current illness, including the incidence and duration of symptoms (e.g., location of the pain as well as its duration and intensity; presence of mass, warmth, tenderness; neurological changes; hematuria), fatigue, and family history (e.g., *p53* dilution, neurofibromatosis).
- A complete physical examination to assess for the presence of a mass (warmth, tenderness); proptosis, rhinorrhea; hematuria; pallor; lymphadenopathy; neurological changes; and signs of increased intracranial pressure.
- A CT or MRI of the affected area to define the mass.
- A Technetium-99m bone scan to rule out metastasis.
- A CT of the chest to rule out metastasis.
- Bilateral bone marrow aspirates and biopsies.
- A radiograph of the affected part for a baseline evaluation.
- A CBC with differential, creatinine, liver function tests, blood urea nitrogen (BUN), electrolytes, calcium, phosphorus, magnesium, uric acid.
- A tumor biopsy, which is necessary for diagnosis.
- A blood sample for molecular diagnostic tests to determine characteristic abnormalities—polymerase chain reaction techniques (PCR).
- Baseline coagulation studies (prothrombin time, activated partial thromboplastin time, fibrinogen).

Prognostic Considerations

The stage, site, age, histology, surgical respectability, and absence or presence of nodal disease or metastatic disease all contribute to the final outcome of patients with RMS. The presence of metastatic disease is the greatest prognostic indicator (**Table 2-19**). Genetics and the molecular biology of tumors are also being considered as prognstic indicators of RMS. Alveolar histology and more than two metastatic sites of disease also indicate a poor prognosis for a child with RMS.

Treatment and Prognosis

The Intergroup Rhabdomyosarcoma Study (IRS) group was formed in 1972, and today, the majority of children with RMS are enrolled in IRS studies. There are three recognized modalities with which to treat children with RMS: surgical removal (if feasible), radiation, and chemotherapy.

Surgery: A surgical resection should always be performed if it is feasible. A second surgery may be necessary if residual disease is present after the initial surgery.

Resection is often feasible for head and neck tumors. Routine node sampling is not necessary because the incidence of regional node involvement is low.

A radical inguinal orchiectomy and a resection of the spermatic cord are performed to treat paratesticular tumors. Routine node sampling is controversial.

Vulvar and vaginal tumors tumors often respond to induction chemotherapy; thus, initial widespread excision can be avoided.

Uterine and proximal vaginal tumors may require hysterectomy, but oophorectomy often is avoided. Distal vaginal

Table 2-19. Intergroup Rhabdomyosarcoma Studies (IRS) Grouping and Staging Criteria

IRS Clinical Group

Group I: Tumors that are completely removed by surgery
Group II: Tumors that are removed, but with tumor at the edge of the surgical margin and/or in regional lymph nodes
Group III: Local tumors that cannot be removed by surgery
Group IV: Distant metastatic disease present at diagnosis

IRS Modified TNM Stage

Stage I: Localized tumor involving the orbit (the area near the eye), head and neck area except for parameningeal sites (next to the membranes covering the brain), or genitourinary tract tumors except bladder and prostate.
Stage II: Localized small tumors of any site not in Stage 1. The tumor must be less than 5 cm (about 2 inches) and there must not be regional lymph node spread.
Stage III: Localized tumor at any site not included in Stage 1 which is greater than 5 cm (2 inches) in diameter and/or spread to regional lymph nodes.
Stage IV: Distant metastatic tumor is present at diagnosis.

Source: Data from National Cancer Institute NCI–PDQ

preservation usually is possible. Second-look surgery is performed for patients with gross residual disease.

Previously, radical surgical procedures were performed to excise bladder and prostate tumors resulting in high morbidity. A total cystectomy and pelvic exenteration are now performed only when patients do not achieve local control by chemotherapy and radiation.

An initial complete resection is recommended for extremity tumors if limb function will not be greatly impaired; amputation is rarely required. Regional node sampling is recommended.

A complete resection is difficult for pelvic, retroperitoneal, and intrathoracic tumors.

With metastatic disease, the value of pulmonary nodule resection is unclear.

Radiation therapy: Radiation therapy is used for most patients, except for those with Group I tumors who have undergone a complete resection. A cumulative dose of 41.4 to 45 Gy is usually used for microscopic disease, with a higher cumulative dose of 50 to 59 Gy given to patients with unresectable or gross total disease. Radiation therapy is usually begun after 9 weeks of chemotherapy, unless it is needed at diagnosis on an emergency basis to relieve spinal cord compression or to reduce intracranial meningeal extension. Intraoperative radiation or radiation implants occasionally are used.

Chemotherapy: Chemotherapy is used for all patients except a small subset of patients with Group I tumors. Vincristine (Oncovin), dactinomycin (actinomycin-D), doxorubicin (Adriamycin), cyclophosphamide (Cytoxan), ifosfamide (Ifex), and etoposide (VP-16) are the most commonly used agents. Topotecan (hycamtin) and irinotecan (CPT-11) are newer agents that are being used in combination with other chemotherapy agents in an attempt to increase cure rates.

Treatment results: IRS-III, the third IRS study, found that orbital, nonbladder, and nonprostate genitourinary tumors have the best prognosis. Intermediate results have been obtained for other head and neck sites, as well as for bladder and prostate tumors. The worst prognosis is associated with tumors in these sites: extremity, cranial parameningeal, truncal, pelvic, retroperitoneal, and paravertebral.

The fourth IRS study identified ifosfamide plus doxorubicin as a significant drug pairing for improving outcomes in patients with metastatic RMS. Although certain groups of patients appear to have benefited from the increased alkylator intensity of IRS-IV, this strategy did not improve the outcome for the majority of patients when it was compared with the IRS-III treatment. IRS-V, the currently accruing protocol for treating RMS, has two major objectives: to evaluate the activity of irinotecan in patients with newly diagnosed metastatic RMS, and to evaluate the efficacy of adding topotecan to the standard 3-drug VAC (vincristine, dactinomycin, cyclophosphamide) regimen for patients with intermediate-risk tumors.

Recurrent Disease

Although rare 3 or 4 years after diagnosis, recurrence can take place many years after treatment is completed. Treatment for a local recurrence consists of surgical excision and chemotherapy with agents that have not previously been used. Cure rates are low, but cures are possible.

It is almost impossible to cure metastatic recurrence. Current research is examining ways to overcome drug resistance as well as exploring the potential role of bone marrow or peripheral stem cell transplantation. Tumor vaccines and immune therapy targeted to specific tumor pathogenesis, as well as antiangiogenic therapy, are also currently being investigated.

Nursing Assessment and Interventions

Goal: The patient will experience minimal complications related to the onset of tumor.

Assessment:

- Know the type of malignancy, location and extent of disease, and presenting symptoms.
- Obtain a complete history, including incidence and duration of symptoms (e.g., pain, fatigue, presence of mass, hematuria, neurological changes) and family history (e.g., p53, neurofibromatosis).
- Perform a complete physical examination to establish the presence of mass (location, tenderness), proptosis, rhinorrhea, pallor, petechiae, lymphadenopathy, hepatosplenomegaly, and neurological changes.
- Review laboratory findings.
- Review radiological imaging studies, as indicated.
- Review surgical and pathology reports, as indicated.
- Assess the child's degree of pain.

Interventions:

- Provide comfort measures.
- Provide pain medication, as needed.
- Explain all tests, procedures, and results to the patient and the family.

Goal: The patient will experience minimal complications related to treatment.

Assessment:

- Assess the child for toxicity related to specific chemotherapy agents (see the discussion of chemotherapy in Section IV, "Childhood Cancer Treatment").
- Assess the child for toxicity related to radiation therapy, if it is given (see the discussion of radiation therapy in Section IV, "Childhood Cancer Treatment").
- Assess the child for complications related to surgery, if performed (see discussion of surgery in Section IV, "Childhood Cancer Treatment").
- Assess for signs of infection.
- Assess the child for evidence of fatigue, bleeding, pain, and nutritional deficits.
- Monitor fluid intake and output and electrolytes.
- Determine the type of intravenous access that is needed.
- Assess for the possibility of emergency complications.
- Assess the patient's response to therapy (i.e., a decrease in the size of the mass or enlarged lymph nodes, changes in any metastatic disease).

Interventions:

- Refer the child for central intravenous access, as needed.
- Provide comfort measures.
- Provide pain medication, as needed.
- Provide instruction on proper mouth care, nutrition, and hygiene.
- Educate the family regarding neutropenia, anemia, thrombocytopenia, signs and symptoms of infection, and fever precautions.
- Obtain cultures and radiological examinations, as ordered, when infection is suspected, and initiate antibiotics, if it is indicated.
- Provide alternative methods of nutrition (e.g., oral supplements, NG or parenteral supplements).
- Review all findings of laboratory studies and radiological studies with the patient and the family.

Goal: Both the patient and the family will be adequately informed regarding the diagnosis, disease, and treatment.

Assessment:

- Assess the level of knowledge of the patient and family about the diagnosis and disease.
- Assess their level of knowledge about treatment (i.e., surgery, radiation therapy, chemotherapy).
- Assess their learning styles (see Section VIII, "Patient and Family Education").
- Assess their understanding of the role of the multidisciplinary team in treating rhabdomyosarcoma.

Interventions:

- Communicate with the patient and the family in an appropriate style.
- Provide them with appropriate educational resources and review the material with them.
- Ensure that the family is aware of when and how to contact the healthcare team.
- Encourage both the patient and the family to ask questions related to the diagnosis, disease, and treatment.
- Clarify information provided by various members of the multidisciplinary team.

Goal: The patient and the family will cope adequately with the diagnosis.

Assessment:

- Assess the family's communication and coping styles in general.
- Assess the family's adjustment to the diagnosis.

Interventions:

- Provide the patient and the family with honest answers to their questions.
- Provide emotional support.
- Anticipate the need for referral services (e.g., social work, chaplain, Candlelighters, American Cancer Society, Leukemia Society).
- Offer the child age-appropriate "hospital play."
- Offer to introduce a contact family who has dealt with a similar malignancy to talk with the patient and the family.

Expected Patient and Family Outcomes

The child and family can do the following:

- Describe the type of rhabdomyosarcoma and the plan of care.
- List the expected and possible toxic side effects of therapy.
- Outline methods for preventing infection.
- Describe the schedule of treatment, procedures, and follow-up care.

- Describe available community resources.
- Demonstrate the skills needed to care for the child at home.
- Explain how and when to contact the healthcare team if problems or questions arise.

RETINOBLASTOMA

Brittany Hardiman

Definition

Retinoblastoma is the most common intraocular tumor seen in children.

Pathophysiology

This tumor consists of a chalky, white intraocular mass, often containing calcified foci and large areas of necrosis. It most commonly originates in the posterior retina, arising from the inner layers of the retina and growing into the vitreous humor (endophytic), or arising from the outer layers of the retina and growing toward the subretinal space (exophytic). It can originate from one or more foci in one or both eyes, or, in rare cases, it can present as trilateral disease with an additional focus of tumor in the pineal gland.

Histology: Retinoblastoma is characterized by cells with scant cytoplasm and hyperchromic nuclei of various sizes, arranged in tight bouquet-like clusters called rosettes.

Metastatic disease: Retinoblastoma can occur as the result of local intraocular extension into the vitreous distal spread through the optic nerve or hematogenous dissemination.

Incidence and Etiology

There are 200 new cases of retinoblastoma in the United States each year; 70%–80% of these are unilateral. No differences in incidence based on race or gender have been noted. Eighty percent of children who present with this disease are under 4 years of age. Retinoblastoma can occur as a familial form (40%) or as a spontaneous form (60%).

Familial form: This form presents as either bilateral or multifocal unilateral disease. Bilateral disease, which can present asynchronously, occurs at a younger age (median age–7 months) than the spontaneous form (median age–23 months). The familial form is associated with deletion, translocation, or errors in transcription affecting chromosome 13, band ql4 and is inherited as an autosomal dominant trait. The retinoblastoma gene, RB1, is contained in chromosome 13q14. Mutations of RB1 are seen in patients with hereditary and nonhereditary retinoblastoma.

The prototype for analysis of inherited cancer syndromes is explained by Knudson's two-hit theory. One chromosomal mutation is inherited from a parent and a second mutation occurs after conception and affects a somatic retinal cell. Errors in transcription occur more often in the paternal allele, suggesting that germline mutations occur more frequently during spermatogenesis than oogenesis. The familial form of retinoblastoma predisposes affected patients to secondary malignant neoplasms.

Clinical Presentation

Leukocoria ("cat's eye reflex"), lack of the normal red reflex of the eye, is the most common presentation. Strabismus, esotropia, exotropia, or decreased vision in one eye, as well as painful eyes and erythmatous conjunctivae, are other symptoms.

Diagnostic

The diagnostic includes an evaluation of the extent of the disease before therapy is begun. An evaluation should include the following:

- A complete history of the current illness, including information about familial incidence of retinoblastoma, ocular loss of unknown etiology, decreased vision in one eye, and changes in the appearance of the eyes (e.g., strabismus, leukocoria).
- A complete physical examination, including an assessment of the patient's visual acuity or tracking, strabismus, esotropia, exotropia, and leukocoria.
- Direct and indirect funduscopic examination under anesthesia by a retinal surgeon.
- Ultrasound and CT of the brain and orbits are the most common radiologic tests completed to confirm diagnosis, and the extent of disease, and ectopic disease of the pineal gland.
- MRI of orbits is a superior method of localizing the intraocular extent of the disease.
- Examination of bone marrow aspirate and cerebrospinal fluid for dissemination of tumor. Staging is determined by the Reese-Ellsworth classification for the extent of intraocular disease (**Table 2-20**) or by the St. Jude Children's Research Hospital Staging System, which evaluates the extraocular extension and dissemination of disease.

Prognostic Considerations

The overall prognosis is excellent; 96% of patients have a disease-free, 5-year survival rate. The extent to which the tumor invades the optic nerve affects prognosis in metastatic disease. The spread of the disease to the central nervous system (CNS) is associated with a poor outcome. The potential for preservation of useful vision depends on the stage of the disease at diagnosis and the treatment that has been given.

Treatment and Prognosis

Treatment and diagnosis depend on the form (i.e., familial or spontaneous) and the stage of the retinoblastoma. The goal is to preserve useful vision without compromising the patient's chances for survival. Treatment includes one or more of following:

- Enucleation—removal of the affected eye.
- External beam radiation—high level rays delivered by a machine outside the body.

Table 2-20. Reese-Ellsworth Classification of Retinoblastoma

Reese-Ellsworth Staging for Retinoblastoma

Group I: Very Favorable

A. Solitary tumor; <4 disc diameters (dd*) in size at or behind the equator

B. Multiple tumors; no tumor >4 dd in size at or behind the equator

Group II: Favorable

A. Solitary tumor; 4 to 10 dd in size at or behind the equator

B. Multiple tumors; 4 to 10 dd in size at or behind the equator

Group III: Doubtful

A. Any lesion anterior to the equator

B. Solitary tumors >10 dd in size behind the equator

Group IV: Unfavorable

A. Multiple tumors; some >10 dd in size

B. Any lesion extending anteriorly to the ora serrata

Group V: Very Unfavorable

A. Tumors involving more than half of the retina

B. Vitreous seeding

*1 dd = 1.5 mm

From *Nursing Care of Children and Adolescents with Cancer* (3rd ed., p.593), by C.R. Baggott, K.P. Kelly, D. Fochtman and G.V. Foley, 2002, Philadelphia: W.B. Saunders.

- Cryotherapy—use of cold temperatures to kill cancer cells.
- Thermotherapy—use of heat to kill cancer cells.
- Laser photocoagulation—use of lasers to destroy blood vessels that go to the cancer cells.
- Plaque radiation therapy—applying radioactive material directly into or near the cancer cells.
- Chemotherapy—use of drugs to kill cancer cells.

It is important to remember that bilateral familial retinoblastoma can occur asynchronously; therefore, conservative management of a neonate with unilateral presentation of retinoblastoma is indicated. Enucleation is indicated when retinal damage is so extensive that useful vision is unlikely. Bilateral enucleation is justified in patients with advanced disease. Exenteration of the orbital contents is necessary in cases of scleral eruption of the disease. Chemotherapy is being utilized more often as treatment for patients with intraocular retinoblastoma. The major objective of current clinical trials is to decrease tumor size so that surgical options are more likely to be an option rather than radiotherapy; therefore, decreasing the risk of secondary cancers and orbital or facial abnormalities. Infants with bilateral familial retinoblastoma may benefit from chemotherapy with vincristine (Oncovin), carboplatin (CBDCA), teniposide (VP-16), and cyclosphosphamide (Cytoxan). All patients must be followed with frequent funduscopic examinations to detect recurrent or new disease.

Recurrent Disease

Recurrent disease portends a poor prognosis. Radiation therapy or systemic chemotherapy provide palliation.

Nursing Assessment and Interventions

Goal: The patient will experience minimal complications related to the onset of tumor.

Assessment:

- Know the type of malignancy, location, and extent of disease.
- Obtain a complete history, including familial incidence of retinoblastoma or ocular loss of unknown etiology, decreased vision in one eye, and other changes in the appearance of the eye.
- Perform a complete physical examination, including an assessment of visual acuity or tracking in infants, strabismus, esotropia, exotropia, and leukocoria.
- Review laboratory findings.
- Review radiological imaging studies, as indicated.
- Review surgical and pathology reports, as indicated.
- Assess the child's degree of pain.

Interventions:

- Provide comfort measures.
- Provide pain medication, as needed.
- Explain all tests, procedures, and results to the patient and the family.

Goal: The patient will experience minimal complications related to treatment.

Assessment:

- Assess the child for toxicity related to specific chemotherapy agents (see the discussion of chemotherapy in Section IV, "Childhood Cancer Treatment").
- Assess the child for toxicity related to radiation therapy, if given (see the discussion of radiation therapy in Section IV, "Childhood Cancer Treatment").
- Assess the child for complications related to surgery, if performed (see the discussion of surgery in Section IV, "Childhood Cancer Treatment").
- Assess for signs of infection.
- Assess the child for evidence of fatigue, bleeding, pain, and nutritional deficits.
- Monitor fluid and electrolytes.
- Determine the type of intravenous access that is needed.
- Assess for the possibility of emergency complications.
- Assess for a response to therapy (i.e., a decrease in the size of the mass or enlarged lymph nodes, evaluation of any metastatic disease).

Interventions:

- Refer the child for central intravenous access, as needed.
- Provide comfort measures.
- Provide pain medication, as needed.
- Provide instruction on proper mouth care, nutrition, and hygiene.
- Educate the family about neutropenia, anemia, thrombocytopenia, the signs and symptoms of infection, and fever precautions.
- Obtain cultures and radiological examinations, as ordered, when infection is suspected, and initiate antibiotics, if indicated.
- Provide alternative methods of nutrition (e.g., oral supplements, NG or parenteral supplements).
- Review all findings of laboratory studies and radiological studies with the patient and the family.

Goal: Both the patient and the family will be adequately informed regarding the diagnosis, disease, and treatment.

Assessment:

- Assess the level of knowledge of the patient and the family about the diagnosis and disease.
- Assess their level of knowledge about treatment (i.e., surgery, radiation therapy, chemotherapy).
- Assess their learning styles (see Section VIII, "Patient and Family Education").
- Assess their understanding of the role of the multidisciplinary team in treating children with retinoblastoma.

Interventions:

- Communicate with the patient and the family in an appropriate style.
- Provide them with appropriate educational resources and review the material with them.
- Ensure that the family is aware of when and how to contact the healthcare team.
- Encourage both the patient and the family to ask questions related to the diagnosis, disease, and treatment.

Goal: The patient and the family will cope adequately with the diagnosis.

Assessment:

- Assess the family's communication and coping styles in general.
- Assess the family's adjustment to the diagnosis.

Interventions:

- Provide the patient and the family with honest answers.
- Provide them with emotional support.
- Anticipate the need for referral services (e.g., social work, chaplain, Candlelighters, American Cancer Society, Leukemia Society and National Resources for the Visually Impaired (i.e., Lighthouse Inc., Helen Keller International World Headquarters, Prevent Blindness America).
- Offer the child age-appropriate "hospital play."
- Offer to introduce a contact family who has dealt with a similar malignancy to talk with the patient and the family.

Expected Patient and Family Outcomes

The parents and child (as appropriate) can do the following:

- Describe the type of retinoblastoma and the plan of care.
- List the expected and possible toxic side effects of therapy.
- Outline methods for preventing infection.
- Describe the schedule of treatment, procedures, and follow-up care.
- Describe available community resources.
- Demonstrate the skills needed to care for the child at home.
- Explain how and when to contact the healthcare team if problems or questions arise.

Rare Tumors of Childhood

Lisa Thomas

Certain malignancies are classified as rare tumors in pediatric oncology because they originate from epithelial tissues, the source of most adult cancer, rather than embryonal tissues, the origin of most childhood cancers. These rare cancers are diagnosed more commonly in the 15- to 19-year-old age group. (**Figure 2–9**)

Children and their families who are affected by the diagnosis of a rare cancer need additional support because there is often little information available about these particular cancers. It is therefore important for a pediatric oncology nurse to identify resources and to reduce the isolation felt by these children and their families.

Fibrosarcoma

Definition: Fibrosarcoma is a malignancy of fibrous tissue.

Incidence and etiology: Fibrosarcoma is one of the most common soft-tissue sarcomas (non-rhabdomyosarcoma) in children and adolescents and is the most common soft-tissue sarcoma that occurs in children under the age of 1 year. Two peak incidences occur, the first in children younger than 5 years of age and the second in those 10–15 years of age. These two types are referred to as congenital, or infant, and adult forms of fibrosarcoma. Tumors in infants usually are benign. The adult form of this disease has been associated in some patients with previous exposure to radiation.

Clinical presentation: The most common site for fibrosarcoma is an extremity, especially its distal segments. Fibrosarcoma also can occur in the trunk or in the head and neck. Presenting symptoms are variable, depending upon the site of the primary tumor.

Treatment and prognosis: The treatment for infant fibrosarcoma is wide surgical excision (conservative surgical approach). Late local recurrences have been noted in

Figure 2–9. Cancer Among Adolescents 15–19 Years Old

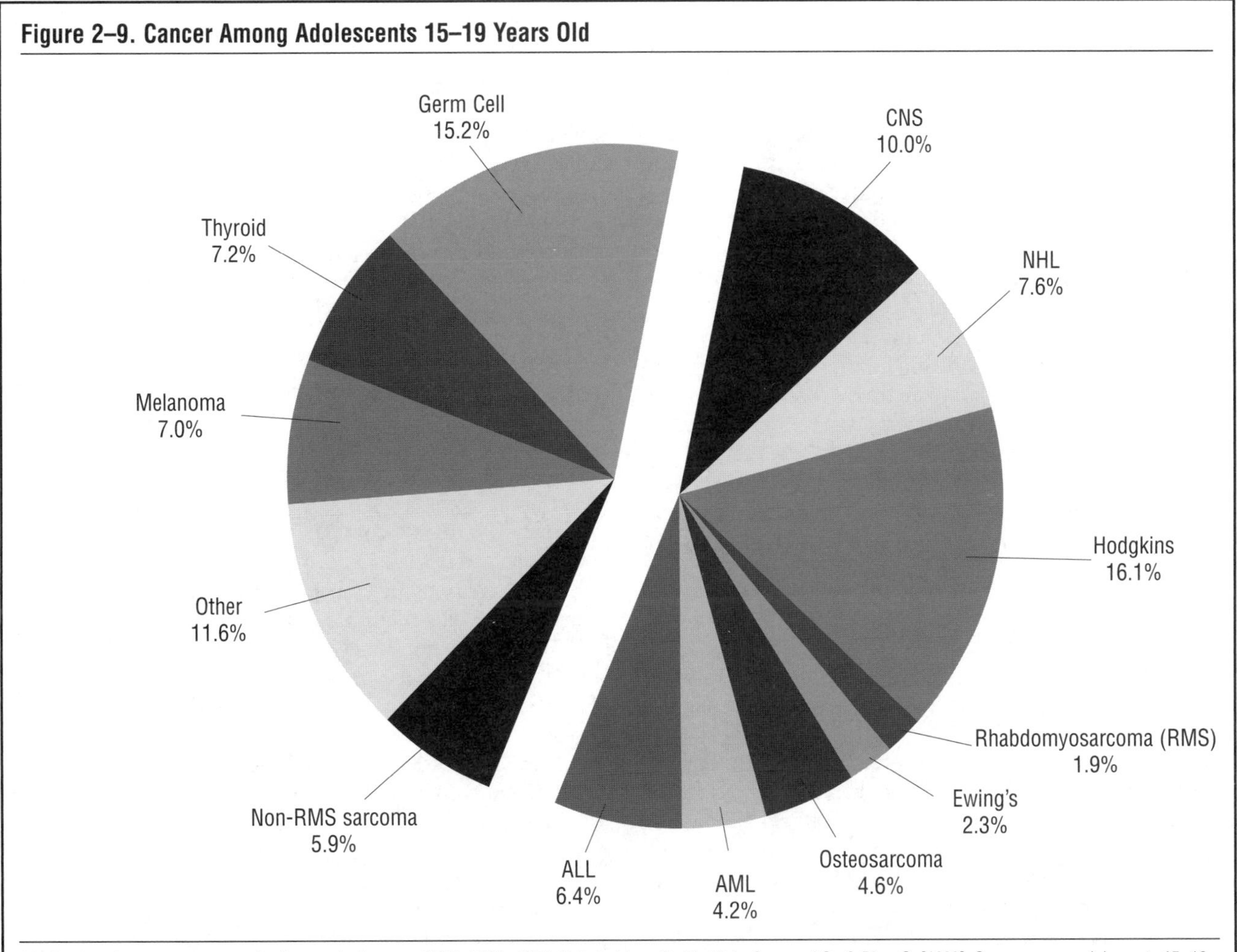

Distribution of cancer types, age <5, all races, both sexes, SEER, 1986–1995. (Adapted from Smith, M.A., Gurney, J.G., & Ries, G. [1999]. Cancer among adolescents 15–19 years old. In L.A.G. Ries, M.A. Smith, J.G. Gurney, et al. [Eds.], *Cancer incidence and survival among children and adolescents: United States SEER Program 1975–1995* [p. 159]. Bethesda, MD: National Cancer Institute, NIH Pub. No. 99–4649.)

17%–43% of cases; however, this does not appear to affect overall survival for this population.

Older children (10–15 years old) usually require preoperative chemotherapy to reduce tumor size before surgical resection, as well as to prevent metastases. The purpose of surgery is to achieve a wide local excision, or amputation if necessary. Chemotherapy treatment is similar to that for rhabdomyosarcoma, including doxorubicin (Adriamycin), ifosfamide (Ifex), etoposide (VP-16), vincristine (Oncovin), dactinomycin, cyclophosphamide (cytoxan), and dacarbazine in various combinations. Prognosis is dependent upon the site of the primary lesion and extent of disease. Congenital fibrosarcoma has a 5-year survival rate of 95%; an older child has a 5-year survival rate of approximately 60%. The prognosis for recurrent or progressive disease, with the exception of infants, is poor, with the most common site of metastasis being the lung.

Synovial sarcoma

Definition: Synovial sarcoma is a tumor of fibrous and epithelial origins.

Incidence and etiology: This type of tumor is most commonly seen in older children and young adults, with approximately 31% of cases occurring in patients younger than 20 (median age–13). Incidence is slightly higher in males than in females (1.2:1.0).

Clinical presentation: Synovial sarcoma most often occurs in a lower extremity, especially in the knee and thigh. It also occurs in the upper extremities as well as in the trunk, head, and neck. The lung is the most common site of metastatic disease, and it also can spread to regional lymph nodes.

Treatment and prognosis: Because this tumor is rare in children, the guidelines for optimal treatment are not firmly established. Wide local excision is the treatment of choice for the primary tumor. Radiation may be used to control microscopic residual disease. This tumor is chemoresponsive; however, the role of adjuvant chemotherapy is still being investigated. Poor prognosis is related to the presence of metastases; a tumor that is larger than 5cm; tumor invasiveness; a primary site other than the hand, foot, or knee; older age at diagnosis; bone or neurovascular invasion; and poor histologic differentiation.

Alveolar Soft-Part Sarcoma

Definition: Alveolar soft-part sarcoma is a soft-tissue sarcoma of unclear histogenesis.

Incidence and etiology: This rare type of sarcoma is usually seen in patients who are 15– 35 years of age.

Clinical presentation: This sarcoma, seen most often in the orbit and in the head and neck in children, is often a slow-growing, asymptomatic mass that does not produce symptoms. In adults, it is most commonly seen in the extremities. The lung is the most common site of metastasis, followed by the brain, bone, and lymph nodes.

Treatment and prognosis: Complete local excision is the most common initial therapeutic treatment. Alveolar soft-part sarcoma grows slowly, but recurrent disease is common and difficult to treat. Despite the fact that more than 80% of patients with this type of sarcoma are alive 2 years after diagnosis, most patients die of this disease, sometimes as long as 20 years after diagnosis. Radiation and chemotherapy (anthracycline-based regimen) often are used for recurrent disease and are increasingly being used during initial treatment.

Malignant Hepatic Tumors

Definition: Malignant hepatic tumors are malignant tumors of the liver. Most are hepatoblastomas and hepatocellular carcinomas.

Incidence and etiology: Approximately 50% of hepatic tumors are malignant, whereas other hepatic lesions may be hemangiomas or hamartomas. The median age of patients with hepatoblastoma is 1 year, and the median age for patients with hepatocellular carcinoma is 12 years. Hepatocellular carcinoma in patients under the age of 15 years is associated with the hepatitis B virus. Hepatocellular carcinoma also is associated with the prolonged use of anabolic steroids.

Clinical presentation: Hepatoblastoma most often presents as an asymptomatic abdominal mass. Pallor, weight loss, and jaundice are rare. Many patients with hepatoblastoma present with osteopenia, which regresses with tumor resection. Hepatocellular carcinoma often presents with abdominal distention and mass in the patient's right upper quadrant. Abdominal pain, nausea, and vomiting are common. The patient may be jaundiced and have associated splenomegaly. The patient's levels of alpha-fetoprotein may be elevated.

Treatment and prognosis: A complete resection may be made possible by preoperative chemotherapy in hepatoblastoma and hepatocellular carcinoma. The most common agents used for hepatoblastoma are fluorouracil (5-FU), vincristine (Oncovin), doxorubicin (Adriamycin), and cisplatin (Platinol). The cure rates are high for hepatoblastoma. Overall survival rates for children who have complete resection of their primary tumor exceed 75%. The following characteristics are correlated with a poor prognosis: tumor involvement in both lobes of the liver; multifocal, disseminated liver metastasis; distant metastasis; vascular invasion; embryonal differentiation; and serum alpha-fetoprotein (<100,000 ng/ml or >100,000 ng/ml). Recurrent disease most often appears in the liver or lungs. Cure is possible for metastatic disease if metastases are surgically resected.

The survival rate for patients with hepatocellular carcinoma is between 10%–20%. A variant form of hepatocellular carcinoma known as fibrolamellar is associated with a high rate of surgical respectability and improved overall survival, compared with typical hepatocellular carcinoma. Hepatocellular carcinoma is difficult to resect and is difficult to cure, even with complete resection. Radiation is of little benefit in treating hepatic tumors. The efficacy of liver transplantation is being investigated.

Nasopharyngeal Carcinoma

Definition: Nasopharyngeal carcinoma is a primary malignancy of the nasopharyngeal epithelium.

Incidence and etiology: It is rare in children—only 9% of all nasopharyngeal carcinomas occur in children who are less than 15 years of age. It is the second most common tumor (after rhabdomyosarcoma) of the upper respiratory tract in children, and is associated with Epstein-Barr virus (EBV). EBV titers may be used as tumor markers. There is a high incidence of EBV-associated tumors in Asia.

Clinical presentation: Nasopharyngeal carcinomas develop in the pharyngeal recesses and spread to the cervical lymph nodes. Lymphadenopathy is often the first and only presenting symptom. Other symptoms include epistaxis, nasal obstruction, tribmus, hearing loss, ear pain, headache, and chronic otitis media. Fifty percent of all patients have cranial nerve involvement. Nasopharyngeal carcinomas metastasize locally to lymph nodes and to the lungs, vertebrae, long bones, or liver.

Treatment and prognosis: Treatment includes radiation therapy to extended fields (6,000–7,000 cGy) and frequently has long-term effects such as xerostomia and fibrosis of the neck muscles. Chemotherapy, including cisplatin (Platinol), fluorouracil (5-FU), methotrexate (Mexate), bleomycin (Blenoxane), vincristine, cyclophosphamide, doxorubicin, and etoposide, is often used. Patients with small tumors have a more favorable prognosis than patients with tumors that extend outside of the nasopharynx. The overall survival rate is 78%.

Germ Cell Tumors

Definition: Germ cell tumors are tumors arising from primitive germ cells, or embryonal cells, and can occur in the gonads or in sites along the migratory path of the germ cells from the yolk sac to the gonads. The morphological type varies according to the site and the patient's age. It is not uncommon for one tumor to include more than one cell type. The classifications of these tumors include: teratomas, germinomas, endodermal sinus tumors, choriocarcinomas, and embryonal carcinomas.

Types of ovarian tumors include dysgerminoma, teratoma (these are often benign), malignant mixed germ cell tumor, endodermal sinus tumor (also called yolk sac tumor), gonadoblastoma, choriocarcinoma, embryonal carcinoma, and polyembryoma.

Types of testicular tumors include endodermal sinus tumor, embryonal carcinoma, teratoma (often benign), tertocarcinoma, gonadoblastoma, seminoma, choriocarcinoma, and mixed germ cell tumor.

Types of extragonadal germ cell tumors include teratoma, endodermal sinus tumor (also called yolk sac tumor), and embryonal carcinoma.

Incidence and etiology: Germ cell tumors, which account for 1% of all childhood tumors, are associated with abnormal sex chromosomes, central nervous system (CNS) and genitourinary abnormalities, and malformations of the low spine. Most sacrococcygeal teratomas occur in girls; most ovarian tumors occur in postmenarchal girls. The incidence for testicular tumors has two peaks—one in infancy and the other postpubertal—and is higher in males with a history of cryptorchidism.

Clinical presentation: The most common sites of metastasis for germ cell tumors are the lungs, liver, regional nodes, and CNS. They rarely spread to the bone marrow. Alpha-fetoprotein and β-human chorionic gonadotropin levels are often elevated.

The most common germ cell tumor is teratoma, which in infants often appears with large external masses (often sacrococcygeal). Other primary sites include the cervical neck, upper jaw, nasopharynx, intracranium, retroperitoneum, mediastinum, and gonads. Patients with ovarian tumors often have abdominal pain and swelling, palpable mass, nausea, vomiting, constipation, or genitourinary symptoms. Most testicular tumors present as painless irregular scrotal masses, often with hydroceles or inguinal hernias.

Treatment and prognosis: Individualized multimodal treatment is necessary because of the variety of germ cell tumors. Surgical resection is the treatment of choice for benign germ cell tumors such as teratoma. In malignant tumors, removal is indicated if it can be done without sacrificing vital structures and or organs. Otherwise, debulking or biopsy only is appropriate.

Chemotherapy is given initially in an attempt to debulk the tumor so that a second surgical procedure can be done. It is recommended that malignant lesions with microscopic residual, lymph node disease, or metastatic disease receive platinum-based chemotherapy. Drugs frequently used include cisplatin, bleomycin, vincristine, etoposide, dactinomycin, cyclophosphamide, and doxorubicin. Cisplatin, etoposide, and bleomycin are the standard drugs used in current studies.

Site, stage, and alpha-fetoprotein (AFP) level have prognostic significance for germ cell tumors. Current survival for stages I and II gonadal sites approaches 100%, and survival for stages III and IV gonadal sites is approximately 95%. Survival for extragonadal tumors is approximately 90% for stages I and II and 75% for stages III and IV. Retroperitoneal and testicular primary sites of disease have been associated with an improved prognosis. Sacrococcygeal and mediastinal tumors have a poorer prognosis.

Nursing Assessment and Interventions

Goal: The patient will experience minimal complications related to the onset of a rare tumor.

Assessment:

- Know the type of rare malignancy, its location, and the extent of the disease.
- Obtain a complete history, including the incidence and duration of symptoms (e.g., fatigue, epistaxis, weight loss, full abdomen, neurological changes), predisposing factors (e.g., exposure to radiation, cytotoxic drugs, anabolic steroids, genetic abnormalities), and family history.
- Perform a complete physical examination that includes an assessment for the presence of mass (warmth, tenderness), pallor, jaundice, ascites, lymphadenopathy, hepatosplenomegaly, and neurological changes.
- Review laboratory findings.
- Review radiological imaging studies, as indicated.
- Review surgical and pathology reports, as indicated.
- Assess the child's degree of pain.

Interventions:

- Provide comfort measures.
- Provide pain medication, as needed.
- Explain all tests, procedures, and results to the patient and the family.

Goal: The patient will experience minimal complications related to the treatment.

Assessment:

- Assess the child for toxicity related to specific chemotherapy agents (see the discussion of chemotherapy in Section IV, "Childhood Cancer Treatment").
- Assess the child for toxicity related to radiation therapy, if given (see the discussion of radiation therapy in Section IV, "Childhood Cancer Treatment").
- Assess the child for complications related to surgery, if performed (see the discussion of surgery in Section IV, "Childhood Cancer Treatment").
- Assess for signs of infection.
- Assess the child for evidence of fatigue, bleeding, pain, and nutritional deficits.
- Monitor fluid intake and output and electrolytes.
- Determine whether there is a need for intravenous access.
- Assess for the possibility of emergency complications.
- Assess for the child's response to therapy (i.e., a decrease in the size of the mass or enlarged lymph nodes, evaluation of any metastatic disease).

Interventions:

- Refer the child for central intravenous access, as needed.
- Provide comfort measures.
- Provide pain medication, as needed.
- Provide instruction on proper mouth care, nutrition, and hygiene.
- Educate the family regarding neutropenia, anemia, thrombocytopenia, as well as the signs and symptoms of infection and fever precautions.

- Obtain cultures and radiological examinations, as ordered, when infection is suspected, and initiate antibiotics if indicated.
- Provide alternative methods of nutrition (e.g., oral supplements, NG or parenteral supplements).
- Review all findings of laboratory studies and radiological studies with the patient and the family.

Goal: Both the patient and the family will be adequately informed about the diagnosis, disease, and treatment.

Assessment:

- Assess the level of knowledge of the patient and the family about the diagnosis and disease.
- Assess their level of knowledge about treatment (i.e., surgery, radiation therapy, chemotherapy).
- Assess their learning styles (see Section VIII, "Patient and Family Education").
- Assess their understanding of the role of the multidisciplinary team in treating children with rare tumors.

Interventions:

- Communicate with the patient and the family in an appropriate manner.
- Provide them with appropriate educational resources and review the material with them.
- Ensure that the family is aware of when and how to contact the healthcare team.
- Encourage both the patient and the family to ask questions related to the diagnosis, disease, and treatment.

Goal: The patient and the family will cope adequately with the diagnosis.

Assessment:

- Assess the family's communication and coping styles in general.
- Assess the family's adjustment to the diagnosis.

Interventions:

- Provide the patient and the family with honest answers.
- Provide them with emotional support.
- Anticipate the need for referral services (e.g., social work, chaplain, Candlelighters, American Cancer Society, Leukemia Society).
- Offer the child age-appropriate "hospital play."
- Offer to introduce a contact family that has dealt with a similar malignancy to talk with the patient and the family.

Expected Patient and Family Outcomes

The child and the parents can do the following:

- Describe the type of rare malignancy and the plan of care.
- List the expected and possible toxic side effects of therapy.
- Outline methods for preventing infection.
- Describe the schedule of treatment, procedures, and follow-up care.
- Describe available community resources.
- Demonstrate the skills needed to care for the child at home.
- Explain how and when to contact the healthcare team if problems or questions arise.

Bibliography

Overview of Childhood Cancer

Bleyer, W. A. (1996). The adolescent gap in cancer treatment. *Journal of Registry Management, 23,* 114-115.

Bleyer, W. A., Tejeda, H., Robinson, L. L., Ross, J. A., Pollack, B. H., et al. (1997). National cancer clinical trials: Children have equal access; adolescents do not. *Journal of Adolescent Health, 21,* 366-373.

Foley, G. V., & Fergusson, J. H. (2002). History, issues, and trends. In C. R. Baggott, K. P. Kelly, D. Fochtman, & G. V. Foley (Eds.), *Nursing care of children and adolescents with cancer* (pp. 2-23). Philadelphia: W. B. Saunders.

Smith, M. A., & Ries, L. A. G. (2002). Childhood cancer: Incidence, survival, and mortality. In P. A. Pizzo & D. G. Poplack (Eds.), *Principles and practice of pediatric oncology* (4th ed.). (pp.1-12). Philadelphia: Lippincott Williams & Wilkins.

Epidemiology of Childhood Cancer

American Cancer Society. (2003). *Cancer facts and figures.* Retrieved March 1, 2003 from http://www.cancer.org/downloads/STT/CAFF2003PWSecured.pdf

American Society of Clinical Oncology. Weber, B.L. (Ed.) (2000). *ONCOSEP: Genetics, an oncology self-education program curriculum text.* Dubuque, IA: Kendall.

Benedict, W. F., Murphree, A. L., Banerjee, A., Spina, C. A., Sparkes, M. C., & Sparkes, R. S. (1983). Patient with 13 chromosome deletion: Evidence that the retinoblastoma gene is a recessive cancer gene. *Science, 219,* 973-975.

Buckley, J. D., Buckley, C. M., Breslow, N. E., Draper, G. J., Robertson, P. K., & Mack, T. M. (1996). Concordance for childhood cancer in twins. *Medical and Pediatric Oncology, 26,* 223-229.

Cavenee, W. K., Dryja, T. P., Phillips, R. A., Benedict, W. F., Godbout, R., Gallie, B. L., et al. (1983). Expression of recessive alleles by chromosomal mechanisms in retinoblastoma. *Nature, 305,* 779-784.

Cavenee, W. K., Hansen, M. F., Nordenskjold, M., Kock, E., Maumenee, I., Squire, J. A., et al. (1985). Genetic origin of mutations predisposing to retinoblastoma. *Science, 228,* 501-503.

Human Genome Project. Major events in the U.S. Human Genome Project and related projects. Retrieved March 1, 2003 from http://www.ornl.gov/TechResources/Human_Genome/project/timeline.html

Knudson, A. G. Jr. (1971). Mutation and cancer: Statistical study of retinoblastoma. *Proceedings of the National Academy of Sciences of the United States of America, 68,* 820.

Lertola, J. (2003). How DNA works. *Time,* February 17, 2003. Retrieved March 1, 2003 from http://www.time.com/time/covers/1101030217/#

Malkin, D. (1998). The Li-Fraumeni syndrome. In B.Vogelstein & K. W. Kinzler, (Eds.), *The Genetic Basis of Human Cancer* (pp. 393-407). New York: McGraw-Hill.

Philip, S. (2000). Angiogenesis inhibitors in oncology: The research continues. *Cancer Practice, 8,* 148-150.

Ruccione, K. S. (2002). Biologic basis of cancer in children and adolescents. In C. R. Baggott, K. P. Kelly, D. Fochtman, & G. V. Foley, (Eds.), *Nursing care of children and adolescents with cancer* (pp. 24-63). Philadelphia: W. B. Saunders Company.

Leukemia

Golub, T.R., & Arceci, R.J. (2002) Acute myelogenous leukemia. In In P. A. Pizzo & D. G. Poplack (Eds.), *Principles and practice of pediatric oncology* (4th ed.). *Principles and practice of pediatric oncology* (4th ed., pp. 545-589). Philadelphia: Lippincott Williams & Wilkins.

Margolin, J.R., Steuber, C.P., & Poplack, D.G. (2002) Acute lymphoblastic leukemia. In In P. A. Pizzo & D. G. Poplack (Eds.), *Principles and practice of pediatric oncology* (4th ed., pp.489-544). Philadelphia: Lippincott Williams & Wilkins.

Silverman, L.B., & Sallan, S.E. (2003) Acute lymphoblastic leukemia. In R. I. Handin, S. E. Lux & T. P. Stossel (Eds.), *Blood principles and practice of hematology* (2nd ed., pp.779-804). Philadelphia: Lippincott Williams & Wilkins.

Smith, M., Arthur, D., Camitta, B., Carrol, A.J., Crist, W., Gayon, P., et al. (1996). Uniform approach to risk classification and treatment assignment for children with acute lymphoblastic leukemia. *Journal of Clinical Oncology, 14*(1), 18-24.

Westlake, S.K., & Bertolone, K.L. (2002). Acute lymphoblastic leukemia. In C.R.Baggott, K.P. Kelly, D. Fotchman, G.V. Foley (Eds.), *Nursing care of children and adolescents with cancer* (3rd ed., pp. 466-490). Philadelphia: W.B. Saunders Co.

Non-Hodgkin's Lymphoma

Hussong, M.R. Non-Hodgkin's lymphoma. In C.R. Baggott, K.P. Kelly, D. Fochtman, & G.V. Foley, (Eds.), (2002). *Nursing care of children and adolescents with cancer* (3rd ed., pp. 536-544). New York: W.B. Sauders Company.

Magrath, I.T. (2000) Malignant Non-Hodgkin's lymphoma in children. In P.A. Pizzo & D.G. Poplack, (Eds.) *Principles and practice of pediatric oncology* (4th ed., pp. 661-705). Philadelphia: Lippincott-Raven.

Murphy, S.B. (1999). Non-Hodgkin's lymphoma and Hodgkin's disease. In C. Herzog & C. Pratt (Eds.), *Therapy of cancer in children* (pp. 11-13). Houston, TX: University of Texas M.D. Anderson Cancer Center.

Sandlund, J. T., Downing, J.R., & Crist, W.M. (1996). Non-Hodgkin's Lymphoma in childhood. *NEJM, 334*, 1238-1248.

Hodgkin's Disease

Donaldson, S.S., Hudson, M.M., Lamborn, K.R., Link, M.P., Kun, L., Billett, A.L., et al. (2002). VAMP and low-dose, involved-field radiation for children and adolescents with favorable, early-stage Hodgkin's disease: Results of a prospective clinical trial. *Journal of Clinical Oncology, 20*, 3081–3087.

Friedmann, A.M., Hudson, M.M., Weinstein, H.J., Donaldson, S.S., Kun, L., Tarbell, N.J., et al. (2002). Treatment of unfavorable childhood Hodgkin's disease with VEPA and low-dose, involved-field radiation. *Journal of Clinical Oncology, 20*, 3088–3094.

Horning, S.J., Williams, J., Bartlett, N.L., Bennett, J.M., Hoppe, R.T., Neuberg, D., et al. (2000). Assessment of the Stanford V regimen and consolidative radiotherapy for bulky and advanced Hodgkin's disease: Eastern Cooperative Oncology Group pilot study E1492. *Journal of Clinical Oncology, 18*, 972–980.

Hudson, M.M., & Donaldson, S.S. (2002). Hodgkin's disease. In P.A.Pizzo & D.G. Poplack (Eds.), *Principles and practice of pediatric oncology* (4th ed., pp. 637–660). Philadelphia: Lippincott Williams & Wilkins.

Central Nervous System Tumors

Betak, M. (2001). Epidemiology of brain tumors. In R. Keating, J.Goodrich, & R. Packer (Eds.). *Tumors of the pediatric central nervous system* (pp. 14–21). New York: Thieme.

CBTRUS (2002-2003). *Statistical report: Brain tumors in the United States, 1993-1999*. Chicago: Central Brain Tumor Registry of the United States.

Halperin, E., Constine, L., Tarbell, N., & Kun, L. (1999). Tumors of the posterior fossa and the spinal canal. In *Pediatric radiation oncology* (3rd ed., pp. 80–125). Philadelphia: Lippincott Williams & Wilkins.

McComb, J., Liker, M., & Levy, M. (2001). Spinal cord tumors. In S. Weistein (Ed.). *The pediatric spine – Principles and practice* (2nd ed., pp. 709–716, 725–731). Philadelphia: Lippincott Williams & Wilkins.

Packer, R. (1999). Brain tumors in children. *Archives of Neurology, 56*, 421-425.

Ryan-Murray, J. & Petriccione, M. (2002). Central nervous system tumors. In C. Baggott, K. Kelly, D. Fochtman, & G. Foley (Eds.). *Nursing care of children and adolescents with cancer* (3rd ed., pp. 503–523). Philadelphia: W.B. Saunders.

Shiminski-Maher, T., Cullen, P., & Sansalone, M. (2002). Posterior fossa syndrome. In *Childhood brain & spinal cord tumors – A guide for families, friends and caregivers* (pp. 157–158), Sebastopo, CA: O'Reilly.

Strother, D., Pollack, I., Fisher, P., Woo, S., Pomeroy, S., & Rorke, L. (2002). Tumors of the central nervous system. In P.A. Pizzo & D.G. Poplack (Eds.). *Principles and practice of pediatric oncology* (4th ed., pp. 751–824). Philadelphia: Lippincott Williams & Wilkins.

Wiestler, D., Schiffer, Coons, S., Prayson, R., & Rosenblum, M. (2001). Ependymomas. In P. Kleihuer & W.K. Cavanee (Eds.). *World Health Organization classification of tumors: Pathology & genetics – tumors of the central nervous system* (pp. 71–81). Lyon, France: IARC Press.

Neuroblastoma

Brodeur, G.M., & Maris, J.M (2002). Neuroblastoma. In P.A. Pizzo & D.G. Poplack (Eds.), *Principles and practice of pediatric oncology* (4th ed., pp. 895–937). Philadelphia: Lippincott Williams & Wilkins.

Dadd, G. (2002). Neuroblastoma. In C.R. Baggott, K.P. Kelly, D. Fochtman, & G.V. Foley (Eds.), *Nursing care of children and adolescents with cancer* (3rd ed., pp. 545–554). Philadelphia: W.B. Saunders.

Lemieux, B., & Woods, W.G. (2000). Mass screening for neuroblastoma: The North American experience. In G.M. Brodeur, T. Sawada, Y. Tsuchida, & P.A. Voute (Eds.), *Neuroblastoma* (pp. 265–279). Amsterdam: Elsevier.

Mugishima, H., & Sakurai, M. (2000). Symptoms of neuroblastoma: Paraneoplastic syndromes. In G.M. Brodeur, T. Sawada, Y. Tsuchida, & P.A. Voute (Eds.), *Neuroblastoma* (pp. 293–301). Amsterdam: Elsevier.

Osteosarcoma

Ferrari, S., Briccoli, A., Mercuri, M., Bertoni, F., Picci, P., Tienghi, A., et al. (2003). Postrelapse survival in osteosarcoma of the extremities: Prognostic factors for long-term survival. *Journal of Clinical Oncology, 21*, 710–715.

Lane, J.M., Christ, G.H., Khan, S.N., & Backus, S.I. (2001). Rehabilitation for limb salvage patients: Kinesiological parameters and psychological assessment. *Cancer, 92*, 1013–1019.

Link, M.P., Gebhardt, M.C., & Meyers, P.A. (2002). Osteosarcoma. In P.A.Pizzo & D.G. Poplack (Eds.), *Principles and practice of pediatric oncology* (pp. 973–1016). Philadelphia: Lippincott, Williams & Wilkins.

Ewing's Sarcoma of Bone and Soft Tissue and Peripheral Primitive Neuroectodermal Tumors

Ginsberg, J.P., Woo, S.Y., Johnson, M.E., Hicks, M.J., & Horowitz, M.E. (2002). Ewing's sarcoma family of tumors: Ewing's sarcoma of bone and soft tissue and the peripheral primitive neuroectodermal tumors. In P.A. Pizzo & D.G. Poplack (Eds.), *Principles and practice of pediatric oncology* (4th Ed., pp. 973–1016). Philadelphia: Lippincott Williams and Wilkins.

Grier, H.E., Krailo, M.D., Tarbell, N.J., Link, M.P., Fryer, C.J., Pritchard, D.J., et al. (2003). Addition of ifosfamide and etoposide to standard chemotherapy for Ewing's sarcoma and primitive neuroectodermal tumor of bone. *New England Journal of Medicine, 348*, 694-701.

Shankar, A.G., Ashley, S., Craft, A.W., & Pinkerton, C.R. (2003). Outcome after relapse in an unselected cohort of children and adolescents with Ewing's sarcoma. *Medical and Pediatric Oncology, 40*, 141–147.

Tumors of the Kidney

Breslow, N., Olshan, A., Beckwith, J.B., & Green, D.M. (1993). Epidemiology of Wilms' tumor. *Medical and Pediatric Oncology, 21*, 172–181.

Breslow, N., Olshan, A., Beckwith, J.B., Moksness, J., Feigl, P., & Green, D. (1994). Ethnic variation in the incidence, diagnosis, prognosis and follow-up of children with Wilms' tumor. *Journal of the National Cancer Institute, 86*, 49–51.

Crist, W.M., & Kun, L.E. (1991). Common solid tumors of childhood. *New England Journal of Medicine, 324*, 461–471.

Drigan, R., & Androkites, A.L. (2002). Wilms' tumor. In C.R. Baggott, K.P. Kelly,. D. Fochtman, & G.V. Foley (Eds.), *Nursing care of children and adolescents with cancer* (3rd ed., pp. 568–574), Philadelphia: W.B. Saunders.

Grundy, P.E., Green, D.M., Breslow, N.E., Ritchey, M.L., Perlman, E.J., & Macklis, R.M. (2002). Renal tumors. In P.A. Pizzo & D.G. Poplack (Eds.), Principles and practice of pediatric oncology (4th ed., pp. 895-937). Philadelphia: Lippincott Williams & Wilkins.

Petruzzi, M.J., & Green, D.M. (1997). Wilms' tumor. *Pediatric Clinics of North America, 44*, 939-952.

Rhabdomyosarcoma

Breneman, J.C., Lyden, E., Pappo, A.S., Link, M.P., Anderson, J.R., Parham, D.M., et al. (2003). Prognostic factors and clinical outcomes in children and adolescents with metastatic rhabdomyosarcoma—A report from the Intergroup Rhabdomyosarcoma Study IV. *Journal of Clinical Oncology*, 21, 78–84.

Kotsubo, C.S. (2002). Rhabdomyosarcoma. In C.R. Baggott, K.P. Kelly, D. Fochtman, & G.V. Foley (Eds.), *Nursing care of the child with cancer*, (3rd ed., pp. 555–567).

Pakakasama, S., & Tomlinson, G.E. (2002). Genetic predisposition and screening in pediatric cancer. *The Pediatric Clinics of North America, 49*, 1393-1413.

Pappo, A.S., Anderson, J.R., Crist, W.M, Wharam M.D., Breitfeld P.P., Hawkins D., et al. (1999). Survival after relapse in children and adolescents with rhabdomyosarcoma; A report from the Intergroup Rhabdomyosarcoma Study Group. *Journal of Clinical Oncology*, 17, 3487.

Wexler, L.H., Crist, W.M., & Helman, L.J. (2002). Rhabdomyosarcoma and the undifferentiated sarcomas. In P.A. Pizzo & D.G. Poplack (Eds.), *Principles and practice of pediatric oncology* (4th ed., pp. 939–971). Philadelphia: Lippincott Williams & Wilkins.

Retinoblastoma

Effective new treatment strategy for retinoblastoma avoids removal of the eye and radiation for selected patients. http://www.cancerconsultants.com

Hurwitz, R.L., Shields, C.L., Shields, J.A., Chevez-Burrios, P., Hurwitz, M.Y., & Chintagumpala, M.M. (2002). Retinoblastoma. In P.A. Pizzo & D.G. Poplack (Eds.), *Principles and practice of pediatric oncology* (4th ed., pp.825–841). Philadelphia: Lippincott Williams & Wilkins.

Kingston, J., Haddad, G., Chan, H.S.L., DeBoer, G., Thiessen, J.J., Budning, A.E., et al. (1996). Combining cyclosporin with chemotherapy controls intraocular retinoblastoma without requiring radiation. *Clinical Cancer Research, 2*, 1499–1508.

Knudson, A.G. (1971). Mutation and cancer: Statistical study of retinoblastoma. *Proceedings of the National Academy of Science USA, 68*, 820–823.

Zhu, X.P., Dunn, J.M., Phillips, R.A., Goddard, A.D., Paton, K.E., Becker, A., et al. (1989). Preferential germline mutation of the parental allele in retinoblastoma. *Nature, 340*, 312–313.

Rare Tumors of Childhood

Hockenberry, M.J. & Kline, N.E. (2002). Nursing support of the child with cancer. In P.A. Pizzo & D.G. Poplack (Eds.), *Principals and practice of pediatric oncology* (4th ed., pp. 1333–1349). Philadelphia: Lippincott Williams & Wilkens.

Miser, J.S., Pappo, A.S., Triche, T.J., Merchant, T.E., & Rao, B.N.(2002). Other soft tissue sarcomas of childhood. In P.A. Pizzo & D.G. Poplack (Eds.), *Principles and practice of pediatric oncology* (4th ed., pp. 1017–1043). Philadelphia: Lippincott Williams &Wilkens.

O'Neill J.B., (2002). Rare tumors. In C.R. Baggott, K.P. Kelly, D. Fotchman, G.V. Foley, *Nursing care of children and adolescents with cancer* (3rd ed., pp. 598–617). Philadelphia: W.B. Saunders Co.

Soule, E.H. & Pritchard D.J. (1977). Fibrosarcoma in infants and children: A review of 110 cases. *Cancer, 40*, 1711–1721.

Thomlinson, G.E. & Finegold, M.J. (2002). Tumors of the liver. In P.A. Pizzo & D.G. Poplack (Eds.), *Principles and practice of pediatric oncology* (4th ed., pp 847–859). Philadelphia: Lippincott Williams & Wilkens.

SECTION III

OVERVIEW OF HEMATOLOGY

Robbie Norville

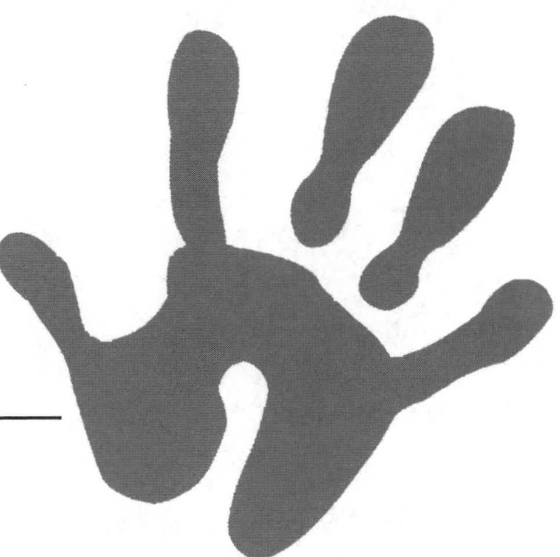

SECTION OUTLINE

Origin of Blood Cells

Tamara E. Scott

Definition

There are two major components of whole blood: plasma (the fluid portion) and formed elements (the cellular portion). Plasma is about 90% water and 10% solutes. Albumin, electrolytes, and proteins are the main solutes. Clotting factors, globulins, circulating antibodies, and fibrinogen are the proteins in the plasma. White blood cells (WBCs), red blood cells (RBCs), and platelets are the cellular elements of blood.

The major blood-forming organs (hematopoietic organs) of the body are the bone marrow (myeloid tissue) and the lymphatic system. The lymphatic system consists of lymph (fluid), lymphatic vessels, and lymphoid structures (lymph nodes, spleen, thymus, and tonsils). After birth, the bone marrow, spleen, and liver are the primary organs for hematopoiesis and cell removal.

Pathophysiology

All formed elements of the blood are formed in the bone marrow and are believed to originate from a primitive cell called a pluripotent stem cell (see **Figure 3-1**).

Recent research suggests that bone marrow stem cells also may be useful in the repair of other organs. Experiments in animals and people suggest possible applications in cardiac repair after myocardial infarction, spinal cord and central nervous system repair after injuries or strokes, and even liver cell replacement (Krause, 2002).

RBCs (erythrocytes) survive approximately 120 days in the peripheral circulation. As they age, their membranes become fragile and eventually rupture. Hemoglobin is broken down into hemosiderin (iron) and bilirubin. Most of the iron (hemosiderin) is reused by the bone marrow for production of new RBCs or stored in the liver and other tissues for future use. The bilirubin is excreted by the liver in the bile.

Figure 3-1. Bone Marrow and Stem Cell Systems

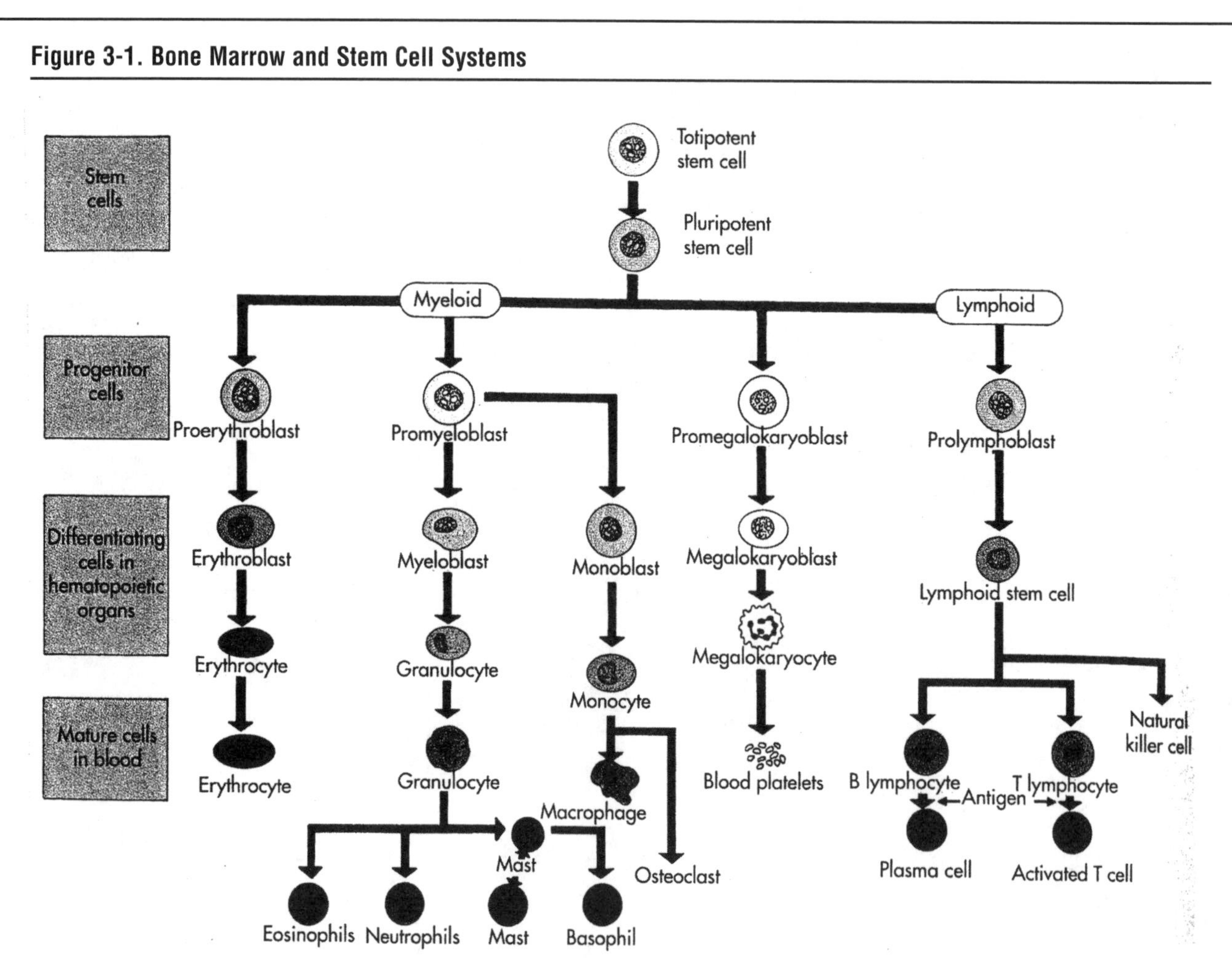

Note: From *Pathophysiology: The Biologic Basis for Disease in Adults and Children* (3rd ed., p. 854), by K.L. McCance and S.E. Huether (Eds.), 1998, St. Louis: Mosby-Year Book.

Normally there is a homeostatic balance between RBC production and destruction. The production of erythropoietin by the kidneys in response to tissue hypoxia is the basic regulator of erythrocyte production. When erythropoietin is released into the bloodstream, the bone marrow is stimulated to make new RBCs. During this time, there is a rapid increase in red cell production; therefore, not all of the circulating erythrocytes will be totally mature, which accounts for an increase in the reticulocyte count. If a rise in the reticulocyte count does not occur at times of tissue hypoxia or with increased destruction of red cells, bone marrow failure could be the reason.

When tissues are adequately oxygenated, erythropoietin production ceases. The RBCs transport oxygen to tissues in response to their needs, not in response to the circulating numbers of erythrocytes. Oxygen transport depends on the number of circulating RBCs and the amount of normal hemoglobin in the cell. (See the subsection titled "Anemia" for a discussion of hemoglobin, hematocrit, and RBC indices.)

White blood cells/leukocytes are produced in both the bone marrow and the lymph tissue. They are categorized as granulocytes and agranulocytes. The granulocytes (neutrophils, basophils, and eosinophils) survive 12–14 hours in blood and about 5 days in tissues. Agranulocytes (monocytes and lymphocytes) can survive for years in tissues. Platelets (thrombocytes) have an average life span of 7–10 days in the blood.

Normal Blood Cell Parameters

Normal blood values vary during infancy, childhood, and adolescence. **Table 3-1** indicates mean normal blood values from infancy through adulthood.

Function of Red Blood Cells

The major function of RBCs is to transport hemoglobin, which, in turn, carries oxygen to all cells of the body. RBCs catalyze the reaction between carbon dioxide and water, allowing large quantities of carbon dioxide to react with blood that is transported to the lungs. The hemoglobin serves as an acid-base buffer, which, when combined with carbon dioxide, maintains the blood pH at a constant level.

Function of White Blood Cells

Neutrophils: Neutrophils are the primary defense in bacterial infection. Neutrophils are able to phagocytize and kill bacteria.

Monocytes: Monocytes are large phagocytic cells that are involved in the early stage of inflammatory reaction.

Lymphocytes: Lymphocytes are involved in the development of antibodies and delayed hypersensitivity and are of two types: B cells, which synthesize and secrete an antibody, and T cells, which are lymphocytes that have circulated through the thymus gland; when exposed to an antigen, they rapidly divide and produce large numbers of new T cells that are sensitized to the antigen. Some are called "killer cells" because they secrete certain compounds and assist B cells in destroying foreign proteins. T cells also play

Table 3-1. Mean Normal Blood Values in Infancy and Childhood*

Age	Hemoglobin (g/dl)	RBC (x 10^{12}/L)	Hematocrit (%)	MCV (fl)	MCH (pg)	MCHC (%)	Reticulocytes (%)
Cord blood	16.6	5.25	63	120	34.0	31.7	3.2
1 day	19.0	5.14	61	119	36.9	31.6	3.2
3 days	18.7	5.11	62	116	36.5	31.1	3.8
7 days	17.9	4.86	56	115	36.2	32.0	0.5
2 weeks	17.3	4.80	54	112	36.8	32.1	0.5
3 weeks	15.6	4.20	46	111	37.1	33.9	0.8
4 weeks	14.2	4.00	43	105	35.5	33.5	0.6
2 months	10.7	3.40	31	93	31.5	34.1	1.8
3 months	11.3	3.70	33	88	30.5	34.8	0.7
6 months	12.3	4.60	36	78	27.0	34.0	1.4
8 months	12.1	4.60	36	77	26.0	34.0	1.1
10 months	11.9	4.60	36	77	26.0	34.0	1.0
1 year	11.6	4.60	36	78	25.0	33.0	0.9
2 years	11.7	4.70	38	79	25.0	33.0	1.0
4 years	12.6	4.70	38	80	27.0	34.0	1.0
6 years	12.7	4.70	39	81	27.0	33.0	1.0
8 years	12.9	4.70	40	83	27.0	33.0	1.0
10-12 years	13.0	4.80	40	83	27.0	33.0	1.0
Men	16.0	5.40	47	87	29.0	34.0	1.0
Women	14.0	4.80	42	87	29.0	34.0	1.0

*Based on standard sources.

Note: From *Blood Diseases of Infancy and Childhood* (p. 37), by D.R. Miller and R.L. Bachner (Eds.), 1995, St. Louis: Mosby-Year Book. Copyright 1995 by Mosby-Year Book. Reprinted with permission.

a significant role in the body's resistance to the proliferation of cancer cells.

Eosinophils: Eosinophils seem to have parasiticidal properties and can selectively destroy parasites, but their function is not completely known. They may also function in the immediate type of allergic or anaphylactic hypersensitivity reactions. They are also thought to release a substance called profibrinolysin, which, when activated to form fibrinolysin, digests fibrin, thereby helping to dissolve a clot.

Basophils: Basophils are seen in increased amounts during the healing phase of inflammation and during prolonged inflammation, but their function is not completely understood. They exit the blood vessels and become mast cells in the tissue. They are responsible for histamine release, which results in increased permeability of the vessels to allow WBCs to exit the vessels at the site of injury.

Function of Platelets

Platelets adhere to the endothelium to form a plug to stop bleeding. The first platelets to arrive at the site of an injury release substances that attract other platelets to the site. They release serotonin at the site of injury, which causes vasoconstriction.

Reference

Krause, D.S. (2002). Plasticity of marrow-derived stem cells. *Gene Therapy, 9,* 754–758.

ANEMIA

Shawn Elliott

Definition

Anemia is a reduction of the circulating hemoglobin, resulting in a decrease in the oxygen-carrying capacity of the red blood cells.

Pathophysiology

The hemoglobin within red blood cells carries almost all of the oxygen to the tissues throughout the body. When the hemoglobin concentration is decreased, tissues, muscles, and organs receive less oxygen. Anemia can be caused by an impaired or decreased production of red blood cells, nutritional deficiencies, or metabolic disturbances or by increased erythrocyte destruction. Any of these four causes can occur in combination.

Clinical Presentation

A review of systems should include the following:

- General: change in behavior, fatigability, inactivity, malaise
- Skin: onset of pallor, jaundice, petechiae, ecchymoses, rashes, ulcerations
- Head: headaches, dizziness, trauma
- Eyes: scleral jaundice, diplopia, blurring, spots, cataracts
- Ears: tinnitus, vertigo
- Nose: epistaxis
- Mouth and throat: stomatitis, swelling, bleeding gums, ulceration of buccal mucosa, change in the texture of the tongue
- Neck: adenopathy
- Cardiopulmonary: palpitations, dyspnea, edema, dizziness
- Gastrointestinal: bleeding, diarrhea, melena, vomiting, anorexia
- Genitourinary: hematuria, menstrual irregularities, urinary frequency
- Musculoskeletal: muscle pain or cramps, joint pain, swelling, stiffness, weakness, numbness, coldness, discoloration of extremities
- Nervous system: loss of consciousness, syncope, paresthesia, seizures, decreased mental concentration
- Endocrine: temperature intolerance, polyuria, polydipsia, polyphagia.

The physical examination should be carefully assessed for the following:

- General: performance status, mental activity and concentration, general appearance, height and weight for age, rate of growth
- Skin: color of skin or pallor, jaundice, pigmentation, pinkness of the palmar creases, nailbeds, conjunctiva, mucous membranes and lips, petechiae, ecchymoses, leg ulcers
- Head and neck: circumference, shape of skull, ecchymoses, bumps, hair texture and pattern
- Eyes: scleral jaundice
- Ears: abnormal hearing screen
- Nose: bleeding
- Mouth: pallor of the mucosa, ulcerations, bleeding, hematoma
- Tongue: texture and color, swelling
- Neck: adenopathy, thyroid enlargement
- Heart: tachycardia, increased pulsations, heart murmur
- Lungs: increased rate and depth of respirations
- Abdomen: splenomegaly, hepatomegaly
- Genitalia: inflammation, ulcerations, bleeding, edema
- Rectum: ulcerations, bleeding, hemorrhoids
- Musculoskeletal: painful swollen joints, stiffness, discoloration of extremities, spoon nails, triphalangeal thumbs
- Lymph nodes: swelling, tenderness
- Nervous system: parasthesias, decreased mental concentration.

Diagnostic Work-up

An evaluation of anemia in a child includes a comprehensive history and physical examination as outlined above. Children with anemia should have a complete blood cell count, RBC indices, reticulocyte counts, and a review of the peripheral smear. All values must be compared with age-matched normal values.

Hemoglobin and hematocrit: Hemoglobin is a true indicator of the physiological potential of blood to transport oxygen to tissue. Hematocrit indicates the percentage of the volume of circulating packed red cells of the total blood and is approximately three times the concentration of hemoglobin in g/dl.

Reticulocyte count: The reticulocyte count is a direct measurement of production of RBCs by the bone marrow and indicates the activity of the bone marrow.

Red blood cell indices: RBC indices (mean corpuscular volume [MCV], mean corpuscular hemoglobin [MCH], mean corpuscular hemoglobin concentration [MCHC]) are based on ratios of RBC volume, RBC count, and hemoglobin concentration.

ABO and Rh type: Prior to transfusion, the patient's blood type must be cross-matched for ABO and Rh type against the donor's red cells to determine the presence or absence of agglutination. Antibody screening, using the Coombs' tests, also must take place. The direct Coombs' test identifies antibodies on the surface of the red cell, whereas the indirect Coombs' test identifies antibodies in serum.

Treatment

Children often tolerate a decreased hemoglobin concentration without symptoms of anemia. However, when they are symptomatic, scheduled for surgery or radiation therapy, or entering a myelosuppressive period, treatment is indicated. The standard treatment for anemia is a leukocyte-reduced, irradiated, packed RBC transfusion of 10 ml/kg. Although criteria for transfusion vary widely, most institutions recommend transfusion when hemoglobin values reach at least 6 to 7 g/dl, if the child is symptomatic. Children receiving radiation therapy need to maintain hemoglobin levels of 10g/dl or higher to get the maximum benefit from the therapy.

The U.S. Food and Drug Administration (FDA) has approved the use of recombinant human erythropoietin (rHuEPO, epoetin alfa) in children. Buyukpamukcu, Varan, Kutluk, and Akyuz (2002) found that epoetin alfa is effective during myelosuppression to boost hemoglobin levels or in place of transfusion and is safe in pediatric cancer patients. Epoetin alfa could be particularly helpful for those families with religious objections to blood transfusions.

Nursing Assessment and Interventions

The nurse must be knowledgeable about the signs and symptoms of anemia and be able to perform a comprehensive history and assessment (see the heading titled "Clinical Presentation," which is presented earlier in this subsection). Nursing interventions for a child with anemia can include the following:

- Observe laboratory data for evidence of a decrease in hemoglobin and notify the healthcare team.
- Monitor for complications related to anemia.
  - Assess skin for pallor, decreased capillary refill, or prolonged redness.
  - Assess for decreased energy, fatigue, lethargy, or irritability.
  - Assess for tachycardia, tachypnea, and dyspnea.
  - Assess for headache, hypotension, or syncope.
  - Assess level of consciousness.
- Monitor patient for transfusion reactions.
- Monitor patient for signs and symptoms of volume overload.
- Maximize the child's physical tolerance.
  - Provide oxygen, as ordered, when decreased oxygen creates difficult breathing.
  - Provide quiet play activities that promote physical and intellectual development.
  - Promote times for rest and sleep.
- Teach the family about anemia.
  - Discuss anemia as the cause of the child's irritability, short attention span, and changing moods.
  - Review ways to save energy and decrease fatigue.
  - Describe signs and symptoms for parents to observe, including a change in color, increased heart rate and respirations, dyspnea, and diaphoresis.
- Administer erythropoietin, if needed.

Expected Patient Outcomes

- Family members are able to report the signs, symptoms, and complications of anemia or treatment for anemia to the healthcare team.
- The healthcare team's interventions minimize physical activity and promote oxygenation.
- The child has minimal complications related to anemia.

Reference

Buyukpamukcu, M., Varan, A., Kutluk, T., & Akyuz, C. (2002). Is erythropoietin alfa a treatment option for chemotherapy-related anemia in children? *Medical and Pediatric Oncology, 39*, 455–458.

Neutropenia

Tamara E. Scott

Definition

Neutropenia is usually defined as a reduction in circulating neutrophils of less than 1,000 absolute neutrophil count (ANC) in infants 2 weeks to 1 year of age or less than 1,500 in children older than 1 year. The risk of serious bacterial infection is increased when the ANC is below 500. The ANC is calculated by multiplying the total WBC count by the percentage of neutrophils and bands in the differential.

Some institutions use the absolute granulocyte count, which is calculated by multiplying the total WBC count by the percentage of monocytes, neutrophils, and bands in the differential.

Pathophysiology

There are many types of neutropenia seen in children. Neutropenia may be a presenting sign of malignancy involving the bone marrow. It occurs most commonly in children with acute lymphoblastic leukemia or acute nonlymphocytic leukemia. It also can be seen as a presenting sign in patients with neuroblastoma and lymphoma. Neutropenia also can be a sign of relapse in patients with leukemia, if it persists for longer than expected after chemotherapy.

This discussion will focus on neutropenia secondary to chemotherapy, radiation therapy, or both for treatment of a childhood malignancy. The administration of chemotherapy results in suppression of the bone marrow and circulating WBCs. This immunosuppression results from an interruption of the normal replication of the bone marrow cells. Cytotoxic drugs that commonly cause neutropenia are listed in **Table 3-2**.

Irradiation also results in suppression of the bone marrow. Its effects, like chemotherapy, are transient; however, ablating doses are given when preparing patients for hematopoietic stem cell transplantation. Bactrim and dapsone, two of the drugs used for pneumocytis prophylaxis, are also known to cause neutropenia in some children.

Clinical Presentation

A child with neutropenia often is asymptomatic. If a child with cancer presents with an ANC below 1,000, a complete review of systems, with attention to the following, should be done:

- Skin: erythema, edema, ulcerations
- Lungs: cough, tachypnea
- Ears, nose, and throat: rhinorrhea, ear pain, throat pain, sinus tenderness
- Mouth: stomatitis, erythema of gums, ulceration of buccal mucosa, difficulty swallowing
- Gastrointestinal: perirectal pain, diarrhea

The physical examination should meticulously assess for the following:

- Skin: integrity of the area of central venous access (if present), any venipuncture or fingerstick site, any open lesion
- Lungs: tachypnea, presence of cough, presence of adventitious sounds in the lung fields
- Ears, nose, and throat: rhinorrhea (color and consistency), sinus tenderness, erythematous tympanic membranes, erythema of the pharynx
- Mouth: ulcerations, stomatitis, erythema of the gums
- Gastrointestinal: perirectal erythema and/or tenderness, perirectal laceration.

Diagnostic Work-up

An evaluation of neutropenia is dependent upon several factors, such as time since the patient's last chemotherapy, presence of fever, and signs of infection, among others. (See Section V, "Side Effects of Treatment," for a more complete

Table 3-2. Chemotherapy Agents that Cause Neutropenia

Drug	Nadir	Recovery
Severe		
Carboplatin	21–24 days	28–35 days
Cytarabine	14–18 days	21–28 days
Daunomycin	10–14 days	21–28 days
Etoposide	7–10 days	21–28 days
Nitrogen mustard	14 days	28 days
Teniposide	5–15 days	24–28 days
Topotecan		
Mild		
BCNU	21–35 days	42–50 days
Busulfan	14–21 days	28 days
CCNU	40–50 days	60 days
Cisplatin	14–23 days	21–39 days
Cyclophophamide	10–14 days	21 days
Dactinomycin	14–21 days	21–28 days
Doxorubicin	10–14 days	21–28 days
Hydroxyurea	10 days	21 days
Melphalan	10–14 days	42–50 days
Mercaptopurine	14 days	21 days
Methtrexate	7–14 days	14–21 days
Thiotepa	14 days	21 days
Vinblastine	5–9 days	14–21 days

discussion of children with fever and neutropenia.) All febrile (38.3°C or 101°F) neutropenic patients should have the following done:

- a history and physical examination (as outlined above in "Clinical Presentation")
- blood cultures from all lumens of indwelling venous catheters (peripheral cultures may be obtained with a new temperature spike)
- urinalysis and urine culture
- stool culture (if diarrhea is present)
- chest X ray (at the discretion of the provider seeing the patient).

Nonfebrile neutropenic patients do not need to have any special studies or diagnostic work-up unless some other sign of infection is present.

Treatment

Many childhood cancer treatment regimens, especially those expected to cause a high degree of myelosuppression, now use granulocyte colony-stimulating factor (G-CSF) starting 1–5 days after chemotherapy and before the onset of neutropenia. The recommended dosage is 5–10(μ)g/kg administered subcutaneously once a day for 10–14 days.

Nursing Assessment and Interventions

The nurse must be knowledgeable about the signs and symptoms of neutropenia and be able to perform a comprehensive history and assessment (see the earlier discussion in "Clinical Presentation"). The nurse should assess for signs of infection (fever; oral lesions; erythema at central venous access site; open skin lesion; perirectal irritation or laceration; cough; rhinorrhea; tachypnea; complaints of ear or throat pain, or both; and diarrhea).

Nursing interventions for a child with neutropenia depend upon the severity of the condition. These interventions can include the following:

- Observe laboratory data for evidence of a decrease in the ANC and notify the physician or responsible healthcare provider.
- Monitor for complications related to neutropenia (watching for signs and symptoms of septic shock).
- Protect the child from exposure to infection by advising the child and family to take the following measures:
  - Wash hands well.
  - Decrease the child's exposure to crowds when the ANC is less than 500.
  - Keep the child away from individuals known to have infections.
  - Use no rectal thermometers or suppositories.
  - Avoid exposure to molds (e.g., digging in soil).
  - Practice good mouth care.
- Teach families about neutropenia.
  - Instruct family members on how to protect the child from infection (as listed above).
  - Teach family members to monitor for signs and symptoms of infection.
  - Instruct parents to notify their physician or a responsible healthcare provider immediately if the child develops a fever higher than 101°F (38.3°C) or any signs of infection.

Expected Patient Outcomes

- There is an early identification of complications related to neutropenia.
- Parents and the child are knowledgeable about neutropenia, the signs and symptoms of infection, and ways to avoid exposure to infection.
- The child has minimal complications related to the neutropenia.

Thrombocytopenia

Shawn Elliott

Definition

Thrombocytopenia is a quantitative decrease in the number of circulating platelets in the peripheral blood and is defined as a platelet count of less than 100,000/mm^3.

Pathophysiology

There are many causes of thrombocytopenia in a child with a malignancy. Bone marrow replacement of malignant cells or bone marrow suppression induced by intense chemotherapy or radiation therapy can cause thrombocytopenia. Chemotherapy causes destruction of rapidly dividing normal hematopoetic cells and malignant cells. This results in a decrease in the number of platelet precursors. This usually occurs within 7 days or as late as 21 days after administration of chemotherapy agents. Radiation therapy causes the destruction of rapidly dividing normal hematopoetic cells in radiation treatment fields such as the pelvis, sternum, and proximal ends of long bones.

In addition to chemotherapy agents as a cause of a decrease in platelets, other pharmacological agents may be associated with platelet dysfunction. Aspirin inhibits platelet aggregation. Penicillin G, ampicillin, carbenicillin, and ticarcillin can also cause transient dysfunction. Amphotericin B has also been implicated as a cause of platelet dysfunction.

Clinical Presentation

Approximately 75% of all children with leukemia are symptomatic with thrombocytopenia at the initial diagnosis. These symptoms include the following:

- Skin: bruising, petechiae, purpura
- Nose and mouth: bleeding from the gums, nose, or both
- Genitourinary and gastrointestinal (GI): blood (whether microscopic or obvious) in urine, stool, or emesis
- Eyes: scleral bleeding

- Neurological: intracranial bleeding (This may be seen especially if the WBC is > 300,000/mm^3. This is a result of ruptured intracerebral vessels damaged by leukocyte sludging or by nodules or leukemic cells). The patient's physical examination should assess for the signs and symptoms listed above.

Diagnostic Work-up

An evaluation of thrombocytopenia is initiated by obtaining a complete blood count with platelets. In addition to the platelet count, a complete history and physical are done to assess for symptoms of thrombocytopenia (e.g., bruising, bleeding, petechiae, ecchymoses). The severity of the thrombocytopenia dictates the type of treatment or even if treatment is warranted.

Treatment

When the platelet count drops below 20,000/mm^3, minor bleeding episodes generally occur; spontaneous internal hemorrhage does not occur until the platelet count is 10,000/mm^3 or less. Treatment is indicated if there is active bleeding. The standard treatment for thrombocytopenia is a random-donor, leukocyte-reduced platelet transfusion of 1 unit of platelets per 10 kg of body weight. Matched ABO and Rh platelet transfusions are usually preferred. Although A and B antigens are only slightly expressed on platelets, the transfusion of incompatible platelets could result in low-grade hemolysis due to plasma antibodies or erythrocyte contamination.

Policy regarding the use of prophylactic platelet transfusion, including the specific platelet values used as criteria for transfusion before procedures, varies. The American Society of Clinical Oncology (ASCO) adopted guidelines based on a study by Schiffer et al. (2001), which recommended that the threshold for platelet transfusions in children be set at a platelet count of 10,000/mm^3. Higher thresholds may be considered for certain comorbidity factors and invasive procedures. Howard et al. (2000) demonstrated that there was no evidence of serious complications from lumbar punctures when the platelet count was between 11,000/mm^3 and 20,000/mm^3. Platelet transfusion should be avoided to decrease the likelihood of alloimmunization. The use of recombinant thrombopoietin has been successful in initial clinical trials and may reduce the use of platelet transfusions in the future.

Nursing Assessment and Interventions

The nurse must be knowledgeable about the signs and symptoms of thrombocytopenia and be able to perform a comprehensive history and assessment (see "Clinical Presentation," which is presented earlier in this subsection). Nursing interventions for a child with thrombocytopenia can include the following:

- Review laboratory information for the platelet count and alert the healthcare team.
- Monitor for complications related to thrombocytopenia.
  - Assess skin, stools, urine, gums, emesis, sputum, and nasal secretions for blood.
- Monitor for transfusion reactions.
- Prevent and decrease the risk of bleeding by
  - applying pressure directly to all needle puncture sites for 5 minutes
  - reducing the risk of constipation by administering a prescribed stool softener
  - encouraging the use of a soft-bristle toothbrush and avoiding dental floss and sharp food items, such as chips and ice, to decrease gum irritation
  - encouraging the patient to avoid contact sports or activities that might cause injury
  - advising sexually active adolescent patients to take precautions to avoid trauma during sexual relations
  - providing safe environments (e.g., using helmets, knee pads, and padded cribs)
  - administering hormonal therapy to inhibit menses if necessary
  - keeping invasive procedures to a minimum
  - instructing the patient and the family about how to treat epistaxis (The child's nostril should be pinched against the nasal septum by applying constant pressure for at least 10 minutes. The child should not lie down while the nose is bleeding because excess blood can drip into the nasopharynx and cause nausea and vomiting.)
  - ensuring that no rectal temperatures are taken or other manipulations (enemas and suppositories) are done
  - advising that adolescents use electric razors.
- Teach families about thrombocytopenia. Families should be instructed on how to decrease the risk of complications of thrombocytopenia and should be taught to report the signs and symptoms to the healthcare team.

Expected Patient Outcomes

- The patient is protected from bleeding.
- The patient and the family verbalize an understanding of how to reduce the risk and complications of thrombocytopenia.
- The patient and the family identify the signs and symptoms of thrombocytopenia to report to medical staff.

References

Howard, S.C., Gajjar, A., Ribeiro, R.C., Rivera, G.K., Rubnitz, J.E., Sunderland, J.T., et al. (2000). Safety of lumbar puncture for children with acute lymphocytic leukemia and thrombocytopenia. *JAMA: The Journal of the American Medical Association, 284,* 2222–2224.

Schiffer, C.A., Anderson, K.C., Bennett, C.L., Bernstein, S., Elting, L.S., Goldsmith, M., et al. (2001). Platelet transfusion for patients with cancer: Clinical practice guidelines of the American Society of Clinical Oncology. *Journal of Clinical Oncology, 19,* 1519–1538.

BIBLIOGRAPHY

Origin of Blood Cells

Abshire, T.C. (2001). Sense and sensibility: Approaching anemia in children. *Contemporary Pediatrics, 18*(9), 104–113.

Norville, R., & Bryant, R. (2002). Blood component deficiencies. In C.R. Baggott, K.P. Kelly, D. Fochtman, & G.V. Foley (Eds.), *Nursing care of children and adolescents with cancer* (pp. 347–364). Philadelphia: W. B. Saunders.

Sieff, C.A., Nathan, D.G., & Clark, S.C. (1998). The anatomy and physiology of hematopoiesis. In D.G. Nathan & S.H. Orkin (Eds.), *Nathan and Oski's hematology of infancy and childhood* (pp. 161–236). Philadelphia: W.B. Saunders.

Anemia

Norville, R., & Bryant, R. (2002). Blood component deficiencies. In C.R. Baggott, K.P. Kelly, D. Fochtman, & G.V. Foley (Eds.), *Nursing care of children and adolescents with cancer* (pp. 347–364). Philadelphia: W. B. Saunders.

Panzarella, C., Baggott, C.R., Comeau, M., Duncan, J.M., Groben, V., Woods, D.A., et al. (2002). Management of disease and treatment-related complications. In C.R. Baggott, K.P. Kelly, D. Fochtman, & G.V. Foley (Eds.), *Nursing care of children and adolescents with cancer* (pp. 279–318). Philadelphia: W.B. Saunders.

Neutropenia

Alexander, S.W., Walsh, T.J., Freifeld, A.F., & Pizzo, P.A. (2002). Infectious complications in the pediatric cancer patient. In P.A. Pizzo, & D.G. Poplack (Eds.), *Principles and practice of pediatric oncology* (pp. 1239–1283). Philadelphia: Lippincott Williams & Wilkins.

Kline, N.E. (2002). Prevention and treatment of infections. In C.R. Baggott, K.P. Kelly, D. Fochtman, & G.V. Foley (Eds.), *Nursing care of children and adolescents with cancer* (pp. 266–278). Philadelphia: W. B. Saunders.

Norville, R., & Bryant, R. (2002). Blood component deficiencies. In C.R. Baggott, K.P. Kelly, D. Fochtman, & G.V. Foley (Eds.), *Nursing care of children and adolescents with cancer* (pp. 347–364). Philadelphia: W. B. Saunders.

Taketomo, C.K., Jodding, J.H., & Kraus, D.M. (2002). *Pediatric dosage handbook* (9th ed.). Hudson, OH: Lexi-Comp, Inc.

Thrombocytopenia

Demetri, G.D. (2001). Targeted approaches for the treatment of thrombocytopenia. *The Oncologist, 6*, 15–23.

Norville, R., & Bryant, R. (2002). Blood component deficiencies. In C.R. Baggott, K.P. Kelly, D. Fochtman, & G.V. Foley (Eds.), *Nursing care of children and adolescents with cancer* (pp. 347–364). Philadelphia: W. B. Saunders.

Panzarella, C., Baggott, C.R., Comeau, M., Duncan, J.M., Groben, V., Woods, D.A., et al. (2002). Management of disease and treatment-related complications. In C.R. Baggott, K.P. Kelly, D. Fochtman, & G.V. Foley (Eds.), Nursing care of children and adolescents with cancer (pp. 279–318). Philadelphia: W.B. Saunders.

SECTION IV

CHILDHOOD CANCER TREATMENT

Robbie Norville

SECTION OUTLINE

Diagnostic and Staging Procedures

Patti Rubino and Jennifer Harley

Principles of Treatment

Diagnostic and staging procedures provide the tools for an accurate diagnosis of childhood cancer. Prompt and accurate diagnosis of a malignancy is essential to begin appropriate treatment, achieve remission, and optimize long-term survival.

Role in Childhood Cancer

Diagnostic procedures enable a healthcare team to determine the type and location of a malignancy as well as the extent of metastasis. Accurate diagnosis allows for planning and the initiation of treatment.

Diagnostic Procedures

History and physical assessment: A history and physical assessment are the most basic and inexpensive diagnostic tools, yet they are highly important. Parents often are the first to detect physical changes in their child. Symptoms such as fatigue, malaise, anorexia, recurrent infections or fevers, lymphadenopathy, bone or joint pain, enlarged abdomen, headache, and bleeding are suggestive of childhood cancers (**Table 4-1**). A detailed physical history that includes information on the child's growth and development, a family history, and a physical assessment will help to determine how to proceed with a diagnostic evaluation.

Laboratory tests: A child with a suspected cancer will have routine blood work and urinalysis done upon arrival at a clinic or admission to a hospital. A CBC with a differential and serum chemistries are commonly performed. If a patient is being evaluated for a particular malignancy, additional tests will be ordered.

CBC with a differential. A significantly elevated white blood cell count with the presence of lymphoblasts can be indicative of leukemia. Malignancies that have bone marrow involvement (e.g., neuroblastoma) may cause the hemoglobin, hematocrit, and platelets to be low.

Serum chemistries. This routine study will help evaluate the body's response to the cancer process. It reflects metabolic compensation and organ function and usually includes an assessment of electrolytes as well as liver and renal functions.

Urinalysis. A routine urinalysis will provide general information regarding renal function.

Tumor markers. A tumor marker is a characteristic or substance that can indicate the presence of a specific tumor. Testing for tumor markers can be useful at diagnosis and in follow-up treatment (**Table 4-2**).

Immunophenotyping and cytogenetics. Tumor cells can be identified, classified, and described using immunophenotyping of monoclonal antibodies. Cytogenetic studies can determine whether there are any chromosomal abnormalities within the tumor.

Nursing Assessment and Interventions

Assessment:

- Determine if the patient has had prior experience with phlebotomy procedures.
- Assess the patient's and the family's knowledge of the blood test to be performed.

Interventions:

- Prepare the patient and the family for the blood test by explaining it in developmentally appropriate terminology.
- Position the child for phlebotomy work.
- Use comforting strategies (e.g., performing a venipuncture on "the count of three" to help a child feel ready for the discomfort and serve as a distraction).
- Tell the family when the test results will be ready.

Expected Patient and Family Outcomes

- The family will display an understanding of the laboratory tests that are being performed.
- The patient will not feel traumatized.

Invasive Diagnostic Procedures

Bone marrow aspiration (BMA) and biopsy: A bone marrow aspiration is performed when leukemia is suspected, the tumor has possibly spread to the bone marrow, or a CBC suggests malfunctioning bone marrow. This procedure is done using an aseptic technique. A topical anesthetic is used to anesthetize the skin, and an injectable anesthetic is used to anesthetize the bone.

The sites most frequently chosen for aspiration are the posterior or anterior iliac crest; the sternum generally is not used because of its close proximity to the vital organs. A needle with a stylet is inserted though the bony cortex into the bone marrow cavity. The stylet is removed, a syringe is connected to the needle, and bone marrow is aspirated. The collected specimen is used to prepare slides for a microscopic examination to determine the cell type and morphology. If leukemia is suspected, the following tests will be performed: flow cytometry and immunophenotyping, karyotyping, and cytogenic analysis. Bone marrow that is packed with leukemic cells may be difficult to aspirate, causing increased discomfort to and anxiety in the patient and the family (more than one site may have to be used).

A bone marrow biopsy is performed if leukemia or metastasis to the bone marrow from a solid tumor is likely. It is done using an aseptic technique. A local anesthetic usually is used to anesthetize the skin and bone. The biopsy is similar to a BMA except that a large Jamshidi needle is used to remove an actual core of bone and bone marrow. The Jamshidi needle is turned and rocked as it is inserted into the bone. The needle is then removed with the core of bone marrow inside.

Lumbar puncture (LP): An LP is performed to determine if cancer (e.g., leukemia, lymphoma, or brain tumor) is present in the cerebral spinal fluid (CSF). A patient who has symptoms indicative of increased intracranial pressure at diagnosis also may have the CSF pressure measured. For

Table 4-1. Symptoms Suggestive of Childhood Cancers

Symptoms	Possible Malignancy	Possible Nonmalignant Condition
Pallor, fatigue, or malaise	Leukemia, lymphoma, neuroblastoma	Iron-deficiency anemia
Bleeding, bruising, petechiae	Leukemia, neuroblastoma	Coagulopathy, ideopathic thrombocytic purpura
Weight loss, night sweats	Hodgkin's lymphoma	Viral illness, tuberculosis
Edematous face and neck	Non-Hodgkin's lymphoma, leukemia	Thrombus in superior vena cava
Pancytopenia	Leukemia, neuroblastoma	Infection, aplastic anemia
Lymphadenopathy	Hodgkin's or non-Hodgkin's lymphoma	Infection
Bone pain and fevers	Leukemia, Ewing's sarcoma	Osteomyelitis, trauma
Limping	Bone tumors, leukemia, neuroblastoma	Osteomyelitis, trauma
Vaginal bleeding	Yolk sac tumor, rhabdomyosarcoma	Trauma, menses
Chronic drainage from the ear	Rhabdomyosarcoma, histiocytosis	Otitis media, otitis externa
Cat's eye reflex	Retinoblastoma	Coats's disease, severe uveitis
Abdominal mass	Wilms' tumor, neuroblastoma, hepatoblastoma	Viral illness
Headache, morning vomiting	Brain tumors	Migraine headaches

Table 4-2. Tumor-Associated Laboratory Studies

Laboratory Test	Normal Range	Associated Malignancies
Alkaline phosphate	20–150 U/l	Bone tumors; NOTE: nonspecific elevations can occur in normal settings.
α-fetoprotein (AFP)	< 20 ng/mL	Heptoblastoma, teratoma, germ cell tumors
β human chorionic gonadotropin (β-hCG)	5 mlu/ml	Hepatoblastoma Germ cell tumors
Carcinoembryonic antigen (CEA)	2.5 ng/ml	Gastrointestinal cancers
Catecholamines (urine):		Neuroblastoma (elevations may occur in one or all)
Epinephrine	0–5 g/24 hr	
Homovanillic acid (HVA)	0–10 mg/24 hr	
Metanephrine	0–300 g/24 hr	
Norepinephrine	0–20 g/24 hr	
Normetanephrine	50–800 g/24 hr	
Vanillymandelic acid (VMA)	2–10 mg/24 hr	
Copper	80–160 g/dl	Hodgkin's disease
Ferritin	7–150 g/l	Neuroblastoma
Lactate dehydrogenase (LDH)	60–170 U/l	Nonspecific Non-Hodgkin's lymphomas, acute lymphocytic leukemia (ALL), osteosarcoma, neuroblastoma, germ cell tumors, Ewing's sarcoma
Neuron-specific enolase (NSE)	15 ng/ml	Neuroblastoma

Data from Malarkey, L.M., & McMorrow, M. (1996). *Nurse's manual of laboratory tests and diagnostic procedures.* Philadelphia: W.B. Saunders; McFarland, M.B. (1995). Nursing implications of laboratory tests. Albany, NY: Delmar.

this aseptic procedure, the patient is placed in a position that exposes the vertebrae. The two most common positions are lying on the side with knees pulled up and back arched or sitting cross-legged with back arched. A topical anesthetic is administered; a local anesthetic also may be used, if necessary. A needle with a stylet is inserted between the lumbar vertebrae at the level of the iliac crest. The stylet is removed, and the CSF is collected in tubes to be tested for glucose, protein, cell differential, and cytology. Additional tests may be ordered, if necessary. This can be a quick procedure if the patient is kept calm and positioned properly. A moving child can lead to a traumatic LP, resulting in a bloody specimen or harm to the patient.

Nursing Assessment and Interventions

Assessment:

- Assess the patient's and the family's knowledge of LP and BMA or biopsy.
- Assess the patient's platelet count if the patient has to have an LP; consult the physician or nurse practitioner if the platelet count is less than 50,000; if the patient is symptomatic, consider a platelet transfusion.
- Assess the child's and family's level of fear and anxiety.

Interventions:

- Prepare the child and the family for the procedure by explaining it ahead of time in a developmentally appropriate manner (see preparation for procedures in Section VI, "Supportive Care").
- Assure the patient and the parents that the patient will be kept as comfortable as possible and that the patient may even fall asleep if sedation is used.
- Apply topical anesthetic to the BMA and/or LP sites at least 60–90 minutes prior to the procedure.
- Administer conscious sedation as ordered (see conscious sedation in Section VI, "Supportive Care").
- Position the patient properly.
  - Bone marrow aspiration and biopsy: Place the patient in a prone position, with the patient's face turned away from the practitioner (the sight of large needles is frightening even to a sleepy child).
  - Lumbar puncture: Place the patient so that his or her vertebrae are exposed, as described earlier in this section under "Invasive Diagnostic Procedures: Lumbar Puncture" to separate the vertebrae for easy entry into the subarachnoid space. Maintain the patient's shoulder alignment and do not allow the shoulders to fall forward, as doing so could close off the lumbar spaces. On rare occasions, it may work best for the patient to be in a sitting position, leaning on the assisting nurse, with the patient's back facing the practitioner. As the practitioner inserts the needle for the lumbar puncture, the assistant should provide counterpressure by pushing inward on the patient's abdomen.
- Follow the guidelines for distracting and preparing patients for procedures (see Section VI, "Supportive Care," for information on preparing patients prior to procedures).
- Use universal precautions when handling specimens.
- Apply pressure to the LP or BMA site after the procedure. A BMA site may need pressure applied for 5 minutes.
- Apply a sterile bandage to the LP site. A pressure dressing may be required for a BMA site).
- Remove the dressing during the first 24 hours after the procedure to examine the site for bleeding and signs of infection. A saturated dressing is a medium for bacterial growth and can lead to infection of the site.

Expected patient and family outcomes:

- The patient and the family will be prepared for a BMA, biopsy, or LP.
- The procedure will not cause the child to feel traumatized and distrustful.
- The BMA, biopsy, or LP site will remain free of infection.
- The patient will be able to cope with procedures that have to be done in the future.

Imaging Studies

Imaging tests are used to locate tumors and metastases and to stage malignancies. Advances in technology have decreased the need for more invasive procedures. Tests are done on the basis of a suspected malignancy and common sites of metastasis (**Table 4-3**).

Radiological studies: Various structures of the body have different densities. X rays allow for visualization of the skeleton and internal organs. The patient is required to remain still to have a clear picture. Sedation is not necessary as it is painless and quick. The most common X rays performed for diagnostic purposes are a chest X ray, which is used to look for tumor in the lungs, mediastinum, or chest wall, and a skeletal survey, which is an X ray of the entire skeleton that allows for visualization of metastases to bone. X rays of specific areas of the body can be done to determine if further imaging is needed.

Computerized tomography (CT) scan: CT, sometimes called *computerized axial tomography*, provides images of planes of the body. A CT scan takes serial X rays of each plane of the area studied, stores this information, and then completes a three-dimensional view. The scanner does this by rotating the X-ray beam completely around the patient. The patient is required to remain still throughout the test, which usually takes 30 minutes.

Either IV or oral contrast dye may be ordered. An IV contrast may be used to help illuminate malignancies. Oral contrast is used for abdominal CT scans to help visualize all aspects of the GI tract. The patient usually drinks contrast dye the night before the test and again 2 hours before the test. The dye usually is mixed in clear fluids, and the patient is given nothing to eat or drink until the test is completed. If the patient is not willing to drink the dye mixture, a nasogastric tube may be placed to administer the contrast dye.

Table 4-3 Diagnostic Imaging Studies for Various Malignancies

Disease	Primary Tumor	Metastatic Search
Leukemia	Bone marrow aspirate and biopsy*	Lumbar puncture* Chest X ray
Neuroblastoma	Computed tomography (CT) scan (abdomen, chest, pelvis)	Bone marrow and biopsy* Magnetic resonance imaging (MRI) for paraspinal lesion
Wilms' tumor	Abdominal CT scan Abdominal ultrasound Pelvic ultrasound	Chest X ray Chest CT scan Bone scan (unfavorable histology) Head CT/MRI scan (unfavorable histology) Skeletal survey (unfavorable histology)
Non-Hodgkin's lymphoma	CT scan of primary tumor area (abdomen, chest, pelvis)	Bone marrow aspirate and biopsy and lumbar puncture* Chest X ray Chest CT scan Bone scan Skeletal survey Gallium scan SPECT scan Head CT scan, if indicated
Hodgkin's disease	CT scan (chest, abdomen, neck, pelvis)	Chest X ray Chest CT scan Bone marrow aspirate and biopsy* Gallium scan SPECT scan
Rhabdomyosarcoma	CT scan or MRI of primary tumor	Chest X ray Chest CT scan Retroperitoneal CT scan (abdomen/pelvic tumor) Bone scan SPECT scan Head MRI or CT scan and lumbar puncture (for parameningeal tumors)
Bone tumors Osteosarcoma Ewing's sarcoma	Extremity or involved bone MRI Bone X-ray	Chest CT scan Chest X ray Bone scan Bone marrow aspirate or biopsy for Ewing's sarcoma* Thallium scans
Hepatoblastoma	Abdominal CT or MRI scan	Chest X ray Chest CT scan
Germ cell tumors	CT scan or MRI of primary site	Chest X ray Chest CT scan Abdominal CT scan Bone scan
Brain tumors	Brain CT scan or MRI with or without enhancement	MRI of spine Lumbar puncture* Bone marrow aspirate or biopsy* (medulloblastoma)

*Not an imaging study; included for completeness.

Data from Malarkey, L.M., & McMorrow, M. (1996). *Nurse's manual of laboratory tests and diagnostic procedures.* Philadelphia: W.B. Saunders; McFarland, M.B. (1995). *Nursing implications of laboratory tests.* Albany, NY: Delmar.

Magnetic resonance imaging (MRI): This scan uses radio waves and magnets to produce a highly defined, computerized image of the body. Radio waves are emitted toward the body and various tissue types absorb the energy. The magnets then pick up the signals produced from the body tissue, and a computer scan is done. All metal items must be detached from the body, including IV poles and pumps. If a patient is suspected of having a metastatic brain tumor or spinal masses, a gadolinium contrast dye may be administered. The patient must remain still for up to 1 hour while the scan is being performed; therefore, sedation may be required.

Bone scan. A bone scan detects the presence, size, and location of a malignancy or metastases in the bone. A radioisotope dye is injected intravenously 2-4 hours prior to the scan. Although the dye is radioactive, it emits about the same amount of radiation as an X ray. Any areas of disease will have an increased uptake of the dye. During the scan, the patient must remain still and may have to be secured to the table. Sedation may be necessary.

Positron emission tomography (PET) scan. A PET scan is an extremely effective, efficient technique in the diagnosis and evaluation of neuroblastoma, Hodgkin's disease, non-Hodgkin's lymphoma, bone tumors, lung and colon cancer, and brain tumors. Positron emission tomography uses isotopes of 18 fluorodeoxyglucose (FDG) to obtain images of physiologic and metabolic activity. Viable tumors can be distinguished from necrotic tissue neoplasm and scar tissue on a PET scan (Kushner, Yeung, & Larson, 2000). The patient must fast prior to the scan to allow for maximum tissue uptake of FDG, which is administered intravenously. The availability of PET scans once was limited because few facilities could afford to purchase and maintain the PET camera; however, Medicare, Medicaid, and a growing number of insurance companies now are reimbursing for the use of PET imaging.

Ultrasound: An ultrasound projects the body structures by using sound waves. An ultrasound transducer is placed on the patient's skin; a transducing gel is used on the skin. Sound waves are emitted to the body tissues, which produce echoes. The returned echoes are then processed and recorded on film, which provides an image on a monitor. This can be used to help visualize an abdominal mass. The patient may be required to ingest fluids orally before the test is conducted because a full bladder enables visualization of certain organs. The length of the procedure is approximately 30 minutes. The child must remain still for an ultrasound; however, sedation usually is not needed.

Echocardiogram: An echocardiogram, which is an ultrasound of the heart, displays the chambers of the heart, contractility, integrity of the septa, and valve function. It also measures cardiac blood flow and the ejection fraction. It can detect a tumor, vegetation, thrombus, or pericardial effusions. An echocardiogram may be done at the time of diagnosis if the patient has abnormal heart sounds. It is performed routinely on patients who are receiving anthracyclines to evaluate for cardiotoxicity. The patient is kept calm and still for this procedure, which lasts 15–30 minutes.

Nursing assessment and interventions

Assessment:

- Assess the patient's developmental level and ability to follow instructions (i.e., ability to remain still).
- Assess the need for sedation and for IV access.
- Assess the patient's and the family's understanding of the test to be done.

Interventions:

- Explain the radiological study to be performed, including what it will be like, the length of time required for the test, and the results, and explain that the test does not hurt but that the patient will have to remain still.
- Remain supportive of the patient and the family because awaiting the diagnosis of a malignancy is a stressful and life-changing time.
- Do not give the patient anything to eat or drink before sedation, while following institutional guidelines.
- If the patient is scheduled to have an abdominal CT, administer an oral contrast dye as ordered (usually mixed with a clear fluid of the patient's choice). Do not give the patient anything to eat or drink, and explain the reason for this to the patient and the family.
- If the patient is to be given an IV contrast dye, explain to the patient and the family why this is required, what it feels like (the patient may experience a sensation of warmth or flushing), and establish IV access.
- Use a heparin (Liquaemin) flush to prepare the venous access device if the patient is to have an MRI; remove the IV tubing, pump, and pole; remove any metal objects from the patient's body.
- Assist the patient with positioning during the test, as needed.

Expected patient and family outcomes

- The patient and the family will feel adequately prepared for the diagnostic studies.
- The patient will not feel traumatized by the studies.
- Optimal studies will be obtained.

Reference

Kushner, B.H., Yeung, H.W., & Larson, S.M. (2000). Extending positron emission tomography scan utility to high risk neuroblastoma: Fluorid-18 fluorodexyglucose positron emission tomography as sole imaging modality in follow-up of patients. *Journal of Clinical Oncology, 19,* 3397–3405.

History of Chemotherapy

Elizabeth Randall

Chemotherapy was originally defined as the treatment of a disease with medications or chemical compounds. The earliest known use of chemotherapy to treat malignancies occurred in the Middle Ages, when heavy metal agents were used. The term *chemotherapy* was first used by Paul Ehrlich in the early 1900s. Ehrlich observed that certain substances were selectively concentrated in microorganisms and speculated that if these substances were toxic to the cells, they could be used therapeutically. There was limited success in developing chemotherapy until the discovery of penicillin. That discovery led to a wide array of bacteria-specific chemotherapy. In recent years, chemotherapy has become associated almost exclusively with the use of antineoplastic agents to treat malignancies.

In the 1890s, Dr. William Coley, a surgeon at Simms Hospital (now known as Memorial Sloan-Kettering Cancer Center), invented Coley's toxins to treat sarcomas. Coley's toxins, an early form of immunotherapy, were a combination of two bacterial agents: *Streptococcus pyogenes* and *Serratia marcescens*.

Early attempts at treating cancer with drugs involved the use of arsenic, benzyl, and urethane, which were able to decrease the number of circulating leukemic cells. These drugs made researchers hopeful that drugs could be used in cancer treatment. With rare exceptions, the continued development of effective chemotherapy thus far has been through luck and trial and error. The metabolism of a cancer cell is so similar to that of a normal cell that minuscule differences must be targeted to develop effective therapy.

The 1940s

During the 1940s, there were several important discoveries in the field of cancer chemotherapy, including the discovery of antitumor antibiotics and the use of folic acid antagonists to treat leukemia. Mechlorethamine (nitrogen mustard) evolved from a chemical weapon (mustard gas, used in World Wars I and II) to an antineoplastic agent. After World War II, Drs. Louis Goodman, Alfred Gilman, and David Karnofsky of the Army's Division of Biological Warfare administered mechlorethamine to patients with advanced lymphoma, and the treatment resulted in significant benefits (Sidell, Takafuji & Franz, 1997). In the late 1940s, Dr. Sydney Farber observed that high concentrations of folic acid inhibited the growth of sarcomas in mice. He also noted that children with leukemia often were deficient in folic acid; paradoxically, he found that supplementation of folic acid resulted in an acceleration of disease. Dr. Farber began to study folic acid antagonists and treated a child with leukemia with one of these agents (aminopterin) in 1947. The child achieved a complete remission, the first remission ever induced in childhood leukemia (Wells, Elion, & Laszlo, 1997).

The 1950s

Significant progress was made in the development of new chemotherapeutic drugs in the 1950s, many of which are important components of cancer treatment today. These drugs include fluorouracil (5-FU), 6-thioguanine (6-TG), mercaptopurine (Purinethol), dactinomycin (Actinomycin-D), methotrexate (Mexate), cyclophosphamide (Cytoxan), melphalan (Alkeran), and busulfan (Myleran). In 1954, the Cancer and Leukemia Group B and the Children's Cancer Group were formed. In 1955, the first randomized clinical trial began, and Congress provided funding for the National Chemotherapy Program. (Wells, Elion, & Laszlo, 1997).

The 1960s and 1970s

Almost all chemotherapeutic agents drugs in use today were discovered by the end of the 1960s. In addition, more cooperative groups of researchers were formed. It was discovered that methotrexate (Mexate) could be injected intrathecally into the cerebrospinal fluid to control the spread of leukemia to the meninges.

In the early 1960s, the concept of multiple agent multimodal therapy in the treatment of acute lymphocytic leukemia was introduced. Vincristine (Oncovin) and prednisone (Deltasone) was used for induction therapy, central nervous system (CNS) prophylaxis, and maintenance therapy, along with mercaptopurine (Purinethol), cyclophosphamide (Cytoxan), and vincristine (Oncovin) or methotrexate (Mexate) (Kardinal, 1993).

A significant advance in combination chemotherapy came with the initiation of the vincristine (Oncovin)-doxorubicin (Adriamycin)-methotrexate (Mexate)-prednisone (Deltasone) program for acute leukemia initiated by Dr. Emil Freireich. For the first time, a combination of four drugs, each with different mechanisms of action, were given as intensive intermittent therapy. The design allowed dosing that produced maximum effectiveness and time for recovery of normal cells after each course. The success of this regimen set a precedent for the intermittent, intensive combination chemotherapy regimens used today (Kardinal, 1993).

Drug development slowed in the 1970s, yet important discoveries about cancer biology were made. Until then, cancer researchers believed that a tumor first developed locally, spread to regional lymph nodes, and then metastasized widely. Wide surgical resection was thought to ensure a better chance of cure; however, analysis showed that in many cases, less radical surgery provided the same, if not improved, outcome. Adjuvant chemotherapy was introduced, and it was found that systemic therapy could improve survival. In other cases, surgery and radiation therapy were used to complement chemotherapy. The National Cancer Institute set up a screening program designed to screen all types of compounds for antitumor activity. The 1960s and 1970s also saw the first use of platinum agents and of MOPP therapy (mechlorethamine, Oncovin, prednisone, and procarbazine) as a successful treatment for Hodgkin's disease. Phase I trials for Adriamycin began in the 1970s.

The 1980s

The 1980s introduced a new series of chemotherapeutic agents: the topoisomerase inhibitors and paclitaxel (Taxol). The 1980s also saw the emergence of therapies to address side effects that had greatly affected the cancer patient's quality of life: cardiotoxicity, hemorrhagic cystitis, nausea, and low blood counts.

The 1990s

In the 1990s, the use of clinical trials became widespread. Scientists continued to develop and study new drugs and drug families, such as the taxane family of drugs, and vinorelbine. Gene- and biologically based therapies were studied. Bone marrow or cord blood transplantation, stem cell rescue, and growth factors allowed the delivery of higher doses of chemotherapy. In pediatric oncology, prognostic indicators were used to tailor therapies to a patient's specific needs. The goal was to promote continued improvement in survival rates while delivering the least amount of therapy possible. This strategy allowed better control of long-term complications.

The 2000s

The monoclonal antibody Mylotarg received approval from the U.S. Food and Drug Administration (FDA). Other biological agents (e.g., antiangiogenic factors, other monoclonal antibodies, and cytokines) have become a major focus of research. The Children's Cancer Study Group and the Pediatric Oncology Group merged to form the Children's Oncology Group (COG).

References

Kardinal, C. G. (1993). Cancer chemotherapy in historical perspective. *Journal of the Louisiana State Medical Society, 145,* 175–177.

Sidell, F. R., Takafuji, E. T. & Franz, D. R. (1997). *Textbook of military medicine: Medical aspects of chemical and biological warfare (Part 1).* Office of the Surgeon General; Washington, DC: TMM Publications; Borden Institute Walter Reed.

Wells, W., Elion, G. & Laszlo, J. (1997). *Beyond discovery: The path from Research to human benefit; Curing childhood leukemia.* Washington, DC: National Academy of Sciences.

Clinical Trials

Jami S. Gattuso

Principles of Treatment

A clinical trial is a scientific experiment designed to answer a specific medical question, usually about the therapeutic effect of a specific treatment. A well-designed clinical trial should answer the medical question with certainty and provide information that is reliable and easy to analyze and interpret. The procedure for conducting a clinical trial, as well as all pertinent background information, is compiled into a protocol. The protocol ensures that the trial is carried out in a systematic manner and that all of the participating investigators provide consistent treatment.

Phases of Clinical Trials

Clinical trials are divided into four phases of research. Each phase has a unique purpose as well as some general characteristics that are common to protocols in that phase.

Phase I: Phase I determines the maximally tolerated dose (MTD) of an investigational agent or combination of agents using a strict administration schedule that is then recommended for use in efficacy studies. The starting dose in children is usually 80% of the MTD in adults. The toxicities related to the therapy and the pharmacokinetic profile of the agent also are described from Phase I data that are collected. Phase I studies usually involve a small trial that includes 15–25 patients with refractory cancer for which no other effective therapies are known. Patients must have adequate organ function as well as a reasonable life expectancy and ability to function. In addition, all standard therapeutic options for curative treatment must have been exhausted. Patients and families choose Phase I trials hoping for a possible cure, disease response, or control of symptoms, or to help future patients by contributing to scientific knowledge.

Phase II: Phase II is designed to determine the efficacy of a new agent in treating specific types of cancer. Studies are disease-specific and based on biochemical data, pharmacological data, or both, preclinical screening in human tumor cell lines, or a suggestion of the agent's antitumor activity in Phase I trials.

All patients must have measurable disease and normal major organ function as well as a reasonable life expectancy and functional status. Patients who have not received intensive treatment already are the best candidates for Phase II trials. The number of patients varies and is based on the number of patients required to allow meaningful statistical conclusions to be drawn about the treatment; the sample size should minimize the chance that a potentially ineffective drug will be accepted or that a potentially effective drug will be rejected. When clinical trials are used to evaluate a treatment regimen rather than a specific agent, Phase I and Phase II trials can be combined; they then are referred to as a pilot study.

Phase III: Phase III is used to assess the role of a new treatment in terms of overall response, survival, and quality of life of newly diagnosed patients with a specific diagnosis. The goal of the trial is to determine whether the treatment is equivalent with or superiority to the current or standard treatment. Randomization between the experimental group and the control group to avoid systematic bias as well as stratification by specific prognostic factors is a key element. Phase III trials require large numbers of patients, and therefore protocols usually must be implemented at a number of institutions or through cooperative groups.

Phase IV: Phase IV is meant to further investigate the long-term safety and efficacy of a treatment and takes place after the new treatment is approved for standard use. These trials are less common in pediatric oncology than trials in other phases, but their goal is to decrease side effects, toxicities, and late effects of treatment while continuing to provide acceptable cure rates.

Regulatory Requirements

To conduct clinical research, investigators must comply with federal guidelines compiled by the FDA. The guidelines are as follows:

- All research with human subjects must be approved by an institutional review board, which serves to protect the rights of research subjects. Institutional review board approval must be obtained before the protocol may be implemented, the approval must be renewed at least annually, all changes (amendments) to the protocol must also be approved, and all unexpected serious toxicities (called adverse drug reactions or serious adverse events) and the deaths of all subjects in the study must be reported.

- All patients or their parents or legal guardians must sign an informed consent document that has been approved by an institutional review board before beginning treatment. Although it is not legally necessary to obtain consent from the children themselves, children who are of an appropriate age should be informed about their participation in the trial and their assent must be obtained. In a clinical trial, the informed consent document must describe in lay terms the research, the purpose of the research, and the risks, benefits, duration of, and alternatives to the research. The document should also describe any compensation, explain how confidentiality will be ensured, and note the responsibilities of the researcher in the case of adverse effects and the financial implications and voluntary nature of the treatment. In a randomized study, the patient, the parent, or both must give informed consent before the randomized assignment is given, thereby agreeing to any of the treatment methodologies in the protocol.
- The subjects' medical records should contain complete documentation of their eligibility, the treatment and any modifications, outcome, toxicities, and the results of the studies required by the protocol. These records must be kept for at least 7 years after the new drug application has been filed with the FDA.
- All investigational drugs require strict record-keeping. Drug accountability logs, which detail the disposition of every dose of drug, must be maintained. These logs are subject to audits and must match the available supply of the drug in the study.

Nursing Assessment and Interventions

Nurses play a vital role in treating patients in clinical trials.

Assessment:

- Ensure that a patient is eligible for a protocol before beginning investigational therapy, all required studies are completed, consents are signed, and compliance with the protocol is maintained.
- Ensure that investigational drugs or therapies are given safely; pay special attention to checking doses, as they may vary throughout the study or be considerably different from a standard dosing regimen; ensure that all lab work and follow-up evaluations are done as stated; assess the patient carefully for adverse side effects; and thoroughly document any side effects in the medical record.

Interventions:

- Serve as an advocate for the patient and family (this is the role of the nurse who has rapport with the patient and the family and is able to assess their concerns about an investigational therapy), help the patient and the family ask questions of the treating physician, and ensure that issues are addressed and the patient and family are comfortable and are proceeding with the investigational therapy. (Patients and families who do not wish to participate in clinical trials may require support and assurance that their care will not be compromised if they choose not to participate.)
- Provide support for the family. Be respectful of choices that families make and support their decisions regardless of the outcome for the child. The families, not the health-care providers, are the ones who must live with the consequences of the decisions they make.
- Provide education for the patient. This is an important responsibility of the nurses who are involved in clinical research. The investigator should give the patient and the family initial information concerning the treatment plan as well as the risks, benefits, and alternatives to the investigational therapy. After this initial discussion, the nurse can reinforce education regarding all aspects of the treatment plan, for example, how drugs will be delivered, how many injections will be required, and methods for controlling side effects. The nurse also should be prepared to discuss clinical research in general and direct patients and families to clinical trial Web sites and registries, thus allowing a patient or a parent to make an informed decision about participation.

Expected Patient and Family Outcomes

The patient or the family or both are able to make an informed decision regarding treatment for cancer.

Chemotherapy

Christine Sullivan

Principles of Treatment

The purpose of using chemotherapy to treat cancer is to prevent the cancer cell from dividing, metastasizing, and ultimately resulting in the death of the patient. Chemotherapeutic agents are designed to treat cancer by preventing the proliferation of cancer cells; however, their cytotoxic effects indiscriminately interfere with the proliferation of normal cells as well. To fully understand how chemotherapy works, it is important to look at how a normal cell reproduces and to compare this to cancer cell growth.

Normal cellular division, the cell cycle: The cell cycle consists of four periods, or phases, of cellular growth and a resting phase (G_0). For cellular proliferation to occur, there must be duplication of the cellular genetic material, DNA, followed by mitosis (M phase), or the phase of the cell cycle that results in the division of the cell into two identical daughter cells. These are the phases of the cell cycle (**Figure 4-1**):

Figure 4-1. Cell Cycle and Cell Division

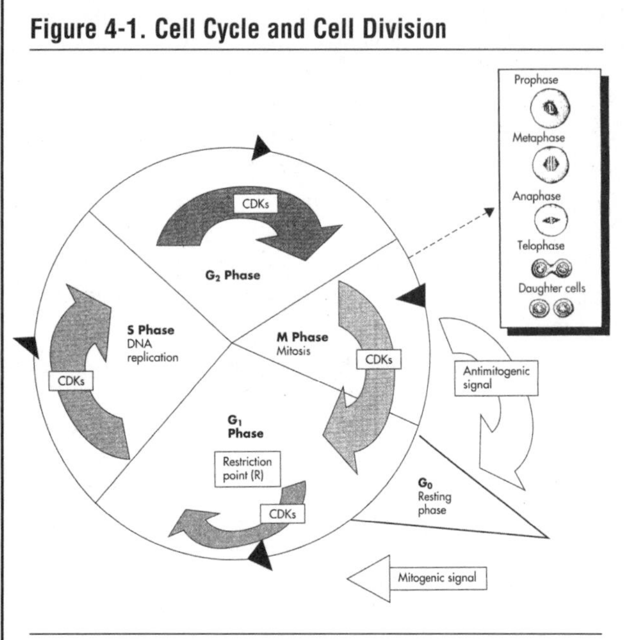

Note: From *Nursing Care of Children and Adolescents with Cancer (3rd ed.)* (p. 134), C.R. Baggott, K.P. Kelly, D. Fochtman, and G.V. Foley, (Eds.), (2002). Philadelphia: W.B. Saunders. Reprinted with permission.

- G_1, the first gap, is the first phase that a cell enters when it leaves the resting phase. This is the phase during which RNA synthesis and protein synthesis occur. G_1 has a widely varied time span, during which cells spend the largest proportion of their dividing lives.
- S is the synthesis phase in which the DNA is replicated.
- G_2, the second gap, is the premitotic phase in which RNA synthesis is completed.
- M is the phase in which mitosis occurs.

Normal cells proceed through the cell cycle in a consistent manner in response to feedback mechanisms and are protected by tumor suppressor genes. They have a defined number of cell divisions and are programmed for cell death, or apoptosis, as they age or are damaged.

Malignant cellular division: A primary characteristic of a cancer cell is that it has lost the usual mechanisms to control growth that a normal cell exhibits. A cancer cell experiences unchecked growth due to the following deviations from normal cellular behavior:

- Cancer cells do not seem to have a preset number of divisions before death, avoiding apoptosis.
- Cancer cells do not appear to be inhibited by contact, but rather, they continue to divide into an unorganized mass.
- Cancer cells do not require the usual amount of growth factors, and some cancer cells even produce their own growth factor.

Role in Childhood Cancer

Since the introduction of chemotherapy, survival statistics for childhood cancers have improved dramatically. Prior to the advent of chemotherapy, treatment consisted of surgery and radiation that primarily addressed local disease. Chemotherapy offers a means of controlling systemic disease and provides a more comprehensive approach to cancer treatment. Chemotherapeutic agents are now included in disease-specific treatment protocols based upon their synergy and improved treatment responses when used in combination.

Chemotherapy is used in several different ways to achieve total destruction of the cells of a given malignancy:

- Multimodal therapy involves the use of chemotherapy in combination with another type of therapy, such as radiation, surgery, or both.
- Adjuvant chemotherapy is the use of chemotherapy as well as surgery and/or radiation to address residual disease or suspected metastases.
- Combination chemotherapy is the use of a multidrug regimen that employs several agents found to be effective against a specific tumor.
- Neoadjuvant chemotherapy is the use of chemotherapy preoperatively to debulk a tumor prior to its surgical excision.
- Sanctuary therapy, or regional chemotherapy, is delivered directly to an area where malignant cells may not be fully eradicated by systemic chemotherapy alone (e.g., intrathecal chemotherapy for central nervous system [CNS] prophylaxis in the treatment of leukemia). Sanctuary and regional chemotherapy also may refer to high-dose chemotherapy administered intra-arterially to decrease systemic effects.

Classification of Chemotherapy Agents

Chemotherapeutics typically are divided into several different classes, each of which has several types of agents. A class of drugs can be defined according to the mechanism of action, the molecular structure, or the physiological action of the agent. An agent's mechanism of action determines whether it is classified as being cell-cycle specific or nonspecific. Cell-cycle-specific agents are most effective during active phases of the cell cycle, whereas cell-cycle-nonspecific agents are effective during all phases of the cell cycle (**Table 4-4**). Agents are selected for combination use to achieve maximum cell kill. Chemotherapeutic agents can be classified as follows (specific agents are described in more detail in **Table 4-5**):

Alkylating agents: These drugs contribute their alkyl group to sites on DNA or other macromolecules, causing DNA disruptions that interfere with replication and transcription.

Antibiotics: Antitumor antibiotics are natural agents synthesized by a variety of bacteria and fungi. They interfere with cellular metabolism by numerous mechanisms. In general, they form stable complexes with DNA, interfering with the synthesis of DNA and RNA.

Antimetabolites: These drugs appear to be similar to naturally occurring metabolites that are used by cells to make nucleic acids; they act by inhibiting essential enzymes or by causing the nucleic acids to produce nonfunctional end products.

Plant alkaloids: These drugs are derived from natural sources or manufactured from compounds extracted from plants. The natural products include mitotic inhibitors such as vincristine (Oncovin) and vinblastine (Velban). They work by inhibiting mitosis.

Epipodophyllotoxins and camptothecins: Theses agents inhibit topoisomerase II and I, respectively, causing DNA breaks.

Hormones (corticosteroids): These steroidal drugs enter the cell and bind with macromolecules in the cytoplasm. Ultimately, they enter the cell nucleus, bind with DNA, and interfere with transcription.

Miscellaneous: Included in this category are drugs whose mechanisms of action are not understood or do not fit into any other category. Examples include enzymes such as L-asparaginase (Elspar).

Delivering the most effective chemotherapy with the least amount of damage to normal cells, and ultimately to the patient, remains the primary challenge of chemotherapy treatment for cancer. **Table 4-6** (page 95) provides a list of methods used to overcome chemotherapy resistance and normal cell damage.

Table 4-4. Classification of Chemotherapy Agents

Cell-Cycle Specific Agents			
Plant Alkaloids		*Antimetabolites*	
Etoposide		Cytarabine	
Paclitaxel		5-Fluorouracil	
Teniposide		Mercaptopurine	
Topotecan		Methotrexate	
Vinblastine		Thioquanine	
Vincristine			
Cell-Cycle Non-Specific Agents			
Alkylating Agents	*Antitumor Antibiotics*	*Hormones*	*Miscellaneous*
Busulfan	Bleomycin	Dexamethasone	Asparaginase
Carboplatin	Dactinomycin	Hydrocortisone	Hydroxyurea
Carmustine	Daunorubicin	Prednisone	Procarbazine
Cisplatin	Doxorubicin		
Cyclophosphamide	Idarubicin		
Ifosfamide	Mitoxantrone		
lomustine			
Mechlorethamine			
Melphalan			
Thiotepa			

Method of Delivery

Chemotherapeutic agents are delivered by oral, subcutaneous, intramuscular, intravenous, intrathecal and intraarterial routes. The administration route is selected based on the chemical properties of the agent and the desired effect.

Potential Side Effects

Most chemotherapeutic agents have a variety of side effects related to their mechanism of action. A goal of combination chemotherapy is to use agents that have either different types of toxicities or different timing of toxicities (see Section V, "Side Effects of Treatment").

These are among the general toxicities of chemotherapy:

- Gastrointestinal: nausea, vomiting, diarrhea, constipation, impaired liver function, pancreatitis, anorexia, and electrolyte imbalances
- Skin/mucosal: mucositis, stomatitis, rashes, discoloration, increased sensitivity to sunlight, alopecia
- Hematologic: anemia, neutropenia, and thrombocytopenia
- Immunosuppression
- Other: pulmonary, renal, neurological, or cardiac damage, possible sterility.

Nursing Assessment and Interventions

The responsibilities of a pediatric oncology nurse surrounding the safe administration of chemotherapy are daunting. Few other nursing responsibilities are associated with such a small margin for error. In light of this fact, institutions that provide chemotherapy to children should have a well-educated team, including pediatric oncologists, pharmacists, and registered nurses responsible for ordering, dispensing, and administering these agents.

Assessment: The nurse should have a thorough understanding of the drug being given and should be able to discuss with the patient and the family the drug's mechanism of action and its potential side effects. The following factors also should be included in a baseline assessment before giving a chemotherapeutic agent to a patient:

- Ensure that the patient and the parents understand the treatment protocol.
- Review the patient's history relative to receiving a particular drug (e.g., determine side effects the patient experienced in the past and the presence of relevant allergies).
- Determine the usual premedication the patient has been given to control nausea and vomiting and its effectiveness.
- Be aware of any drug-specific concerns. For example, is it necessary to check when the patient had his or her last bowel movement? Must the patient have any tests done before taking the drug? Is the drug likely to cause an allergic or anaphylactic reaction?.
- Know the "five rights" of the drug (right patient, right schedule, right dose, right drug, and right rate) as well as the right sequence of the drug in the protocol.
- Determine the patient's ability to take the drug as ordered. For instance, can or will this patient take medicine by mouth? Is the patient's platelet count high enough for an injection or lumbar puncture? Is the IV line adequate for chemotherapy, particularly a vesicant?

Table 4-5. Chemotherapeutic Agents

Drug	Classification	Route	Side Effects	Special Considerations
Asparaginase (Elspar) Erwinia asparaginase PEG-asparaginase (pegaspargase, Oncaspar)	Enzyme from *Escherichia coli* or *Erwinia carotovora* PEG-asparaginase is *E. coli* asparaginase conjugated with polyethylene glycol Inhibits protein synthesis by hydrolyzing serum asparagine to nonfunctional aspartic acid and ammonia Cell cycle nonspecifc	Intramuscular (IM), IV	Common: local allergic reaction, hyperammonemia, low fibrinogen Occasional: rash, hyperglycemia, abnormal liver function tests, coagulation abnormalities Rare: hypersensitivity with anaphylaxis, nausea, vomiting, anorexia, somnolence lethargy, pancreatitis, convulsions, thrombosis, edema, CNS ischemic attack, renal compromise	IV administration is associated with increased risk of anaphylaxis. Have emergency equipment and drugs available. Observe patient for at least 1/2 hr after dose. Coagulation abnormalities place child at risk for thrombus formation or bleeding.
Bleomycin sulfate (Blenoxane)	Antibiotic	IV, IM, subcutaneous (SQ)	Common: none Occasional: hyperpigmentation, pneumonitis, high fever 2–6 hr after administration Rare: anaphylaxis, fever, hypotension, nausea, vomiting, anorexia, skin rash, mucositis, pulmonary fibrosis, renal failure	High fevers may occur without anaphylaxis; give earlier in the day so does not occur at night. Rare, lethal anaphylactoid reactions with severe fever and hypotension—have emergency equipment available. If test dose require, administer 1–2 Units IM; wait 1 hr and give remaining dose. Lower dose may need to be given when pulmonary radiotherapy is used. Pulmonary function tests are done as baseline, throughout course of therapy, and for a period of time after therapy; patients can develop fibrosis with decreased diffusion capacity.
Busulfan (Myleran)	Alkylating agent	By mouth (PO)	Common: myelosuppression, mild nausea, vomiting, "bronzing" of the skin Occasional: seizures with high dose, oral mucositis, skin breakdown, decreased adrenal function Rare: skin rashes, veno-occlusive disease (VOD), amenorrhea, testicular atrophy, gynecomastia, myasthenia symptoms, cataract, atrophic bronchitis	Prophylactic anticonvulsant therapy may be useful in patients receiving high doses of the drug.

continued

Table 4-5. Chemotherapeutic Agents *continued*

Drug	Classification	Route	Side Effects	Special Considerations
Carboplatin (Paraplatin)	Heavy metal alkylating agent	IV infusion	Common: nausea, vomiting, myelosuppression Occasional: electrolyte disturbances, anaphylaxis Rare: metallic taste, peripheral neuropathy, hepato toxicity, renal toxicity, ototoxicity, secondary leukemia	IV infusion over 15 min or longer. Aluminum reacts with carboplatin, causing precipitate formation and loss of potency; therefore do not allow needles or IV sets containing aluminum parts to come in contact with the drug. Elimination dependent upon glomerular filtration rate (GFR) and may be prescribed based on GFR and area under the curve (AUC) desired. Premedicate, or consider desensitization if previous hypersensitivity reaction has occurred.
Carmustine (BCNU, BiCNU)	Nitrosourea Lipid-soluble alkylating agent that crosses blood-brain barrier Cell cycle nonspecific	IV	Common: burning with peripheral administration, nausea, vomiting, myelosuppression, alopecia, late pulmonary dysfunction Occasional: marked facial flushing, liver dysfunction, thrombophlebitis at injection site Rare: brownish discoloration of skin, renal dysfunction, pulmonary fibrosis, secondary malignancy	Avoid extravasation or local contact with skin or conjunctiva. Avoid rapid infusion, which is associated with burning and/or hypotension. Use glass containers and polyethylene-lined administration sets for stability.
Cisplatin (Platinol)	Heavy metal alkylating agent Inhibition of DNA synthesis	IV	Common: nausea, vomiting, anorexia, myelosuppression, hypomagnesemia, high-frequency hearing loss, nephrotoxicity Occasional: metallic taste, electrolyte disturbances, hearing loss in the normal hearing range Rare: peripheral neuropathy, tinnitus, seizure, liver, toxicity, secondary malignancy	Synergistic with radiation therapy. Aluminum reacts with cisplatin, causing precipitate formation and loss of potency; therefore do not allow needles or IV sets containing aluminum parts to come in contact with drug. Premedicate with antiemetics; continue throughout and beyond course of therapy, causes delayed nausea and vomiting. During course of therapy carefully monitor input and output (I&O). Maintain urinary output at least at 2 ml/kg/hr. Administer furosemide (Lasix) or mannitol as ordered to ensure adequate urinary output. Intensifies aminoglycoside toxicity and should be used with caution when administered concurrently. To decrease risk of hypomagnesemia, supplement with magnesium.

continued

Table 4-5. Chemotherapeutic Agents *continued*

Drug	Classification	Route	Side Effects	Special Considerations
Corticosteroids (prednisone, dexamethasone, hydrocortisone, methylprednisolone)	Lympholytic Decreases edema produced by tumor or caused by tumor necrosis	IV, PO Intrathecal (IT) Equivalent potency: • Cortisone 5 • Hydrocortisone 4 • Methylprednisolone 0.8 • Dexamethasone 0.15	Common: hyperphagia, immunosuppression, personality changes, Cushing's syndrome, pituitary-adrenal axis suppression, acne Occasional: poor wound healing, stomach upset, hyperglycemia, gastritis, muscle weakness, osteonecrosis Rare: pancreatitis, electrolyte imbalance, gastrointestinal (GI) bleeding, increased intraocular pressure, hypertension, aseptic necrosis of femoral head, growth retardation, striae, osteopenia, peptic ulcer, cataracts	Decrease salt intake; protect from infection; observe for hyperglycemia.To decrease or prevent GI upset, take with meals or snacks; may need to take with histamine H_2-receptor antagonist such as cimetidine, ranitidine.
Cyclophosphamide (Cytoxan)	Alkylating agent	IV, PO	Common: anorexia, nausea, vomiting, myelosuppression, alopecia, gonadal dysfunction/sterility Occasional: metallic taste, hemorrhagic cystitis, syndrome of inappropriate antidiuretic hormone (SIADH) Rare: transient blurred vision, cardiac toxicity with arrhythmias (in higher doses), myocardial necrosis, pulmonary fibrosis, secondary malignancy, bladder fibrosis	Maintain adequate hydration, urinary output. Check urine for blood frequently. Outpatient therapy should be given early in the day when possible so that toxic metabolites do not accumulate in bladder overnight. Encourage patient to urinate before going to bed at night to empty bladder completely. Administration of high doses of cyclophosphamide should be preceded and followed by IV fluids and mesna.
Cytarabine (ara-C, cytosine arabinoside, Cytosar-U)	Antimetabolite	IV, IM, SQ, IT	Common: nausea, vomiting, anorexia, conjunctivitis with higher doses, myelosuppression, stomatitis, alopecia Occasional: flulike symptoms with fever, diarrhea Rare: encephalopathy, cerebellar dysfunction, or pulmonary capillary leak with higher doses; rash, hepatotoxicity, VOD, pneumonitis, gonadal dys function With intrathecal administration: Nausea, vomiting, headache, pleocytosis, fever, learning disability, rash, somnolence, meningismus, convulsions, paresis, myelosuppression, ataxia	Administer steroid eyedrops to prevent conjunctivitis with high dose.

continued

Table 4-5. Chemotherapeutic Agents *continued*

Drug	Classification	Route	Side Effects	Special Considerations
Dactinomycin (actinomycin D, Cosmegen)	Antineoplastic antibiotic	IV	Common: nausea, vomiting, local ulceration if extravasated, myelosuppression, alopecia, skin photosensitivity or hyperpigmentation Occasional: diarrhea, mucositis, immune thrombocytopenia, radiation recall Rare: hepatotoxicity	Vesicant—severe tissue damage if extravasation occurs. Protest from light. Avoid preservatives. Do not filter. Radiation recall may occur in an area of previous radiotherapy.
Daunorubicin (daunomycin, Cerbidine) and Doxorubicin (Adriamycin)	Anthracycline antibiotic	IV	Common: subclinical cardiac arrhythmias, nausea, local ulceration if extravasated, pink or red color to urine, myelosupporession, alopecia Occasional: stomatitis, hepatotoxicity, mucositis, cardiomyopathy (cumulative and dose dependent) Rare: anaphylaxis, allergic reaction, rash, secondary malignancy	Vesicant—severe tissue damage if extravasation occurs. Warn patient and family about urine discoloration. Cardiac studies with echocardiogram or multigated angiography (MUGA) scan should be done periodically to monitor cardiac function—must have acceptable cardiac ejection/monitor cumulative dose.
Etoposide (VP-16, VePesid)	Plant alkaloid Epipodophyllotoxin	IV, PO	Common: nausea, vomiting, myelosuppression Occasional: alopecia, enhanced damage due to radiation, diarrhea Rare: hypotension, anaphylaxis, skin rash, peripheral neuropathy, stomatitis, secondary malignancy	Severe hypotension can occur with rapid infusion. Concentrations above 0.4 mg/ml have unpre dictable stability in solution. Do not refrigerate intravenous solution, PO capsules must be refrigerated.
5-Fluorouracil (5-FU, fluorouracil, Adrucil)	Antimetabolite	IV, PO	Common: nausea, vomiting, metallic taste, immunosuppression, myelosuppression Occasional: diarrhea, stomatitis, sun sensitivity, hyper pigmentation, dry skin, palmar-plantar erythrodysesthesia (red painful skin irritation) Rare: hypotension, angina, electrocardiogram (ECG) changes, tearing, conjunctivitis and blurred vision, partial loss of nails, headache, visual disturbances, cerebellar ataxia, proctitis	Take on empty stomach (at least 1 hr before or 2 hr after food). For oral administration mix parenteral solution of 5-FU with flavored water or carbonated beverage; avoid acidic fruit juice.
Hydroxyurea (Hydrea)	Antimetabolite	PO	Common: myelosuppression with rapid drop in WBC count Occasional: nausea, vomiting, stomatitis, anemia Rare: rash, facial erythema, dysuria, renal tubular damage, headache, dizziness, jaundice, radiation recall, hallucination, convulsions, nail changes	Take on empty stomach (1 hr before or 2 hr after meals). Dose often titrated to WBC count. Do not add to solutions that are acidic or carbonated, alkaline solutions preferred.

continued

Table 4-5. Chemotherapeutic Agents *continued*

Drug	Classification	Route	Side Effects	Special Considerations
Idarubicin (Idamycin)	Anthracycline	IV	Analogue of daunorubicin with similar activity and side effects	Vesicant—severe tissue damage if extravasation occurs. Protect from light. See daunomycin. Perhaps less cardiotoxicity than doxorubicin and daunorubicin.
Ifosfamide (isophosphamide, Ifex)	Alkylating agent	IV	Analog of cyclophosphamide Common: nausea, vomiting, anorexia, myelosuppression, alopecia Occasional: somnolence, confusion, weakness, seizure, SIADH, hemorrhagic cystitis, cardiac toxicities with arrhythmias as high dosages, myocardial necrosis, Fanconi's renal failure Rare: encephalopathy, peripheral neuropathy, acute renal failure, pulmonary fibrosis, secondary malignancy, bladder fibrosis	Risk of severe hemorrhagic cystitis if given without uroprotection from mesna. Can be mixed with mesna. More severe symptoms may occur at higher doses and after rapid injection. Must receive PO or IV hydration beginning 3–6 hr before and 24 hr after dose. Must monitor I&O and urinary specific gravity. Fanconi's renal failure more common with history of cisplatin, prior kidney damage, and greater than 70–100 g/m^2 cumulative dose. May require electrolyte supplementation with magnesium (Mg), potassium (K+), and phosphorous (PO^4).
Interferon (Intron A, Roferon-A)	Protein produced by recombinant DNA technology	IV, IM, SQ	Common: none Occasional: fever, headache, fatigue, anorexia, nausea, myalgia, arthralgia, diarrhea, depression, confusion Rare: vomiting, chills, stomatitis, somnolence, psychosis, elevated transaminases, myelosuppression, peripheral neuropathy, sinus tachyarrhythmias, hypocalcemia, hyperkalemia, anaphylaxis, dyspnea, hypotension, rash, dizziness, impotence, alopecia, menstrual disorder	Premediation with magnesium choline salicylate, acetaminophen, or, if not contraindicated, nonsteroidal anti-inflammatory drugs (NSAIDS), may reduce fever and myalgias.
Irinotecan (CPT-11, Camptosar)	Topoisomerase I inhibitor	IV	Common: transient early diarrhea, nausea, vomiting, abdominal pain, anorexia, fever, dehydration, alopecia, asthenia, myelosuppression, later diarrhea, alopecia Occasional: elevation in transaminases, alkaline phosphatase, bilirubin, creatinine, constipation, pain at infusion site Rare: dermatitis, tremor, hematuria, hypoproteinemia, glucosuria, mucositis, headache, dizziness, disorientation/confusion, facial hot flushes, colitis, pulmonary infiltrates, pneumonitis	May require antidiarrheal for control of diarrhea: atropine for early diarrhea, loperamide for delayed diarrhea.

continued

Table 4-5. Chemotherapeutic Agents *continued*

Drug	Classification	Route	Side Effects	Special Considerations
Lomustine (CCNU, CeeNU)	Nitrosourea	PO	Common: nausea, vomiting, myelosuppression Occasional: anorexia Rare: elevation of liver enzymes, pulmonary toxicity, renal toxicity, cumulative myelosuppression	PO in one dose on an empty stomach, 1 hr before meals or 2 hr after meals.
Mechlorethamine (nitrogen mustard, Mustargen, HN2)	Alklylating agent	IV	Common: nausea, vomiting, anorexia, metallic taste, phlebitis, alopecia, diarrhea, myelosuppression, gonadal dysfunction/sterility, necrosis if extravasated	Vesicant—can also cause skin irritation with local contact (use sodium thiosulfate and ice). Use within 1 hr after reconstitution. May cause thrombosis, phlebitis, and discoloration of vein.
Melphalan (Alkeran, L-PAM, L-sarcolysin)	Alkylating agent	PO, IV	Common: anorexia, ulceration if extravasated, nausea, vomiting, myelosuppression, mucositis, diarrhea, alopecia Occasional: lethargy Rare: hypotension, diaphoresis, hypersensitivity reaction, pulmonary fibrosis, sterility, secondary malignancy	Infusion over 15–30 min. Good hydration for 24 hr after IV dose. Furosemide may be given to maintain urinary output after IV dose. Take daily dose at one time. Take on empty stomach.
Mercaptopurine (Purinethol, 6-MP)	Antimetabolite	PO	Common: myelosuppression Occasional: anorexia, nausea, vomiting, diarrhea, mucositis Rare: anaphylactic reaction, urticaria, hepatic fibrosis, hyperbilirubinemia	Reduce oral dose 75% if give with allopurinol. Take daily dose at one time, preferably at bedtime on an empty stomach (2 hr after meals).
Methotrexate (amethopterin, MTX)	Antimetabolite	IV, IM, PO, IT	Common: transaminase and bilirubin elevations Occasional: nausea, vomiting, anorexia, diarrhea, myelosuppression, stomatitis, photosensitivity, learning disability Rare: dizziness, malaise, blurred vision, allergic reaction, peeling, redness and tenderness of skin—especially soles and palms, alopecia, folliculitis, renal toxicity, leukoencephalopathy, seizures, acute neurotoxicity, lung damage, liver damage, hyperpigmentation, osteoporosis, osteonecrosis and soft tissue necrosis, progressive CNS deterioration Intrathecal administration: nausea, vomiting, headache, pleocytosis, fever, convulsion, learning disability, rash, somnolence, meningismus, convulsions, paresis, myelosuppression, somnolence, ataxia, leukoencephalopathy, progressive DNS deterioration	Renal impairment will enhance toxicity. Advise patients to use sunscreen; severe sunburn can occur even with low weekly doses. When intermediate or high-dose methotrexate is given, leucovorin is administered as a rescue agent. Avoid vitamins containing folic acid to avoid the metabolic block caused by methotrexate. Hydration and urine alkalinization are used with higher dose infusions. Methotrexate readily enters body fluids; patients with effusions may have delayed clearance. Do not give concomitant trimethoprim and sulfamethaxozole, NSAIDs, aspirin because delayed clearance and increased toxicities may occur.

continued

Table 4-5. Chemotherapeutic Agents *continued*

Drug	Classification	Route	Side Effects	Special Considerations
Mitoxantrone (Novantrone, DHAD)	Topoisomerase II inhibitor	IV	Common: cardiac arrhythmias, nausea, vomiting, worsening side effects due to radiation, local ulceration if extravasated, bluish-green color to urine, myelosuppression, immunosuppression, alopecia Occasional: stomatitis, hepatotoxicity, mucusitis, cardiomyopathy (dose dependent) Rare: anaphylaxis, allergic reactions, rash, secondary malignancy	Vesicant—severe tissue damage if extravasation occurs. Not recommended for patients who have received full doses of anthracycline. Do not give IV push. May discolor urine; educate patient and family
Paclitaxel (Taxol)	Plant alkaloid	IV	Common: pain, swelling, erythema if extravasated, myelosuppression, diminished or absent deep tendon reflexes, alopecia, fatigue Occasional: acute anaphylactic reaction, nausea, vomiting, headache, skin rash, mucositis, diarrhea, fiver, glove and stocking numbness, hyperesthesia with burning sensation, mild to severe myalgias, increased triglyceride levels	Irritant—avoid extravasation. Premedicate with diphenhydramine, dexamethasone, and an H^2 receptor blocker. Do not administer in any bag or tubing containing polyvinyl chloride (PVC). Use filters because small fibers can appear after dilution.
Procarbazine (Matulane)	Aklylating agent	PO	Common: nausea, vomiting, diarrhea, anorexia, inhibits monoamine oxidase (MAO) activity, myelosuppression, alopecia Occasional: headache, flulike syndrome, gonadal dysfunction/sterility Rare: nightmare, hallucinations, hemolytic anemia, pruritis, rash, depression, insomnia, convulsions, coma, stomatitis, pulmonary reaction, hypertension, secondary malignancy	Hypotension and/or CNS depression may occur in the presence of alcohol, narcotics, antihistamines, phenothiazines, phenytoin (Dilantin), tricyclic antidepressants, barbiturates, sympathomimetic drugs and tyramine-rish foods such as aged cheese, wine, bananas, yogurt. Take 1 hr before or 2 hr after meals
Retinoic acids (13-*cis*-retinoic acid, isotretinoin All-*trans* retinoic acid (tretinoin [Vesanoid])	Differentiating agents Vitamin A and its derivatives stimulates clonal proliferation of erythroid and myeloid progenitor cells and play a roll in growth, reproduction, epithelial cell differentiation, and immune function	PO	Common: dry skin, dry mucosa, inflammation of the lips Occasional: nausea, vomiting, rash, conjunctivitis, musculoskeletal pains, fatigue, headache, triglyceride elevation, cholesterol elevations, transaminase elevations, retinoic acid syndrome with hyperleukocytosis Rare: changes in skin pigmentation, nonspecific GI complaints, dizziness, pseudotumor cerebri, anemia, leukopenia, respiratory distress, fever, hypotension, skeletal hyperostosis	Take with food or meals to enhance absorption. Monitor lipid levels. Avoid sun exposure, use good lubricant for skin and lips. Monitor nutritional status Use saline eye drops, as needed.

continued

Table 4-5. Chemotherapeutic Agents *continued*

Drug	Classification	Route	Side Effects	Special Considerations
Teniposide (VM-26, Vumon)	Plant alkaloid Epipodophyllotoxin	IV	Common: nausea, vomiting, myelosuppression Occasional: alopecia, enhanced damage due to radiation, diarrhea Rare: hypotension, anaphylaxis, skin rash, peripheral neuropathy, stomatitis, secondary malignancy	Irritant—avoid extravasation. Do not use PVC-containing bags or tubing to administer. Do not refrigerate diluted solutions. Heparin can precipitate; must be flushed from lines. Anaphylaxis or hypotensive reaction with rapid infusion. Flush vein before and after administration.
Thioguanine (6-thioguanine, 6-TG)	Antimetabolite	PO	Common: myelosuppression Occasional: anorexia, nausea, vomiting, diarrhea, mucositis Rare: anaphylactic reaction, urticaria, hematuria, crystalluria, hepatic fibrosis, hyperbilirubinemia	Take oral dose at one time, preferably at bedtime on empty stomach (2 hr after meals).
Thiotepa (Triethylenethio-phosphoramide, Thioplex)	Alklyating agent	IV, IM, SQ, IT Intracavitary Intratumor	Common: nausea, vomiting, anorexia, myelosup pression, mucositis and esophagitis at higher doses in conditioning regimens for bone marrow transplant (BMT), gonadal dysfunction/infertility Occasional: pain at injection site, dizziness, headache; inappropriate behavior, confusion, somnolence, increased liver transaminase, increased bilirubin, hyperpigmentation of the skin at higher dose in conditioning regimens for BMT Rare: hives, skin rash, febrile reaction	Use 0.22-micron filter to eliminate haze with IV infusions; solutions that are grossly opaque or contain obvious precipitation should not be used. Dilute reconstituted solutions with NS before use. Should be used within 8 hr. of reconstitution
Topotecan (Hycamtin)	Plant alkaloid Topoisomerase I inhibitor	IV, IT	Common: myelosuppression, alopecia Occasional: nausea, vomiting, diarrhea, mucositis, flulike symptoms, headache, rash, elevated transaminases, elevated alkaline phosphatase, elevated bilirubin, asthenia Rare: abdominal pain, rigors, microscopic hematuria Intrathecal: Nausea, vomiting, headache, fever, back pain, possible leukoencephalopathy, seizures, or paralysis	Administer IT doses over 5 min to avoid potential adverse reactions.

continued

Table 4-5. Chemotherapeutic Agents *continued*

Drug	Classification	Route	Side Effects	Special Considerations
Vinblastine (VLB, vincaleukoblastine, Velban)	Plant alkaloid	IV	Common: myelosuppression, alopecia Occasional: constipation, loss of deep tendon reflexes, paresthesias Rare: nausea, vomiting, anorexia, bone pain, allergic reaction, stomatitis, peripheral neuropathy, hoarseness, ptosis, double vision	Vesicant—severe tissue damage if extravasation occurs. Administer stool softeners; increase bulk and fiber in diet.
Vincristine (VCR, Oncovin)	Plant alkaloid	IV	Common: local ulceration if extravasated, hair loss, loss of deep tendon reflexes Occasional: jaw pain, weakness, constipation, numbness, tingling, clumsiness Rare: paralytic ileus, ptosis, vocal cord paralysis, myelosuppression, CNS depression, seizures, SIADH	Vesicant—severe tissue damage if extravasation occurs. Refrigerate and protect from light. Stool softeners may be given prophylactically or for constipation. Liver dysfunction or concomitant radiation therapy to the liver may enhance toxicity. Must have special overwrap label that bears the statement, "Do not remove covering until moment of injection. Fatal if given intrathecally. For intravenous injection only." Infants may have difficulty feeding because of jaw pain. Maximum single dose: 2 mg regardless of BSA or weight
Miscellaneous Drugs				
Allopurinol (Zyloprim)	Enzyme inhibitor; blocks uric acid production by inhibiting xanthine oxidase	IV, PO	Common: rash, fever Occasional: granulomatous hepatitis, ocular lesions, alopecia, slight bone marrow suppression, drowsiness, peripheral neuropathy, GI complaints Rare: agranulocytosis, toxic epidermal necrolysis, severe systemic vasculitis, exfoliative dermatitis	Dose reduction is required in moderate to severe renal impairment. Increased toxicities may occur when used with 6-MP or azathioprine—use with great caution. With cyclophosphamide, warfarin, oral antidiabetic drugs, ampicillin, amoxicillin, or thiazide diuretics, use with caution. Maintain adequate hydration. Physically incompatible with methotrexate—do not give in same IV fluid.
Amifostine (Ethyol)	Organic thiophosphate cytoprotective agent	IV	Common: nausea, vomiting, flushing, hypotension, hypocalcemia (with multiple daily or multiple day dosing) Occasional: sleepiness, dizziness, sneezing	If multiple doses are administered within a 24-hr period, monitor serum calcium levels and supplement, as needed. Administer with patient lying down. Have normal saline bolus available

continued

Table 4-5. Chemotherapeutic Agents *continued*

Drug	Classification	Route	Side Effects	Special Considerations
			Rare: hiccups, chills	Monitor blood pressure frequently during infusion (every 3–5 min). Hypotension often occurs toward the end of the infusion. If hypotension develops, place patient in Trendelenberg's position and administer NS bolus (20 ml/kg over 20 min). If blood pressure normalizes, resume infusion. Doses are given immediately before radiation therapy or chemotherapy. Inspect parenteral solutions for particulate matter or discoloration. Do not use if cloudiness or precipitate is observed. Use with NS solutions only. Compatibility with other solutions has not been examined.
Dexrazoxane (Zinecard)	Iron chelator that interferes with iron-mediated free radical generation	IV	Common: Pain on injection, phlebitis, myelosuppression Occasional: transient increases in triglycerides, amylase, and alanine transaminase (ALT), mild nausea, vomiting, and diarrhea Rare: neurotoxicity (headache, constipation)	Recommended dose ratio of dexrazoxane:doxorubicin is 10:1. Doxorubicin must be given before elapsed time of 30 min from beginning of dexrazoxane infusion.
Leucovorin calcium (Wellcovorin, citrovorum factor, folinic acid)	Antidote Bypasses the inhibitor action of folic acid antagonist (methotrexate)	IV, IM, PO	Rare: allergic sensitization, rash	Used as cellular rescue when intermediate- or high-dose methotrexate is given. May be given as a single dose after IT methotrexate. Must be given exactly at the times ordered.
Mesna (Mesnex)	Uroprotective agent	IV, PO	Common: bad taste with oral use Occasional: nausea, vomiting, stomach pain Rare: headache; pain in arms, legs and joints; fatigue; rash; transient hypotension; allergy; diarrhea	False positive test for urinary ketones. Not compatible with cisplatin. May be mixed with cyclophosphamide or ifosfamide. Must be given exactly at the times ordered. IV dose may be given orally at a higher dose, orally has a foul taste. Do not use the multidose vial in young infants or neonates because preservative benzyl alcohol is used.

continued

Table 4-5. Chemotherapeutic Agents *continued*

Drug	Classification	Route	Side Effects	Special Considerations
Trimethoprim and sulfamethoxazole (Bactrim, Septrax, Co-Trimoxizole)	Antibiotic used prophylactically to prevent *Pneumocystis carinii* pneumonia	IV, PO	Occasional: neutropenia, anorexia, nausea, vomiting, diarrhea, GI upset, hepatic dysfunction, rash Rare: Stevens-Johnson syndrome, toxic epidermal necrolysis	May be given as a prophylaxis for *P. carinii* on a schedule of 3 consecutive days weekly. If allergic to Bactrim, may use intravenous or aerosolized pentamidine or PO dapsone. Must be diluted in 5% dextrose in water (D_5W) solution for IV administration; infuse parenteral solution over 60–90 min; monitor for hyponatremia. Not compatible with other drugs in IV solution. Avoid use during methotrexate infusion; delays methotrexate clearance and increases risk of toxicities. Use sunscreen during use because Trimethoprim increases sensitivity to sun.

Data from Almuete, V., Brisby, J., Delman, B., et al. (2000). 2000 Guide for the administration and use of cancer chemotherapeutic agents. *Oncology Special Edition, 3,* 51–55; Balis, F., Hocenberg, J., & Poplack, D.G. General principles of chemotherapy. In P.A. Pizzo & D.G. Poplack (Eds.). *Principles and practice of pediatric oncology* (3rd ed., pp. 215–272). Philadelphia: Lippincott-Raven; Henry, D., Cartwright, J., & Sinsabaugh, D. (2000). *Children's Oncology Group pharmacology manual.* Arcadia, CA: Children's Oncology Group Operations Center; Renick-Ettinger, A. (1993). Chemotherapy. In G.V. Foley, D. Fochtman, & K.H. Mooney (Eds.), *Nursing care of the child with cancer* (2nd ed., pp. 81–116). Philadelphia: W.B. Saunders.

- Assess the patient's CBC with a differential and other required lab tests to determine, among other concerns, whether the results are within the protocol's parameters.
- Ensure that the chemotherapy doses and drugs are correct by following the institution's policies for double-checking the orders and doses, identify the correct patient by looking at the armband, and review the patient's allergy profile as well.
- Prepare IV chemotherapy according to Occupational Safety and Health Administration (OSHA) guidelines for handling cytotoxic or hazardous drugs, or both. (It is important to remember that oral chemotherapy tablets should be crushed in the pharmacy under a hood to prevent inhalation of the dust.)
- Prepare the appropriate and necessary protective equipment based on the potential for exposure before entering the patient's room (refer to OSHA guidelines for the handling of chemotherapeutic agents later in this section).
- Monitor the IV site during and after the administration of the chemotherapy.
- Teach the family and the patient about drug-specific side effects that may be immediate (e.g., doxorubicin [Adriamycin] can turn urine an orange-to-red color).
- Teach the family about the side effects that the patient will experience after administration of the drug (e.g., bone marrow suppression and alopecia).

Interventions: Nursing interventions should be specific to the type of chemotherapy being administered. Care must be taken to accurately assess and document the occurrence of any side effects, particularly if the patient is in a research study. These are some general considerations:

- Administer appropriate premeditations based on the assessment.
- Monitor and document the effectiveness of the antiemetic regimen and any expected side effects.
- Ensure that the chemotherapy is given as ordered and that if the patient is given an IV, the site is carefully monitored for evidence of local irritation or reaction.
- Discuss the potential side effects and the expected side effects of the drug, and ensure that the caregiver understands any home care that is necessary after administration of the drug.
- Teach the family to anticipate side effects that may occur days or weeks after administration of chemotherapy.
- Follow the institution's policy for handling chemotherapy wastes, including the patient's body fluids, to protect people and the environment from exposure to the cytotoxic drugs.

Table 4-6. Overcoming Chemotherapy Resistance

Methods to Overcome Chemotherapy Resistance	Advances to Offset Normal Cell Damage
1. Development of multidrug resistance (MDR) modulators 2. Administration of chemotherapy at maximum dose intensity (maximum tolerated dose and shortest possible interval between doses) 3. Development of combination chemotherapy regimens (multiple alternating agents used to prevent the development of resistance) Characteristics of agents selected for combination chemotherapy regimens: –differing side effect profiles –action at different phases of cell cycle –show synergy with other agents–nonoverlapping toxicities –conform to dose intensity principles 4. Utilization of pharmacokinetics and pharacodynamics in the development of therapeutic protocols	1. Investigation of drugs that have shown the ability to modulate MDR by inhibiting P-glycoprotein. 2. Normal cell return is improved with supportive care measures, such as the use of growth factors, aggressive antibiotic/regimens for infection, safer transportation practices, and early symptom management. 3. Dose adjustments are made to offset toxicities and biochemical modulators are used to improve chemotherapy tolerance –Use of leucovorin calcium with high-dose methotrexate to rescue normal cells –Use of cryoprotective agents (mesna to prevent bladder toxicity, amifostine to prevent ototoxicity, and dexrazoxane to prevent cardiac toxicity) –Use of asparaginase as a rescue drug after methotrexate and cytarabine 4. Children's physiological differences may provide an advantage in terms of drug absorption, distribution, metabolism, excretion, and, ultimately, drug tolerance.

Expected Patient and Family Outcomes

- The patient successfully completes the course of chemotherapy with effective management of side effects.
- The patient, the family, or both understand the home care that is necessary after the chemotherapy.
- The patient, the family, or both are aware of the concerns about bone marrow suppression after chemotherapy and are able to verbalize the proper steps to take to deal with any episodes of fever, bleeding, or excessive fatigue.
- The patient and the family are aware of the resources available to help the patient make a transition back into the school system, if applicable.
- The patient, the family, or both are aware of the patient's next follow-up visit.

OSHA Guidelines for Handling Chemotherapy

Susanne B. Conley

Nurses who administer chemotherapy may have questions about the risks associated with repeated exposure to these agents. In 1986, these questions prompted OSHA to publish its first set of guidelines for the preparation, administration, and disposal of chemotherapeutic agents. OSHA placed antineoplastic agents into a category labeled "cytotoxic drugs." However, as drug research increased, OSHA revised its guidelines in 1995 and included another category of drugs labeled "hazardous." OSHA does not maintain a set list of drugs that fall into the category of hazardous drugs.

The purpose of these guidelines is to provide recommendations consistent with current scientific knowledge. The recommendations apply to all care settings, such as hospitals, outpatient clinics, physicians' offices, and home care companies. According to OSHA (1995), safe levels of occupational exposure to cytotoxic agents cannot be determined, and no reliable method of monitoring exposure exists. Research indicates that compliance with established safety guidelines offers adequate protection to those healthcare workers involved in handling and administering chemotherapy agents or caring for the patients receiving them (Ritchie, McAdams, & Fritz, 2000).

With today's rapid expansion of chemotherapy services, the need for specialized instruction in the safe handling of cytotoxic drugs has become increasingly apparent. An established procedure manual standardizes safe work practices for use in training new personnel and evaluating staff exposure to cytotoxic drugs.

Classification

Hospitals and clinics use OSHA guidelines as a basis for developing their own policies for administration and disposal of cytotoxic and hazardous drugs. Chemotherapy cannot always be prepared for administration by a pharmacist in a protected area of a hospital pharmacy especially since more chemotherapy is being given in outpatient and clinic settings than in the past. Consequently, chemotherapy preparation and administration guidelines must provide optimal protection for the small oncology office and home care settings as well.

The following is a summary of the OSHA recommendations (the policies of individual institutions may differ slightly):

- Staff should wear gowns with back closures, nitrile gloves, and eye protection during preparation and drug administration. If there is a risk of aerosolization during administration, a mask should be worn as well. During preparation, a safety hood with appropriate ventilation must be used.

- IV tubing should have Luer-lock connections, and the connection sites should be taped. An absorbent pad with a plastic back is necessary for collecting any spill from the tube when the tubing is being attached to the patient.
- IV tubing should be primed under a hood. If priming occurs at the administration site, IV tubing should be primed with a nondrug fluid or using the backflow method.
- It is important to remember that oral agents can cause exposures, too. The precautions taken with oral drugs should be based on the potential for exposure that exists. For example, a young child may spit out a pill that has been crushed and mixed with liquids. Also, tablets should be crushed only under a hood to prevent inhalation of the dust.
- Potential health risks are associated with biotherapeutic agents. OSHA has identified interferons as hazardous agents.
- Staff should wear appropriate protection to shield them from blood and body fluid for up to 48 hours after chemotherapy has been completed because patients excrete the drugs in their urine and feces.
- Any unused drugs should be returned to the pharmacy for disposal.
- IV tubing should be disposed of intact as a single unit. Needles used for withdrawing medication should be placed in a puncture-resistant container.
- Gloves and gowns should be disposed of before leaving the room. If either of these items becomes soiled before administration or preparation of a drug is complete, they must be removed and replaced with clean items.
- Soiled tubing, gloves, and gowns should be disposed of in designated containers. These containers must be labeled in accordance with the Hazard Communication Standard, as directed by OSHA guidelines.
- Patients' soiled linens, diapers, or emesis basins should be disposed of in the same manner as other equipment and materials if the patient has received chemotherapy within the previous 48 hours.

Nursing Assessment and Interventions

Assessment:

- Review the institution's policies before handling or administering cytotoxic or hazardous drugs.

Interventions:

- Prepare protective equipment before entering the patient's room and be aware of clean-up procedures and the location of spill kits.
- Prepare patients and their families for the precautions that will be taken before entering their room wearing protective equipment. It can be frightening for them to see staff enter with a gown, gloves, and eyewear.
- Prepare patients and their families for home administration of chemotherapy. Caregivers in the home should be given written instructions and personal protective equipment whenever there is a risk of cytotoxic drugs being released into the environment. Prescriptions for chemotherapy gloves, masks, and spill kit should be given to patients and parents as appropriate.
- Home care workers should be instructed to
  - Dispose of unused agents in designated containers labeled "hazardous."
  - Designate a workplace for handling cytotoxic agents.
  - Work below eye level.
  - Use detergent and water to wash surfaces that come into contact with cytotoxic drugs.
  - Institute universal precautions when handling the blood, vomitus, or excreta of a patient who has received chemotherapy within the previous 48 hours.

Expected Patient and Family Outcomes

- Chemotherapy is administered safely, in accordance with OSHA guidelines.

References

Occupational Safety & Health Administration. (n.d.). *OSHA technical manual: Controlling occupational exposure to hazardous drugs.* Retrieved May 7, 2003, from http://www.osha.gov/dts/osta/otm/otm_vi/otm_vi_2.html

Ritchie, M., McAdams, C. & Fritz, N. (2000). Exposure risk in the handling and administration of chemotherapy agents: A review and synthesis of the literature. *Online Journal of Knowledge Synthesis for Nursing, 7*(4). Retrieved February 1, 2003, from http://www.stti.iupui.edu/ library/ojksn/

Administration of Vesicants

Christine Sullivan

Principles of Treatment

Vesicants are agents that cause significant tissue necrosis when extravasation occurs. Despite the risk associated with the delivery of vesicants, they are crucial to the success of many treatment regimens. The risk of extravasation is lessened to some degree by the use of central access devices. However, if these devices are improperly managed, extravasation can still occur. Vesicants can be categorized as either DNA-binding or non-DNA-binding.

DNA-binding agents: DNA-binding agents (e.g., anthracyclines, including doxorubicin [Adriamycin], daunomycin [Cerubidine], idarubicin [Idamycin], and dactinomycin [Actinomycin-D]) produce more damage as they spread through tissue; therefore, minimizing dilution of a vesicant and applying a cold compress to the extravasation site is in the patient's best interest.

Non-DNA-binding agents: Non-DNA-binding agents (e.g., vinca alkaloids such as vincristine [Oncovin] and vinblastine [Velban]) cause less tissue damage when the extravasated drug is diluted and diffused. In these situations, the ideal actions to take are to administer warmth to the site and the appropriate antidote.

Although a list of agent-specific antidotes has been developed for use in the event of extravasation, the effectiveness of such antidotes has been marginal at best. This is particularly true of the antidotes to DNA-binding agents, because DNA-binding agents cause ongoing damage beyond the site of initial insult. Often, the full extent of the injury is not known for days or even weeks. The non-DNA-binding agents cause much less damage because the injury is confined to the tissues directly affected at the time of the extravasation.

Role in Childhood Cancer

Vesicants are an integral part of most systemic therapy protocols because of their effectiveness against a wide variety of malignancies.

Classifications/Method of Delivery

Practice guidelines emphasize the importance of preventing extravasations. The guiding principle should be, if in doubt, thoroughly assess the situation prior to vesicant administration. For example, if a central venous catheter does not have a blood return despite flushing easily, institutional policy will require a radiographic study to assess the line prior to administration. Fibrin sheaths on catheter tips have been known to cause vesicants to track retrograde outside of the catheter, resulting in severe extravasations. When peripheral access is used, careful site selection must be practiced. Ideally, the vessel chosen is large enough to sustain adequate blood flow and is in an area that allows stabilization of the needle during administration. Joints and ligaments should be avoided.

Two-syringe technique: This technique involves choosing an appropriate vein, accessing the vein, flushing with 3–5 ml of normal saline (NS), and assessing blood return and any other signs of infiltration. After adequate access has been established, the NS syringe should be removed and the chemotherapy syringe should be attached. The drug should be injected slowly while checking for blood return after each 1–2 cc of injected drug, should be followed with 3–5 cc, and should be flushed with saline (as in the sidearm technique described in the next section).

Sidearm technique: Adequate IV access should be obtained (as described earlier in the discussion of the two-syringe technique). Free-flowing IV fluids should be connected to the catheter, and an assessment for blood return should be made by pinching off the tubing. While the IV fluids are being infused, the drug should be injected into the IV line via a side port. An assessment for blood return should be made throughout administration by pinching the tubing, and the needle should be flushed with saline upon completing the push.

Vesicant extravasations can be treated with drugs that act as antidotes. If extravasation is suspected, infusion should be stopped immediately. Generally the patient will complain of pain and burning, and slight infiltration close to the site might be seen. The antidote that is chosen is based on the drug classification. **Table 4-7** gives a summary of the available antidotes and a description of how to administer these drugs.

Nursing Assessment and Interventions

Assessment:

- Assess the patient's IV access. (For a peripheral IV, staff must know their institution's policy about using an existing IV or whether there is a need to establish new access. The peripheral IV must be located away from joints and tendons, have a good blood return, and be able to be flushed easily. In children, the hand and forearm are generally used. For a central venous access device, blood return should be verified, the catheter should be flushed to determine patency, and the dressing should be dry and secure. If there is no blood return but the IV flushes well, a vesicant should not be given. The institution's policy for assessing a blocked catheter should be followed.)

Interventions:

- Gather the equipment needed to administer the drug and establish IV access.
- Ask the patient, if the patient is old enough to do so, to communicate any pain, burning, or other discomfort experienced during or after administration of the drug.
- Stop the administration of a vesicant *immediately* if any burning, swelling, or tenderness occurs.
- Notify a physician immediately if extravasation occurs.
- Obtain an extravasation kit and administer an antidote if necessary. (Each institution should have a kit where chemotherapy is administered, and it usually determines what is in this kit and where it is located.)
- Apply heat or a cold compress as indicated in **Table 4-7**.
- Document the extravasation in the nurses' notes.

Expected Patient and Family Outcomes

- The patient has minimal complications related to extravasation.

Table 4-7. Vesicant and Irritant Chemotherapeutic Agents and Extravasation Antidote

Chemotherapeutic Agents	Antidote	Local Care	Comments
Vesicant Agents			
Dactinomycin (Actinomycin D)	None	Ice as comfort measure Elevate extremity and do not use for several days	More pronounced if receiving or previously received radiotherapy May need surgical consult
Daunorubicin (Daunomycin)	None	Apply ice for 15 min every 3–4 hr, as tolerated, for 24–48 hr	May need surgical consult
Doxorubicin (Adriamycin)			
Epirubicin			
Idarubicin (Idamycin)			
Mitomycin C (Mutamycin)			
Mechlorethamine (Nitrogen Mustard)	Isotonic sodium thiosulfate	Mix 4 ml 10% sodium thiosulfate with 8.4 ml sterile H_2O Inject 1–4 ml through existing IV line or subcutaneously (SQ) at extravasation site	
Vinblastine (Velban) Vincristine (Oncovin) Vindesine (Eldisine) Vinorelbine (Navelbine)	Hyaluronidase	Mix 150 units/ml hyaluronidase with 1 ml of normal saline (NS) Inject 1.4 ml through existing IV line of SQ at extravasation site	
Irritant Agents			
Irritant agents cause pain, venous irritation, and/or chemical phlebitis		Apply cold pack to IV site and along vein	Slowing infusion rate and/or increasing diluent may decrease pain associated with administration of irritant agents
Carboplatin Carmustine (BCNU)			
Dacarbazine (DTIC)			
Etoposide (VP-16)			
Ifosfamide			
Teniposide (VM-26)			

Data from Goodman, M. (2000). Chemotherapy: Principles of administration. In C.H. Yarbro, M.G. Frogge, M. Goodman, et al. (Eds.), *Cancer nursing: Principles and practice* (5th ed., pp. 385–443). Sudbury, MA: Jones & Barlett; Tortorice, P.V. (2000). Chemotherapy: Principles of therapy. In C.H. Yarbro, M.G. Frogge, M. Goodman, et al. (Eds.), *Cancer nursing: Principles and practice* (5th ed., pp. 352–384). Sudbury, MA: Jones & Barlett.

Surgery

Cathy Burks

Surgery is an important component of a multidisciplinary treatment approach to childhood cancer, which also may include chemotherapy, radiation, or both.

Principles of Treatment

Surgical treatment of childhood cancer is indicated for the following reasons:

- diagnostic biopsy
- staging and "second-look" procedures
- complete resection of tumor
- debulking of tumors that are not fully resectable
- debridement of necrotic tissue
- surgery will help while being minimally invasive
- complications (obstruction, infection)
- palliation of symptoms
- supportive care, such as long-term venous access.

Types and Classification of Surgeries

Biopsies: Biopsies include fine-needle aspirations, True Cut needle biopsies for larger tissue specimens, and open procedures to remove entire lymph nodes and sections of tumor tissue.

Staging: Staging is indicated when treatment depends on the location of the cancer and the extent of disease involvement. "Second-look" procedures are used to assess a patient's response to nonsurgical treatment.

Complete resection: A resection is indicated for tumors that can be fully removed without compromising vital structures.

This may be done before chemotherapy, radiation, or both or during the course of these therapies. Tumors such as rhabdomyosarcoma have higher cure rates when resection includes "clean" margins that are free of tumor. Resection in a limb may be done to salvage the limb or to amputate it.

Debulking: Debulking involves removing a portion of the tumor mass when it is not possible to remove the entire mass. This may be done as a first-line therapy or after several courses of chemotherapy or radiation.

Minimally invasive surgery: Thorascopic and laparoscopic techniques in which instruments directed through cannulas achieve resection or debulking smaller wounds, minimal manipulation of organs or tissues, and decreased recovery time.

Surgery due to complications: This type of surgery may be done to decompress structures such as the bowel, bladder, or spinal cord.

Debridement: Debridement is the removal of necrotic tissue that impairs wound healing.

Palliation: Palliative surgery is done to relieve the symptoms caused by tumors that have been unresponsive to medical therapy. It also may be done to relieve pain and bleeding.

Placement of venous access devices: Surgery may be performed to place tunneled external catheters or implanted venous access devices.

Method of Delivery

Surgery in children is almost always performed under general anesthesia to ensure the safety and comfort of the child during the procedure. Exceptions would include a mediastinal mass with compression of the trachea or a vena cava, for which general anesthesia would be dangerous. In cases such as these, a combination of local anesthesia, sedation, and positioning would be used instead to maintain and protect the airway and venous return while promoting comfort.

Preoperative Management

Children should be in the best possible condition for surgery. Their hydration, nutritional status, and electrolyte balance should be as close as possible to normal levels. Hemodynamically, there should be adequate platelets ($\geq$50,000 mm^3 is preferred), clotting factors, hemoglobin ($\geq$8 g/dl for adequate oxygenation), and white blood cells. Children may receive intravenous hydration fluids with electrolyte supplementation, as indicated, or total parenteral nutrition. Transfusions of blood products and antibiotics should be given preoperatively, if indicated. Additional laboratory studies and radiologic studies may need to be ordered on the basis of the patient's specific diagnosis. Preoperative planning may include measures such as vaccinations. In the case of splenectomy, vaccines against *Haemophilus influenza* and pneumococcal and meningococcal infections should precede the surgery (by 4–6 weeks, if possible).

Parental preparation should include providing informed consent and an opportunity to ask questions. Children should be given age-appropriate explanations, including the opportunity to handle medical equipment and a tour of operating room, if time permits.

Postoperative Management

Airway/breathing: Following anesthesia, it is important to protect against postoperative atelectasis. Atelectasis may be evidenced by fever, labored breathing, or decreased breath sounds.

Fluid shifts: Patients will experience fluid shifts for the first few days. These are evidenced by facial edema, general puffiness, weight gain, and decreased urine output.

Fever: Fevers during the first 3 days after surgery are almost always related to atelectasis. Wound infections usually do not occur for at least 5 days after surgery.

Tube management: Drainage tubes that function properly promote healing by evacuating fluids that accumulate in operative sites. These fluids can stress suture lines and compress blood vessels that bring nutrients to the surgical site.

Antibiotics: Almost all surgical patients will have antibiotics "on call" for the operating room. They may or may not have antibiotics ordered postoperatively, usually depending upon the surgery and the structures involved. "Dirty" cases (such as a bowel resection) will always require postoperative antibiotics, whereas "clean" cases (such as a liver resection) might not.

Pain management: Intravenous or epidural medications are indicated for the first 2–5 days after surgery. Oral medications should be given as needed after IV or epidural medications are discontinued.

Nursing Assessment and Interventions

Airway/breathing:

Assessment.

- Monitor vital signs with close attention to increase in respiratory rate or fever.
- Ausculte breath sounds for rhonchi, rales, or diminished air movement.
- Monitor oxygen saturation.

Interventions.

- Use incentive spirometry.
- Encourage position changes, early ambulation, and deep breathing and cough.
- Perform chest physiotherapy as indicated to help reexpand the patient's lungs and decrease atelectasis.

Fluid status:

Assessment.

- Assess skin turgor, mucous membranes, and perfusion.
- Monitor blood chemistries when large volume of drainage occurs.

Interventions.

- Keep accurate measures of intake and output.
- Replace any drainage (i.e., nasogastric tube), as necessary.

Fever:

Assessment.

- Ausculte breath sounds for rhonchi, rales, or diminished breath sounds.

- Monitor patients who have compromised immune systems and who also may require blood cultures, a chest X ray, and antibiotics.
- Assess incision for redness, swelling, drainage, or increased tenderness.

Interventions.
- Administer antipyretics, as indicated, to promote comfort.
- Administer antibiotics, as ordered.

Tube management:
Assessment.
- Assess tubes for patency and irrigate them, as ordered.

Interventions.
- Document the amount and characteristics of drainage.
- Make sure the tubes are well secured.

Antibiotics:
Assessment.
- Monitor the serum level of aminoglycosides.
- Watch for evidence of side effects and drug reactions.

Intervention.
- Administer postoperative antibiotics, as ordered.

Pain management:
Assessment.
- Monitor pain, judging manifestations according to patient age.
- Monitor changes in vital signs, especially increases in heart rate, respiratory rate, or blood pressure.
- Monitor the patient for side effects of the administered medications.

Interventions.
- Use an age-appropriate, objective, pain-rating system for evaluating postoperative pain and the effectiveness of analgesic and behavioral interventions.
- Administer pain medication, as indicated, for discomfort.
- Consider administering pain medication prior to ambulation, a dressing change, or other potentially uncomfortable activities.

Wound care: Some surgeries will require extensive wound care and management.
Assessment.
- Monitor the dressing for drainage and circle the drainage on the dressing.
- Assess the appearance of the wound and document it in the medical record.
- Monitor wound size and granulation of tissue and monitor for any drainage.

Intervention.
- Change the dressing, as ordered.

Education:
Assessment.
- Assess the learning needs of the patient and the family and adjust the teaching plan accordingly.

Intervention.
- Instruct the patient and family to report any symptoms of infection.

Follow-up:
Assessment.
- Decide with the family whether home care will be required for home management.
- Ensure that the family knows whom to call in the event of complications or questions.
- Ensure that the patient keeps appointments for follow-up visits.

Intervention.
- Make the appropriate referrals.

Expected Patient and Family Outcomes

- The patient, the family, or both feel competent and can demonstrate the skills required to care for the child at home.
- The patient, the family, or both demonstrate competence in any specialized skills (e.g., for stoma care) related to the child's surgery.
- The patient, the family, or both know the signs and symptoms of fever as well as wound infections and complications and what to do if these should occur.
- The patient's family is able to provide emotional support to help the child deal with fears and anxieties about the surgery.
- The patient's wound heals properly, thus enabling the child to resume chemotherapy and radiation.
- The patient views the surgery in either a neutral or a positive way.

Radiation Therapy

Joy Hesselgrave

Principles of Treatment

Radiation therapy (RT) uses high-energy particles or waves to destroy cancer cells while sparing adjacent tissues. The unit of absorbed radiation dose is called the Gray (Gy), and 1 centigray (cGy) is equal to <1/100> Gy. RT kills tumor cells by preventing cell replication through radiation of the tumor. RT is most effective when the tissues are well oxygenated. Oxygen is essential to the production of the free radicals that lead to the chemical changes resulting in cell destruction.

Role in Childhood Cancer

RT is a treatment modality used for many different types of pediatric cancers. It may be used in combination with chemotherapy, surgery, or both. Many solid tumors and lymphomas are radiosensitive. RT can be used to prevent central nervous system disease in children with leukemia or lymphoma. RT also may be used emergently to treat tumors that may be causing superior vena cava syndrome, spinal cord compression, or airway compromise or interfering with other vital organ functions. Palliative RT may be helpful in managing pain and other symptoms that are not responsive to medications.

Radiation Therapy Process

The RT process includes a consultation with a radiation oncologist who will evaluate the patient, discuss the side effects of RT, obtain informed consent, and develop a treatment plan. As a part of the treatment planning process, most patients undergo radiation simulation prior to starting treatment to determine the radiation field. (This is done by using computed tomography (CT) or magnetic resonance imaging (MRI). During the simulation the exact areas to be irradiated are identified and the necessary markings, immobilization devices, and blocks are created. This helps ensure that the radiation will be consistently delivered to the same location at each RT session.

Children younger than 4 years old often will need sedation for their simulation session and radiation treatments. As a general rule, a child who requires sedation for an MRI will probably need it for radiation therapy. Children requiring sedation usually will need some form of central venous access. Children between 4 and 6 years old may be able to tolerate the procedure without sedation if they receive adequate support. Child life intervention for education, relaxation, and distraction is invaluable for children receiving RT (see Section VI, "Supportive Care"). Children older than 7 years are usually able to cooperate when receiving radiation treatments (Cullen et al., 2002).

Types of Radiation Therapy

External beam: A well-defined beam of radiation is aimed toward a specific anatomic site or tumor volume. X rays, gamma rays, or electrons are the most common types of external beam radiation.

Fractionation: Fractionation refers to the division of a dose of radiation into daily doses, or fractions, usually delivered on a Monday–Friday schedule.

Hyperfractionation: Hyperfractionation refers to the use of smaller doses given more frequently, usually two fractions a day. Total body irradiation is an example of radiation that is often given in hyperfractionated doses (see "Hematopoietic Stem Cell Transplantation").

Brachytherapy: Brachytherapy is the direct application of radionuclides in a high-dose volume to anatomic sites. Implantation into body cavities, tissue, and the skin surface has been used in adults for many years. Pediatric applications have been primarily in children who have soft tissue tumors, retinoblastoma, and central nervous system tumors. Brachytherapy may be done as a boost to the tumor bed in conjunction with external-beam RT.

Conformal: In three-dimensional conformal RT, the contours of the tumor and area to be treated are identified in the planning process, and radiation is delivered precisely to conform to the affected area, sparing healthy tissue.

Intensity modulated radiation therapy (IMRT): In IMRT, the radiation dose is delivered by many small beams entering the site from different angles. The maximum dosage is delivered to the target area, while the surrounding healthy tissue is spared. IMRT also can be used to treat multiple sites with varying doses of radiation at the same time. Consistent positioning is imperative to deliver these precise doses (Swift, 2002).

Intraoperative radiation therapy (IORT): IORT is delivered in the operating room as a single dose to the tumor bed and surrounding area while the patient is in surgery. This enables the patient to receive radiation only at the affected site, preserving healthy tissue. The delivery of this single dose has the biologic effect of several daily fractions.

Proton: Proton RT is a type of external beam therapy using proton-charged particles that deliver energy over a short distance known as the Bragg peak (Tarbell & Koov, 2002). A low dose is delivered in front of the tumor, and a high dose is delivered to the entire tumor, with minimal exit radiation. The advantage of this type of radiation is that it can be directed to conform to the tumor, minimizing radiation to normal tissue.

Stereotactic radiosurgery: This treatment is especially appropriate for small tumors. A rigid frame is attached to the patient, usually to the cranium, and is used to deliver a dose of radiation to the affected area. A CT or MRI is used for three-dimensional planning. This method may be used to deliver a single high dose or multiple fractions.

Potential Side Effects

A dose of radiation to an organ may be associated with a certain probability of a radiation-induced complication. This concept is referred to as the minimum tissue tolerance dose (TTD). Different organs have variable TTD values. The following section discusses some of the acute toxicities associated with RT. (For information on chronic toxicities related to RT, see Section X, "Late Effects of Childhood Cancer.")

Central nervous system: In general, RT is not recommended for children under 3 years of age because myelination is incomplete at this age and RT could cause significant functional impairment.

Brain. Headache, nausea, and vomiting may occur. Somnolence syndrome, which can occur from a few weeks to 3 months after cranial irradiation, is characterized by a prolonged period of fatigue and slowed mentation. It generally is resolved completely without intervention within 4–6 weeks.

Spinal cord. Transient radiation myelopathy can occur 2–4 months after spinal RT. Symptoms are characterized by an electrical shock-like sensation following neck flexion. The syndrome is usually self-limiting and frequently is resolved without treatment; corticosteroids are rarely used to manage symptoms.

Eyes: Low doses of RT can produce total lens opacification. The TTD to the eye is 6–12 Gy (Halperin, Constine, Tarbell, & Kun, 1999).

Digestive tract:

Salivary glands. The salivary glands may swell and become painful after the first one or two RT treatments. Radiation parotitis usually is resolved quickly. Increased viscosity of the saliva and a decrease in its volume often occur. Patients may complain of a dry mouth. RT to the parotid gland may be accompanied by an elevated serum amylase.

Oral mucosa. Erythema of the oral mucosa occurs at dosages of approximately 20 Gy. At dosages greater than 40 Gy, desquamation may develop. Regeneration of the oral mucosa occurs about 2–3 weeks after completion of RT. Children who receive head and neck irradiation may experience dental problems, including abnormal tooth formation and early loss of their permanent teeth.

Esophagus. Dysphagia and odynophagia occur at dosages of 20 Gy. Symptoms usually are resolved 2–3 weeks after RT has been completed.

Stomach. Acute nausea and vomiting may occur. Ulceration of the stomach can occur with dosages of 45 Gy, but this would be an unusual complication related to pediatric RT because a dosage this high is rarely, if ever, given.

Liver. Hepatic enlargement, tenderness, and elevation of serum liver function tests can occur. The TTD for RT to the liver is 35–40 Gy (Halperin et al., 1999). Radiosensitivity of the liver is increased by combination chemotherapy that includes doxorubicin (Adriamycin), dactinomycin (Actinomycin-D), cyclophosphamide (Cytoxan), and vincristine (Oncovin).

Small intestine. Nausea and vomiting can occur after RT. Diarrhea and cramping occur after 20–30 Gy of RT. Obstruction of the small bowel, malabsorption, and fistula formation can occur but are usually late side effects (see Section X, "Late Effects of Childhood Cancer").

Large intestine. Frequent diarrhea and tenesmus can occur after administration of 25–50 Gy of RT. Persistent proctitis, rectal ulceration, or stenosis are seen with RT dosages higher than 60 Gy.

Pulmonary: Dosages greater than 20 Gy to both lungs can produce radiation pneumonitis. This is characterized by dyspnea, dry cough, tachypnea, tachycardia, and radiographic pulmonary infiltrates. The TTD for RT of the whole lung is 20 Gy. The incidence of radiation pneumonitis increases if some types of chemotherapeutic agents are used (e.g., bleomycin [Blenoxane] and dactinomycin [Actinomycin-D]).

Cardiac: Postirradiation pericarditis can occur 2 months to 2 ½ years after therapy and is characterized by fever, dyspnea, pleuritic chest pain, and a pericardial friction rub. Steroids may be used to relieve symptoms. Pericarditis rarely progresses to a chronic condition. The TTD for the heart is 55–65 Gy (Halperin et al., 1999).

Urinary tract:

Kidney. Acute radiation nephritis can occur 6–12 months after RT, and symptoms are similar to nephrotic syndrome (e.g., hypertension, proteinuria). Medical management usually prevents significant complications. Late symptoms can occur and include hypertension, edema, proteinuria, and azotemia (see Section X, "Late Effects of Childhood Cancer"). TTD for the kidney is 23–28 Gy (Halperin et al., 1999).

Bladder. Acute radiation cystitis can occur as a result of pelvic RT. This is characterized by urinary frequency and pain on urination. With RT dosages higher than 60 Gy, urinary abnormalities may be permanent. Because hemorrhagic cystitis is a common complication of cyclophosphamide (Cytoxan) therapy, RT to the bladder is not given concurrently with cyclophosphamide therapy.

Reproductive organs: (See Section X, "Late Effects of Childhood Cancer.") *Testes.* At doses of 1 Gy, patients may temporarily experience low sperm count, and with RT of 4–6 Gy, azoospermia can persist for 5 years.

Ovaries. Administered dosages greater than 6 Gy may result in sterilization.

Hematopoietic: Circulating lymphocytes are acutely sensitive to the effects of RT. Even when little or no bone marrow is included in the RT field, the peripheral lymphocyte count can fall. White blood cells other than lymphocytes and platelets are less sensitive; however, the bone marrow precursors of these cells are quite sensitive. RT to a large area of bone marrow will produce significant declines in the circulating blood count.

Bones: An RT dosage of 6–10 Gy will result in slow bone growth at the epiphyseal plate. A dosage higher than 20 Gy will arrest growth, and hypoplastic changes in muscle and tissue are often more apparent than the alterations in the bone (see Section X, "Late Effects of Childhood Cancer," for a further discussion of this effect).

Skin: An RT dosage higher than 20 Gy will produce erythema. Desquamation of the skin is seen at dosages of approximately 40 Gy and moist desquamation occurs at 50 Gy. These reactions are resolved within a few weeks after completion of RT. Temporary alopecia develops after dosages of 25–30 Gy. Hair regrowth occurs within 3–4 months after RT. Permanent hair loss occurs with RT dosages higher than 55 Gy (Cullen et al., 2002).

Endocrine glands: Changes in endocrine glands are delayed effects (see Section X, "Late Effects of Childhood Cancer," for a discussion).

Nursing Assessment and Interventions

The patient will usually receive daily fractions of RT Monday through Friday for consecutive weeks until the entire dose has been delivered. Most RT is delivered on an outpatient basis. Some side effects, such as stomatitis, nausea, vomiting, diarrhea, neutropenic fever, and increased intracranial pressure, may require hospitalization. During hospitalization, the radiation oncologist and the primary oncologist must determine whether the patient should continue with RT or should discontinue therapy until the symptoms improve.

When radiation therapy and chemotherapy are given together, it is the nurse's responsibility to be aware of the interaction between the two treatment modalities and to monitor for side effects. Acute side effects occur within the first 2–3 weeks, whereas late effects occur at least 3 months after the completion of radiation therapy.

Assessment: Side effects experienced as a result of RT are related to the site that was irradiated. These are among the side effects that should be assessed:

- Central nervous system—headache, nausea and vomiting, somnolence syndrome, malaise, fatigue
- Head and neck—mucositis, pain, xerostomia, dysphagia, esophagitis
- Abdomen—liver tenderness, nausea and vomiting, diarrhea, cramping, tenesmus
- Lungs—dyspnea, chest pain, dry cough
- Heart—chest pain, dyspnea, fever
- Genitourinary—urinary frequency, pain on urination, hematuria
- Hematologic—myelosuppression, fatigue, bruising and bleeding
- Skin—redness, desquamation, alopecia, pruritis, and pigment changes. Hair loss usually occurs around the third week of RT, with regrowth beginning within 3 months of completion of therapy. Radiation recall is a phenomenon that may be seen when chemotherapy follows radiation. The affected skin may have a painless erythematous area where the patient previously received radiation. This effect also can occur when radiation follows chemotherapy.

Interventions: Interventions are implemented to decrease the specific side effects caused by RT.

Central nervous system.

- Educate the patient and the parents regarding somnolence syndrome.
- Encourage the child to rest during the day.
- Recommend earlier bedtimes.

Head and neck.

- Offer pain medications, as necessary.
- Treat mucositis (see Section V, "Side Effects of Treatment"). For severe mucositis, hospitalization for parenteral narcotics, hydration, and nutrition may be required.
- Offer nutritional supplements, if indicated.
- Provide agents to increase saliva.

Abdomen.

- Provide antiemetics for nausea and vomiting.
- Prevent dehydration and reinforce the importance of oral intake of liquids.
- Treat diarrhea by administering fluids and giving antidiarrheal agents, if indicated.
- Monitor intake and weight changes closely.
- Provide sitz baths to keep perirectal area clean.
- Instruct patients and families not to use enemas or rectal suppositories or thermometers.

Lungs and heart.

- Monitor for dyspnea, hacking cough, and low-grade fever, which may indicate pulmonary changes.
- Monitor for pneumonitis, which may require oxygen, systemic corticosteroids, and cough suppressants.
- Teach deep breathing exercises.
- Report symptoms to the physician.

Genitourinary.

- Monitor for urinary frequency, pain on urination, and hematuria.
- Reinforce the patient's oral intake.
- Report symptoms to the physician.

Hematologic.

- Monitor blood counts during RT. Monitoring frequency depends on the site being irradiated and whether there is any concurrent chemotherapy. Some patients may require packed red blood cell transfusions during RT to keep hemoglobin above 10 g/dl.
- Report symptoms of fever or increased bruising to the physician.

Skin.

- Observe skin changes closely.
- Prevent infections.
- Emphasize the importance of keeping the patient's skin clean and dry.
- All skin care products should be completely washed off before RT. During RT, use only skin products recommended by the radiation staff, which may include water-soluble moisturizers and aloe vera and lanolin products. After the course of RT is completed, use moisturizers liberally.
- Use sun screens with sun protection factor (SPF) 30 on skin, and have patient avoid prolonged sun exposure.
- Address hair loss and use of head covering or wig.

Expected Patient and Family Outcomes

- The patient and the family are knowledgeable about RT.
- The patient and the family understand what to expect during the RT treatments.
- The patient experiences minimal side effects during RT.
- The patient and the family understand the specific short-term and late effects that may be experienced after RT.

References

Cullen, P.M., Derrickson, J.D., & Potter, J.A. (2002). Radiation therapy. In C.R. Baggott, K.P. Kelly, D. Fochtman, & G.V. Foley (Eds.), *Nursing care of children and adolescents with cancer* (pp. 116–132). Philadelphia: W.B. Saunders.

Halperin, E.C., Constine, L.S., Tarbell, N.J., & Kun, L. (1999). *Pediatric radiation oncology* (3rd ed.). Philadelphia: Lippincott Williams & Wilkins.

Swift, P. (2002). Novel techniques in the delivery of radiation in pediatric oncology. *Pediatric Clinics of North America, 49,* 1107–1129.

Tarbell, N.J. & Koov, H.M. (2002). General principles of radiation oncology. In P.A. Pizzo & D.G. Poplack (Eds.), *Principles and practice of pediatric oncology* (pp.369–380). Philadelphia: Lippincott Williams & Wilkins.

Hematopoietic Stem Cell Transplantation

Robbie Norville, Rebecca Monroe, and Kathy Forte

Principles of Treatment

The purpose of hematopoietic stem cell transplantation (HSCT) is to replace diseased, damaged, or absent hematopoietic stem cells with healthy stem cells. In general, allogeneic transplants are used if the patient's bone marrow is diseased. The new immune system from the donor also may be effective in preventing a recurrence of disease by providing a graft-versus-leukemia effect. Allogeneic transplants also are used to replace damaged or absent cells for a number of hematologic and immunodeficiency disorders. An autologous transplant is used to provide a stem cell rescue after higher doses of chemotherapy or radiation therapy. In some circumstances, autologous stem cells may be used, even if there is a history of disease in the bone marrow. These stem cells are usually treated or purged to remove residual tumor cells before the infusion.

Role in Childhood Cancer

Children with malignancies may not always be cured with conventional chemotherapy, surgery, and radiation therapy. Higher doses of chemotherapy and radiation therapy, which might prove to be curative, can cause myelosuppression as a dose-limiting toxicity. Infusing stem cells that were previously collected from the patient or stem cells from a healthy donor allows the bone marrow to recover after intensive therapy. In addition, patients who have tumor invasion of the bone marrow benefit from the transplantation of healthy cells from a donor. HSCT has proved to play an important role in treating children who have aggressive malignancies in first remission or have recurrent disease.

Types of Hematopoietic Stem Cell Transplantation

Allogeneic: The stem cells are collected from someone other than the recipient.

Matched related. This involves a 6/6 antigen match (usually a sibling).

Mismatched related. This involves a 3/6–5/6 antigen match (usually a sibling or a parent).

Matched unrelated. This type involves a 5/6 or a 6/6 antigen match from an unrelated donor.

Cord blood (related or unrelated). This type involves a 3/6–6/6 antigen match from cord blood.

Autologous: The stem cells are collected from the recipient (see **Table 4-8** for an overview of the advantages and disadvantages for each type of stem cell source).

HLA typing: Human leukocyte antigen (HLA) refers to a complex series of proteins on the surface of human cells. These proteins, called antigens, make up the major histocompatibility complex, which helps the body recognize cells that are foreign. The antigens of primary concern for typing include A, B, and DR. The DR antigens are among the predictors for the risk of graft-versus-host disease (GVHD). Each individual inherits one set of antigens from each parent. A biological parent is always at least a 3/6 match for the child (see **Figure 4-2** for an example of HLA typing). Through the growth and diversity of national and international donor registries, more patients are being provided matched related donors.

Diseases Treated with a Hematopoietic Stem Cell Transplant

See **Table 4-9** for a list of diseases treated using HSCT and the rationales for treatment.

Collection of Stem Cells

Stem cells are the immature progenitor cells that mature in the bone marrow. Upon maturation, they are released into the circulation as white cells, red cells, or platelets. Stem cells can be collected from the bone marrow, peripheral blood, or blood from the placenta and umbilical cord that is obtained postpartum.

Bone marrow harvest: Stem cells are removed from the donor's posterior and, possibly, the anterior iliac crest. This procedure is performed under general anesthesia at most medical centers. Cells are mixed with heparin (Liquaemin) and filtered to remove bone chips, spicules, fat cells, and blood clots. The advantages are that this is a relatively quick and well-tested method of collection. The risks to the donor are associated with general anesthesia, infection, and mild-to-moderate pain at the harvest site.

Peripheral stem cell collection: Stem cells are collected through a large catheter by a pheresis machine, which selects the stem cells from the circulating blood on the basis of weight. The remaining cells are reinfused into the patient. Stem cells are mobilized into the peripheral blood circulation through the use of granulocyte colony-stimulating factors (G-CSF) or granulocyte-macrophage colony-stimulating factor (GM-CSF) or high-dose priming chemotherapy, such as cyclophosphamide (Cytoxan) (for autologous patients only). The stem cells are then mixed with heparin (Liquaemin) and a preservative prior to being frozen (i.e., cryopreservation).

The advantages to this collection method are that there is no need for general anesthesia for the donor, engraftment is faster, and there is presumed to be a decreased risk of tumor contamination compared with autologous marrow harvest. The risks to the donor are associated with bone pain as a consequence of growth factor administration, reaction to citrate (i.e., numbness and tingling in the fingers and lips or hypotension) during collection, and catheter placement.

Cord blood collection: Stem cells are collected from a newborn's cord and placenta immediately after birth. The advantages of this practice are quick and easy collection and a decreased chance of transmission of viral disease. There is no risk to the donor.

Table 4-8. A Comparison of the Advantages and Disadvantages of Donor Sources

Type of Stem Cell Transplant	Advantages	Disadvantages
Matched related	Healthy source of cells Easy access to the donor	Some graft-versus-host disease (GVHD) 30% likelihood of a sibling match
Mismatched related	Healthy source of cells Easy access to the donor Availability of a donor for most patients	Greater risk of GVHD Risk of graft failure
Matched unrelated	Healthy source of cells	Risk of GVHD 3–6-month waiting time for donor procurement Few ethnic minority donors Expensive donor charges
Cord blood	Healthy source of cells Easy procurement of cells No risk to the donor Decreased chance of viral transmission More diverse HLA types	Limited number of cells per unit Increased time to platelet engraftment Potential transmission of genetic diseases
Autologous	Easy access to the donor No GVHD	No graft-versus-leukemia effect (increased risk of relapse) Possible tumor contamination

Figure 4-2. An Example of HLA Typing

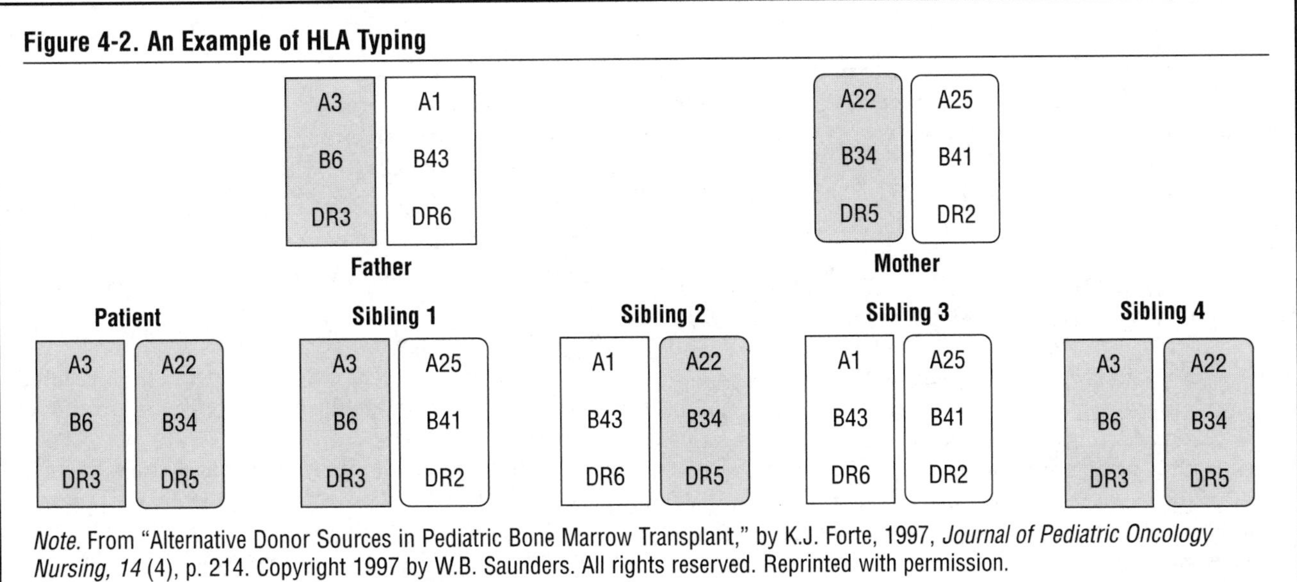

Note. From "Alternative Donor Sources in Pediatric Bone Marrow Transplant," by K.J. Forte, 1997, *Journal of Pediatric Oncology Nursing, 14* (4), p. 214.

Stem Cell Purging and T-Cell Depletion

Purpose: The purpose of stem cell purging is to remove any remaining tumor cells before autologous stem cell transplantation. The purpose of T-cell depletion is to decrease the number of T lymphocytes to help decrease the risk of GVHD (before allogeneic stem cell transplantation). The purpose of CD34+ (very young stem cells that are not lymphocytes) selection is to collect specific progenitor cells for infusion in either autologous or allogeneic stem cell transplantation.

Methods:

Immunologic technique. A monoclonal antibody specific for a type of tumor or T lymphocytes is added to the stem cells.

Pharmacological technique. A chemotherapeutic analog is added to the stem cells to kill the remaining tumor cells. An example is 4HC, a derivative of cyclophosphamide (Cytoxan).

Lymphocyte depletion. Lymphocytes are removed by several different techniques: elutriation, a method that uses a centrifuge to select cells based on size; anti-T-cell monoclonal antibodies, a method in which antibodies bind with and remove lymphocytes; E-rosetting, a technique in which red blood cells from sheep are added to marrow to bind with T lymphocytes; and CD34+ stem cell selection, a method that

Table 4-9. Diseases for Which Hematopoietic Stem Cell Transplantation Is a Treatment Option

Disease	Rationale for Hematopoietic Stem Cell Transplantation
Leukemias, lymphomas	Chemotherapy, with or without total body irradiation, is used to eradicate tumor cells and to make room for engraftment of healthy cells. Irradiation is often used in mismatched and unrelated transplants.
Solid tumors: neuroblastoma, sarcoma, brain tumor	High doses of chemotherapy or radiation therapy are given to kill tumor cells. An autologous "rescue" is given to prevent prolonged myelosuppression.
Hematologic diseases: thalassemia, sickle-cell disease, severe aplastic anemia, Fanconi's anemia	Chemotherapy is given to eradicate cells in the bone marrow and to make space for engraftment of healthy allogeneic cells. The new donor cells will produce normal white cells, red cells, and platelets.
Immunodeficiency diseases: Wiskott-Aldrich syndrome, severe combined immunodeficiency syndrome (SCIDS)	Chemotherapy is given to eradicate cells in the bone marrow and to make space for engraftment of healthy allogeneic cells. In the case of SCIDS, chemotherapy may not always be used.
Genetic diseases: adrenoleukodystrophy, metachromatic leukodystrophy, Hurler's syndrome	Chemotherapy is given to eradicate cells in the bone marrow. Donor cells, which will eventually produce the deficient enzyme, are infused.

involves the addition of a monoclonal antibody that is specific for CD34+ stem cells, which results in significant T-cell reduction in the final product.

Evaluation of a Donor and a Recipient

Evaluation of a donor: A donor must have healthy stem cells and be able to tolerate the harvest procedure. The acceptable age range is 4 months to 65 years. The evaluation should include a physical examination, a complete health history to rule out genetic diseases, and serological testing that includes a CBC with differential, chemistry profile, coagulation screen, infectious disease testing (hepatitis profile, HIV, cytomegalovirus [CMV], herpes simplex virus [HSV], Epstein-Barr virus), crossmatching (to determine if the donor is ABO-compatible with the patient), confirming HLA typing, and a pregnancy test, if appropriate. Donors may be asked to donate an autologous unit of blood prior to harvest. Issues, such as testing procedures, health risks, and psychological sequelae, should be discussed with donors, especially child donors. Consultation with child life specialists, social workers, and clergy may be beneficial.

Evaluation of a patient: The patient should have a more extensive evaluation. In addition to the items listed for the donor, the work-up should include organ function tests, such as a chest X ray, echocardiogram, pulmonary function test (if the patient's age is appropriate), creatinine clearance/glomerular filtration rate, audiogram (if the patient has a history of hearing loss or has previously received ototoxic agents), an eye exam (if the patient is to receive total body irradiation), and a dental exam. Other serological tests are thyroid function tests and serum immunoglobulins. Disease staging evaluations depend on the type of disease and previous areas of involvement, including scans, bone marrow aspiration, and lumbar puncture. Neuropsychological testing may be performed as a baseline for late effects monitoring. Information regarding sperm banking and egg harvesting should be provided to age-appropriate patients.

Preparative Regimens

The preparative regimen serves the following purposes:

- eradicates tumor cells (malignancies only)
- immunosuppresses the patient to prevent rejection of the graft
- prepares the bone marrow space to allow for the growth of healthy cells.

In general, the preparative regimen is given for 4–9 days prior to the stem cell infusion. The type and timing of therapy offered depends upon the patient's disease and the type of stem cells to be infused.

Chemotherapy: Chemotherapeutic agents are the mainstay of therapy and are used for most HSCTs. Commonly used agents include the following:

- alkylating agents such as cyclophosphamide (Cytoxan), busulfan (Myleran), melphalan (Alkeran), thiotepa (Thiotepa)
- antimetabolites such as cytarabine (Cytosine Arabinoside)
- nitrosoureas (carmustine [BCNU])
- heavy metals (carboplatin [CBDCA], cisplatin [Platinol])
- plant alkaloids (etoposide [VP-16]).

Radiation therapy (RT): Radiation therapy is used to eradicate tumor cells in the central nervous system and sanctuary sites, which may not be able to be treated by chemotherapy alone. It is also used to provide increased immunosuppression for patients who are receiving an unrelated or mismatched transplant and to decrease the risk of graft failure and graft-versus-host disease (GVHD).

Total body irradiation. This type of RT is usually given in fractionated doses twice a day for 4–5 days.

Local control irradiation. This type of RT may be given before or after a transplant to patients with solid tumors or to patients who have a history of central nervous system disease.

Immunotherapy: Immunosuppressive agents such as antithymocyte globulin (ATG) are used to bind with and destroy the patient's circulating T lymphocytes in an attempt to decrease the incidence of graft rejection. Antithymocyte globulin usually is given once a day for 3 days during the preparative regimen. Newer monoclonal antibodies, such as Campath (alemtuzumab) and CD45, are being used to deplete the patient's circulating lymphocytes, also in an attempt to decrease the incidence of graft rejection.

Infusion of Stem Cells

Stem cells harvested from bone marrow, peripheral blood, and cord blood can be frozen and infused at a later time.

Types of infusion:

Frozen. Frozen stem cells are most often used in autologous transplants (i.e., transplants in which cells are collected from the patient). Stem cells are frozen or cryopreserved, most commonly with a preservative called dimethyl sulfoxide (DMSO). DMSO has a garlic-like odor that is excreted through the lungs of the patient for 1–2 days after the transplant. DMSO can cause transient cardiac arrhythmias, most commonly bradycardia. Many centers require some form of cardiac monitoring during and immediately after the infusion. Rapid IV infusion is recommended. Stem cells should not be irradiated or filtered.

Fresh. Stem cells used for allogeneic transplants usually are fresh when infused, generally within 48 hours of collection. The ABO status and volume of donor cells will dictate the need for red cell or volume depletion. The method of infusion is slow intravenous infusion over 2–4 hours. Stem cells should not be irradiated or filtered.

Nursing assessment:

- Know the potential side effects and adverse reactions associated with each type of hematopoietic stem cell transplantation.
  - For infusion of frozen stem cells, the side effects include a bad taste in the mouth, nausea, vomiting, arrhythmia (bradycardia), hypertension, hemoglobinuria, flushing, allergic reaction (anaphylaxis), renal failure, micropulmonary emboli, fluid overload, and infection.
  - For infusion of fresh stem cells, the side effects include allergic reaction (anaphylaxis), hemolytic transfusion reactions, fluid overload, micropulmonary emboli, and infection.
- Assess the patient's and the family's understanding of the infusion and monitoring procedures.
- Assess the patient's vital signs before, during, and after the infusion (an EKG and pulse oximetry monitoring may be required).

Nursing interventions:

Base nursing interventions on the type of stem cell infusion done.

- For infusion of frozen stem cells, patients are premedicated with an antihistamine, an antiemetic, a corticosteroid and/or antipyretic, and diuretic. Prehydration fluids with an alkaline base added are administered 4–12 hours before the infusion. During the infusion, which is done through a central venous access device, the patient should be monitored for evidence of adverse reactions. After infusion, the patient should be monitored for adverse reactions according to the institution's policy. Postinfusion fluids (12–24 hours) may be infused, diuretics may be administered to ensure renal perfusion, adequate urine output should be maintained, and alkaline urine should be maintained for 12–24 hours.
- For infusion of fresh stem cells, the premedications include an antihistamine, a corticosteroid, an antipyretic and/or a diuretic may be given if there is an ABO incompatibility or the patient has a history of transfusion reactions). Prehydration fluids are indicated when there is an ABO incompatibility (12–24 hours before the infusion). During the infusion, the patient should be monitored for evidence of adverse reactions, and stem cells should be infused through a central venous access device. After the infusion, the patient should be monitored for adverse reactions according to the institution's policy. Postinfusion fluids should be administered if there is an ABO incompatibility, and brisk urine output should be maintained for 12 hours.

Expected Patient and Family Outcomes

- The patient, the family, or both can verbalize the infusion and monitoring procedures.
- The patient tolerates an infusion without adverse reactions.

Complications of Hematopoietic Stem Cell Transplantation

Complications related to HSCT can occur at any time during the transplant process. **Table 4-10** reviews the time sequence of complications with a HSCT.

Bone marrow suppression: All cell lines in the bone marrow will be eradicated, causing low levels of hemoglobin, platelets, and white blood cells and an absolute neutrophil count (ANC) of 0. It occurs 7–10 days after the preparative regimen is started.

Engraftment is the term used to indicate that the new stem cells have taken hold and are starting to reproduce. The timing of engraftment depends on the stem cell source, the patient's history of prior therapy, and the patient's condition. An ANC of 500 and a platelet count of 20,000/mm^3 without transfusions indicate engraftment. In general, white blood cells engraft before platelets. As red cells engraft, the recipient's blood type will change to that of the donor. The average number of days after a transplant for white blood cell and platelet engraftment is listed in **Table 4-11**.

Neutropenia: The risk of infection is significantly increased when the ANC is less than 500. Measures for preventing infection include air filtration, hand washing, and screening visitors. Isolation policies vary from institution to institution. Prophylactic antimicrobials may be used to prevent herpes, cytomegalovirus, and/or fungal and bacterial infections.

Anemia: Transfusions often are given when hemoglobin levels fall below 8 g/dl. There is a potential for cardiac and respiratory compromise when hemoglobin levels fall below 7 g/dl.

Nursing assessment.

- Inspect the patient's mouth, rectum, IV sites, and all wounds for infection.
- Assess for signs and symptoms of infection: dysuria, sore throat, rectal pain, and cough.
- Check the patient's vital signs every 4 hours.
- Assess the patient for signs and symptoms of anemia: pallor, fatigue, tachycardia, shortness of breath, and dizziness.
- Test the urine, emesis, and stool for blood.
- Assess for bruising, petechiae, epitaxis, or oozing from the patient's gums or the central venous line.
- Assess the patient for signs and symptoms of bleeding or blood loss.
- Check the WBC, ANC, hemoglobin and hematocrit, and platelet count daily.

Nursing interventions.

- Initiate bleeding precautions.
- Call a physician if the patient is febrile or has other signs and symptoms of infection, anemia, or bleeding.
- Administer antimicrobial therapy and monitor the patient's response to treatment.
- Teach the patient, the family, or both how to provide meticulous oral and perineal hygiene.
- Administer red blood cell transfusions and platelet transfusions as needed (maintain a Hgb of greater than or equal to 8.0 and a platelet count of greater than or equal to 20,000/mm^3 [all blood products except for stem cells should be irradiated and leukocyte depleted]).
- Administer oxygen to prevent tissue hypoxia, if needed.
- Teach the patient, the family, or both the signs and symptoms of infection, anemia, and thrombocytopenia.

Expected patient and family outcomes.

- The patient will experience minimal complications related to infection or blood loss.
- The patient, the family, or both will understand the signs and symptoms of infections, anemia, and bleeding.
- The patient, the family, or both will perform self-care activities to prevent infection and bleeding.

Infectious complications: Infections occur because of the absence of circulating white blood cells after the preparative regimen, the use of immunosuppressive therapy to prevent or treat graft-versus-host disease, and the prolonged absence of donor immunoglobins after initial engraftment. All of the infections listed **Table 4–12** can occur later, particularly if the patient is being treated with immunosuppressive therapy, such as steroids.

Prevention. If the patient or the donor is HSV-positive, acyclovir (Zovirax) should be administered. If the patient or the donor is CMV-positive, a higher dose of acyclovir or valacyclovir should be administered starting on the day before stem cell transfusion and ganciclovir (Cytovene) or foscarnet (Foscavir) should be administered after engraftment of the stem cells occurs. There is controversy about the efficacy of

Table 4-10. The Timing Sequence of Complications Associated with Hematopoietic Stem Cell Transplantation

Immediate (First Week)	Delayed (First 100 Days)	Late Effects (After 100 Days)
Nausea/vomiting	Bone marrow suppression	Immunosuppression
Diarrhea	Mucositis	Chronic graft-versus-host disease
Hemorrhagic cystitis	Hemorrhagic cystitis	Cataracts
Parotitis	Anorexia	Endocrine dysfunction: thyroid, gonadal growth
	Capillary leak syndrome	Pulmonary restrictive disease
	Veno-occlusive disease	Secondary malignancies
	Graft failure	Recurrence of disease
	Graft-versus-host disease	Infections: encapsulated bacteria, cytomegalovirus, varicella zoster virus, other latent viruses, Pneumocystis carinii pneumonia
	Pneumonitis	Sun sensitivity
	Pulmonary hemorrhage	
	Acute renal failure	
	Infections: bacterial, viral (herpes simplex, adenovirus cytomegalovirus), fungal	

Table 4–11. Average Number of Days After HSCT for Engraftment to Occur

Type of HSCT	Average Number of Days: ANC > 500	Average Number of Days: Platelets > 20,000
Autologous: peripheral blood stem cells	+12	+21
Autologous: purged marrow	+28	+35
Allogeneic: matched sibling	+16	+28
Allogeneic: matched unrelated	+23	+28
Allogeneic: unrelated cord blood	+23	+56
Allogeneic: peripheral blood stem cells	+12	+16

Table 4–12. Infectious Complications of HSCT

The Types of Possible Infection	Time of Occurrence
Bacterial (gram-positive and gram-negative)	2–3 weeks after HSCT
Viral: herpes simplex virus	2 weeks after HSCT
Viral: cytomegalovirus	2–4 months after HSCT
Fungal: *Candida, Aspergillus*	1–2 months after HSCT
Protozoa: *Pneumocystis*	2–4 months after HSCT
Viral: varicella zoster	1–6 months after HSCT

immunoglobin therapy. Some centers infuse immunoglobin (IgG) every 2–4 weeks; other centers treat only patients with low IgG levels. Many centers use fluconazole (Diflucan) or low-dose amphotericin B (Fungizone) as prophylaxis for fungal infections.

Nursing assessment.

- Check the patient's temperature every 4 hours and as needed.
- Assess the patient for signs and symptoms of infection every 8 hours.

Nursing interventions. Treatment varies according to institutional policies and sensitivity data.

- Draw blood cultures and start broad-spectrum antibiotics as soon as possible for a first fever; get a chest X ray and take a throat or urine culture, if applicable.
- Draw blood cultures once a day for subsequent fevers; if the patient appears ill, alter the therapy to provide the broadest coverage. (Patients who continue to be febrile for more than 5 days should be placed on a treatment dose of amphotericin B [Fungizone]. CT scanning to assess for areas of infection should be considered.)

Expected patient and family outcomes.

- The patient will experience minimal infectious complications.
- The patient, the family, or both will understand the signs and symptoms of infection.

GI toxicity: Nausea or vomiting can begin within the first 24 hours of starting the preparative regimen and continue through the first week after the transplant. Vomiting can recur after a transplant due to antibiotics, infections, graft-versus-host disease, or slow mucosal healing.

Diarrhea can begin any time during the preparative regimen and can continue as long as 2 weeks after HSCT. Causes of delayed diarrhea include infection, refeeding syndrome, or graft-versus-host disease.

Anorexia can start during the preparative regimen and can continue for several months after HSCT. Causes include a change in taste sensation, dry mouth, damaged mucosa, nausea and vomiting due to the preparative regimen, and GVHD.

Mucositis usually starts by the 3rd day after the HSCT, peaks by the 7th through the 10th day and starts to heal by the 12th day (healing often occurs with engraftment of WBCs).

Nursing assessment.

- Assess the patient for nausea, vomiting, diarrhea, and pain.
- Check the patient's weight on a daily basis.
- Assess the patient's intake and output during every shift.

Nursing interventions.

- Give scheduled antiemetic agents, such as ondansetron (Zofran) or granisetron (Kytril) (serotonin antagonists), during the preparative regimen; add steroids for breakthrough vomiting.
- Stop the serotonin antagonists 1–2 days after transplant. Continue other agents, such as benzodiazapenes, as long as needed for nausea and vomiting.
- Administer fluids or total parenteral nutrition, as needed.
- Discontinue total parenteral nutrition and start nasogastric feedings if the gut has healed and the patient is still unable to eat by mouth.
- Offer nutritional counseling and supplements.
- Send a specimen for a stool culture if the patient develops diarrhea.
- Promote good oral hygiene, perirectal hygiene, and skin care.

- Administer opioids IV for pain associated with mucositis.

Expected patient and family outcomes.

- The patient will experience minimal discomfort due to nausea, vomiting, diarrhea, and mucositis.
- The patient will receive adequate fluids and caloric intake.

Capillary leak syndrome: Tissue damage from the preparative regimen causes the release of cytokines (IL-2, TNF). This, in turn, causes increased capillary permeability, which can lead to weight gain, fluid retention, ascites, or pulmonary edema. The highest risk for its occurrence is 7–14 days after HSCT.

Nursing assessment.

- Assess the patient for signs and symptoms of fluid overload (intake greater than output, weight gain, high blood pressure, "wet lungs").

Nursing interventions.

- Notify a physician if the patient has signs and symptoms of fluid overload.
- Administer diuretics, as needed.
- Administer a renal dose of dopamine (Intropin) to increase renal perfusion.

Expected patient and family outcome.

- The patient will experience minimal complications associated with capillary leak syndrome.

Veno-occlusive disease: The preparative regimen and previous liver damage may cause the veins of the liver to become narrow and fibrotic, which can lead to obstruction of blood flow, liver enlargement, and ascites. The classic presentation of veno-occlusive disease includes elevated bilirubin, 5% weight gain, and painful hepatomegaly. It occurs 7–21 days after HSCT.

Nursing assessment.

- Measure strictly the patient's intake and output.
- Assess the patient's weight and abdominal girth twice each day.
- Check the patient's liver and kidney function studies.
- Assess the patient for evidence of ascites, pain in the right upper quadrant, and jaundice.
- Check the platelet count and other coagulation studies (coagulation profile, antithrombin III [ATIII] level), as needed. (The use of anticoagulants is controversial. Some centers advocate the replacement of ATIII if the serum level is low.)

Nursing interventions.

- Administer diuretics and pain medications as needed.

Expected patient and family outcomes.

- The patient will have minimal complications associated with veno-occlusive disease.
- The patient will have adequate pain control.
- The patient and the family will understand the signs and symptoms and the management of veno-occlusive disease.

Graft failure: Primary graft failure can occur if the stem cell dose is too low or if the patient's immune system has not been completely ablated, thereby allowing the body to recognize the donor cells as foreign. Other causes of graft failure include myelosuppressive medications, viral or fungal infections, or recurrence of tumor.

Primary graft failure occurs within the first 100 days after hematopoietic stem cell transplantation. Secondary graft failure can occur within 1 year of HSCT.

The use of immunosuppressants prior to HSCT is used to prevent graft failure. To treat graft failure, another infusion of donor cells can be administered with or without additional immunosuppression.

Nursing assessment.

- Check the CBC with a differential on a daily basis.

Nursing interventions.

- Provide supportive care measures to prevent or treat infection.
- Help the patient and the family identify coping strategies if engraftment does not occur.

Expected patient and family outcome.

- The patient will experience minimal complications throughout the period of pancytopenia.

Acute graft-versus-host disease (AGVHD): AGVHD occurs within the first 100 days after HSCT; it usually coincides with engraftment. The donor cells recognize that the patient's body is foreign and mount an attack. The target organs include the skin, liver, and gut. A red maculopapular rash typically starts on the palms and soles and spreads down from the head to the trunk and, lastly, down the lower extremities. A severe rash includes blister formation and desquamation. An elevated bilirubin count indicates liver involvement. Watery green diarrhea that contains pieces of bowel tissue is most characteristic of gut involvement (see **Table 4-13** for staging and grading).

Preventive measures include administration of agents such as cyclosporine (Sandimmune), tacrolimus (Prograf), methotrexate (Mexate), steroids, or monclonal antibodies. T-cell depletion prior to stem cell infusion may also prevent or limit AGVHD.

Nursing assessment.

- Assess the patient for clinical signs and symptoms of AGVHD (e.g., skin rash, diarrhea, abdominal pain, and elevated bilirubin).
- Measure strictly the patient's intake and output and assess the patient's fluid and electrolyte status if the patient has diarrhea.
- Assess the patient for right upper quadrant pain, diffuse abdominal pain, and generalized skin pain.

Nursing interventions.

- Prepare the patient and the family for the patient's skin or rectal biopsy (the patient may also need an endoscopy).
- Administer immunosuppressive therapy. First-line therapy is usually administration of high-dose steroids. Second-line therapy varies according to institutional priorities. (See

Table 4-14 for the mechanisms of action and the toxicities of immunosuppressive agents used to prevent and treat AGVHD.)

- Provide symptom management for skin AGVHD, including the use of hypoallergenic skin moisturizers, gel dressings, or porcine dressings for severe desquamation.
- Provide adequate pain control.
- Teach the patient and the family about the signs, symptoms, and treatment associated with AGVHD.
- Teach the patient and the family self-care measures for controlling symptoms.

Expected patient and family outcomes.

- The patient will experience minimal complications associated with AGVHD.
- The patient and the family will identify the signs and symptoms associated with AGVHD and its treatment.
- The patient and the family will describe self-care measures for symptom control.

Chronic graft-versus-host disease (CGVHD): CGVHD is a chronic autoimmune syndrome that resembles collagen vascular disease. The symptoms include dry eyes and mouth, oral ulcerations, hair loss, brittle nails, thin skin with lichenoid and sclerodermatous changes, weight loss, malabsorption of food, elevated liver enzymes and bilirubin, obstructive lung disease, contractures, immunosuppression, and thrombocytopenia. CGVHD can occur from 100 days to 2 years after BMT.

Treatment consists of immunosuppressant therapy that includes many of the same agents used to treat acute graft-versus-host disease. Most patients are treated with cyclosporine (Sandimmune) or tacrolimus (Prograf) and steroids on an every-other-day schedule that is slowly tapered over several months. Several new agents are now available for the treatment of CGVHD (see **Table 4-14**).

Nursing assessment.

- Assess the patient for clinical manifestations of CGHVD.
- Assess the patient's nutritional status.
- Assess for evidence of infection or bleeding (particularly if the patient is taking steroids).
- Check the patient's CBC and electrolytes as needed.

Nursing interventions.

- Administer immunosuppressive therapy and monitor the side effects.
- Maintain measures to prevent infection.
- Use products to lubricate the patient's eyes and mouth, as needed.
- Teach the patient and the family to apply skin moisturizers and protect the patient's skin from sunlight; emphasize the need to use sunscreen.
- Teach the patient and the family the signs and symptoms, therapeutic agents, and symptom management strategies associated with CGVHD.

Table 4-13. GVHD Stage and Grading Systems

Staging of Individual Organ System(s)

Organ	Stage	Description
Skin	+1	Maculopapular (M-P) eruption over <25% of body area
	+2	Maculopapular eruption over 25%–50% of body area
	+3	Generalized erythrodema
	+4	Generalized erythrodema with bullous formation and often with desquanmation
Liver	+1	Bilirubin 2.0–3.0 mg/dl; SGOT 150–750 IU
	+2	Bilirubin 3.1–6.0 mg/dl
	+3	Bilirubin 6.1–15.0 mg/dl
	+4	Bilirubin >15.0 mg/dl
Gut	+1	Diarrhea >30 ml/kg or >500 ml/day
	+2	Diarrhea >60 ml/kg or >1,000 ml/day
	+3	Diarrhea >90 ml/kg or >1,500 ml/day
	+4	Diarrhea >90 ml/kg or >2,000 ml/day; or severe abdominal pain and bleeding with or without ileus

Overall Grading of Acute GVHD

Grade	Skin Staging	Liver Staging		Gut Staging
I	+1 to +2	0		0
II	+1 to +3	+1	and/or	+1
III	+2 to +3	+2 to +4	and/or	+2 to +3
IV	+2 to +4	+2 to +4	and/or	+2 to +4

Adapted from Chao, N.J. (1999). *Graft-versus-host disease* (2nd ed.). Austin, TX: R.G. Landes.

Table 4-14. Immunosuppressive Agents Used in GVHD Prevention and Treatment

Agent/Treatment	Mechanism of Action	Possible Side Effects
Antithymocyte globulin (Atgam)	Eliminates antigen reactive T lymphocytes	Fever, chill, hypotension, rash, anaphylaxis, serum sickness
Azathioprim (Imuran)	Inhibits synthesis of DNA and RNA	Fever, chills, rash, vomiting, myelosuppression, hepatotoxicity
Corticosteroids	Suppresses immune system and inflammation	Myelosuppression, mood swings, hypertension, hyperglycemia, GI bleeding, osteoporosis, acne, cushingoid syndrome, muscle wasting
Cyclosporine (Sandimmune, Neoral)	Inhibits production and release of IL-2; inhibits IL-2-induced activation of T lymphocytes	Renal toxicity, hypertension, magnesium wasting, hyperkalemia, tremors, seizures, gingival, hypertrophy, hirsutism, cortical blindness
Daclizubab (Zenapax)	Inhibits IL-2-mediated activation of lymphocytes	Hypertension, headache, diarrhea, vomiting, edema
Hydroxychloroquine (Plaquenil)	Impairs complement-dependent antigen-antibody reaction	Ocular toxicity, nausea, diarrhea, rash, headache, myelosuppression, photosensitivity
Infliximab (Remicade)	Binds with TNFα	Fever, chills, rash, hypotension, headache, nausea
Methotrexate (Mexate)	Inhibits DNA synthesis by competitively binding with dihydrofolate reductase	Renal toxicity, hepatotoxicity, mucositis
Mycophenolate Mofetil (Cellcept)	Inhibits T- and B-cell proliferation, cytotoxic T-cell generation, and antibody secretion	Myelosuppression, abdominal pain, vomiting, headaches, hypertension, renal toxicity
Muromonab-CD3 (Orthoclone, OKT3)	Modulates T lymphocyte antigen CD3 complex, inactivating T lymphocytes	Reaction to first dose: (cytokine release) fever chills, diarrhea, dizziness, chest pain, wheezing, tremor
Pentostatin (Nipent)	Inhibits DNA synthesis	Fever, chills, rash, vomiting, myelosuppression
Psoralen and ultraviolet radiation (PUVA)	Causes apoptosis of T lymphocytes	Tanning or darkening of skin, itching, stinging sensation
Sirolimus (Rapamune)	Inhibits T lymphocyte activation and proliferation	Hypertension, diarrhea, peripheral edema, rash
Tacrolimus (Prograf, Protopic)	Inhibits T-cell activation	Renal toxicity, hypertension, magnesium wasting, hyperkalemia, tremors, seizures, gingival hypertrophy, hirsutism, cortical blindness
Thalidomide	Decreases the number of helper T cells; increases the number of suppressor T cells	Peripheral neuropathies, constipation, sedation, rash, birth defects

Expected patient and family outcomes.

- The patient will experience minimal complications associated with CGVHD.
- The patient and the family will identify the signs and symptoms and self-care measures associated with CGVHD.

Pulmonary complications:

CMV pneumonitis. CMV pneumonitis is bilateral interstitial pneumonia caused by cytomegalovirus. The signs and symptoms include tachypnea, cough, and low-grade fever. It can occur 2–4 months after HSCT. Treatment consists of ganciclovir (Cytovene) and high-dose immunoglobulin therapy.

Pulmonary hemorrhage. Pulmonary hemorrhage is diffuse bleeding in the lungs, thought to be caused by the release of cytokines at the time of engraftment. It occurs at the time of engraftment. Treatment consists of platelet transfusions, ventilation, and high-dose steroid therapy.

Pulmonary edema. Pulmonary edema is increased capillary permeability leading to fluid leaking into the lungs. It occurs 1–2 weeks after HSCT. Treatment consists of the aggressive use of diuretics; intubation may be necessary.

Nursing assessment.

- Assess the patient's vital signs and respiratory status every 4–8 hours.
- Send surveillance blood cultures or other studies to the lab to test for CMV.
- Check pulse oximetry or a blood gas if the patient is in respiratory distress.

Nursing interventions.

- Administer antiviral therapy, diuretics, or steroids, as needed.
- Administer blood products as needed.
- Administer supplemental oxygen or ventilation, as needed.
- Provide anticipatory guidance to the patient, the family, or both, if the patient requires intensive respiratory support.

Expected patient and family outcomes.

- The patient will experience minimal pulmonary complications.
- The patient, the family, or both will understand the signs and symptoms and treatment associated with CMV pneumonitis, pulmonary hemorrhage, or edema.

Renal toxicity:

Acute renal failure. Acute renal failure is due to damage to the epithelial cells of the lining of the renal tubules because of medications that are toxic to the kidneys or decreased blood flow. The creatinine and BUN increase, and there is decreased ability to excrete fluid and metabolic waste. Dialysis may be required if the toxicity is severe. Increased incidence is associated with medications that are toxic to the kidneys.

Nursing assessment.

- Monitor the patient's blood chemistries on a daily basis.
- Monitor the levels of medications that are toxic to the kidneys (e.g., cyclosporine [Sandimmune], vancomycin [Vancocin], amphotericin B [Fungizone]).
- Assess the patient's intake and output during every shift.
- Check the patient's weight every day.

Nursing interventions.

- Adjust the dose and frequency of medications that are toxic to the kidneys, as ordered.
- Administer a renal dose of dopamine (Intropin) to promote renal perfusion.
- Use dialysis if the renal failure is severe.

Hemorrhagic cystitis. A metabolite of cyclophosphamide (Cytoxan) irritates the bladder mucosa and causes bleeding. Viruses such as adenovirus and BK virus also can cause cystitis. Hemorrhagic cystitis can occur within 24 hours of administration of the chemotherapy and as late as 2 months after HSCT.

Nursing assessment.

- Measure the patient's intake and output.
- Test the patient's urine for blood at least once a day.
- Culture the urine for viruses if hematuria occurs.
- Assess the patient frequently to determine if there is pain with urination.

Nursing interventions.

- Administer vigorous hydration (i.e., 1.5 times the maintenance level), and encourage the patient to empty the bladder frequently.
- Administer mesna (Mesenex) in conjunction with cyclophosphamide (Cytoxan).
- Provide continuous bladder irrigation if the cystitis is severe.
- Administer pain medications as needed.

Expected patient and family outcomes.

- The patient will experience minimal renal toxicity and complications associated with hemorrhagic cystitis.
- The patient, the family, or both will understand the supportive care measures used to prevent or treat renal toxicity or cystitis.

Discharge Planning

General discharge criteria can include the following:

- The patient has an absolute neutrophil count of 500.
- The patient is afebrile and preferably is off intravenous antibiotics.
- The patient is able to take oral medications (especially immunosuppressant therapy).
- The patient's oral intake of calories and fluids is 50% of his or her caloric need (or is on total parenteral nutrition or nasogastric feedings).
- The family is able to care for the central venous line and any nutritional support that is needed.
- The family understands the discharge instructions, including the purposes of medications and infection precautions.

Parents should receive education about the following issues prior to discharge:

- the importance of calling a member of the transplant team immediately when there are signs or symptoms of fever, bleeding that does not stop within a few minutes, severe vomiting or diarrhea, change in level of consciousness, breathing difficulty, skin rash, or exudate at the central venous line site
- the importance of communicating the signs or symptoms related to decreased appetite or weight loss; intermittent nausea, vomiting, or diarrhea; mild headache; mild cough; or fatigue at the next clinic visit
- how to take a temperature accurately
- how to care for the central venous line at home
- the importance of protecting the skin from sunlight
- the importance of talking with the bone marrow transplantation team before taking medications or immunizations
- swimming, pets, and the child's reentry to school.

Outpatient Follow-Up

Outpatient follow-up appointments are tailored to meet the needs of the patient. If the patient has not engrafted platelets, clinic visits may be as frequent as five times a week, including weekend visits. In general, it is necessary to check the blood counts, serum chemistries, and medication levels (cyclosporine [Sandimmune] or tacrolimus [Prograf]) frequently for the first 3 months after HSCT. Patients who receive an autologous transplant usually do not have to be followed as closely as patients who receive allogeneic transplants, and care may be transferred to the referring oncologist when engraftment has occurred and HSCT complications have been resolved. Patients who receive an allogeneic transplant are followed closely by the HSCT team for the first 100 days and are seen regularly for the first year after transplant and annually thereafter.

Significant tests to be done 1 year after hematopoietic stem cell transplantation:

- CBC with differential
- chemistry panel
- immunoglobulin levels
- immune function testing
- thyroid function tests
- follicle-stimulating hormone, lutenizing hormone, estradiol for girls, and testosterone for boys
- pulmonary function testing
- cardiac function testing
- ophthalmologic examination
- bone marrow aspiration (if indicated by the protocol or clinical scenario)
- creatinine clearance/glomerular filtration rate
- neuropsychological evaluation

Reasons for readmission to the hospital: Readmission to the hospital can occur for any of the following reasons:

- fever
- infection that requires intravenous antibiotics
- new onset or flare-up of graft-versus-host disease
- active bleeding
- respiratory distress
- uncontrolled hypertension
- uncontrolled vomiting, diarrhea, and dehydration
- alteration in mental status or seizures

Late Effects

Chronic graft-versus-host disease (CGVHD): CGVHD is a chronic immune disorder that occurs between 100 days and 2 years after HSCT. Organs that can be involved include the skin, mouth, gastrointestinal tract, liver, lungs, eyes, and vaginal mucosa. It is most common for patients to present with sicca syndrome (e.g., dry, burning, itching eyes), a dry mouth with ulcerations and changes in taste, and skin changes (e.g., dyspigmentation, desquamation, and lichenoid changes).

Immunosuppression: Patients who have had an autologous or allogeneic HSCT without chronic GVHD will have few infectious complications 100 days after the HSCT. Patients who experience chronic GVHD are profoundly immunosuppressed from the disease itself as well as from the therapy used to treat it. Infectious complications can include the following: varicella zoster, CMV, pneumocystic pneumonia, and other latent viruses such as adenovirus and parainfluenza virus.

Cataracts: Posterior cataracts, which are usually bilateral, occur in 20% of patients who receive total body irradiation; the average peak onset of formation is 3 years after HSCT. Glucocorticosteroids also can increase the risk of cataract formation. The treatment is surgical removal of the cataracts.

Endocrine dysfunction: Endocrine dysfunction is manifested in the following complications (in general, none of the complications listed occur in children who are treated with cyclophosphamide [Cytoxan] alone):

- *thyroid dysfunction*—due to increased thyroid stimulating hormone and decreased thyroxine levels, caused by total body irradiation; treatment is thyroid replacement therapy
- *growth and developmental delays*—occur in most children who receive total body irradiation or steroid therapy or who have GVHD; treatment may include growth-hormone therapy
- *ovarian dysfunction*—involves more permanent infertility and menopausal symptoms in females who receive chemotherapy after puberty than in those who receive chemotherapy before puberty; total body irradiation may result in primary gonadal failure in females regardless of their age
- *testicular dysfunction*—includes sterility, azoospermia, and premature ejaculation in males who are treated with total body irradiation; treatment can include hormone replacement therapy; total body irradiation results in primary gonadal failure in males regardless of their age.

Pulmonary complications: Pulmonary complications can include interstitial pneumonitis, restrictive disease, and less commonly, obstructive disease. Possible causes include total body irradiation, cytotoxic agents, chronic GVHD, and infectious pathogens (pneumonitis only).

Secondary malignancies: Secondary malignancies are reported to occur at a rate up to seven times higher than normal. Possible causes include cytotoxic chemotherapy, total body irradiation, viral infection, high-dose steroid therapy, and genetic predisposition.

Recurrence of disease: Relapse is seen more often in patients who have had more aggressive disease before HSCT. In general, patients with acute myeloblastic leukemia or acute lymphocytic leukemia who receive transplants while they are in remission are reported to have relapse rates of 5%–30%. Those who receive transplants during a more advanced stage of disease have relapse rates of 40%–80%. Unfortunately, the prognosis is quite poor for patients who have relapses, especially those that recur within 1–2 years after HSCT.

Biologic Response Modifiers

Sandy Call

Principles of Treatment

Biologic response modifiers (BRMs) are agents or therapeutic approaches that stimulate the body's immune system to eliminate tumor cells. The two major categories of BRMs are antibodies and cytokines. Surgery, radiation therapy, and chemotherapy have been the standard approaches to cancer treatment. Use of BRMs is recognized as the fourth cancer treatment modality.

Role in Childhood Cancer

BRMs are used for the treatment and diagnosis of various pediatric diseases, including cancer. The three major ways that BRMs affect the host-tumor response include modifying the immune response to the tumor, acting directly against the tumor by suppressing tumor growth or killing the tumor cell, and altering other biological activities that can directly or indirectly influence the viability of the tumor.

Types and Classification

Monoclonal antibodies: Monoclonal antibodies (MABs) are immunoglobulin molecules produced for a single clone of cells that bind to a unique target site on a specific antigen. The identification of tumor antigens provides a new method for diagnosis and treatment of malignancies. More than 20 MABs are available commercially, and many more are in development (See **Tables 4–15** and **4–16**). Those that have demonstrated some utility in pediatric malignancies include Mylotarg for acute myelogeneous leukemia (AML) and Rituximab for non-Hodgkin's lymphoma and Epstein-Barr virus-lymphoproliferative disease (EBV-LPD). Others (Daclizumab, Infliximab, Etanercept) have been found useful in the treatment of AGVHD but require further study, and still others (e.g., Palivizumab) may prove useful in the treatment of respiratory syncytial virus (RSV) in immunocompromised patients.

Use as diagnostic indicators. Radioactive isotopes can be attached to MABs that aid in the detection of cancer cells. MABs are being used to confirm the diagnosis of gliomas and lung, kidney, prostate, and breast cancers. Examples include bectumomab (ImmuRaid-LL2, LymphoScan) for imaging non-Hodgkin's lymphoma; ibritumomab tiuxetan bound to In-111 (Zevalin) for imaging B-cell non-Hodgkin's lymphoma, capromab pendetine (ProstaScint) for imaging prostate cancer, Tc-99 oregovomab (OvaRex) for imaging ovarian cancer, and In-111 satumomab (OncoScint) and Tc-99 votumumab (HumaSPECT) for imaging colorectal cancer.

Use as therapeutic treatment modalities. MABs can be used alone or with drugs, toxins, or radionuclides, often termed "magic bullets," to combine a MAB with another agent. Because the MAB targets a desired tumor-associated antigen, treatment can be administered directly to the malignant cells. MABs are administered intravenously.

Cytokines: Cytokines are nonantibody proteins that regulate the immune response. The cells of the immune system are their primary source, and immunoregulation is their primary function. Classes of cytokines include interferons, interleukins, and the hematopoietic growth factors.

Interferons. Interferons are cytokines that are recognized for their direct antiproliferative effects on tumor cells and for their ability to activate natural killer cells. Three classes of interferons exist: alpha interferon (IFN[alpha]) and beta interferon (IFN[beta]) play a more important role as antiviral and antiproliferative proteins, whereas gamma interferon (IFN[gamma]) has more potent immunoregulatory properties. Interferons have subcutaneous, intramuscular, and intravenous routes of administration.

Interleukins. Interleukins are natural proteins produced by macrophages or activated T cells that function as messengers between the cells of the immune system. Interleukins are named with an IL, followed by a number based on the order of their discovery (e.g., IL-1, IL-2, IL-3). IL-2, which has shown clinical activity in patients with renal cell cancer and melanoma, is under investigation in combination with other cancer treatment modalities. Interleukins have subcutaneous and intravenous routes of administration.

Hematopoietic growth factors. Hematopoietic growth factors are responsible for the differentiation and maturation of blood cells. Hematopoietic growth factors shorten the myelosuppression associated with disease or chemotherapy regimens, can facilitate an increase in the dose and/or the intensity of the chemotherapy regimen, reduce the risk of infections, serve as an adjunct to peripheral stem cell harvest, and accelerate bone marrow transplant recovery. They are classified according to the major cell line they affect.

- *Epoetin (Epogen, Procrit)*: Erythropoietin, which is normally produced by the kidneys, regulates and controls production and maturation of red blood cells. Epoetin, the synthetic version of erythropoietin, is used primarily to treat chemotherapy-related anemia and anemia related to chronic renal failure. It is administered subcutaneously.
- *Darbepoetin alfa (Aranesp)*: Darbepoetin alfa is a long-acting form of epoetin used to treat chemotherapy-related anemia and anemia related to chronic renal therapy. A major advantage of darbepoetin alfa is that it has a longer half-life than epoetin and requires less frequent dosing. One disadvantage is that darbepoetin alfa has a higher incidence of subcutaneous pain than epoetin.
- *Granulocyte-macrophage colony-stimulating factor (Leukine):* GM-CSF is produced by a variety of immune cells and affects multiple cell lineages, including early myeloid, erythroid, and megakaryocytic progenitors. It is also capable of activating mature granulocytes, eosinophils, and monocytes and macro-phages. It has subcutaneous and IV routes of administration.
- *Granulocyte colony-stimulating factor (Neupogen):* G-CSF is produced primarily by monocytes and macrophages. It increases the number of granulocytes (mainly neutrophils)

Table 4-15. MABs Used in Pediatric Malignancies and Hematopoietic Stem Cell Transplantation

MAB (brand)	Target Receptor	Clinical Application
Alemtuzumab (Campath-1H)	CD-52	B-cell chronic lympocytic leukemia, investigational for prevention of graft-versus-host disease in patients receiving HSCT
Daclizumab (Zenapax)	CD-25	Investigational for prevention of graft-versus-host disease
Etanercept (Enbrel)	TNF-alpha	Investigational for treatment of graft-versus-host disease
Gemtuzumab ozogamicin (Mylotarg)	CD-33	CD33 + AML, investigational for MDS and chronic myeloid leukemia
Ibritumomab [Au: Ibritumomab tiuxetan?] +Y90 (Zevalin)	CD-20	B-cell lymphoma
Iodine I-131 tositumomab (Bexxar)	CD-20	Non-Hodgkin's lymphoma
Infliximab (Remicade)	TNF-alpha	Investigational for treatment of graft-versus-host disease
Muromonab-CD3 (Orthoclone)	CD-3	Prophylaxis and treatment of acute graft-versus-host disease
Rituximab (Rituxan)	CD-20	B-cell non-Hodgkin's lymphoma, investigational for post trans plant LPD, and immune mediated thrombocytopenia

Table 4-16. MABs in Development

Investigational MAB	Target Receptor	Potential Clinical Application
Ch14.18	GD2	Neuroblastoma
MTP-PE		Osteosarcoma
ImmTher	Macrophage stimulating agent	Ewing's sarcoma

and also may increase phagocytic activity and antibody-dependent killing. It has subcutaneous, IV, and oral routes of administration.

- *Pegfilgrastim (Neulasta):* Pegfilgrastim is the long-acting form of filgrastim. Whereas filgrastim is administered in daily injections, pegfilgrastim is administered via subcutaneous injection every 3 weeks.

Other (investigational): Muramyl tripeptide phosphatidylethanolamine (MTP-PE) is a biologic response modifier currently being investigated in the treatment of newly diagnosed osteosarcoma. Early animal studies have demonstrated that systemic administration of MTP-PE eradicated microscopic metastases in the lungs and lymph nodes. MTP-TE is a synthetic lipophilic molecule derived from a component of the bacterial cell wall that is capable of stimulating an immune response. Once ingested by phagocytosis, MTP-PE activates the cell that then seeks out and destroys tumor cells without harming normal cells. It has an IV route of administration.

Potential Side Effects

Monoclonal antibodies: MABs are associated with potential allergic reactions, fever, chills, rigors, malaise, nausea, vomiting, and hypotension.

Cytokines:

Interferons. The incidence and severity of side effects increase with dosage; they include flulike syndrome (e.g., fever, chills, myalgias, arthralgias, and headache), fatigue and malaise, anorexia, diarrhea, changes in mental status (e.g., poor concentration, somnolence, depression, forgetfulness, irritability), abnormal liver function tests, neutropenia, thrombocytopenia, skin irritation, and bone pain.

Interleukins. The side effects of interleukins are flulike syndrome (e.g., fever, chills, myalgias, arthralgias, and headache), vascular leak syndrome that involves shifts from intravascular or intracellular areas to extravascular or extracellular areas, skin and mucosal changes, nausea, vomiting, CNS changes, and altered laboratory values.

Hematopoietic growth factors. The side effects of erythropoietin (Epogen) are hypertension, headaches, fever, myalgia, and rashes. The side effects of GM-CSF are flulike symptoms (e.g., fever, fatigue, bone pain, myalgias, and arthralgias, headache, pain or erythema at the injection site), "first-dose" phenomena (i.e., flushing, hypoxia, tachycardia, and oxygen desaturation). The side effects of G-CSF are bone pain, joint pain, fever, rashes, and pain at the injection site.

Nursing Assessment and Interventions

Assessment:

- Know the risks associated with the use of each biologic response modifier in order to assess for side effects.
- Assess the patient's and the family's understanding of the drug to be given and their readiness to learn.

Interventions:

- Maximize the safety of the administration of biologic response modifiers in patients by taking the following measures:
  - ensuring aseptic preparation and administration
  - identifying the location of emergency supplies
  - obtaining the patient's baseline pulse, respiration, blood pressure, and temperature prior to administration of BRMs

- administering premedications (e.g., acetaminophen [Tylenol], diphenhydramine [Benadryl], and hydrocortison) when they are warranted
- teaching patients and their families about the signs and symptoms of adverse reactions to BRMs (e.g., fever of more than 103°F, shortness of breath, significant weight gain)

- Monitor for these complications of BRM therapy:
  - increased pulse rate, orthostatic blood pressure changes, fever patterns, and critical changes in laboratory values
  - excessive fatigue, weight gain or loss of more than 10% in 1 week, changes in mental status (e.g., confusion, somnolence, psychosis), chest pain, arrhythmias, hypotension, dyspnea, and edema
  - local inflammation or severe allergic reactions
- Intervene to decrease the incidence and severity of complications associated with BRM therapy.
  - by encouraging measures to maintain skin integrity (e.g., getting out of bed, changing position, applying lubricants after bathing, avoiding any scrubbing of the skin)
  - by assessing changes in mental status at regular intervals, teaching the family to monitor for behavioral changes, and evaluating the impact of changes in mental status on the patient's functional status
  - by administering supportive medical therapy (e.g., albumin, diuretics, fluids, vasopressors), as needed, for capillary leak syndrome, instructing the patient to change positions slowly to avoid dizziness, and reporting decreased urinary output, hypotension, dyspnea, and weight gain of more than 10% over 1 week
  - by teaching the patient and the family essential self-care skills for continuing BRMs after discharge and providing available literature on BRMs
  - by teaching strategies for managing any chronic side effects of therapy (e.g., fatigue, anorexia, changes in mental status)

Expected Patient and Family Outcomes

- The patient and the family can describe the type of treatment with BRMs and the rationale for therapy.
- The patient and the family know about the immediate and long-term complications associated with the type of biotherapy and self-care measures to decrease the incidence and severity of the complications of biotherapy.
- The patient and the family demonstrate the self-care skills required for administration of biotherapy.
- The patient and the family can list changes in the patient's condition that should be reported to the healthcare team.

Gene Therapy

Robbie Norville and Beth Hasenauer

Principles of Treatment

Gene therapy can be defined as the introduction, with therapeutic intent, of new genetic material into cells. Gene therapy can involve enhancement, restoration, or introduction of a novel cell function. Gene therapy represents a new and different way of thinking about cancer and cancer treatment. It focuses on the cause of the cancer (i.e., the genetic dysfunction) in contrast with the treatment and control of the disease process. Even though more than 800 clinical protocols for gene therapy have already been approved, this treatment remains an experimental approach to cancer that is still in its infancy.

There are four major approaches to incorporating gene therapy into the treatment of childhood cancers (Brenner, 2002):

- The tumor itself can be modified, either by repairing the genetic defects associated with the malignant process, by introducing a gene that triggers an antitumor immune response, or by delivering a prodrug-metabolizing enzyme that renders the tumor sensitive to the corresponding cytotoxic agent.
- The immune system response to the tumor can be modified by altering the specificity of immune system cells.
- The drug sensitivity of normal host tissues can be decreased by delivering cytotoxic drug-resistance genes to marrow precursor cells.
- The efficacy of therapies can be monitored closely by "marking" normal or malignant cells to help distinguish the targeted cells.

Successful gene therapy requires

- identification of the responsible gene and successful replications (i.e., manufacturing) of normal copies of this gene
- development of effective methods for inserting the normal gene into a sufficient number of the patient's appropriate cells
- the expression of the inserted gene's normal gene product at a level adequate for treatment of the disease without toxicity or interference with normal cell functioning.

The duration of the therapeutic response to gene therapy depends upon the cell population targeted for gene transfer. Dividing cell populations (e.g., hematopoietic cells, skin fibroblasts) allows for modified genes to pass to successive cell generations, thereby producing a long-term therapeutic effect. In nondividing mature cell populations (e.g., kidney, brain), the effect of modified genes is limited to the life span of the target cells, producing a temporary response that requires repeated applications of gene therapy to maintain a long-term therapeutic effect.

If gene therapy is to become a viable option, it must be accomplished in a cost-efficient manner and in a manner that gives acceptable risk-benefit ratios.

Role in Childhood Cancer

The ultimate role of gene therapy in treating childhood cancer remains unclear, though the results of early clinical trials using this approach have shown promise. Future options for cancer treatment likely will involve some form of gene therapy. This therapy should be useful in the treatment of cancer because cancers are the result of genetic mutations or the loss of genetic material. However, like chemotherapy, gene therapy is unlike to prove to be a cure-all for childhood cancer. Limitations to the widespread application of gene therapy for cancer treatment include limited technical ability to transfer and express new genes in target cells, lack of vector (carrier) specificity, limited antitumor effect of the transgene (gene transferred from one cell to another), and the inability to target every tumor cell.

Type or Classification

Gene transfer: Gene transfer is the process of inserting one or more genes into a cell. All approaches to gene therapy depend on techniques for gene transfer. There are two gene-transfer techniques:

- *Ex vivo*, or indirect gene transfer, involves a transfer of genetic material to target cells that have been removed from the host and manipulated in the laboratory. After the transfer of the genetic material, the modified cells are reimplanted in the host.
- *In vivo*, or direct gene transfer, is the transfer of genetic material directly to target cells located within the host.

Both gene transfer techniques require a vector that can be used to transfer the required genes into the target cells of the host (see the discussion in "Method of Delivery," the subsection that immediately follows this subsection).

Somatic-cell gene transfer: Somatic-cell gene transfer is the insertion of corrected or altered genes into nonreproductive human cells. It is the only form of gene therapy approved for clinical trials.

Germ-cell gene transfer: Germ-cell gene transfer involves the insertion of genetic material into reproductive cells (either sperm or egg cells). Germ-cell gene therapy has controversial ethical and societal implications.

Application to Cancer Therapy

Gene transfer techniques currently are applied to cancer therapy through modification of the tumor by inserting genetic material into the tumor to correct the specific genetic defects causing the malignancy, by inserting genes that encode enzymes able to convert harmless prodrugs into lethal cytotoxins, or by enhancing immune recognition of tumors. The polyclonal nature of most pediatric malignancies makes tumor correction especially problematic; it is hoped that certain individual genetic abnormalities that are amenable to correction will prove to be key to the malignant process. Transfer of prodrug-metabolizing genes is being explored in the Phase I treatment of retinoblastoma. In this strategy, the tumor is directly injected with a vector carrying the herpes simplex virus-1 thymidine kinase (HSV-TK) gene, which converts ganciclovir into a metabolite that acts as a "suicide gene," killing dividing cells (tumor cells). In some tumors, neighboring cancer cells that have not taken up the transgene also are killed by the "bystander effect." It is believed that this effect occurs when channels between cells, known as gap junctions, allow the toxic metabolite to spread from the transduced cell in which it was produced to neighboring nontransduced cells.

Tumor vaccine studies are being evaluated to enhance immune recognition of tumors with poor immunogenicity. Transduced tumor cells are being used as vaccines in adjuvant therapy to prevent relapse in patients with presumed minimal residual disease. Phase I studies of tumor vaccines for neuroblastoma and leukemia are currently being evaluated by a variety of investigators. Modification of the immune system to modulate the response of the immune system to tumor cells also are being considered. Adoptive transfer of cytotoxic T lymphocytes (CTLs) directed at viral or tumor antigens is an example of this strategy. Clinical studies have demonstrated the feasibility and safety of administering Epstein-Barr virus (EBV) CTLs to prevent and treat Epstein-Barr virus-lymphoproliferative disease (EBV-LPD) in postallogeneic transplant patients. Clinical studies using EBV-specific gene-marked CTLs for relapsed EBV + Hodgkin's disease are underway (Biagi, Bollard, Rousseau, & Brenner, 2003), and further genetic modifications will likely make the cells more effective in vivo.

Modification of the sensitivity of normal host cells to cytotoxic drugs, thus increasing the therapeutic index of these agents, is another therapy. The multidrug-resistant-1 (MDR-1) gene is the most widely studied drug-resistant gene to date. This gene, once inserted, acts as a drug efflux pump and prevents the accumulation of small toxic molecules, including a range of cytotoxic drugs. Transfer of drug resistant genes into hematopoietic stem cells would exert a protective effect, attenuating drug-induced myelosuppression. Researchers are studying other drug resistant genes, including dihydrofolate reductase, which protects against methotrexate, and the bacterial nitroreductase, which protects against thiotepa (Abernathy & Wilson, 2000; Biagi et al., 2003).

Although not directly therapeutic, gene marking of hematopoietic progenitor cells provides information that can be used to improve therapies that incorporate autologous stem cell transplantation. Gene marking has been used to address questions regarding cancer biology and clinical issues, specifically to determine the source of relapse after autologous stem cell transplant, to learn more about normal marrow reconstitution, and to evaluate ways to accelerate the reconstitution process.

Method of Delivery

A gene transfer vector is the mechanism by which the gene is transferred into the cell. The process of introducing a transgene into a cell is called transduction. There are two types of vectors: viral vectors and nonviral vectors.

Viral vectors: Viral vectors use the inherent ability of viruses to carry foreign genetic material into cells. The virus to be used as the vector, modified so that it will not replicate, infects the desired cell by introducing the new genetic material into its cytoplasm or genome. If the vector also enters the DNA of the transduced cell, this information is passed to its daughter cells through mitosis. Otherwise, the new gene (transgene) exists as an extra chromosomal episome and is diluted out during cell division.

Retroviral vectors. Retroviral vectors are RNA viruses that convert their RNA to DNA in the cells they infect and then insert their DNA directly into the cell genome (i.e., chromosomes), which contains all of the genetic material of the cell. They require dividing cell populations so the genetic material can be inserted into the genome of the host cell. The limitations of the use of retroviral vectors are the risk of random insertion of the genetic material into any of the chromosomes of the target cell (i.e., lack of specificity), the risk of insertional mutagenesis (mutation of the chromosome), and the risk that the virus could retain the ability to replicate itself, which could result in viremia, which is rare but possible.

Adenoviral vectors. Adenoviral vectors are DNA viruses that are carried into the cytoplasm of the host cell but do not integrate their DNA into the genome of the cell. Because they do not require cell division to introduce DNA into the host cell, adenoviral vectors can enter a wide variety of dividing and nondividing cell populations. Limitations to the use of adenoviral vectors are their ability to stimulate a host immune response and their lack of long-term persistence in the host cell, requiring repeated applications of the vector to maintain a constant therapeutic response.

Nonviral vectors: Nonviral vectors rely on the transfer of genetic material into host cells by chemical or physical methods. This genetic material does not become integrated into the host genome.

Liposomes. Liposomes are the most common nonviral vectors in use. DNA is contained within the lipid structure of their biodegradable fatty droplets and is delivered directly to the cell when the liposome fuses with the cell membrane. Cell division is not required to introduce the DNA. Liposomes can enter into a wide variety of dividing and nondividing cell populations.

The advantages of liposomes are that they are nontoxic, the extensive safety testing necessary for viral vectors is not required, and they have the potential to insert multiple copies of the transferred gene into the host target cells. Their limitations include their limited targeting ability and short-term persistence in the host cell, thus requiring repeated applications of the vector to maintain the therapeutic response in the host target cells.

Potential Side Effects

Due to the experimental status of gene therapy, the risks associated with patient safety and toxicity are not well defined. The ratio of relative risk to the potential benefit to the patient must be carefully evaluated. All gene therapy protocols require stringent review by institutional review boards, the FDA, and the National Institutes of Health Recombinant DNA Advisory Committee (RAC) prior to their implementation in human subjects. Long-term monitoring strategies must be ongoing for all clinical trials with gene therapy.

Risk of retroviral viremia infection of healthcare providers and patients: Viral vectors are modified to make them incompetent for replication. Rigorous safety testing and quality control in the manufacturing of retroviral vectors is ongoing to ensure the safety of the vectors. Healthcare providers should follow universal precautions in direct care situations. Patients should be monitored over the long term for the possibility of developing retroviral viremia.

Risk of insertional oncogenesis for patients receiving retroviral gene therapy: Random insertion of genetic material by retroviral vectors could alter normal cellular function leading to malignant transformation. Ongoing patient monitoring and safety testing to define this risk should continue.

Side effects of overall gene-transfer protocols: Gene transfer protocols are well tolerated with minimal short-term toxicity. Specific side effects include the following:

Viral therapy. The constitutional symptoms experienced by patients in studies of retroviruses are fever, chills, fatigue, nausea, vomiting, and anorexia. Localized symptoms of retrovirus studies are cutaneous reactions, induration, erythema, pruritus, pain, and skin irritation; CNS symptoms are meningeal inflammation, headache, and seizure. The following are the symptoms experienced by patients in adenovirus studies: fatigue, fever, hypoxemia, pulmonary infiltrates, and abnormalities in lung function (transient).

Nonviral therapy. The symptoms associated with liposome studies are pain at the time of injection and transient pneumothorax.

Nursing Assessment and Interventions

Assessment: The nurse's role in gene therapy trials parallels the nurse's role in traditional Phase I and Phase II clinical drug trials. Gene therapy can be a component of a larger therapeutic trial with a documented toxicity profile. Patients can receive gene therapy in a variety of patient care settings. The direct caregiver is required to provide careful planning of patient care as well as monitoring and documentation of expected and unexpected short- and long-term toxicities.

- Be knowledgeable about the clinical trial, treatment schema, the known and potential toxicities, and symptom management.
- Establish safe parameters for administration of treatments.
- Identify, through an assessment of the patient, past treatment or symptom management problems and current medical problems that could affect the patient's tolerance to therapy.
- Identify, monitor, and record the patient's subjective and objective responses to the investigational therapy and symptom management.

- Assist with long-term monitoring of the patient's response to therapy and identification of trends related to toxicities, benefits of the therapy, or both.
- Be fully informed in order to be viewed as an essential member of the research team and to function effectively in the role of patient advocate and educator.
- Have a basic understanding of genetics and its relationship to cancer and the concepts of gene therapy (i.e., the unique nature of genetic information).
- Understand the goals and limitations of the clinical trial process as it applies to gene therapy and the participants in gene therapy.
- Appreciate the ethical, societal, and cultural concerns aroused by the implications of the molecular genetic revolution, the concept of gene therapy, and the specific implications this has for participating patients and healthcare providers.

Interventions:

- Provide accurate, understandable information that allows for meaningful participation by the patient and the family during the informed-consent process and for future care.
- Provide ongoing clarification of the procedures, toxicities, and expectations related to the patient's participation in the clinical trial with the patient and the family.
- Uphold and advocate for patients' rights during the clinical trial process.
- Maintain ongoing communication and dialogue with the research team in relation to the patient's and the family's concerns.
- Discuss the financial considerations, including third-party funding, of the patient's participation in the clinical research trials.
- Protect and uphold the patient's and the family's rights to privacy and confidentiality.

Expected Patient and Family Outcomes

- The patient and the family are able to explain their understanding of the purpose, procedures, limitations, and risks of the treatment plan and their decision about participating.
- The patient and the family recognize the importance of unusual symptoms and their potential relationship to the experimental treatment and are able to establish ongoing communication patterns with the healthcare team.
- The patient and the family express satisfaction that their needs are being met and their basic rights are respected and being supported by the healthcare team.

References

Abernathy, E., & Wilson, H.B. (2000). Gene therapy: Overview and implications for peripheral stem cell transplantation. In P.C. Buchsell & P.M. Kapustay (Eds.), *Stem cell transplantation: A clinical textbook* (pp. 11.3–11.17). Pittsburgh: Oncology Nursing Press.

Biagi, E., Bollard, C., Rousseau, R., & Brenner, M. (2003). Gene therapy for pediatric cancer: State of the art and future perspectives. *Journal of Biomedicine and Biotechnology, 1,* 13–24.

Brenner, M.K. (2002). Gene transfer and the treatment of pediatric malignancy. In P. Pizzo & D.G. Poplack (Eds.), *Principles and practice of pediatric oncology* (pp. 453–464). Philadelphia: Lippincott Williams & Wilkins.

Complementary and Alternative Treatments

Janice Post-White

Principles of Treatment

Also referred to as integrative therapies or integrated health care, complementary and alternative medicine (CAM) encompasses practices and therapies outside of conventional medicine. CAM is recommended as an adjunct to standard treatment and not as a replacement for conventional care. The focus of CAM research in childhood cancer is to evaluate the safety and efficacy of therapies in children, provide evidence-based therapies that improve supportive care, and promote the patient's participation in the care of his or her body, mind, and spirit.

Types of Complementary and Alternative Therapies

The National Center for Complementary and Alternative Medicine of the National Institutes of Health designates five major domains of CAM (NCCAM, 2003).

Alternative medical systems: These systems involve philosophies and practices independent from conventional Western medicine. Traditional Chinese medicine relies on acupuncture, herbal medicine, oriental massage (i.e., shiatsu), *qi gong,* and *tai chi* to maintain or restore the proper balance of *qi* or vital life energy. Ayurvedic medicine, which originated in India, emphasizes restoring the innate harmony of the body, mind, and spirit through diet, exercise, meditation, herbs, massage, exposure to sunlight, and controlled breathing. Naturopathic medicine also relies on innate healing and emphasizes health restoration through diet, acupuncture, herbal medicine, chiropractic, ultrasound, light therapy, counseling, and homeopathy. Homeopathic medicine is based on the principle that "like cures like." Homeopathic remedies contain minute doses of substances that, in greater quantities, would actually cause the symptoms they are intended to relieve.

Mind-body interventions: These interventions use the mind to influence symptoms or physical responses and are considered the most "mainstream" CAM technique. Evidence exists for effectiveness of cognitive-behavioral therapies, imagery, and support and educational groups. Less studied are the effects of art and music therapy, dance and movement therapy, some forms of hypnosis, and prayer.

Biologically based therapies: The therapies encompass ingestible or injectable agents and include herbal therapies, dietary supplements, special diets, and pharmacologic treatments, such as antineoplastons, shark cartilage, and L-carnitine (the last for cardiac protection) Vitamins and herbs are among the most frequently used CAM therapies in cancer; they also have the greatest potential to interact with conventional treatment (Richardson & Strauss, 2002). The role of antioxidants as adjuncts to treatment is controversial and is being intensely studied. Current recommendations are to avoid antioxidants on the days of chemotherapy or radiation therapy because of potential interactions.

Manipulative and body-based methods: These methods encompass chiropractic, massage, and osteopathy to reduce fatigue and restore the structure and function of the musculoskeletal and nervous systems.

Energy therapies: These therapies channel spiritual or healing energy to manipulate or interrupt energy fields either within the body (biofields) or external to the body (electromagnetic fields). *Qi gong, reiki,* therapeutic touch, and healing touch involve identifying and correcting energy imbalances and promoting energy flow.

Role in Childhood Cancer

The use of CAM in children with cancer is prevalent across the world, with reported use of 31% to 84% in various settings and countries (Post-White, Sencer, Fitzgerald, 2002) Parents primarily choose CAM to help their child manage side effects, cope with emotional effects, or feel more hopeful (Post-White, Sencer, Fitzgerald, & Miranda, 2000). Some parents report using CAM to boost the immune system, though there is little evidence to support this use. Use of CAM in long-term childhood cancer survivors is under investigation in the National Cancer Survivors Study.

Many mind-body therapies are well documented for use in pediatric cancer populations. Imagery and hypnosis have been used for two decades to reduce procedural pain, anxiety, nausea, and distress (Columbia University, 2001). Biologically based therapies, however, carry a greater risk of side effects and have not undergone rigorous scientific testing. There currently are no standards for recommended pediatric dosages and little oversight of the herbal or nutritional industries, resulting in products with uneven quality and purity. No known published research exists on energy therapies or alternative medical systems for children with cancer.

Potential Side Effects

Side effects are specific to the type of CAM therapy used, with few adverse responses to mind-body interventions, touch therapies, or energy therapies. The most common adverse response in adults is the surfacing of distressing emotions. Children may be distrustful of strangers touching them. Practitioners should be trained in the therapy provided and have experience in treating children. Based on occasional reports of bleeding or tissue swelling from pressure point massage or shiatsu, only light touch therapies should be used with patients with low platelet counts or bleeding disorders.

Biologically based therapies carry the greatest risks: potential interference (interactions) with treatments (e.g., chemotherapy, radiation therapy) or liver, cardiac, or renal toxicities. Some heavy-metal impurities in products also carry a greater risk to children because of their smaller body size and developing organs.

Nursing Assessment and Interventions

Assessment: The most important role of the healthcare provider is to discover what CAM therapies, if any, are being used or considered. In a study of 120 families of children with cancer using some form of CAM, 28% did not tell their provider because they were never asked (Post-White et al., 2000). Use of CAM and potential interactions with treatment should be assessed at diagnosis, during each hospitalization, and at every phase of medical treatment. If parents are instructed to bring medications to clinic visits, they also should be asked to bring vitamins or supplements used by their child. Determining therapies used and the reasons why families use CAM will provide insight into what therapies work for individual patients and symptoms and what patients' emotional or resource needs are.

Interventions: The Oncology Nursing Society's position on the use of CAM requires that nurses assess for CAM use; rely on credible sources and providers when giving information to patients; evaluate CAM for safety, efficacy, cost, third-party payer coverage, ethics, and liability; and evaluate their own beliefs regarding CAM (Oncology Nursing Society, 2000). Misrepresentation of facts or expectations voids informed consent and triggers legal liability (Monaco & Smith, 2002). The bibliography provides resources and Web sites to identify CAM clinical trials and evidence-based research.

- Listen objectively to what therapies parents or adolescents are using or considering using.
- Document what is being used and why, including dosages and frequency.
- Ascertain all known and suspected potential side effects and interactions with treatment.
- Explore how the child, adolescent, or parent expects the therapy to help.
- Offer therapies that can be used at home at any time, such as acupressure, aromatherapy, massage by a parent or friend, music, relaxation, yoga, and meditation.
- Provide a list of local resources, including practitioners who have pediatric experience.
- Provide reliable resources for information on specific therapies, including where to obtain them.
- Ask questions to ensure the family has considered the risks, benefits, and cost.
- Discuss options for insurance reimbursement. Reimbursement typically requires a medical order and inpatient service; however, state laws and insurance policies vary.

- Monitor the patient's response to any CAM therapies used. Ask at each visit if CAM therapies are still being used and whether they have been helpful.
- Assess for negative responses, including allergic reactions, side effects, emotional distress, or financial hardship.
- Periodically assist the family to evaluate the need and value of the therapy.

Expected Patient and Family Outcomes

- The family makes informed decisions regarding choice of CAM therapies for their child.
- Families work with trained providers who have experience with pediatric patients.
- Resources consulted by families are current, reputable, and reliable.
- Families report to their providers their use of CAM, any side effects, and perceived benefits attributable to CAM therapies.

References

Columbia University, Integrative Therapies Program for Children with Cancer. (2001). *Research.* Retrieved February 11, 2003, from http://carolann.hs.columbia.edu/research/index.shtml

Monaco, G.P., & Smith, G. (2002). Informed consent in complementary and alternative medicine: Current status and future needs. *Seminars in Oncology, 29,* 601–608.

National Center for Complementary and Alternative Medicine, National Institutes of Health. (2002, May). *Major domains of complementary and alternative medicine* (NCCAM Publication No. D156). Retrieved February 11, 2003, from http://nccam.nih.gov/health/whatiscam/ index.htm

Oncology Nursing Society. (2000). Oncology Nursing Society position on the use of complementary and alternative therapies in cancer care. *Oncology Nursing Forum, 27,* 749.

Post-White, J., Sencer, S., & Fitzgerald, M. (2002). Complementary and alternative treatments in children with cancer. In C.R. Baggott, K.P. Kelly, D. Fochtman, & G.V. Foley (Eds.), *Nursing care of children and adolescents with cancer* (pp. 256–263). Philadelphia: W.B. Saunders.

Post-White, J., Sencer, S., Fitzgerald, M., & Miranda, M. (2000). Complementary therapy use in pediatric cancer. *Oncology Nursing Forum, 27,* 342–343.

Richardson, M.A., & Strauss, S.E. (2002). Complementary and alternative medicine: Opportunities and challenges for cancer management and research. *Seminars in Oncology, 29,* 531–545.

Bibliography

Diagnostic and Staging Procedures

Braverman, R.M., & Parker, B.R. (2002). Imaging studies in the diagnosis and management of pediatric malignancies. In P.A. Pizzo & D.G Poplack (Eds.), *Principles and practice of pediatric oncology* (4th ed., pp. 205–236). Philadelphia: Lippincott Williams & Wilkins.

Brown, J.G. (2000). Diagnostic evaluation, classification, and staging. In C. H.Yarbro, M.H. Frogge, M. Goodman, & S. Groenwald (Eds.), *Cancer nursing: Principles and practice* (pp. 214–239). Sudbury, MA: Jones and Bartlett.

Hockenberry, M.J., Wilson, D., Winkelstein, M.L, & Kline, N.E. (2003). *Wong's nursing care of infants and children.* St Louis: Mosby.

Leonard, M. (2002). Diagnostic evaluations and staging procedures. In C.R. Baggott, K.P. Kelly, D. Fochtman, & G.V. Foley (Eds.), *Nursing care of children and adolescents with cancer* (pp. 66–89). Philadelphia: W.B. Saunders.

Seymour, J.F., & Hicks, R.J. (2002). Fluorine-18 fluorodexyglucose positron emission tomography, galluim-67 scintigraphy, and conventional staging for Hodgkin's disease and non-Hodgkin's lymphoma. *American Journal of Medicine, 112,* 262–268.

Vietti, T.J., & Steuber, C.P. (2002). Clinical assessment and differential diagnosis of the child with suspected leukemia In P.A. Pizzo & D.G. Poplack (Eds.), *Principles and practice of pediatric oncology* (4th ed., pp. 149–160). Philadelphia: Lippincott Williams & Wilkins.

History of Chemotherapy

Brown, K.A., Esper, P., Kelleher, L.O., O'Neill, J., Polovich, M., & White, J. (Eds.). *(2001). Chemotherapy and biotherapy: Guidelines and recommendations for practice.* Pittsburgh: Oncology Nursing Society Publishing Division.

Khana, C. (2001). Biotherapy of cancer. Retrieved March 13, 2003, from http://www.perseusfoundation.org/page33.html

Tortorice, P. (2001). Chemotherapy: Principles of therapy. In C. Yarbro, M. Frogge, M. Goodman, & S. Groenwald (Eds.), *Cancer nursing principles and practice* (5th ed., pp. 353). Boston: Jones and Bartlett.

U.S. Department of Veterans Affairs. (1999, April). Mustard gas exposure and long term health effects [Fact sheet]. Retrieved March 13, 2003, from http://www.va.gov/pressrel/99mustd.htm

Wheellock, L., & Summers, B. New chemotherapy agents in cancer care. *Oncology Nursing Updates, 3*(4). Retrieved March 13, 2003, from http://www.ons.org/xp6/ONS/Library.xml/ONS_Publications.xml/Oncology_Nursing_Updates.xml/Volume_Three_Number_Four.xml

Wright, J. (2002). Almost famous: E. Clark Noble, the common thread in the discovery of insulin and vinblastine. *Canadian Medical Association Journal, 167,* 1391–1396.

Clinical Trials

Hinds, P.S., Gilger, E.A., Eder, M., & Kodish, E. (2002). The nurse as witness in the research consent/assent process: An inherently problematic role or an ethical obligation? *Journal of Pediatric Oncology Nursing, 19,* 35–40.

Hughes, W. (2000). The importance of clinical trials. In G. Steen & J. Mirro (Eds.), *Childhood cancer: A handbook from St. Jude Children's Research Hospital* (pp. 183–194). Cambridge, MA: Perseus Publishing.

Levi, R.B., Marsick, R., Drotar, D., & Kodish, E. (2000). Diagnosis, disclosure, and informed consent: Learning from parents of children with cancer. *Journal of Pediatric Hematology/Oncology, 22,* 3–12.

McCray, A.T. (2000). Better access to information about clinical trials. *Annals of Internal Medicine, 133,* 609–614.

National Cancer Institute. (n.d.). *Understanding Clinical Trials.* Retrieved October 2001 from http://www.nci.nih.gov/clinicaltrials/understanding

National Library of Medicine. (n.d.). *Understanding Clinical Trials.* Retrieved February 11, 2003, from http://clinicaltrials.gov

Public Welfare, Protection of Human Subjects, 45 C.F.R (s) 46 (1991).

Santana, V. (2000). Medical research in children. In G. Steen & J. Mirro (Eds.), *Childhood cancer: A handbook from St. Jude Children's Research Hospital* (pp. 175–182). Cambridge, MA: Perseus Publishing.

Simon, R. (2001). Clinical trials in cancer. In V.T. DeVita, Jr., S. Hellman, & S.A. Rosenberg (Eds.), *Cancer: Principles and practice of oncology* (pp. 521–538). Philadelphia: Lippincott Williams & Wilkins.

Ungerleider, R.S., Ellenberg, S.E., & Berg, S.L. (2002). Cancer clinical trials: Design, conduct, analysis, and reporting. In P.A. Pizzo & D.G. Poplack (Eds.), *Principles and practice of pediatric oncology* (pp. 463–488). Philadelphia: Lippincott Williams & Wilkins.

Chemotherapy

Balis, F.M., Holcenberg, J.S., & Blaney, S.M. (2002). General principles of chemotherapy. In P.A. Pizzo & D.G. Poplack (Eds.), *Principles and practice of pediatric oncology* (pp. 237–308). Philadelphia: Lippincott Williams & Wilkins.

Brown, K.A., Esper, P., Kelleher, L.O., Brace O'Neill, J.E., Polovich, M., & White, J.M. (2001). *Chemotherapy and biotherapy: Guidelines and recommendations for practice.* Pittsburgh: Oncology Nursing Society Publishing Division.

Children's Oncology Group, COG Pharmacy Discipline Committee. (2003). *COG pharmacology manual.* Retrieved May 20, 2003, from http://members.childrensoncologygroup.org/_files/reference/PharmacologyManual.pdf

Ettinger, A.G., Bond, D.M., & Sievers, D. (2002). Chemotherapy. In C.R. Baggott, K.P. Kelly, D. Fochtman, & G.V. Foley (Eds.), *Nursing Care of Children and Adolescents with Cancer* (pp. 133–176). Philadelphia: W.B. Saunders Company.

Wittes, R.E. (2003). Therapies for cancer in children—past successes, future challenges. *New England Journal of Medicine, 348,* 747–749.

OSHA Guidelines for Handling Chemotherapy

Brown, K.A., Esper, P., Kelleher, L.O., Brace O'Neill, J.E., Polovich, M., &White , J.M. (2001). *Chemotherapy and biotherapy: Guidelines and recommendations for practice.* Pittsburgh: Oncology Nursing Society Publishing Division.

Ettinger, A., Bond, D., & Sievers, T. (2002). Chemotherapy. In Baggott, C.R., Kelly, K.P., Fochtman, D., and Foley, G.V. *Nursing care of children and adolescents with cancer* (pp. 133–176). Philadelphia: W. B. Saunders.

National Association of Children's Hospitals and Related Institutions (NACHRI): Patient Care Focus Groups. (1999). *Enhancing the chemotherapy process in oncology services.* Alexandria, VA: Author.

Occupational Safety & Health Administration. (n.d.). *OSHA technical manual: Controlling occupational exposure to hazardous drugs.* Retrieved May 7, 2003, from http://www.osha.gov/dts/osta/otm/otm_vi/otm_vi_2.html

Administration of Vesicants

Balis, F.M., Holcenberg, J.S., & Blaney, S.M. (2002). General principles of chemotherapy. In P.A. Pizzo & D.G. Poplack (Eds.), *Principles and practice of pediatric oncology* (pp. 237–308). Philadelphia: Lippincott Williams & Wilkins.

Ettinger, A.G., Bond, D.M., & Sievers, D. (2002). Chemotherapy. In C.R. Baggott, K.P. Kelly, D. Fochtman, & G.V. Foley (Eds.), *Nursing care of children and adolescents with cancer* (pp. 133–176). Philadelphia: W. B. Saunders.

Kassner, E. (2000). Evaluation and treatment of chemotherapy extravasation injuries. *Journal of Pediatric Oncology Nursing, 17*(3), 135–148.

Langstein, H.N., Duman, H., Seelig, D., Butler, C.E., & Evans, G. R. (2002). Retrospective study of the management of chemotherapeutic extravasation injury. *Annals of Plastic Surgery, 49,* 369–374.

Schulmeister, L., & Camp-Sorrell, D. (2000). Chemotherapy extravasation from implanted ports. *Oncology Nursing Forum, 27,* 531–540.

Surgery

Ashcraft, K.W., Murphy, P.J., Sharp, R.J., Sigalet, D.L., & Snyder, C.L. (Eds.). (2000). *Pediatric surgery.* Philadelphia: W.B. Saunders.

Bagnall-Reeb, H., & Perry, S. (2002). Surgery. In C.R. Baggott, K.P. Kelly, D. Fochtman, & G.V. Foley (Eds.), *Nursing care of children and adolescents with cancer* (pp. 90–115). Philadelphia: W.B. Saunders.

Carachi, R., Azmy, A.F., & Grosfeld, J.L. (Eds.). (1999). *The surgery of childhood tumors.* New York: Oxford University Press.

Shamberger, R.C., Jaksic, T., & Ziegler, M.M. (2002). General principles of surgery. In P.A. Pizzo & D.G. Poplack (Eds.), *Principles and practice of pediatric oncology* (pp. 351–368). Philadelphia: Lippincott Williams & Wilkins.

Radiation Therapy

Hodgson, D.C., Goumnerova, L.C., Loeffler, J.S., Dutton, S., Black, P.M., Alexander, E., et al. (2001). Radiosurgery in the management of pediatric brain tumors. *International Journal of Radiation Oncology, Biology, Physics, 50,* 929–935.

Levin, V.A. (Ed.). (2002). *Cancer in the nervous system.* New York: Oxford University Press.

Teh, B.S., Mai, W.Y., Grant, W.H., III, Chiu, J.K., Lu, H.H., Carpenter, L.S., et al. (2002). Intensity modulated radiotherapy (IMRT) decreases treatment-related morbidity and potentially enhances tumor control. *Cancer Investigation, 20,* 437–451.

http://www.astro.org The Web site of the American Society for Therapeutic Radiology and Oncology

http://www.abta.org The Web site of the American Brain Tumor Association

http://www.cancer.gov The Web site of the National Cancer Institute.

http://radiologyinfo.org A Web site developed jointly by the American College of Radiology and the Radiological Society of North America.

Hematopoietic Stem Cell Transplantation

Centers for Disease Control and Prevention. (2000). *Guidelines for preventing opportunistic infections among hematopoietic stem cell transplant recipients.* Retrieved April 22, 2003, from http://www.phppo.cdc.gov/cdcrecommends/

Foss, F.M., Gorgun, G., & Miller, K.B. (2002). Extracorporeal photopheresis in chronic graft-versus-host disease. *Bone Marrow Transplantation, 20,* 719–725.

Gonzalez-Ryan, L., Van Syckle, K., Coyne, K.D., & Glover, N. (2000).Umbilical cord blood banking: Procedural and ethical concerns for this new birth option. *Pediatric Nursing, 26,* 105–110.

Gross, T.G., Egeler, R.M., & Smith, F.O. (2001). Pediatric hematopoietic stem cell transplantation. *Hematology/Oncology Clinics of North America, 15,* 795–808.

Heiney, S.P., Bryant, L.H., Godder, K., & Michaels, J. (2002). Preparing children to be bone marrow donors. *Oncology Nursing Forum, 29,* 1485–1489.

Jacobsohn, D.A., & Vogelsang, G.B. (2002). Novel pharmacotherapeutic approaches to prevention and treatment of GVHD. *Drugs 2002, 62,* 879–889.

Kemp, J., & Dickerson, J. (2002). Interdisciplinary modular teaching for patients undergoing progenitor cell transplantation. *Clinical Journal of Oncology Nursing, 6,* 157–160.

Kupst, M.J., Penati, B., Debban, B., Camitta, B., Pietryga, D., & Margolis, D., et al. (2002). Cognitive and psychosocial functioning of pediatric hematopoietic stem cell transplant patients: A prospective longitudinal study. *Bone Marrow Transplantation, 30,* 609–617.

Ryan, L.G., Kristovich, K.M., Haugen, M.S., Coyne, K.D., & Hubbell, M.M. (2002). Hematopoietic stem cell transplantation. In C.R. Baggott, K.P. Kelly, D. Fochtman, & G.V. Foley (Eds.), *Nursing care of children and adolescents with cancer* (pp. 212–255). Philadelphia: W.B. Saunders.

Secola, R. (2001). Hematopoietic stem cell transplantation: A glimpse of the past and a view of the future. *Journal of Pediatric Oncology Nursing, 18,* 171–177.

Takemoto, C.K., Jodding, J.H., & Kraus, D.M. (2002). *Pediatric dosage handbook* (9th ed.). Hudson, OH: LexiComp, Inc.

Zaia, J.A. (2002). Prevention and management of CMV-related problems after hematopoietic stem cell transplantation. *Bone Marrow Transplantation, 29,* 633–638.

http://www.asbmt.org American Society for Blood and Marrow Transplantation

http://www.ibmtr.org International Bone Marrow Transplant Registry

http://www.marrow.org National Marrow Donor Program

Biologic Response Modifiers

Andolina, M., Rabusin, M., Maximova, N., & Di Leo, G. (2000). Etanercept in graft-versus-host disease. *Bone Marrow Transplant, 26,* 929.

Arceci, R.J., & Cripe, T.P. (2002). Emerging cancer-targeted therapies. *Pediatric Clinics of North America, 49,* 1339–1368.

Brown, K.A., Esper, P., Kelleher, L.O., Brace-O'Neill, J.E., Polovich, M., &White , J.M. (2001). *Chemotherapy and biotherapy: Guidelines and recommendations for practice.* Pittsburgh: Oncology Nursing Society Publishing Division.

Cheung, N.V., Kushner, B.H., & Kramer, K. (2001). Monoclonal antibody-based therapy of neuroblastoma. *Hematology/Oncology Clinics of North America, 15,* 853–866.

Edwards, L. (2001). The interferons. *Dermatologic Clinics, 19,* 139–146.

Meijer, E., Dekker, A.W., Weersink, A.J., Rozenberg-Arska, M., & Verdonck, L.P. (2002). Prevention and treatment of Epstein-Barr virus-associated lymphoproliferative disorders in recipients of bone marrow and solid organ transplants. *British Journal of Haematology, 19,* 596–607.

Mihich, E. (2000). Historical overview of biologic response modifiers. *Cancer Investigation, 18,* 456–466.

Mocellin, S., Wang, E., & Marincola, F.M. (2001). Cytokines and immune response in the tumor microenvironment. *Journal of Immunotherapy, 24,* 392–407.

Rosenberg, S.A. (2001). Progress in the development of immunotherapy for the treatment of patients with cancer. *Journal of Internal Medicine, 250,* 462–475.

Uchiyama, M., Iwafuci, M., Yagi, M., Iinuma, Y., Ohtaki, M., & Tomita, Y., et al. (2000). Treatment of childhood renal cell carcinoma with lymph node metastasis: Two cases and a review of literature. *Journal of Surgical Oncology, 75,* 266–269.

van Esser, J.W., Niesters, H.G., van der Holt, B., Meijer, E., Osterhaus, A.D., & Gratama, J.W., et al. (2002). Prevention of Epstein-Barr virus-lymphoproliferative disease by molecular monitoring and preemptive rituximab in high-risk patients after allogeneic stem cell transplantation. *Blood, 99,* 4364–4369.

Wagner, L.M., & Furman, W.L. (2001). Haematopoietic growth factors in paediatric oncology: A review of the literature. *Paediatric Drugs, 3,* 195–217.

Woolery-Antill, M. (2002). Biotherapy. In C.R. Baggott, K.P. Kelly, D. Fochtman, & G.V. Foley (Eds.), *Nursing care of children and adolescents with cancer* (pp. 177–211). Philadelphia: W.B. Saunders.

Worth, L.L., Jeha, S.S., & Kleinerman, E.S. (2001). Biologic response modifiers in pediatric cancer. *Hematology/Oncology Clinics of North America, 15,* 723–740.

Gene Therapy

Beltinger, C., Uckert, W., & Debatin K.M. (2001). Suicide gene therapy for pediatric tumors. *Journal of Molecular Medicine, 78,* 589–612.

Cashion, A. (2002). Genetics in transplantation. *Medical-Surgical Nursing, 11*(2), 91–94.

Fibison, W.J. (2000). Gene therapy. *Nursing Clinics of North America, 35,* 757–772.

Loud, J.T., Peters, J.A., Fraser, M., & Jenkins, J. (2002). Applications of advances in molecular biology and genomics to clinical cancer care. *Cancer Nursing, 25*(2), 110–122.

Rieger, P.T. (2000). The gene genies. *American Journal of Nursing, 100*(10), 87–90.

Rousseau, R.F., Bollard, C.M., & Heslop, H.E. (2001). Gene therapy for paediatric leukaemia. *Expert Opinion in Biol. Ther., 1,* 663–674.

Rousseau, R.F., Height, A.E., Hirschmann-Jax, C., Yvon, E.S., Rill, D.R., & Mei, Z., et al. (2003). Local and systemic effects of an allogeneic tumor cell vaccine combining transgenic human lymphotactin with interleukin-2 in patients with advanced or refractory neuroblastoma. *Blood, 101,* 1718–1726.

http://www.ornl.gov/TechResources/Human_Genome/project/about.html Information on the Human Genome Project

http://cis.nci.nih.gov/fact/7_18.htm Cancer facts from the National Cancer Institute

Complementary and Alternative Treatments

National Center for Complementary and Alternative Medicine, National Institutes of Health. (2002, August). *Are you considering using complementary and alternative medicine (CAM)?* Retrieved February 11, 2003, from http://nccam.nih.gov/health/decisions/index.htm

National Cancer Institute. (n.d.). *PDQ cancer information summaries: Complementary and alternative medicine.* Retrieved March 14, 2003, from http://www.cancer.gov/cancerinfo/pdq/cam

National Institutes of Health Clinical Center. (2002, December 17). *Facts about dietary supplements.* Retrieved March 14, 2003, from http://www.cc.nih.gov/ccc/supplements/intro.html

Weiger, W.A., Smith, M., Boon, H., Richardson, M.A., Kaptchuk, T.J., & Eisenberg, D.M. (2002). Advising patients who seek complementary and alternative medical therapies for cancer. *Annals of Internal Medicine, 137,* 889–903.

http://nccam.nci.nih.gov/health/clearinghouse/Clearinghouse for the National Center for Complementary and Alternative Medicine, National Institutes of Health

http://www3.cancer.gov/occam/Office of Cancer Complementary and Alternative Medicine (OCCAM), National Cancer Institute

http://www.mcp.edu/herbal/Home page of the Longwood Herbal Task Force. Information on herbal medicine from the Massachusetts College of Pharmacy and Health Sciences.

SECTION V

Side Effects of Treatment

Karla Wilson

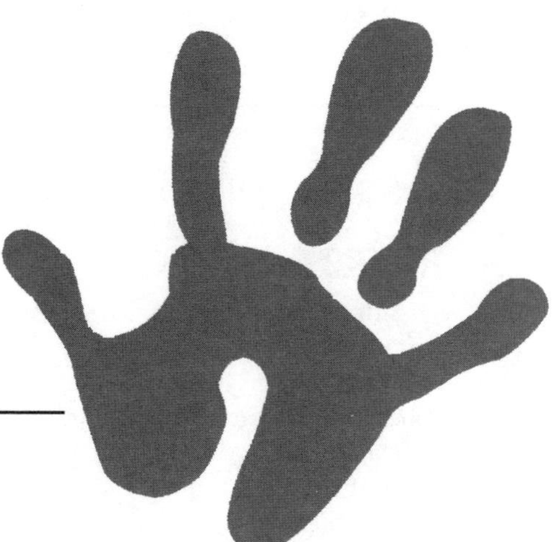

Section Outline

Introduction

Side effects associated with cancer treatment can occur after surgery, chemotherapy, radiation therapy, or supportive care therapy, which includes the administration of antibiotics, colony-stimulating factors, or blood products. The type of cancer, its location, and the age of the child will affect the severity of the side effects. This section describes side effects of treatment in relation to body systems.

Bone Marrow Suppression

Karla Wilson

Bone marrow provides the environment for the formation of red blood cells (RBCs), white blood cells (WBCs), and platelets. Because the hematopoietic system has a rapid turnover, cells are constantly being regenerated. Cancer treatment has a direct impact on this process. Bone marrow suppression is the most common dose-limiting component of cancer therapy. During the nadir, infection and bleeding can occur and can require blood product support and the use of biologic response modifiers to stimulate bone marrow activity. This can include one or more of the following: erythropoietin (Epogen), darbepoietin (Aranesp), granulocyte-colony stimulating factor (GCSF) (Neupogen), granulocyte macrophage-colony stimulating factor (GM-CSF) (Leukine), and interleukin 11 (IL-11) (Neumega) to stimulate bone marrow activity.

Conditions Related to Bone Marrow Suppression

The following conditions are related to bone marrow suppression.

Anemia:

Definition. Anemia is a deficiency in the number of circulating RBCs required for normal tissue and organ oxygenation (see Section III, "Overview of Hematology").

Clinical presentation. The symptoms are fatigue, pallor, tachycardia or gallop heart rhythm, and hemoglobin less than or equal to 7.5 g/dl and hematocrit of 20% or less.

Thrombocytopenia:

Definition. Thrombocytopenia is a decrease in the total number of circulating platelets (see Section III, "Overview of Hematology"). The severity is defined by the following parameters:

Mild: Platelet count = 75,000/mm^3 to within normal limits
Moderate: Platelet count = 50,000–74,900/mm^3
Moderately severe: Platelet count = 20,000–49,900/mm^3
Severe: Platelet count <20,000/mm^3

Clinical presentation. The symptoms can include oozing of the gums, epistaxis, petechiae, ecchymosis, hematuria, and hematochezia.

Neutropenia:

Definition. Neutropenia is a reduction in circulating neutrophils determined by the percentage of segmented neutrophils and band neutrophils that constitute the total WBC (see Section III, "Overview of Hematology"). The absolute neutrophil count (ANC) is calculated as follows:

(% bands + % segmented neutrophils) × total WBC = ANC).

The severity of neutropenia is defined by the following parameters:

Mild: ANC = 1,500–1,900/mm^3
Moderate: ANC = 1,000–1,499/mm^3
Moderately severe: ANC = 500–999/mm^3
Severe: ANC < 500/mm^3

Clinical presentation. Neutropenia can be asymptomatic. If there are signs or symptoms of anemia or thrombocytopenia, a patient frequently also is neutropenic. The symptoms are fever and infection (i.e., bacteremia or viral, fungal, opportunistic [e.g., *Pneumocystis carinii* pneumonia] infection) (see Section VI, "Supportive Care").

Disease-related risk factors. The disease-related risk factors are acute lymphoblastic leukemia (ALL), acute nonlymphoblastic leukemia (ANLL), and metastatic bone marrow involvement from solid tumors.

Treatment-related risk factors. The treatment-related risk factors are myelosuppressive chemotherapy and radiation, including cranial or spinal radiation, radiation involving flat bones such as the ribs, sternum, and pelvis, and total body irradiation.

Supportive care factors. Supportive care measures, such as hyperhydration, can have a dilutional effect on the complete blood count (cbc), and medications such as trimethoprim-sulfamethoxazole (TMP-SMZ) (Bactrim) can cause myelosuppression.

Medical Management

Anemia: Packed RBC transfusions at 10–15 ml/kg of body weight can be given if clinical symptoms are present. Erythropoietin (Epogen) may be given to some patients; the dose is 150–300 units/kg subcutaneously or intravenously every other day. Darbepoietin alfa (Aranesp) is a new, long-acting erythropoietin that is given on a weekly basis; the dose is 1–4 mcg/kg subcutaneously. Erythropoietin and darbepoietin are not widely used in pediatrics, but studies to establish their safety and efficacy are in progress.

Thrombocytopenia: Platelet transfusions are administered at a dose of 6 units/m^2; single-donor units should be given when possible. A medically stable patient who has shown no evidence of bleeding is sometimes transfused when the platelet count is less than 10,000–20,000/mm^3 (or according to institutional practice). A patient who is bleeding, has significant infection, has residual intracranial tumor, or requires surgical intervention may need transfusions to keep the platelet count above 50,000/mm^3. Irradiated, leukocyte-depleted blood products can be given to children receiving cancer treatment; cytomegalovirus (CMV)-negative blood products should be administered to patients who are potential or actual bone marrow transplant candidates, again according to institutional practice.

Interleukin-11 (Neumega) is a thrombopoietic growth factor that stimulates proliferation and maturation of megakaryocytes in the bone marrow resulting in increased circulating platelets. It is administered subcutaneously at 75–100 mcg/kg/day for 10–21 days.

Neutropenia: G-CSF or GM-CSF may be used selectively in some patients (see Section IV, "Childhood Cancer Treatment"), depending upon the treatment protocol or institutional practice. Administration of colony stimulating factors results in an early release of neutrophils from the bone marrow, decreasing the duration of the neutrophil nadir. The dose of G-CSF is 5–10 mcg/kg/day, while the dose of GM-CSF is 250. Either medication may be given subcutaneously or intravenously, though both are thought to have better efficacy if given via the subcutaneous route. Colony stimulating factor therapy is discontinued when the ANC reaches either the value indicated by the treatment protocol or by institutional recommendation.

Potential complications associated with medical management include reactions related to transfusions: hypersensitivity, alloimmunization, or both. Symptoms can include urticaria, fever, chills, rigors, hemolytic reactions, and volume overload. Although the blood supply in the United States is extremely safe, there is still a small risk for the following infections from a contaminated product: hepatitis B, hepatitis C, CMV, human immunodeficiency virus (HIV), and bacteremia. Graft-versus-host disease is a complication that can occur in severely immunocompromised patients who are receiving numerous transfusions (See "Blood Product Support" in Supportive Care, Section V).

Potential complications associated with the granulocyte colony-stimulating factor (Neupogen) are fever, bone pain, and hypersensitivity manifested by an allergic reaction (especially if the patient has a history of allergy to *E. coli* L-asparaginase [Elspar]).

The complications that are associated with erythropoietin (Epogen) are hypertension, seizures, and thrombotic events.

Side effects of treatment with IL-11 (Neumega) include fever, headaches, and flu-like symptoms.

A complication of continued treatment with antibiotics is fungal infection, which can occur particularly when a patient has severe, prolonged neutropenia.

Nursing Assessment and Interventions

Assessment:

- Know the timing of the nadir associated with various types of therapies.
- Review the patient's response to previous therapy.

Interventions:

- Reinforce the need to wash hands thoroughly.
- Teach the patient and the family the importance of knowing the patient's blood counts.
- Teach precautions to the patient and the family. The patient should avoid large crowds or ill persons, limit participation in contact sports, and engage in quiet activities when his or her blood cell count is low. Both the patient and the family should be alert to the signs and symptoms of anemia, which include pallor, fatigue, tachycardia, and shortness of breath. Thrombocytopenia can cause ecchymosis, epistaxis, petechiae, hematuria, and hematochezia. Fever greater than 101° F (38.4° C), is a major concern when the child is neutropenic.
- Discuss the pros and cons of directed donor transfusions. (Transfusion of a blood product from a potential bone marrow donor to the patient may impair engraftment in the patient at the time of bone marrow transplant.)

Expected Patient and Family Outcomes

- The patient and the family understand the implications of bone marrow suppression and can identify the signs and symptoms of anemia, thrombocytopenia, and infection in order to seek early medical intervention as needed.
- The patient and the family comply with prophylactic and supportive-care measures.

Impairment of the Immune System

Karla Wilson

Both the cellular and the humoral components of the immune system are altered when a child has cancer. Lymphocyte function can be affected by either the disease process or the associated treatment. Impairment of T and B lymphocytes results in a deficient production of antibodies and decreased ability to process antigens, thereby altering a patient's ability to resist infection. In an immunosuppressed child, severe neutropenia further enhances the child's susceptibility to bacterial, fungal, and viral infections.

Immunizations

Live attenuated vaccines and inactive or killed vaccines help provide immunity for specific diseases frequently associated with childhood (e.g., measles, mumps, and rubella). In an immunocompromised child, a live vaccine actually can cause the disease and result in a potentially fatal outcome. Inactivated vaccines can be ineffective because the host is unable to develop a cell-mediated response.

Immunization issues for patients, their siblings, and peers: Patients may receive killed (inactivated) vaccines and influenza vaccine while in therapy. All routine immunizations can resume 3–12 months after treatment is completed, depending upon individual situations. Patient-related precautions include not permitting a patient to assist with diaper changes of an infant who has been vaccinated with oral polio vaccine. Conversely, if a patient who is not immune to chickenpox is exposed to someone with a vesicular rash who has received Varivax, it is not considered a varicella exposure. Administration of varicella zoster immune globulin (VZIG) is not indicated in this situation since the risk of transmission is extremely low. It has been suggested that children with ALL in remission be considered for Varivax vaccination. Although the risk of natural varicella outweighs the danger presented by the attenuated vaccine virus, vaccination is currently not standard practice.

It is recommended that all household members receive influenza vaccine. They may also have all routine childhood immunizations, including chicken pox vaccine. Patients' siblings or other children living in the house should receive an inactivated polio virus (IPV) vaccine.

Nursing assessment and interventions

Assessment:

- Review the patient's immunization status with the patient and the family.

Intervention:

- Teach the patient and the family about the issues related to immunizations (**Table 5-1**).

Expected Patient and Family Outcomes

- The patient and the family know the potentially serious side effects of immunizations in an immunocompromised host.

Common Infections Associated with an Impaired Immune System

***Pneumocystis carinii* pneumonia (PCP):**

Definition. Pneumocystis carinii pneumonia is the most common protozoal infection in immunosuppressed children. It is manifested by pneumonitis or pneumonia or both and is frequently fatal. Almost all PCP cases occur in cancer patients who are not compliant with PCP prophylaxis or have not been placed on prophylaxis by their healthcare provider. However, children who are immunocompromised because of HIV infection or AIDS have been infected with PCP despite documented evidence that they have complied with the prophylactic regimen.

Clinical presentation. PCP symptoms can include fever, cough, tachypnea, nasal flaring, intercostal retractions, decreased oxygen saturation, increased respiratory effort, and diffuse bilateral alveolar disease with or without hyperinflation as revealed by chest radiograph. Definitive diagnosis is made through finding *Pneumocystis carinii* organisms in the lung tissue or respiratory secretions obtained by open lung or transbronchial biopsy or by broncoalveolar lavage.

Risk factors. The risk factors are immunosuppression, neutropenia, malignancy, and HIV infection or AIDS.

Medical management. The prophylactic treatment of choice is trimethoprim-sulfamethoxazole (TMP-SMZ, trade names Bactrim, Septra) given by mouth at a dose of 5 mg/kg/day divided b.i.d. for 3 days a week. If a child does not tolerate TMP-SMZ, other prophylactic regimens are available. These include (in order of preference): Dapsone given orally at a dose of 2 mg/kg/day (maximum dose 100 mg/day) once daily, or 4mg/kg (maximum dose 400 mg/week); aerosolized pentamidine isoethionate (Pentam-300) 300mg via Respigard II inhaler, given monthly; or atovaquone 30 mg/kg given orally daily in children 1–3 months of age, and 45 mg/kg orally daily in children more than 2 years old. Treatment for active infection includes therapy with either TMP-SMZ, pentamidine, or atovaquone; and supportive measures that include corticosteroids, oxygen, and mechanical ventilation, as needed.

Potential complications. Complications can include chronic pulmonary disease, prolonged interruption of cancer treatment, or death.

Nursing Assessment and Interventions

Assessment:

- Review the prophylaxis regimen for *Pneumocystis carinii* pneumonia with the patient and the family.
- Assess for symptoms of *Pneumocystis carinii* pneumonia.

Interventions:

- Tell the patient and the family that *Pneumocystis carinii* pneumonia can be prevented with prophylactic treatment.

Table 5-1. Issues Related to Immunizations

Children with Cancer

Children receiving treatment for cancer have decreased immunity and are not able to fight infection in the same way as a child with a normal immune system. For this reason, live-bacteria and live-virus vaccinations are contraindicated for patients with cancer. Inactivated vaccines may be administered, but it should be realized that the child's immune response may be inadequate. Inactivated vaccines include diptheria-tetanus-pertussis (Tri-Immunol), hepatitis B (Engerix-B), inactivated poliovirus (IPV) (Polivax), pneumococcal (Pneumovax) and influenza virus (Fluogen) vaccines.

A definite recommendation for initiation of immunizations after treatment for cancer varies according to the diagnosis and intensity of treatment. Most institutions restart immunizations within 6-12 months after cessation of treatment (American Academy of Pediatrics, 1997).

Siblings and Household Contacts

Siblings can receive live immunizations without harm to their brother or sister with cancer as can other people in the house who have contact with the child with cancer. The exception is that siblings and household contacts should receive the IPV because live polio vaccine strains are transmissible. Varicella vaccine (Varivax) is recommended for these people as well.

Friends, Classmates, and Daycare Contacts

It is unnecessary to avoid or prevent contact with friends or classmates after they have been vaccinated. If a contact develops a vesicular rash after receiving the varicella vaccine (Varivax), physical contact with the child with cancer should be avoided, if possible, until the rash resolves. However, it is not necessary to administer VZIG if exposure inadvertently occurs, as the risk of infection transmission is low. Children with cancer should avoid contact with the stool (i.e., by assisting with diaper changing) of anyone who has received the live polio virus (OPV) because live polio virus is excreted in the stool for several weeks. In rare cases, the oral polio virus has been excreted in the stool for more than 2 months (American Academy of Pediatrics, 1997).

- Inform the patient and the family that prophylaxis must continue for approximately 6 months after treatment ends, or until the patient's absolute lymphocyte count is consistently higher than 1,500.
- Tell the patient and the family that TMP-SMZ (Bactrim) may need to be discontinued briefly since it can prolong neutropenia, should it occur.

Expected Patient and Family Outcomes

- The patient and the family know about the risk factors for contracting *Pneumocystis carinii* pneumonia.
- The patient and the family comply with the prophylactic regimen.

Varicella zoster (chicken pox) and herpes zoster (shingles): Chicken pox is a common childhood illness of the herpes virus group that is manifested by pruritis, fever, and clear vesicular lesions. Although it is rare, a systemic illness that can include pneumonia, hepatitis, or encephalitis can occur. The incubation period is 10–21 days, and the host is infectious approximately 24–48 hours prior to the onset of lesions. The contagious period ends after all lesions are crusted over and no further lesions develop. After an infection, the virus remains latent in the nerve tissues and can be reactivated during times of stress, or if a person is immunocompromised. The subsequent rash is recognized as herpes zoster, a painful, vesicular clustering of lesions along a nerve pathway.

Risk factors. A person is at risk if he or she has had no previous immunity to varicella, is immunocompromised, or is exposed to someone with a varicella infection.

Medical management. Management measures include documenting a patient's immune status by testing for varicella titers. An intramuscular dose of varicella zoster immune globulin (VZIG)(125 units/10 kg [maximum dose of 625 units]) should be given as soon as possible after exposure (but no later than 96 hours afterward). An oral or intravenous course of acyclovir (Zovirax) is given for 7 days when a child develops chicken pox or herpes zoster while receiving treatment, or within 6 months after treatment is ended.

Symptom management. Antihistamine therapy is given for pruritis. Medications for pain management frequently are needed for patients with shingles.

Potential complications. Complications can include systemic (i.e., pulmonary, hepatic, central nervous system) involvement, prolonged interruption of cancer treatment, or death.

Nursing Assessment and Interventions

Assessment:

- Assess the patient's varicella titer.
- Document varicella titer in the patient's medical record.

Interventions:

- Teach the family about what constitutes an exposure and the importance of avoiding exposure (**Table 5-2**).
- Instruct the family about how these diseases are spread by direct contact with patients with varicella or zoster, occasionally by airborne spread of respiratory secretions, and, rarely, from zoster lesions.

Table 5-2. Exposure to Chicken Pox

Chicken pox, also called varicella, is a contagious disease. This means it can be caught by spending *1 hour* or more in the same room with someone who is contagious. Chicken pox is contagious about 24-36 hours before the first spot appears. It continues to be contagious until all the sores have scabs on them. The chicken pox rash usually develops 10-21 days after exposure. In addition, a child who breaks out into a vesicular rash following Varivax immunization is considered to be mildly contagious. Contact should be avoided, when possible, but it is not necessary for the immunosuppressed child to receive VZIG.

Symptoms may be a runny nose, watery eyes, tiredness, and a fever. Within a day or two a rash develops. There are three types of sores: small red spots, raised red areas, or fluid-filled blisterlike sores that break open and scab over. The chicken pox rash usually starts on the stomach, chest, back, or scalp. It then spreads over the rest of the body. A person who has had chicken pox usually develops an immunity to the disease. This means that most people get chicken pox only once.

A child who is receiving chemotherapy has a harder time fighting infections. Therefore, the following information is important to know about their care.

The physician or nurse should be called right away if a child who is receiving chemotherapy was with someone for *1 hour* or longer who has the chicken pox rash or who broke out in a rash 24–36 hours later. **It is very important to call as soon as the child was exposed.** (If the family finds out at night, they can wait until the morning).

Some people who have a low resistance to infections have to get a special medicine after they are exposed to chicken pox. This special medicine, called globulin or varicella zoster immune globulin (VZIG), will lower the risk of a severe infection but may not prevent the person getting the chicken pox. It is important that the person get VZIG within 96 hours of exposure.

After receiving VZIG, a person can take up to 28 days to break out in chicken pox. Also, VZIG may prevent someone from developing an immunity even if the person breaks out in chicken pox. A blood test can be done about 6 weeks after a person has recovered from chicken pox to determine if he or she has immunity. As long as a person does not have immunity, he or she will require VZIG with each chicken pox exposure until the person has been off chemotherapy for 6–12 months.

- Alert authorities at the patient's school to notify the child's parents if there is a chicken pox outbreak.
- Tell the family to notify the child's healthcare provider when an exposure occurs to ensure a timely administration of varicella zoster immune globulin.
- Teach the family to recognize the signs and symptoms of a more serious progression of disease.
- Encourage the habit of washing hands thoroughly.

Expected Patient and Family Outcomes

- The patient and the family know about the potential seriousness of varicella infections.
- The patient and the family comply with the recommendations for treatment related to an exposure or outbreak.

Central Nervous System Complications

Linda Madsen

Central nervous system (CNS) side effects from disease or treatment, or both, offer a significant challenge to patients, families, and healthcare providers. These side effects cause a wide range of symptoms related to the specific location within the CNS that has been injured. A child's age and developmental stage can increase the difficulty healthcare providers have in recognizing and managing these problems.

Diabetes Insipidus

Definition: Diabetes insipidus (DI) is a disorder that causes a decreased production of the antidiuretic hormone (ADH) vasopressin, resulting in the interruption of tubular reabsorption of water by the kidneys (**Figure 5-1**). Osmoreceptors in the brain regulate the synthesis and release of vasopressin in the hypothalamus. Vasopressin travels through the pituitary stalk to the posterior lobe of the pituitary, where it is stored until it is released into circulation. In patients with DI, the hypothalmus may be unable to produce ADH, or the kidneys may be unable to respond.

Risk factors: The risk factors include CNS tumors or surgery that affects the hypothalamic-pituitary axis (HPA). Postoperative swelling occurs 24–48 hours after surgery, influencing the production of vasopressin. Other factors include Langerhans cell histiocytosis; midline, supratentorial, or infratentorial brain tumors (i.e., pituitary tumors, hypothalamic tumors, pineal tumors, craniopharygiomas, germ cell tumors, and third ventricular tumors); CNS leukemia; and radiation therapy to the HPA. Medications associated with DI include furosemide, gentamicin, amphotericin, cisplatin, foscarnet, methicillin, vinblastine, and aminoglycosides.

Clinical presentation: The symptoms of diabetes insipidus are polyuria, nocturia, polydipsia, a specific gravity of less than 1.005, hypernatremia, hypokalemia, and lethargy.

Medical management: A complete history is taken and a physical examination, including neurological assessment, is done. An MRI or CT is done to evaluate the underlying disease. Diagnosis is based on fluid deprivation tests to determine osmolality of serum and urine vasopressin levels. If a patient's urine concentration or osmolality does not increase despite fluid restriction, the diagnosis is confirmed. When the cause is a brain tumor, surgical resection may alleviate pressure, and radiation, chemotherapy, or both are given when possible to reduce the mass. Steroids may be given to reduce inflammation after surgery. Fluid balance should be strictly monitored.

Figure 5-1. The Centers of the Hypothalamus and Pituitary Gland Involved in Water Balance

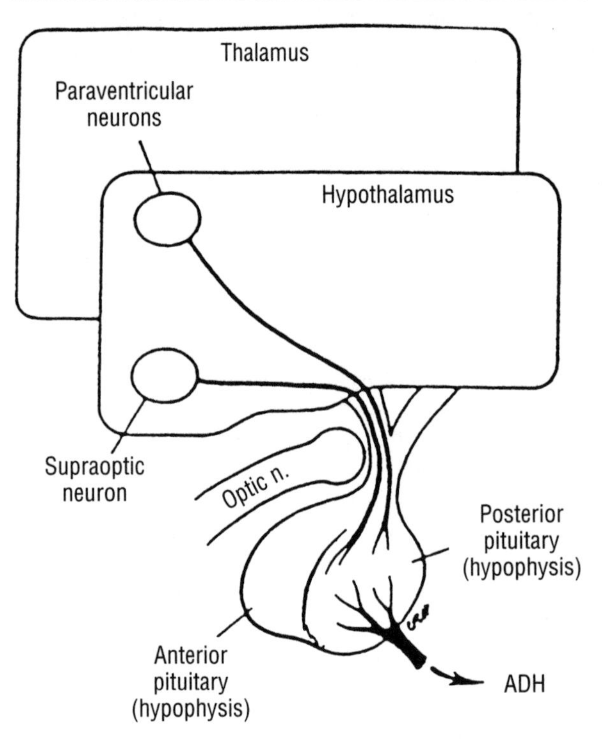

Note. From *Pathophysiology: Concepts of Altered Health States* (3rd ed., p. 487), by C.M. Porth, 1990, Philadelphia: Lippincott. Copyright 1990 by Lippincott. Reprinted with permission.

Potential complications: The potential complications of DI are severe dehydration, hypovolemia, hypernatremia, and hypokalemia.

Nursing Assessment and Interventions

Assessment:

- Monitor the patient's intake and output strictly.
- Weigh the patient twice a day.
- Monitor the patient's serum sodium every 4–6 hours.
- Do a neurological assessment.
- Assess the educational and support needs of the patient and the family.

Interventions:

- Serum sodium and osmolality should be monitored every 4–6 hours. The urine specific gravity and urine osmolality should be monitored every time the patient voids. Fluids should be replaced, as needed, and medications (desmopressin [DDAVP] given orally or intranasally and vasopressin [Pitressin] given subcutaneously) should be administered.

- Educate the patient's parents about the basic pathology and etiology of DI.
- Teach the parents how to administer DDAVP.
- Teach the parents when to give required medications and when to give emergency medications.
- Teach the parents the signs and symptoms of breakthrough diuresis or overdose of medications; help the parents obtain a Med-Alert bracelet for the patient.
- Inform the parents that DDAVP dose adjustments may be needed during illness.
- Emphasize to the family that DI disrupts the normal thirst mechanism and the ability to maintain normal hydration and that the child may be at risk for dehydration.
- Inform the appropriate people at the child's daycare center or school of the absolute necessity that the child has unlimited access to a bathroom and to oral fluids.

Expected Patient and Family Outcomes:

- The patient and the family know about the disease process.
- The patient and the family can adjust independently the patient's DDAVP dose.
- The patient and the family comply with follow-up recommendations.
- Appropriate fluid balance is maintained.

Cranial Nerve Deficits

Definition: A cranial nerve deficit is an impingement or invasion of the nerves arising from the brain stem that results in specific functional deficits (**Figure 5-2**).

Risk factors: The risk factors associated with cranial nerve deficits are primary or metastatic tumors of the CNS (brain stem gliomas, pontine tumors, medulloblastomas, ependymomas, pineal tumors, pituitary tumors, optic gliomas, CNS lymphomas and leukemias, parameningeal or nasopharyngeal rhabdomyosarcomas, soft tissue sarcomas, neuroblastomas, nasopharyngeal carcinoma, neurofibromatosis, and retino-blastoma); resection of the tumor, radiation, and chemotherapeutic agents, including vincristine (Oncovin), vinblastine (Velban), cytarabine (Cytosine Arabinoside), cisplatin (Platinol), and ifosfamide (Ifex).

Clinical presentation: The symptoms include cranial nerve deficits (**Table 5-3**). Parinaud's syndrome, which is manifested by convergence nystagmus, no upward gaze, and increased pupillary reaction to accommodation to light, is often associated with pineal tumors; Horner's syndrome, which is manifested by miosis, ptosis, exophthalmos, anhydrosis (decreased sweating), and constriction of the pupils, is often associated with hypothalamic tumors, tumors of the brain stem or the upper cervical cord and neuroblastoma.

Medical treatment: The patient should have a complete medical history taken and a physical and neurological examination. A CT scan, an MRI, or both should be done to evaluate the underlying cause. When the cause is a mass, surgical resection, when possible, may be done to alleviate pressure on the nerves. Radiation and chemotherapy may be implemented to reduce the mass. Speech and occupational therapy should be implemented to evaluate the effects of the cranial nerve deficits on function and to rehabilitate the patient, or help him or her compensate as needed.

Potential complications: Potential complications include muscle atrophy, facial palsy, persistent deficits that inhibit function (e.g., dysphasia, altered taste resulting in poor nutrition, visual deficits, facial sensation, and mobility and hearing impairment).

Nursing Assessment and Interventions

Assessment:

- Assess the extent of the deficit and its effects on the patient's functioning.
- Assess the chronicity of the deficits.

Figure 5-2 Cranial Nerves: Ventral Surface of the Brain Showing Attachment of the Cranial Nerves

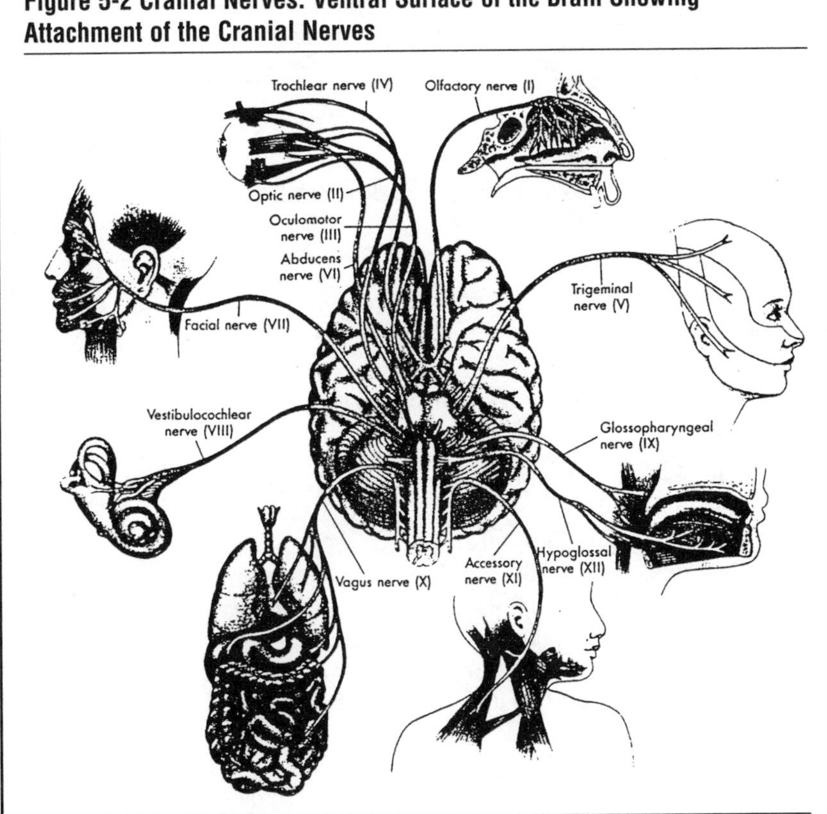

Note. From *Anatomy and Physiology* (p. 345), by G.A. Thibodeau and K.T. Patton, 1992, St. Louis: Mosby. Copyright 1992 by Mosby. Reprinted with permission.

Table 5-3. The Central Nervous System: Cranial Nerves and Their Function

Number	Nerve Name	Function	Deficits and Findings
1	Olfactory	Smell	Loss of smell
2	Optic	Vision	Loss of acuity, optic atrophy, altered visual fields
3	Oculomotor	Pupil constriction, eyelid movement, and extraoccular movements	Ptosis, dilated pupils, altered ocular muscle function, poor near vision, nystagmus
4	Trochlear	Downward and inward eye movement	Altered ocular muscle function-nystagmus
5	Trigeminal	Motor function of the jaw and sensory function of the eye and face	Numbness, poor blink reflex, weakened chewing movements
6	Abducens	Lateral eye movement	Altered ocular muscle function-nystagmus
7	Facial	Movement of the forehead, around eyes and mouth, and taste of the anterior two-thirds of the tongue	Facial paralysis, drooping mouth, sagging lower lid, flat nasolabial fold
8	Acoustic	Hearing and balance	Sensory neuronal hearing loss, vertigo, nausea and vomiting, ataxia
9	Glossopharyngeal	Sensory functions of the pharynx and posterior tongue, including taste	Altered taste and sensation of the throat
10	Vagus	Sensory and motor function of the pharynx and larynx and movement of palate	Hoarseness, altered gag reflex, altered swallowing function
11	Spinal accessory	Motor function of sternomastoid and trapezius muscles	Head tilt to one side, weakness of the shoulder muscles
12	Hypoglossal	Motor function of the tongue	Tongue movement

- Assess the patient's and the family's coping abilities to support a child with deficits.
- Assess the learning needs of the child and the family and their need for safety measures.

Interventions:

- Assist with adaptation of ADLs.
- Assist with occupational and speech therapy to reinforce and support rehabilitation strategies.
- Notify the child's physician if complications develop.
- Provide a safe environment for the patient.
- Provide the patient with nutritional supplements or enteral feeding, if needed.
- Provide home care teaching (i.e., assess and adapt the home environment, as needed; educate the family about necessary adaptations and rehabilitation strategies; provide for ongoing occupational and speech therapy, if needed; intervene when necessary to facilitate the patient's reentry to school; and help with educational planning).

Expected Patient and Family Outcomes

- The patient and the family comply with the recommendations for rehabilitative therapy.
- A safe environment is provided in the home and in modes of transportation.
- The patient shows evidence of good hygiene, skin care, and nutrition.
- The patient focuses on attaining optimal functioning despite deficits.

Cognitive Deficits and Behavioral Changes

Definition: Cognitive deficits are changes in, or loss of, intellectual and developmental ability and functioning. Behavioral changes relate to the patient's personality and to social functioning.

Risk factors: Risk factors are medications that alter mood (e.g., steroids, procarbazine [Matulane], ifosfamide [Ifex]) and supportive care medications that include antiemetics, pain medications, and antidepressants. Intrathecal chemotherapy and cranial radiation can affect intellectual functioning (see Section X, "Late Effects of Childhood Cancer").

Other risk factors include tumors or resections of tumors, including craniopharyngioma (can be associated with memory deficits, personality changes, cognitive abnormalities), pontine tumors (can be associated with personality changes), hypothalamic tumors (can be associated with memory and/or cognitive dysfunction), optic pathway tumors (can be associated with memory and/or cognitive dysfunction), hemispheric gliomas (can be associated with poor academic performance and/or personality changes), posterior fossa tumors (can be associated with emotional lability and declining academic performance),frontal lobe tumors (can be associated with behavioral problems), brain stem gliomas (can be associated with depression and irritability).

Encephalitis and meningitis are additional factors that present an increased risk in younger children. Stress brought on by hospitalization, diagnosis, treatments, and pain also is a risk factor.

Clinical presentation: The signs and symptoms can include a decline in school performance; failure to achieve, or a loss of, developmental milestones; a change in personality and temperament (e.g., irritability, drastic mood swings, fatigue, lethargy, depression, emotional lability, apathy); short-term memory loss; diencephalic syndrome (i.e., failure to thrive, or emaciation in a euphoric infant with an increased appetite or caloric consumption and hyperkinesis); and increased intracranial pressure, which may be manifested by early morning vomiting or headaches.

Medical management: Medical management consists of a complete medical history and physical examination and should include an MRI or CT scan to evaluate the underlying cause. Surgical resection and placement of a ventriculostomy or ventriculo-peritoneal (V-P) shunt may be done when possible to alleviate pressure. Radiation, chemotherapy, or both are given when possible to reduce the mass. Steroids may be given to reduce inflammation after surgery. In addition, there must be a careful evaluation of concomitant medications that can contribute to behavioral changes or cognitive decline. Medications can be ordered to moderate ongoing mood disorders or to regulate behavior. Neuropsychological evaluations should be done regularly to determine the extent of the patient's deficits and to help plan educational or behavioral interventions. The effects of radiation on the developing brain must be considered, and tumor management must be adapted when possible to minimize this complication. Patients should be treated for pain and should be referred for psychological support if it is needed.

Potential complications: Possible complications are a worsening symptomatology; permanent impairment; social isolation, poor peer relationships, or both; a developmental crisis; family stress; and poor self-esteem.

Nursing Assessment and Interventions

Assessment:

- Assess the patient's behavioral and cognitive functioning.
- Assess the impact of the child's behavior on family stress and functioning, as well as on his or her self-image and relationships.
- Assess the impact of cognitive functioning on the child's academic and developmental performance.
- Assess the side effects of medications that can alter behavior or impair learning ability or intellectual performance.

Interventions:

- Plan for the patient's reentry to school to ease his or her adaptation.
- Assess early changes that indicate worsening symptoms or a recurrence of cognitive deficits or changes in behavior.
- Discuss strategies for managing behavior.
- Provide anticipatory guidance for the parents (i.e., review the potential side effects of medications, discuss how to identify symptoms that could indicate the patient's worsening status, and help identify resources to alleviate the family's stress).
- Encourage regular neuropsychological evaluations.
- Educate the child and the parents about school issues and reintegration.
- Encourage early intervention for cognitive and behavioral issues.
- Encourage the patient to interact with both unaffected peers and those who have experienced similar problems.

Expected Patient and Family Outcomes

- The patient and the family know about potential cognitive deficits.
- The patient adopts a healthy lifestyle within the constraints of his or her deficits.
- The patient and the family comply with recommended therapeutic interventions.

Posterior Fossa Syndrome

Definition: Posterior fossa syndrome consists of transient, or occasionally permanent, deficits after posterior fossa surgery. This syndrome often results in mutism or speech disturbance, dysphasia, decreased motor function, weakness, emotional lability, and cranial nerve palsies, which usually present 24–48 hours after surgery and can last for approximately 2–6 months.

Risk factors: Risk factors are posterior fossa tumors (i.e., medulloblastoma or primitive neuroectodermal tumor, astrocytoma, brain stem glioma, ependymoma), large tumor resection, surgical manipulation of the floor of the fourth ventricle, hydrocephalus, cerebellar insult, meningeal spread of tumor, cerebellar atrophy, and vascular disturbances.

Clinical presentation: The signs and symptoms may include, but are not limited to: facial weakness, nystagmus, emotional lability and irritability, mutism or difficulty verbalizing, inability to follow verbal commands, random movements, weakness of the arms and legs, dysphasia, hemiparesis, and/or absence of bladder or bowel control.

Medical management: The patient is given a complete physical and a neurological examination, as well as a thorough examination to assess the patient's swallowing ability and vocal cord function. Hydrocephalus is treated, if needed. Referrals for occupational therapy, physical therapy, and speech therapy may be made. Enteral or parenteral feeding may be necessary if the patient is dysphasic. Patients also may benefit from taking glucocorticoids.

Potential complications: Complications may include permanent impairment, aspiration, muscle atrophy, nutritional deficiency, and family dysfunction.

Nursing Assessment and Interventions

Assessment:

- Assess early changes in the patient's neurological status.
- Monitor the patient's intake and output.
- Weigh the patient on daily basis.
- Assess the patient's gag reflex, voice characteristics, and cognitive and swallowing abilities.
- Assess the effects of the deficits on the patient's personal safety.
- Assess the educational, psychological, and social support needs of the patient and the family.

Interventions:

- Prepare the families of high-risk patients before surgery for the possible onset of the syndrome.
- Provide support for the family.
- Provide reassurance that symptoms typically improve over time, though in some situations they will not totally resolve.
- Implement safety precautions related to preventing aspiration, impaired motor function, and unsteady gait.
- Provide skin care.
- Implement enteral or parenteral feedings as appropriate.
- Support adaptive communication strategies.
- Support rehabilitation strategies.
- Assess and adapt the home environment, as appropriate.
- Educate the family about needed adaptations and support rehabilitation strategies.
- Provide for ongoing occupational therapy and speech therapy, if needed.
- Help plan for the patient's reentry to school, including adaptation to school and remediation, if needed.

Expected Patient and Family Outcomes

- The patient and the family understand the implications of deficits.
- The patient and the family comply with recommended therapeutic interventions.
- The patient and the family can identify and use available resources.

Ototoxicity

Wendy Landier

Definition: Ototoxicity is damage to the hearing organ that is associated with a therapeutic agent, which results in hearing loss or vestibular (balance) changes. The type of hearing loss associated with ototoxic agents is sensorineural (resulting from damage to the cochlea/inner ear) and is usually irreversible (**Figures 5-3** and **5-4**). Ototoxicity has the potential to adversely affect a child's social, emotional, and intellectual development.

Figure 5-3. Normal audiogram

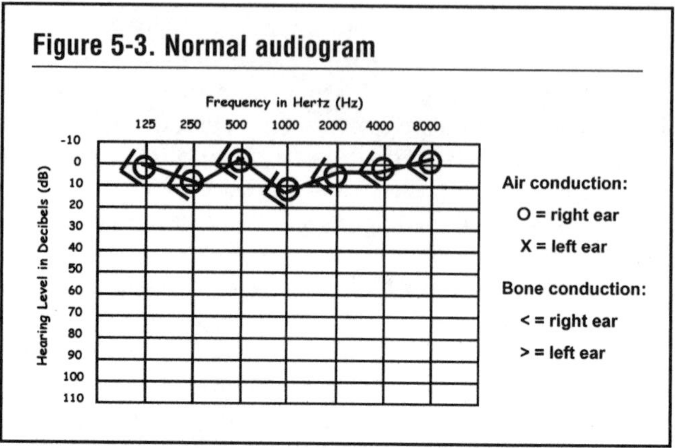

Figure 5-4. Audiogram of child with sensorineural hearing loss (after receiving a platinum-based chemotherapy regimen)

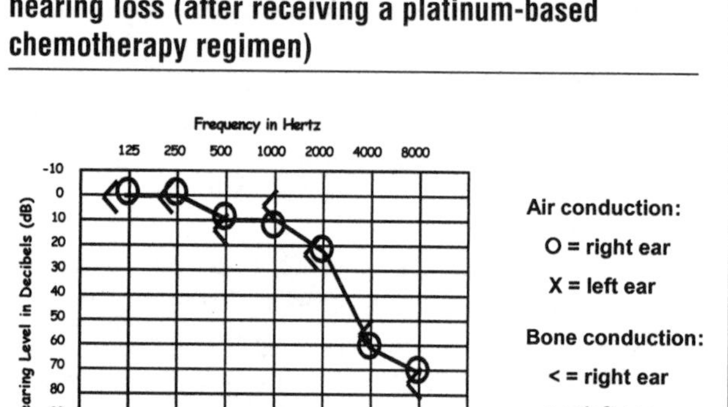

Risk factors: Potentially ototoxic agents commonly used in pediatric oncology including platinum-based chemotherapy (e.g., cisplatin, carboplatin), aminoglycoside antibiotics (e.g., gentamicin, tobramycin, amikacin), loop diuretics (e.g., furosemide), and radiation therapy to the ear, midbrain, or brainstem. Patients who are at increased risk for ototoxicity include those who are younger than 4 years of age when the ototoxic agent is administered, and patients who receive higher cumulative doses of platinum chemotherapy, higher doses of radiation to the cochlea, or therapy with multiple ototoxic agents. Other risk factors include the diagnosis of a CNS tumor, diminished renal function, rapid intravenous administration of the ototoxic agent, and preexisting hearing loss.

Clinical presentation: Symptoms of early hearing loss may include tinnitus and/or vertigo, difficulty in hearing when there is background noise, inattentiveness, or failure to turn toward sounds. However, many children have no symptoms of early hearing loss. Therefore, audiologic monitoring is required for all children receiving potentially ototoxic agents. Methods of audiologic evaluation include pure-tone audiometry (standard audiograms and behaviorally based assessments used with children who can cooperate with testing), or brainstem auditory evoked response (electrophysiologic measurement of hearing used with infants or children who are unable to cooperate with standard testing). All patients who receive ototoxic agents should undergo periodic audiologic evaluations by an experienced pediatric audiologist.

Medical management: Patients with identified hearing loss should be referred to a pediatric otologist or audiologist for evaluation and fitting of appropriate hearing aids. Frequent follow-up assessments (every 6 months) for retesting and refitting of hearing aids are essential, especially for younger, growing children. Since hearing loss associated with ototoxicity usually is irreversible, preventive measures currently are being evaluated, including the use of chemoprotective agents (e.g., amifostine), shielding or modification of radiation fields to limit cochlear exposure, and modification of therapeutic protocols to make possible earlier detection of ototoxicity and subsequent dose reduction or substitution of less ototoxic agents, when feasible.

Nursing Assessment and Interventions

Assessment:

- Assess risk factors for ototoxicity in all patients who are receiving potentially ototoxic agents.
- Ensure that all such patients are being appropriately monitored (e.g., periodic audiologic evaluations, frequent monitoring of aminoglycoside levels).

Interventions:

- Avoid rapid intravenous administration of ototoxic agents, such as loop diuretics, aminoglycosides, platinum chemotherapy.
- Ensure that preventive measures are implemented when medically indicated (e.g., prompt dose modification of aminoglycosides, if indicated, per blood levels; early dose modification of platinum chemotherapy per protocol guidelines if hearing loss is detected; use of chemoprotective agents per protocol guidelines).
- Advise patients and parents about otoprotective strategies (e.g., using earplugs in noisy environments to prevent noise-induced hearing loss, avoiding ototoxic medications when alternatives are available).
- For children with hearing loss:
  - Assure that the patient receives a referral for hearing aid evaluation.
  - Assure that parents and patient learn proper cleaning and care of the hearing aid, including the importance of replacing batteries on a regular basis (most require replacement every 1–2 weeks).
  - Familiarize parents and patient with options regarding communication methods (e.g., auditory/verbal, cued speech), and assistive devices (e.g., FM amplification system, telephone amplifiers, text telephones, adaptive appliances).
  - Familiarize parents and the patient with community and educational resources (e.g., in-home speech therapy, specialized classroom accommodations).

Endocrine Abnormalities

Kathleen E. Marson

Chemotherapy and radiation therapy commonly induce hormone alterations. The primary endocrine effects from cancer treatment are related to the type of drug, dose, duration of treatment, and the age and sex of the patient. Changes in endocrine function as a result of radiation therapy usually occur months or years after treatment and are more common in areas that include the hypothalamic-pituitary axis or thyroid gland.

Hormone Deficits

Definition: Hormone deficits are abnormally low levels of hormones secreted by the body. They occur because of neuroendocrine damage caused by the tumor or cancer treatment and resulting in hypothyroidism, gonadal dysfunction, and growth hormone deficiency (see Section X, "Late Effects of Childhood Cancer").

Risk factors: There are treatment-related and disease-related risk factors.

Treatment-related factors. These risk factors include those associated with radiation therapy (e.g., dose, patient's age, and radiation treatment site) and those associated with chemotherapy (i.e., alkylating agents, nitrosoureas). Alkylating agents can produce gonadal atrophy that can alter permanently reproductive function.

Disease-related factor. Tumor location is the disease-related factor.

Clinical presentation: The signs and symptoms of hormone deficits can include abnormal thyroid levels, fatigue, a change in bowel habits, dry skin, delayed growth and development of secondary sexual characteristics, precocious puberty, irregular menses, amenorrhea, hormone levels (i.e., follicle-stimulating hormone [FSH], luteinizing hormone [LH], testosterone, estradiol, growth hormone) that are abnormal for the patient's age, a decrease in linear growth, and syndrome of inappropriate antidiuretic hormone (SIADH) secretion (see Section X, "Late Effects of Childhood Cancer," for further discussion).

Medical management: The patient should have a complete physical examination and a health history taken, as well as assessments of growth and secondary sexual maturation. Hormone replacement may be indicated after the patient has been evaluated by an endocrinologist.

Potential complications: Complications may include a decrease in hormone levels, alterations in linear growth, precocious puberty or alterations in sexual maturation, hypothyroidism, temporary amenorrhea or irregular menses, and SIADH.

Nursing Assessment and Interventions

Assessment:

- Measure the patient's height and weight throughout therapy and after therapy is concluded.

- Obtain baseline serum hormonal evaluations (e.g., T3, free T4, TSH, LH, FSH) prior to the initiation of radiation therapy to the hypothalamic pituitary axis or thyroid gland.
- Assess the patient's sexual development using the Tanner staging system.
- Assess a female patient's menstrual history at each visit.

Interventions:

- Provide ongoing education about the effects of the disease and its treatment.
- Encourage and support a multidisciplinary approach to endocrine problems related to the disease, the treatment, or both.

Expected Patient and Family Outcomes

- The patient and the family comply with the multidisciplinary plan of care.
- The patient understands the need for long-term compliance and follow-up.

Preservation of Sperm and Ova

Sperm banking: The literature is not definitive on whether semen from patients is adequate for artificial insemination or whether sperm will tolerate cryopreservation. There is controversy among researchers about the technique of cryopreserving sperm—even when the samples appear to be adequate—because of its expense, sperm banks' variable quality controls, and concerns about the viability and integrity of sperm that have been stored for long periods. Sperm banking is an option that should be discussed with an adolescent, and potential complications and the possibility that a sample will be nonviable should be fully explained.

Harvesting of ova and embryos: Currently, the viability and integrity of ova and embryos after cryopreservation is uncertain (see Section X, "Late Effects of Childhood Cancer," for a further discussion).

Cardiac and Pulmonary Complications

Anna Pursell

Cardiac and pulmonary side effects can be directly related to the underlying disease, but they are more commonly associated with specific therapies or an infectious process. A combination of these factors places a patient at greater risk for complications. Acute episodes of cardiopulmonary toxicities frequently evolve into chronic conditions (see Section X, "Late Effects of Childhood Cancer," for more details).

Acute Cardiomyopathy

Definition: Cardiomyopathy is a defect of the heart muscle resulting from damage to cardiac myocytes; it causes loss of muscle fibers and shifts in intracellular calcium (see Section X, "Late Effects of Childhood Cancer").

Risk factors: Chemotherapy-related risk factors include cumulative doses of anthracyclines (the doses must be lowered if radiation treatment also is used), single agents (i.e, cyclophosphamide [Cytoxan]), as well as combination chemotherapy, and combination chemotherapy and radiation. Other risk factors are radiation therapy to the mediastinum, surgery for removal of a tumor in the chest wall or thorax, underlying cardiac disease, administration of IV products that cause fluid overload, anemia, age (particularly when a patient is younger than 4–5 years of age), and the use of glucocorticoids, which can cause hypertension.

Clinical presentation: The signs and symptoms of acute cardiac myopathy can include hypertension or hypotension, chest pain, decreased activity level, fatigue, tachycardia, shortness of breath, nonproductive cough, distention of the neck vein, pedal edema, cardiomegaly, gallop rhythm of the heart, and hepatomegaly.

Medical management: Medical management consists of performing a complete physical examination and taking a health history to review potential risk factors, establish baseline cardiac status, obtain information about prior therapies (including the cumulative dose of radiation and chemotherapy), assess whether there has been routine monitoring of cardiac status, and assess the child's activity level. Pharmacological management comprises adjusting the rate, schedule, and dose of chemotherapy and prescribing any needed antiarrthymic drugs. Blood product transfusions also may be given if the patient is anemic, and oxygen therapy can be given, if necessary. Cardioprotective agents currently are under study to determine their effectiveness in preventing cardiomyopathy.

Potential complications: Complications can include disturbances in the cardiac rhythm, congestive heart failure, or death.

Nursing Assessment and Interventions

Assessment

- Assess the patient's risk factors for developing acute cardiomyopathy.
- Assess the patient for clinical manifestations of congestive heart failure (i.e., tachycardia, shortness of breath, gallop heart rhythm, hepatomegaly, pedal edema, distention of the veins in the neck).
- Monitor the patient's vital signs and assess the heart rate for a normal rhythm and regularity.
- Assess electrocardiogram, echocardiogram, and 24-hour Holter monitoring data, and the results of chest radiograph, according to the treatment protocol or as ordered.

Interventions

- Administer prescribed medications.
- Teach the family medication administration techniques.
- Teach the patient and the family the signs and symptoms of congestive heart failure.

Expected Patient and Family Outcomes

- The patient has minimal complications related to acute cardiomyopathy.
- The patient and the family understand the risk factors associated with acute cardiomyopathy.

Pneumonitis

Definition: Pneumonitis is an inflammation of the lung resulting from infectious agents, irritants, or both.

Risk factors: The risk factors are neutropenia, bacterial agents (i.e., *Pneumocystis carinii, Hemophilus influenza, Streptococcus pneumonia*, mycobacterium), viral agents (i.e., cytomegalovirus, herpes zoster, chicken pox, respiratory syncytial virus, Epstein-Barr virus), chemotherapy (e.g., busulfan [Myleran], melphalan [Alkeran], methotrexate [Mexate], bleomycin [Blenoxane]), radiation therapy to the lungs, and underlying respiratory disease.

Clinical presentation: Patients may present with dyspnea, nonproductive cough, malaise and/or fatigue, fever, moist rales, and a pleural friction rub. Tachypnea, cyanosis, and decreased oxygen saturation are late signs of impaired lung status.

Medical management: Prophylactic trimethoprim-sulfamethoxazole (TMP-SMZ, brand name Bactrim), pentamidine (Pentam-300), or dapsone (Avlosulfon) are used to prevent *Pneumocystis carinii*; antibiotics are given for bacterial infections. Patients should receive an influenza vaccine annually. For symptomatic patients, blood cultures, a chest X ray, pulmonary function tests, and pulse oximetry monitoring are obtained routinely. Bronchodilators may be prescribed. Oxygen and ventilator assistance are given, if needed.

Potential complications: Complications include pulmonary fibrosis or death.

Nursing Assessment and Interventions

Assessment:

- Assess the patient's respiratory rate and effort.
- Assess the patient for signs of pulmonary toxicity.
- Assess the patient for dyspnea, nonproductive cough, rales, and tachypnea.

Interventions:

- Place emphasis on activities the patient can accomplish with minimal exertion.
- Discuss the importance of frequent rest periods, especially during periods of exertion, such as walking.
- Provide measures to decrease dyspnea, such as elevating the head of the patient's bed.

Expected Patient and Family Outcomes

- The patient and the family understand the cause(s) of pneumonitis.
- The patient experiences minimal discomfort.
- The patient and the family take measures to reduce the patient's oxygen expenditure.
- The patient and the family identify symptoms or changes that necessitate an immediate medical evaluation.

Pulmonary Fibrosis

Definition: Pulmonary fibrosis is the formation of fibrous scar tissue in the lungs as a consequence of an inflammation, an injury, or both.

Risk factors: The risk factors are chemotherapy (i.e., busulfan [Myleran], methotrexate [Mexate], melphalan [Alkeran], bleomycin [Blenoxane]), radiation therapy to the lungs, radiation therapy in combination with chemotherapy, previous lung biopsy, underlying pulmonary disease, and smoking.

Clinical presentation: A patient may present with respiratory distress (e.g., tachypnea, dyspnea, cough, hypoxemia, increased respiratory effort), chest pain, or interstitial infiltrates on a chest X ray.

Medical management: A patient should have a complete routine physical examination and a health history taken. These measures establish the patient's baseline pulmonary status, provide information about prior therapies—including cumulative doses of radiation and chemotherapy—and provide a review of potential risk factors.

The patient's pulmonary status including pulmonary function, pulse oximetry, and chest X rays, is routinely monitored. The patient's activity level and respiratory status are assessed. For symptomatic patients, corticosteroids may be used; oxygen therapy may be given, if needed.

Potential complications: Complications include pulmonary hypertension or death.

Nursing Assessment and Interventions

Assessment:

- Maintain complete and current treatment records, including information on prior therapies, doses, and test results.
- Monitor the patient for signs and symptoms of congestive heart disease and respiratory distress.
- Provide laboratory results and information on the patient's status to the physician and the patient's family.
- Monitor the patient's IV fluid rate to avoid fluid overload.
- Strictly maintain intake and output records.
- Weigh the patient daily.

Interventions:

- Teach the family how to modify the patient's activities according to his or her cardiopulmonary status.
- Teach the family the correct use of medications and prescribed therapies and explain their side effects.
- Tell the patient and the family about potential future risk factors during times of increased cardiovascular stress caused by conditions such as pregnancy, illness, heavy weightlifting, or anesthetization.

Expected Patient and Family Outcomes

- The patient and the family understand the potential complications of the disease and the treatment related to the cardiopulmonary system.

- The patient and the family understand the need for long-term follow-up.
- The patient and the family comply with the recommended therapy.

Gastrointestinal Complications

Ruth Landers

Gastrointestinal (GI) complications associated with cancer treatment are common in children. The mucosal cells in children's GI tracts are rapidly dividing cells and are particularly sensitive to chemotherapeutic agents and radiation therapy. The cellular destruction of cancer treatment results in mucositis, an inflammatory response. Disruption of this mucosal barrier places an immunocompromised child at increased risk for pain, ulceration, bleeding, dehydration, malnutrition, and opportunistic infection.

Mucositis and Esophagitis

Definition: Oral mucositis, or stomatitis, is an inflammation or an ulceration of the mucous membranes of the oral cavity (i.e., the lips, tongue, palate, buccal mucosa, gingiva, and floor of the mouth). Esophagitis is mucositis of the esophagus.

Risk factors: Risk factors are trauma to the oral cavity, esophagus, or both because of surgical manipulation; cytotoxic therapy, such as anthracyclines and antimetabolites; radiation therapy to the head, neck, chest wall, and mediastinum (e.g., mantle radiation in lymphoma patients); radiation-induced xerostomia due to mucosal atrophy and fibrosis of the salivary glands; graft-versus-host disease; immunosuppression; local irritants, including alcohol, tobacco, commercial mouthwashes, and spicy or hot foods; malnutrition; dehydration; dental caries; and gastroesophophageal reflux.

Clinical presentation: *Mucositis.* A patient may have pale, ridged, erythematous, ulcerated, or bleeding mucous membranes and gingiva; dry, blistered, or cracked lips; whitish plaques with slightly raised, indurated borders caused by *Candida albicans* fungus; or ulceration of the oral mucosa caused by herpes simplex virus. Oral discomfort may cause difficulty in opening the mouth, speaking, or swallowing. The patient may experience difficulty in eating and drinking because of local discomfort and may develop alterations in taste. In addition, a patient may exhibit psychosocial withdrawal due to pain, an inability to communicate, and loss of oral gratification (especially in infants and toddlers).

Esophagitis. Patients can have burning retrosternal chest pain (heartburn) when stomach acid comes in contact with inflamed esophageal tissue, or if there is *Candida* infection. Other symptoms include nausea, bloating, early satiety, or coughing.

Medical management: Treatment can include oral rinses (e.g., chlorhexidine [Peridex], normal saline solution, baking soda solution) after meals, at bedtime, and as needed to clean the oral mucosa, remove debris, and reduce the incidence of plaque and dental caries (**Table 5-4**). Fluoride rinses and saliva substitutes are used for xerostomia or dry mouth. Antifungal treatments include nystatin (Mycostatin) suspension or frozen treat, clotrimoxazole (Mycelex) troches, and mouthwashes (amphotericin-B, nystatin), as well as fluconazole (Diflucan), or amphotericin B (Fungizone) to treat systemic candidiasis. Acyclovir (Zovirax) is used as a treatment for herpetic lesions and as a prophylaxis in bone marrow transplant patients. Other measures include intravenous fluid therapy in the acute phase when oral therapy is not adequate, parenteral nutrition if mucositis persists and weight loss becomes a problem, and consultation with a dentist and a dietitian.

Pain control. Local palliation can be provided by topical agents such as viscous lidocaine, diphenhydramine (Benadryl), and sucralfate (Carafate). Histamine antagonists and antacids relieve gastric irritation and irritation of the lower esophagus. Centrally acting analgesics range from acetaminophen (Tylenol) to continuous narcotic infusion, with the choice being dependent upon the severity of the mucositis or esophagitis.

Potential complications: Complications include viral, bacterial, or fungal infection, malnutrition, cachexia, dehydration, GI bleeding, and esophageal stricture.

Nursing Assessment and Interventions

Assessment:

- Assess the patient's oral cavity by following the guidelines listed in **Table 5-5**.
- Assess for functional impairment in speech, swallowing, drooling.
- Monitor the patient's fluid and dietary intake.
- Weigh the patient daily.

Interventions:

- Provide care in a nonthreatening manner to optimize compliance.
- Promote meticulous oral care. For younger children, recommend the use of sponges or toothettes (foam brushes) for swabbing affected areas. Recommend that the patient brush his or her teeth with a soft-bristle brush, floss when oral tissues are healthy and platelet count is acceptable, and use toothettes to cleanse, moisten, and apply medications to the oral cavity. (The last recommendation applies especially to thrombocytopenic patients). Swish-and-spit medications are reserved for use by older children.
- When the patient's speech is impaired, use communication methods that are appropriate for his or her age and developmental stage.
- Instruct the patient to avoid food or drink for 30 minutes after using oral rinses or antifungal medications so as to maximize their effects.
- Evaluate the patient's pain frequently and provide topical and systemic analgesia, as indicated.
- Give pain medications before mealtime to decrease pain during dining.
- Encourage the patient to drink fluids unless they are contraindicated.

Table 5-4. A Guide to Oral Care Measures

Indication	Product	Comments
Daily oral care	Warm saline rinses (OTC) (1/2 tsp. salt to I pint water)	Safe, effective, economical, readily available. Thought to aid in formation of granulation tissue and promote healing.
	Sodium bicarbonate rinse (OTC) (I tsp. baking soda to I pint water) Salt and soda solution (OTC) (1/2 tsp. salt and 1 tsp. baking soda in 1 pint water)	Dissolves mucin and loosens debris. Unpleasant taste. Salt improves palatability of sodium bicarbonate. Reduces odor and removes necrotic tissue.
Nonmechanical debridement	Peroxyl (OTC) (1.5% hydrogen peroxide with mint flavoring) (Colgate Oral Pharmaceuticals, Inc, Canton, MA)	Prediluted. May be diluted further if needed. For short-term use only (3 days maximum). Do not use with fresh granulation tissue. Foaming action may cause choking.
	Amosan (OTC) (sodium perborate derivate) (Oral-B Laboratories, Redwood City, CA)	
Antiseptics	Peridex (chlorhexidine gluconate 12%) (Proctor & Gamble, Cincinnati, OH)	Antiplaque and antigingivitis agent. Medicinal taste. Potential to stain teeth.
	ST-37 (OTC) (hexylresorcinol 0.1%, glycerin 28.2% & sodium bisulfate) (Beecham, Inc, Pittsburgh, PA)	Dilute 1:1 with water. Mild topical anesthetic effect. Well tolerated.
Commercial mouthwashes	Cepacol (OTC) (phenol) (Marion, Merrell, Dow, Inc, Kansas City, MO)	Contain alcohol, may cause irritation. NOT RECOMMENDED.
Topical anesthetics	Ulcerease (0.6% phenol, sodium borate, sodium bicarbonate, glycerin and water) (Med Derm, Inc, Kingsport, TN)	Mild anesthetic effect. Phenol also acts as an antiseptic.
	Cepastat Lozenges (OTC) (Marion, Merrill, Dow, Inc)	Contain phenol. May use every 2 hours.
	Chloraceptic (OTC) (Richardson-Vicks, Inc, Cincinnati, OH)	Contain alcohol, may cause irritation. NOT RECOMMENDED.
	Maalox, Kaopectate, or Milk of Magnesia plus diphenhydramine (individual ingredients OTC) (Rhône Polenc Rhorer Pharmaceuticals, Inc, Collegeville, PA; Upjohn, Kalamazoo, MI; and Roxane Laboratories, Inc, Columbus, OH, respectively)	Antacids reduce oral acidity, dissolve mucin film, and have a demulcent effect, softening and soothing the tissues. Benadryl has a mild anesthetic effect. Pectin in Kaopectate forms coating.
	Viscous xylocaine 2% (Roxane Laboratories, Inc)	Give 15 to 20 minutes before meals. Effect is brief and taste unpleasant to some. CAUTION: Limit usage to reduce systemic toxicity. Numbness may increase danger of biting trauma, burns from hot food, or aspiration.
	Dyclonine hydrochloride	Longer anesthetic effect than with other agents. CAUTION: Limit usage to reduce systemic toxicity. Numbness may increase danger of biting trauma, burns from hot food, or aspiration.
	Hurricaine Capsaicin (Beulich LP Pharmaceuticals, Waukegan, IL)	20% Benzocaine topical gel active ingredient in chili peppers. Produces a burning pain that gradually lessens with repeated applications and desensitizes pain receptors. No commercially available product for use in mucositis. Not proven to be tolerated in children.
Coating agents	Orabase (OTC) (with or without Benzocaine) (Colgate Oral Pharmaceuticals, Inc)	Protective paste. Odorless and tasteless. Allergic reactions have been observed.
	Kanka (OTC) (tincture of benzoin, benzocaine 5%, cetylpyridium chloride and flavoring) (Blistex, Inc, Oakbrook, IL)	Provides a protective coating.
	Sucralfate suspension (100 mg/mL)	Cytoprotectant. Soothes and coats.
Lubricants	Xero-lube (artificial saliva) (OTC) (Scherer Corporation, Kenilworth, NJ)	For patients with diminished salivary output. Tasteless. Consistency objectionable to some.

(continued)

Table 5-4. A Guide to Oral Care Measures *(continued)*

Indication	Product	Comments
Lubricants *(continued)*	Moi-Stir (Fiber-tipped swabstick sorbitol, sodium carboxymethylcellulose and electrolytes common in saliva) (Kingswood Laboratory, Inc, Carmel, IN)	Effective cleansing and moistening agents. More acceptable than lemon-glycerin swabs. Does not contain alcohol.
	Petroleum jelly (OTC)	Forms an occlusive oil film preventing moisture evaporation. FLAMMABLE: Avoid use in patients receiving oxygen.
	Nature's Second Skin (lanolin) (OTC) (Lansinoh Laboratories, Oak Ridge, TN)	Retains moisture better than petroleum jelly. Contains no water additives or color.
	Mineral Oil (OTC)	Can inflame trachea and lungs if aspirated. NOT RECOMMENDED.
	KY jelly (OTC) (Johnson & Johnson, Skillman, NJ)	Forms a film on the skin. Water-soluble, can be used in patients receiving oxygen.
Mechanical debridement	Toothbrush	Regular soft toothbrush OK if not neutropenic or thrombocytopenic.
	UltraSuave toothbrush (Periodontal Health Brush, Inc, Osseo, WI)	May be used if patient neutropenic or thrombocytopenic or if regular brushing is too painful. Use nonmechanical cleansing rinses if unable to tolerate these measures.
	Dental floss	Waxed and unwaxed floss equally effective. Mint and cinamon flavoring available.
	Foam swabs Pink Toothettes (Halbrand, Inc, Willoughby, OH)	Less effective than brushing or using gauze around finger. Hygienic (disposable) and effective in stimulating the gums and palate. Also useful for medication application (nystatin, topical anesthetics, etc).
	Foam swabs Green Oraswab (Sage, Inc., Crystal Lake, IL)	Contain hydrogen peroxide with mint flavoring. For short-term use only (3 days maximum). Do not use with fresh granulation tissue or when foaming could cause choking.
	Lemon/glycerin swab	Inefficient in removing debris. Acid may cause pain and decalcify teeth. Effective salivary stimulant and should not be used too often or in dehydrated patients. Glycerin may be somewhat drying. NOT RECOMMENDED.
	Power spray irrigation instruments	Irrigation instrument. Delivers solution (often antibiotic or saline) under high pressure which must be simultaneously suctioned. Best suited for treatment room setting. Expensive.
	Water Pik (OTC) (Teledyne Waterpik, Fort Collins, CO)	Alternative to power sprays. Less expensive, can be used in patient room, suction equipment not needed unless patient is unable to get rid of fluid. Saline cannot be used.
	Enema bag and #14F catheter	Inconvenient, but inexpensive and readily available.

Note. From "Continuing Education: Assessment and Management of Chemotherapy-Induced Mucositis in Children," by L. Kennedy and J. Diamond, 1997, *Journal of Pediatric Oncology Nursing, 14*(3), pp. 170-172. Copyright 1997 by W.B. Saunders. Reprinted with permission.

Table 5-5. Assessment of the Oral Cavity

Site	Grade 1	Grade 2	Grade 3	Grade 4
Lips	Smooth, moist, and intact/pink	Slightly dry, wrinkled, and inflamed	Dry, rough, swollen, and inflamed	Very dry, inflamed, cracked, ulcerated, and bleeding
Tongue	Smooth, firm, pink, and intact	Dry, pink with some reddened areas	Raised red papillae, patchy ulcerations	Confluent ulcerations, inflamed, bleeding
Teeth	Clean without debris	Slightly dull with some debris present	Dull with more than half of teeth covered in debris	Very dull covered in debris; bleeds easily
Gums	Intact, pink	Slightly inflamed with minimal swelling, may have slight bleeding with teeth brushing	Inflamed, swollen, and moderate bleeding with minimal trauma	Very inflamed and swollen, may have continuous oozing without trauma
Saliva	Sufficient quantity, thin	Slightly thickened with decreased quantity	Thick, ropy, mouth may appear dry	Very thick, ropy, or mucoid appearing; mouth very dry

Grade 1 = No mucositis
Grade 2 = Mild mucositis
Grade 3 = Moderate mucositis
Grade 4 = Severe mucositis

Criteria based on NCI Common Terminology Criteria for Adverse Events

- Instruct the patient to avoid hot, dry, spicy foods.
- Educate the patient through gentle reassurance and psychosocial support.
- Encourage routine dental exams and prophylaxis.

Expected Patient and Family Outcomes

- The patient has good oral hygiene habits.
- The patient and the family identify oral medications that are appropriate for the patient's needs.
- The patient and the family recognize situations that require prompt professional intervention (e.g., inadequate oral intake, fever, pain).

Diarrhea

Definition: Diarrhea is an increase in the quantity, frequency, or fluid content of stool that differs from the usual pattern of bowel elimination. Diarrhea is caused by changes in intestinal absorption and motility.

Risk factors: Risk factors include manipulation of the bowel during surgery and resection of a significant portion of the small bowel, which can lead to decreased reabsorption and result in diarrhea and electrolyte loss. Chemotherapy agents that can cause bowel irritation include 5-fluorouracil (5-FU), cisplatin (Platinol), cytarabine (Cytosine Arabinoside), mech-lorethamine (nitrogen mustard), methotrexate (Mexate), and anthracyclines such as doxorubicin (Adriamycin) or daunomycin (Cerubidine), and topoisomerase I inhibitors (irinotecan, topotecan). Radiation to the abdomen, pelvis, or the lower thoracic and lumbar spine increases the incidence of diarrhea. Other risk factors are biologic response modifiers such as interleukin-2 and interferon; intestinal infections secondary to mucositis and neutropenia (e.g., rotavirus, *E. coli*, shigella, salmonella, giardia); medications such as metoclopramide (Reglan), laxatives, antacids, electrolyte supplements, and antibiotics; dietary causes, including lactose intolerance, caffeine, alcohol, spicy and fatty foods, raw vegetables and fruits, tube feedings, and feeding supplements; and conditions such as endocrine tumors, graft-versus-host disease and hyperthyroidism.

Clinical presentation: A patient may have frequent loose stools, perineal irritation, rectal excoriation or ulceration, abdominal cramping, hyperactive bowel sounds, fever, or mucus or blood in the stool. Sloughing of the gastrointestinal lining also may be detected in the stool. The patient may show signs of lethargy and dehydration, electrolyte imbalance, and poor nutrition (e.g., poor skin turgor, weight loss, hypotension, dry mucous membranes, lethargy, and edema).

Medical management: Medical management consists of restoring and maintaining fluid and electrolyte balance, nutrition, normal bowel function, protecting skin integrity, and providing comfort. Parenteral therapy is given as indicated. Antidiarrheal medications (e.g., loperamide, octreotide) are given with caution because the patient may have a bowel obstruction or the diarrhea may be caused by an infection. Stool cultures should be taken if a microorganisim is suspected. Antispasmodic medications may be indicated to relieve abdominal pain, tenesmus, or both. Vancomycin (Vancocin) or metro-nidazole (Flagyl) are the antibiotic therapy for *Clostridium difficile* enteritis. The patient's platelet count may be maintained at more than 50,000 if blood is present in the stool. Sitz baths and barrier creams should be used to protect the perineum and anal/rectal area. The patient should have a diet specific to his or her individual needs.

Potential complications: Complications can include intestinal bleeding and infection, breakdown of rectal tissue, cellulitis or abscess, electrolyte imbalance, dehydration, malnutrition, and social withdrawal because of embarrassment and interruptions to daily functioning.

Nursing Assessment and Interventions

Assessment:

- Monitor the volume, appearance, color, odor, and consistency of the patient's stool.
- Strictly monitor intake and output.
- Assess the patient frequently for signs and symptoms of dehydration and electrolyte imbalance.
- Weight the patient daily or as frequently as his or her circumstances dictate.
- Assess the perianal region carefully for signs of skin breakdown.
- Perform a detailed abdominal assessment, giving attention to pain, bowel sounds, and girth.

Interventions:

- Administer GI and pain medications, as ordered, and monitor their effects.
- Encourage the patient to take fluids orally.
- Encourage the patient to eat a high-calorie, potassium-rich diet with adequate soluble fiber to provide bulk to enhance fluid absorption in the gut.
- Gently and meticulously clean the patient's perianal area; do not rub the skin (it should be patted dry to prevent excoriation).
- Use alternative techniques to reduce the patient's stress and anxiety (e.g., relaxation, distraction, play therapy, and imagery).
- Control noxious odors to decrease nausea and vomiting.

Expected Patient and Family Outcomes

- The patient and the family can identify methods of preventing and treating diarrhea.
- The patient and the family understand proper cleansing and personal hygiene methods to prevent and treat skin breakdown and perirectal cellulitis.
- The patient and the family recognize situations that require medical assistance (i.e., diarrhea unrelieved by usual interventions, dehydration).

Constipation

Definition: Constipation is the infrequent passing of hard, dry stool, often accompanied by straining, abdominal cramping, bleeding, and rectal discomfort.

Risk factors: Risk factors are obstruction or ileus; abdominal or pelvic surgery; postoperative adhesions; surgical trauma to the intestines, the rectum, or both; a treatment-related decrease in activity or immobility; spinal cord decompression; neurotoxic effects of chemotherapy that decrease peristalsis (e.g., vinca alkaloids, vincristine [Oncovin] and vinblastine [Velban]); the side effects of drugs (e.g., narcotics, anticholinergics); poor dietary intake of fiber and fluids; metabolic conditions (e.g., hyperalcemia, hypokalemia, hypothyroidism); and an alteration in the defecation reflex because of discomfort, anxiety, lack of privacy, or change in environment.

Clinical presentation: A patient may have decreased or absent bowel sounds; generalized abdominal tenderness, distention, or both; decreased appetite; nausea; vomiting; pain and fear associated with difficulty in producing a stool; decrease in the normal frequency of stools; and hard, formed, and possibly blood-streaked stools.

Medical management: Surgery may be necessary to relieve an obstruction or to resect an invading tumor. Laxatives and stool softeners are given to relieve constipation and as a prophylaxis when constipation is anticipated. The patient should follow a high-fiber diet, increase fluid intake, and be encouraged to maintain or increase activity. Rectal manipulation, medication, and thermometers are contraindicated because of the increased risk of infection and bleeding.

Potential complications: Complications can include fecal impaction, paralytic ileus or intestinal obstruction, and perirectal abscess.

Nursing Assessment and Interventions

Assessment:

- Monitor the frequency, volume, and consistency of the patient's stool output.
- Examine the patient's rectal area routinely for skin breakdown, fissures, hemorrhoids, swelling, or bleeding.
- Perform a complete abdominal assessment that includes level of pain, auscultation, palpation, and girth.

Interventions:

- Encourage the patient to drink fluids and eat a diet rich in fiber.
- Administer prescribed laxatives.
- Encourage the patient to ambulate and increase activity to alleviate gas pains and facilitate defecation.
- Report all adverse signs, including bleeding, increased abdominal pain, distention, and absent bowel sounds.
- Promote an environment of privacy and relaxation to enhance the patient's ability to maintain a normal bowel pattern.
- Encourage the patient to maintain a home toileting routine (this is especially important to prevent regression in a child who has recently been toilet-trained).

Expected Patient and Family Outcomes

- The patient and the family understand methods for preventing and treating constipation.
- The patient and the family can identify a regular bowel pattern.
- The patient and the family recognize the signs and symptoms of constipation that require medical attention.

Perirectal Cellulitis

Definition: Perirectal cellulitis involves inflammation and edema of the perineal and rectal area. Tears or fissures in the anorectal mucosa can cause perirectal cellulitis. Aerobic gram-negative bacilli and anaerobic bacteria are the most common infective organisms.

Risk factors: Risk factors include constipation or the passage of hard stool, causing trauma to the rectal mucosa; diarrhea involving caustic fluid that causes irritation and breakdown of perirectal tissue; perirectal mucositis associated with chemotherapy, radiation therapy, or both; chronic or profound neutropenia, thrombocytopenia, or both; rectal trauma (e.g., rectal stimulation, thermometers, suppositories); hemorrhoids; and anal fissures.

Clinical presentation: The patient may experience perineal and/or rectal discomfort. The patient also may develop fever and be afraid to defecate because of the resulting pain. A visual perirectal examination may reveal minimal irritation, fissures, gross swelling, and/or inflammation.

Medical management: Antibiotic treatment should be initiated at the first sign of discomfort or tenderness; such treatment includes a specific antianaerobic agent (e.g., clindamycin [Cleocin], metronidazole [Flagyl]) and a broad-spectrum antibiotic. Other measures include administration of antipyretics, pain medications, stool softeners, sitz baths, or perineal irrigation 3–4 times a day. Dietary modifications may been required.

Potential complications: Complications include constipation and fecal impaction, tissue sloughing and necrosis, and infection that begins as a local abscess and leads to systemic sepsis. Mortality ranges from 8%–36%; the primary cause of death is septic shock.

Nursing Assessment and Interventions

Assessment:

- Inspect the patient's perirectal mucosa frequently for signs of irritation or skin breakdown.
- Monitor the patient for signs of infection or deteriorating integrity of tissue in the perirectal area.

Interventions:

- Administer prescribed medications to alleviate symptoms and control pain.
- Provide or encourage meticulous perineal hygiene, especially when the patient is neutropenic.
- Apply prescribed barrier creams and medicated creams.

Expected Patient and Family Outcomes

- The patient, the family, or both can identify the risk factors for perirectal cellulitis.
- The patient practices good perineal hygiene.
- The patient, the family, or both can discuss measures to minimize the risks associated with cellulitis.
- The patient, the family, or both can identify situations that require prompt professional intervention (e.g., pain, fever, erythema, tissue breakdown).

Chemical or Reactive Hepatitis

Definition: Chemical or reactive hepatitis is a nonviral inflammation of the liver caused by exposure to chemical or other environmental toxins, such as chemotherapy, biotherapy, and radiation.

Risk factors: Risk factors can include radiation to the liver or to the right side of the abdomen, chemotherapeutic agents (e.g., methotrexate [Mexate], chlorambucil [Leukeran], mercaptopurine [Purinethol], daunomycin [Cerubidine], doxorubicin [Adriamycin], and thioguanine [6-TG]). Intrahepatic chemotherapy, surgical resection of the liver followed by cancer treatment, underlying liver disease (e.g., infections, hepatitis, or hepatic candidiasis), and supportive care medications, such as antimicrobials, anticonvulsants, and nonsteroidal antiinflamatory agents, also can contribute to the development of hepatitis.

Clinical presentation: Patients may have pain in the right upper quadrant; nausea; vomiting; dyspepsia; anorexia; fever, malaise; flu-like symptoms; jaundice (i.e., yellow sclera and conjunctiva, dark-orange urine, clay-colored stools); malabsorption (accompanied by diarrhea, weight loss, dehydration); bruising, bleeding or both; pruritis; and abnormalities in laboratory tests (e.g., elevated liver enzymes, prolonged prothrombin times).

Medical management: Agents that could cause the hepatotoxicity should be discontinued temporarily or permanently, and the use of additional hepatotoxic drugs should be avoided. Serum chemistries, liver transaminases, complete blood count, and coagulation profile should be monitored regularly. Abdominal ultrasound or liver biopsy may be required for further work-up. Antiemetics and intravenous hydration should be given as needed for nausea and vomiting. Antipruritic agents and glucocorticoids can be given as well. Ursodiol can be used to treat hyperbilirubinemia. The patient also should be put on a low-fat, high-glucose diet with vitamin B and C additives, and physical activity should be limited.

Potential complications: Complications can include veno-occlusive disease, chronic active hepatitis, and cirrhosis.

Nursing Assessment and Interventions

Assessment:

- Perform a routine physical assessment to detect jaundice and to determine the patient's neurological status.
- Monitor the patient for signs of bleeding.
- Assess for pain and discomfort from itching.

Interventions:

- Encourage the patient to rest.
- Apply lotions and encourage the patient to take tepid baths to decrease pruritis.
- Instruct the patient to wear loose, light clothing.
- Encourage the patient to eat a low-fat, high-glucose diet.
- Administer analgesics, antipyretics, and antiemetics, as ordered, and monitor their effects.

Expected Patient and Family Outcomes

- The patient and the family know about potential complications.

- The patient and the family comply with the recommended care.

Pancreatitis

Definition: Pancreatitis is an acute or chronic inflammation of the pancreas.

Risk factors: Risk factors for pancreatitis are chemotherapy agents, specifically L-asparaginase (Elspar); radiation to the pancreas or to the left side of the abdomen; diabetes; tumor lysis syndrome; and use of an intrahepatic catheter.

Clinical presentation: The signs of pancreatitis can include epigastric or abdominal pain that radiates to the flank, back, or substernal area and is unrelieved by vomiting. They also can include abdominal rigidity, fever, tachycardia, hypotension, nausea and vomiting, elevated serum amylase and lipase, metabolic disturbances (e.g., hypoglycemia), signs and symptoms of shock, and hypoactive bowel sounds, or ileus.

Medical management: Any treatment that could be the causative agent should be discontinued temporarily or permanently. Serum lipase and amylase and serum chemistries should be done. An abdominal ultrasound or CT may be obtained. Pain relief is essential but may be problematic, since some analgesics increase pain because of spasms of the sphincter of Odi. The patient should not take anything by mouth and may need a nasogastric tube. He or she should have a bland, low-fat diet when feeding is resumed. Fluid and electrolyte replacement and volume expanders should be given if the patient experiences shock. Physical activity should be limited.

Potential complications: Complications can include pancreatic abscess, pancreatic pseudocyst, and pancreatic necrosis.

Nursing Assessment and Interventions

Assessment:

- Assess the patient's level of pain.
- Monitor the patient's vital signs.
- Assess the patient's level of consciousness and physical condition for signs of shock or electrolyte imbalance.

Interventions:

- Administer the appropriate analgesic and monitor its effect.
- Ensure that the patient receives appropriate oral and nasal care while a nasogastric tube is in place.
- Comfort and reassure the patient.

Expected Patient and Family Outcomes

- The patient, the family, or both recognize the early symptoms of pancreatitis and seek early medical intervention.
- The patient complies with dietary and pharmacological recommendations.

Nausea and Vomiting

Description: Nausea occurs when the vomiting center in the brain is stimulated, causing wavelike feelings of gastrointestinal distress. Vomiting is the forceful expulsion of stomach contents. Nausea and vomiting related to chemotherapy and radiation therapy is mediated by the vomiting center in the brain (**Figure 5-5**). It occurs through several different mechanisms; 1) activation of the chemoreceptor trigger zone (CTZ) in the fourth ventricle of the brain, 2) peripheral stimulation by neurotransmitter receptors in the gut wall, 3) cortical pathway activation by learned response (anticipatory nausea and vomiting), 4) vestibular pathway disruption related to motion and balance.

Nausea and vomiting are among the most common and feared side effects of cancer-related chemotherapy. Poorly controlled nausea and vomiting can result in dehydration, electrolyte imbalances, extended anorexia, esophageal tears, and significant distress. The consequences can include prolonged hospitalization, increased length of time between chemotherapy cycles, and patient-initiated discontinuation of treatment. Clinical research demonstrates that the cycle of nausea and vomiting is difficult to reverse once it has been established. The best form of management is prevention.

Risk factors: All agents used in chemotherapy have the potential to cause nausea and vomiting. The emetogenic potential and patterns of vomiting varies among the different agents (**Table 5-6**). To determine the emetogenic potential, an understanding is required of the agent, the dosage, the duration of infusion, and the combination of drugs used.

Figure 5-5. Pathophysiology of Nausea and Vomiting

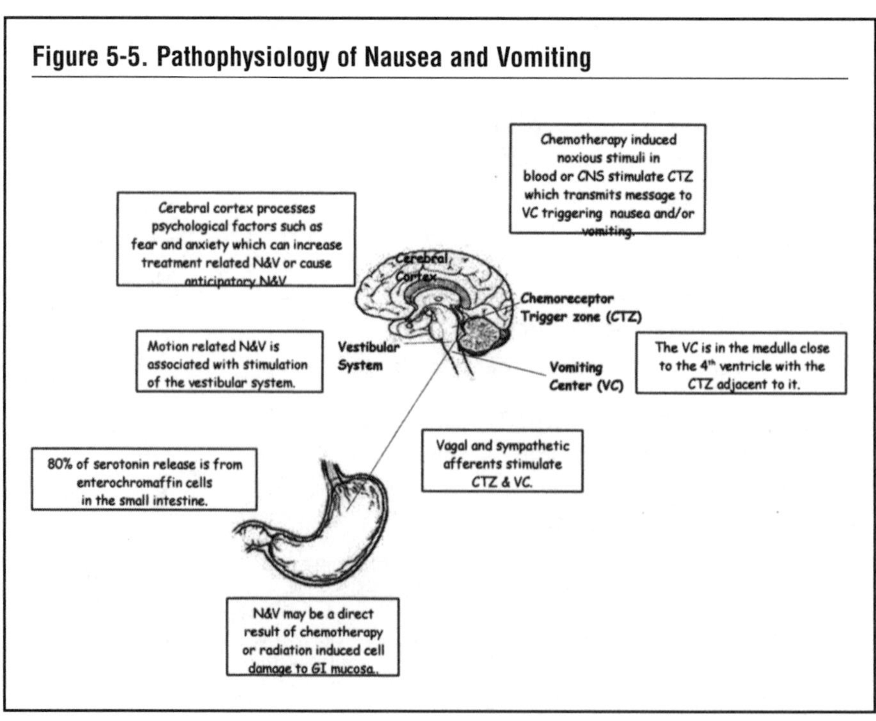

Table 5-6. Emetogenic Potential of Chemotherapeutic Agents

Acute symptoms

Highly emetogenic

Actinomycin-D
Cisplatin (≥40 mg/m^2)
Cyclophosphamide (≥1 g/m^2)
Cytarabine (≥1 g/m^2)
Dacarbazine
Ifosfamide
Mechlorethamine

Moderately emetogenic

Anthracyclines (Daunorubicin, Doxorubicin, Idarubicin)
Carboplatin
Cisplatin (<40 mg/m^2)
Cyclophosphamide (<1 g/m^2)
Cytarabine (IV <1 g/m^2, or IT)
Mercaptopurine (IV)
Methotrexate (IV >1 g/m^2)
Nitrosoureas (Carmustine, Lomustine)

Mildly emetogenic

Bleomycin
Epipodophyllotoxins (Etoposide, Teniposide)
Paclitaxel
Procarbazine
Topotecan
Vonblastine

Nonemetogenic

Asparaginese
Mercaptopurine (PO)
Methotrexate (low-dose IV, IM, PO, IT)
Steroids
Thioguanine
Vincristine

Delayed symptoms

Severe

Cisplatin

Moderate

Cyclophosphamide

Radiation therapy also can cause nausea and vomiting when applied to the total body and to the head and abdomen. Cerebral edema contributes to the nausea associated with cranial radiation. Serotonin release from the intestine is likely to contribute to nausea associated with abdominal radiation.

Other factors that contribute to nausea are increased intracranial pressure secondary to brain tumors, metabolic disturbances, side effects of narcotics, younger age, and female gender.

Patterns of nausea and vomiting: The acute pattern begins within several hours of chemotherapy and produces the most severe symptoms during the first 12–24 hours. It is usually self-limited and is resolved within 24 hours.

The delayed pattern begins after chemotherapy has been administered, and can last up to 2 weeks. It occurs when antiemetic therapy is either insufficient, is being given on a poorly planned schedule, or both.

The anticipatory pattern is a conditioned response and can occur any time after one course of chemotherapy. Risk factors include inadequate control of a previous chemotherapy episode, resulting in nausea and vomiting, age (usually young adults or adolescents), and preexisting anxiety, depression, or both. Triggers can include the sight of the hospital, clinic, or healthcare workers, or hospital-associated odors. The pattern usually is resistant to standard therapy. An oral dose of lorazepam (Ativan), given the night before and the morning of, chemotherapy may decrease the pattern's incidence.

Medical management: Various neurotransmitters (e.g., serotonin, dopamine, histamine, norepinephrine, vasopressin) activate the CTZ and vomiting center. The goal of antiemetic therapy is to identify the emetic pathways and block the neurotransmitter release. The goals of successful antiemetic therapy are to minimize or prevent nausea and vomiting and enhance the patient's quality of life (see Section IV, "Childhood Cancer Treatment," for a description of the pharmacological classification of these agents, and **Tables 5-7** and **5-8**). The principles related to using antiemetics are as follows:

Table 5-7. Pharmacological Classification of Antiemetics

Serotonin receptor antagonists (e.g., ondansetron [Zofran], granisetron [Kytril])

- Are highly selective antagonists of serotonin receptors but have no effect on dopamine receptors
- Have a main site of action thought to be on vagal afferents in the small intestine
- Have two main side effects: headache and a transient elevation of liver enzymes

Dopamine antagonists (e.g., phenothiazines: chlorpromazine [Thorazine] and prochlorperazine [Compazine])

- Alter the effects of dopamine (Intropin) in the central nervous system and block dopamine receptors in the chemoreceptor trigger zone
- Have these main side effects: extrapyramidal effects, athetosis (i.e., involuntary movement of limbs and facial grimacing, oculogyric crisis, rhythmic protrusion of the tongue, bulbar-type speech, dystonic reaction), sedation, hypotension, arrhythmias, constipation, and dry mouth

Glucocorticoids (e.g., dexamethasone [Decadron], prednisolone [Pediapred, Hydeltra-T.B.A.])

- Are thought to interfere with the permeability of the blood-brain barrier to allow other antiemetic agents to act on the chemoreceptor trigger zone
- Have these main side effects: depression, euphoria, hypertension, acne, and a cushingoid appearance

Table 5-8. Antiemetic Agents for Children

Mild-to-Moderate Emetogenic Chemotherapy	Dose	Routes	Frequency	Side Effects
Prochlorperazine (Compazine)	0.5 mg/kg	po, IV	q 4-6 hr	EPS, agitation
Chlorpromazine (Thorazine)	0.5 mg/kg	po, IV	q 4-6 hr	EPS, agitation
Promethazine (Phenergan)	0.5 mg/kg	po, IV	q 4 hr	EPS, agitation
Mild-to-Severe Emetogenic Chemotherapy				
Metoclopramide (Reglan)	1-2 mg/kg	IV	q 2-4 hr	EPS[a], sedation
Ondansetron (Zofran)	0.15 mg/kg if given as three doses, or 0.45 mg/kg as one dose	po, IV	qd, tid	Headache
Granisetron (Kytril)	10 mg	po, IV	qd	Headache
Supplemental Agents				
Diphenhydramine (Benadryl)	1 mg/kg	po, IV	q 4-6 hr,	Sedation
Dexamethasone (Decadron)	6 mg/m^2 as one dose, or divided tid	po, IV	qd, tid	Facial flushing, hyperglycemia, Electrolyte imbalance
Lorazepam (Ativan)	0.025 mg/kg	po, IV	q 6 hr	Sedation

EPS = extra pyramidal symptoms.

- Drugs should be selected on the basis of their sites of action.
- Appropriate doses should be based on the patient's weight.
- Drugs should be scheduled according to their duration of action.
- Drugs should be scheduled according to the pattern of emesis.
- The frequency of emesis and the effectiveness of agents should be evaluated frequently.

Nonpharmacological interventions include relaxation exercises, distraction and guided imagery, self-hypnosis, and music therapy.

Nursing Assessment and Interventions

Assessment:

- Monitor fluid balance.
- Document characteristics of emesis; volume, color, presence of blood.
- Report adverse signs and symptoms to the patient's physician and document findings in the patient's medical record.
- Assess the effectiveness of antiemetics on the basis of the patient's response.

Interventions:

- Formulate an individualized plan of care with the patient and family that is based on previous responses and personal coping skills.
- Explain the possible side effects of chemotherapy.
- Instruct the patient regarding the administration of antiemetics.
- Modify the treatment plan, as needed.

Expected Patient and Family Outcomes

- The patient has minimal nausea and vomiting caused by chemotherapy.
- The patient and the family understand the use of antiemetics and know how to administer them at home.
- The patient and the family know when to call for professional help during an episode of nausea and vomiting.

Renal and Bladder Complications

Kathleen E. Marson

Abnormalities and impairments of renal function that develop during cancer therapy most often are related to the pathophysiology of the disease process, the nephrotoxic chemotherapeutic agents that are used for treatment, abdominal or pelvic irradiation, or a combination of these factors. These side effects can be transient, cumulative, permanent, or progressive.

Kidney Impairment

Definition: Kidney impairment is the decreased ability of a kidney to perform the normal functions of electrolyte balance, elimination of waste products, and maintenance of the acid and base balance.

Risk factors: Risk factors are primary tumors involving the kidney and treatment-related factors such as rapid tumor lysis; increased cellular metabolism; cancer chemotherapy; other medications (e.g., antibiotics); volume depletion, dehydration or both; radiation therapy; and sepsis.

Clinical presentation: The laboratory findings for patients with kidney impairment can include elevated BUN, creatinine, and/or uric acid; proteinuria, hematuria, or both; decreased urine creatinine clearance; and alterations in fluids and electrolytes.

Physical symptoms are increased weight, unbalanced intake and output, elevated blood pressure, tachycardia, tachypnea, oliguria, ascites or abdominal distention, and fatigue.

Medical management: Renal function (e.g., BUN, creatinine and electrolyte results, urinalysis) should be assessed and evaluated before each course of chemotherapy (especially courses that include agents associated with increased renal toxicity). Renal toxicity is increased when the baseline renal function is already reduced. A physical assessment should be made and vital signs should be checked before treatment is started. The patient should have adequate hydration before receiving chemotherapy, and alkalinization, hyperhydration, or both should be instituted when certain agents (e.g., methotrexate [Mexate], cisplatin [Platinol]) are administered. Diuretic therapy should be given when it is indicated. Amifostine may protect against renal damage and is being tested in several protocols for children who are receiving nephrotoxic drugs. Doses of other nephrotoxic agents (e.g., vancomycin [Vancocin]) should be decreased or minimized, when possible. Dialysis is instituted when patients have renal failure.

Potential complications: Complications include the syndrome of inappropriate antidiuretic hormone (SIADH); dehydration; acute tubular necrosis; fluid and electrolyte imbalance; hyperkalemia; hyperuricemia or both; Fanconi's syndrome; and hypocalcemia, hyperphosphatemia, or both.

Nursing Assessment and Interventions

Assessment:

- Assess the patient's vital signs.
- Maintain accurate intake and output (maintain urine output of 1 to 2 ml/kg/hr or more during infusion of chemotherapy).
- Weigh the patient daily and twice a day when he or she is receiving high doses of cyclophosphamide (Cytoxan) and methotrexate (Mexate).
- Assess the patient's urine for specific gravity, pH, and presence of blood.
- Monitor the patient for dehydration.

Interventions:

- Maintain adequate patient hydration.
- Teach the patient and the family about care of the patient at home.
- Educate the patient and the family about the importance of maintaining adequate hydration after discharge.
- Arrange for at-home IV hydration for the patient when it is needed.
- Instruct both the patient and the family to monitor the patient's urine output at home and to report changes in urine color, odor, and amount.

Expected Patient and Family Outcomes

- Both the patient and the family recognize the signs and symptoms of renal failure and seek early intervention.
- Both the patient and the family understand the importance of maintaining adequate hydration through oral intake.

Hemorrhagic Cystitis

Definition: Hemorrhagic cystitis is a condition in which symptoms range from mild dysuria and urinary frequency to severe hemorrhage associated with significant damage to the epithelial lining of the bladder.

Risk factors: Chemotherapy (e.g., ifosfamide [Ifex], cyclophosphamide [Cytoxan]) and radiation therapy to the lower abdomen are risk factors.

Clinical presentation: Symptoms include hematuria and dysuria.

Medical management: Prevention of hemorrhagic cystitis is a major goal and requires adequate patient hydration. Kidney function (i.e., serum BUN, creatinine levels) should be monitored before each course of chemotherapy. Mesna (Mesenex) should be administered in conjunction with cyclophosphamide (Cytoxan) or ifosfamide (Ifex). In addition, furosemide (Lasix) can be given to maintain urine output; serum electrolytes, BUN, and creatinine levels should be monitored daily.

Potential complications: Complications include Fanconi syndrome, SIADH, and renal tubular necrosis. Fanconi's syndrome can persist for years after the patient completes therapy that included ifosfamide or high-dose cyclophosphamide.

Nursing Assessment and Interventions

Assessment:

- Maintain the patient's urine specific gravity at less than 1.010.
- Perform a daily urinalysis when the patient is receiving either cyclophosphamide (Cytoxan) or ifosfamide (Ifex).
- If needed, do dipstick tests on urine; when a sample is positive for blood, send it to the laboratory for a microscopic urinalysis.
- Assess the patient's intake and output accurately.
- Weigh the patient daily and monitor the weight twice a day when the patient is receiving a high dose of cyclophosphamide (Cytoxan).

Interventions:

- Maintain adequate patient hydration.
- Have the patient void every 1–2 hours during the chemotherapy, and have the patient continue this pattern for 12–24 hours after chemotherapy.

- Instruct the patient and the family about hydration before and after chemotherapy.
- Educate the patient and the family about care needed at home.
- Educate the patient and family on the signs and symptoms of hemorrhagic cystitis (e.g., hematuria or dysuria)
- Assess the patient's ability to maintain adequate hydration at home.
- Instruct the patient to void every 1–2 hours during waking hours and just before bedtime.
- Instruct the family to report any changes in urine output, dysuria, or hematuria.

Expected Patient and Family Outcomes

- The patient and the family recognize the signs and symptoms of hemorrhagic cystitis and seek early medical intervention.
- The patient and the family understand the importance of maintaining adequate hydration.
- The patient and the family comply with recommended therapies.

Skin Changes

Anna Pursell

Skin is a natural barrier to infection. A break in this barrier increases the risk for infection. An immunocompromised child with cancer has a risk of developing serious infection from normal flora when a portal of entry is provided. Adequate hygiene and skin protection will help minimize the effect of cancer treatment on the skin.

Altered Skin Integrity

Definition: Altered skin integrity is a disruption of the ability of the skin to serve as a protective barrier.

Risk factors: Risk factors include underlying tumor, radiation therapy, chemotherapeutic agents, antibiotics, corticosteroids, procedures that disrupt skin integrity (e.g., injections, ostomies, excisions, central venous access devices, gastrostomy tubes), prosthetic devices, malnutrition, and immobility.

Clinical presentation: There are numerous potential causes and presentations of alteration in skin integrity. The effects of radiation on skin can include mild erythema, moist and dry desquamation, tenderness, and pruritis at the site of the radiation field. Alopecia, which can occur as a result of chemotherapy, radiation, or both, usually begins 2–3 weeks after treatment. Alopecia can be patchy and is usually temporary, although permanent alopecia almost always occurs with radiation of more than 4,000 cGy. Photosensitivity can occur as a result of treatment with trimethoprim-sulfamethoxazole (TMP-SMZ) (Bactrim) or methotrexate (Mexate). Depigmentation and hyperpigmentation are associated with methotrexate and bleomycin (Blenoxane). Delayed healing or an increased incidence of infection is associated with chemotherapy, radiation or both; poor nutritional status; and glucocorticoid therapy. Skin reactions called *radiation recall* can occur at previous radiation ports when antitumor antibiotics such as doxorubicin [Adriamycin] are administered. Presentation includes warmth, erythema, and dermatitis, which can progress to severe desquamation and ulceration.

Friability of the skin may be a consequence of an underlying tumor and puts the skin at risk of breakdown.

Nursing Assessment and Interventions

Assessment:

- Perform a baseline assessment of the patient's skin, and then assess it daily to determine if there are potential problem areas. Particular attention should be given to any disruption in skin integrity, radiated areas, skin folds and creases, and areas overlying tumor masses.
- Assess the patient's understanding of alopecia, encourage a discussion of altered body image, and, if the patient desires it, refer him or her for a wig.
- Monitor the healing of the patient's wounds, including those caused by central venous access devices and gastrointestinal tubes, incision sites or wounds, and surgical sites, throughout the course of therapy.
- Examine the patient's skin at previously irradiated ports for signs or symptoms of radiation recall after the patient has received antitumor antibiotics; provide appropriate treatment.

Interventions:

- Explain photosensitivity to the patient and the need to avoid excessive sunlight while receiving medications such as trimethoprim-sulfamethoxazole (TMP-SMZ, trade name Bactrim) or methotrexate (Mexate).
- Instruct the patient on the use of sunscreen.
- Teach the child and the family how to assess skin integrity and teach them appropriate skin care techniques.
- Emphasize the importance of a good daily hygiene regimen (**Table 5-9**).
- Report all changes in skin integrity to the child's physician.
- Reposition the patient every 2 hours if his or her mobility is limited.
- Ensure that the patient is receiving adequate nutrition. Consider a nutritional consult if he or she has persistent weight loss (loss of 5% or more of body weight) or poor nutritional status.
- Consult a specialist in enterostomal therapy for patients who have particularly complex wound management needs.

Expected Patient and Family Outcomes

- The patient and the family comply with the requirement that the patient use sunscreen when outdoors.
- The patient's skin remains intact or infection-free.

Table 5-9. Nursing Care of Irradiated Skin

When treatment begins:	Assess skin integrity. Instruct patient to minimize trauma and protect skin within treatment field: Cleanse skin with lukewarm water as needed. Avoid use of soaps, powders, perfumes, and deodorants. Avoid shaving. Protect skin from cold, heat, and sun. Wear loose-fitting clothing over treatment site. Avoid adhesive tape on irradiated skin.
If dry desquamation occurs:	Use a hydrophilic moisturizing lotion two to three times a day (e.g., Aquaphor). Remove excess lotion from skin before daily treatment.
If moist desquamation occurs:	Saline irrigations or cool compresses may be used three to four times a day. Apply hydrocolloid dressing for comfort (e.g., DuoDerm). If treatment is withheld, zinc oxide or silver sulfadiazine may be applied to skin reaction and covered with a nonadherent dressing. Culture suspicious lesions and drainage. Use analgesics as necessary.
When treatment is completed and skin is healed:	Instruct patient to protect irradiated skin by avoiding exposure to sun, heat, or cold. Advise patient to use sunblock when sun exposure is unavoidable.

Note. From *Oncology Nursing* (3rd ed., p. 515), by S.E. Otto (Ed.), 1997, St. Louis: Mosby. Copyright 1997 by Mosby. Reprinted with permission.

- The patient and the family comply with necessary wound and ostomy care for the patient.

Musculoskeletal Alterations

Kathleen E. Marson

Children diagnosed with musculoskeletal malignancies often receive combination therapy (e.g., surgery, chemotherapy, radiation therapy, and immunotherapy) to promote their long-term survival. Surgeons attempt to reduce functional and psychological morbidity in their surgical approach to soft tissue and bone tumors. Primary surgical procedures fall into two main categories: amputation and limb salvage procedures. Advances in surgical techniques involving limb reconstruction make possible limb-sparing procedures in an increasingly greater number of children. Complications of aggressive combination therapy include limitation of movement, asymmetry, and alteration in body image and function related to limb salvage and amputation procedures.

Limitation of Movement and Asymmetry

Decreased range of motion (ROM) can occur in joints because of the location of the malignancy, treatment-associated complications, or both. Asymmetry of the extremity or trunk may result.

Risk factors: Risk factors are the site of the disease itself, the site and dose of radiation therapy, the surgical excision of the tumor and surrounding tissue and bone, and the use of glucocorticoids.

Clinical presentation: The patient can have decreased ROM, direct or indirect (i.e., referred) pain, alteration in gait, scoliosis or kyphosis, changes in functional performance, and changes in skin integrity. There also can be a discrepancy in the length of the patient's limbs.

Medical treatment: Medical treatment consists of a complete history and physical examination, a functional evaluation, a radiological evaluation, and the control of symptoms and pain management. Treatment also can include a rehabilitation consult (e.g., occupational therapy [OT], physical therapy [PT]), use of prosthetic devices (e.g., brace, splint, lift, crutches), or joint replacement.

Potential complications: Complications can include fracture; infection; avascular necrosis; altered gait; limb asymmetr;y alterations in body image; decreased muscle tone; mass, or both; weakness in or atrophy of the muscles; thrombosis; and decreased employment opportunities.

Nursing Assessment and Interventions

Assessment:

- Perform ongoing functional assessments of the patient.
- Perform accurate height and extremity measurements.

Interventions:

- Encourage the patient to comply with the recommended rehabilitation.
- Provide skin care.

- Manage the patient's symptoms.
- Provide psychosocial support for the patient.
- Educate the patient and the family about home care, including coordination of a convenient location and schedule for rehabilitation and necessary adaptations for the patient at school and at home; provide information related to community services.

Expected Patient and Family Outcomes

- The patient and the family understand the needed for long-term follow-up.
- The patient and the family comply with needed therapies.

Amputation and Limb-Salvage Procedures

Definition: Amputation is the surgical removal of tumor-bearing bone with a 6–7 cm margin proximal to the upper limit of the tumor. Limb-salvage procedures include rotational plasties, autologous grafts, vascularized grafts, allografts, endoprostheses, metallic prostheses, arthrodises, and/or allograft prosthetic composites.

Risk factors: Fractures can prevent or delay limb-salvage procedures. In addition, the location and/or size of the tumor can prohibit a limb-salvage procedure. Infections can develop after an amputation or a limb-salvage procedure. The life span of prosthetic devices used in limb reconstruction continues to be problematic. Screening candidates for limb salvage requires careful staging, including high-resolution scanning of the entire involved bone. The degree of primary tumor response to chemotherapy can be a factor in deciding upon a limb-sparing resection.

Medical treatment: The oncology team coordinates care with the surgeon, rehabilitation team, and oncology team. Symptom management and restoration of function are other aspects of medical treatment.

Potential complications: Complications can include fractures, joint dislocations, skin necrosis, wound infections, thrombosis, rejection of a graft, and delayed complications such as arthritis, recurrence of local tumor, nonunion of osseous junctions, and late infections.

Nursing Assessment and Interventions

Assessment:

- Assess the patient's ability to function.
- Evaluate the patient's need for PT, OT, or both.
- Assess the patient's need for assistive devices (e.g., crutches).
- Determine if the patient needs counseling or other support related to the loss of a limb.

Interventions:

- Provide comprehensive preoperative planning and education for the patient.
- Discuss with the patient and the family their participation in creating a rehabilitation program.
- Allow and encourage time for the patient to verbalize his or her emotions about physical changes.
- Support the patient's grief process over the loss of function and change in body image.
- Provide comfort measures (see the discussion of surgery in Section IV, "Supportive Care").
- Support the patient in his or her use of assistive devices (e.g., crutches, a prosthesis).
- Encourage long-term follow-up for the patient.
- Arrange for assessments of the patient's home and school to determine their adaptiveness to assistive devices; anticipate potential changes in the patient's self-care activities; arrange for rehabilitation at the patient's home or school or nearby rehab center; provide information about community resources.

Expected Patient and Family Outcomes

- The patient adjusts to the amputation and prosthetic device, if one is used.
- The patient makes use of appropriate community resources.
- The patient and the family understand the need for long-term follow-up.
- The patient achieves maximum mobility.

Nutritional Complications

Kenneth Lown

Adequate nutrition helps a patient maintain an overall feeling of wellness. Nutritional support during cancer therapy aids in maintaining growth and development, preventing infections, and improving energy levels. Good nutrition is linked directly to a patient's quality of life. Poor nutrition is directly related to the severity of the side effects of treatment, such as wound healing, skin integrity, and infection. The issues are not always biological, and they encompass psychological factors related to control, anxiety, fear, and depression. Children who feel a total lack of control related to their cancer diagnosis frequently use eating as the one aspect of their situation they can control (see Section VI, "Supportive Care").

Alteration in Nutrition

Definition: An alteration in nutrition is a change in intake resulting in weight loss or weight gain (see Section VI, "Supportive Care").

Risk factors: Risk factors include radiation to the head, neck, abdomen, spine, or pelvis. Other risk factors include chemotherapy, use of corticosteroids, pain, constipation, and metastatic and/or recurrent disease. Location of brain tumors also can be a risk factor.

Clinical presentation: Radiation to the head and neck can affect the appetite control center in the brain, normal tissues of the salivary glands, oral mucosa, muscle, and bone. The presenting signs and symptoms can include stomatitis, alteration in taste (i.e., a metallic taste), xerostomia (i.e., decreased saliva production), dysphagia, anorexia, and pain. Radiation to the abdomen or pelvis can lead to intestinal dysfunction; presenting signs and symptoms include nausea, vomiting, anorexia, diarrhea, and acute radiation-related enteritis.

Chemotherapy can cause side effects that interfere with nutrition. These include nausea, vomiting, anorexia, mucositis, pain, alterations in taste, vitamin deficiencies, constipation, and diarrhea.

Glucocorticoids often are used for cancer therapy and for supportive care. Although glucocorticoids offer great benefit, they can also cause nutritional side effects that include weight gain, increased appetite, fluid retention, abnormal serum chemistries, and gastric irritation and ulceration.

Cachexia, which often affects patients with advanced cancer, is a complex metabolic process resulting in a loss of body weight, fat, and muscle. Presenting signs and symptoms include anorexia, weight loss or emaciation, and metabolic abnormalities.

Nutrition management: Management includes giving a patient oral food supplements (e.g., Carnation Instant Breakfast, Ensure, Pediasure), instituting enteral feedings via a nasogastric tube or a gastrostomy tube, or instituting total parenteral nutrition (see also Section VI, "Supportive Care").

Nursing Assessment and Interventions

Assessment:

- Assess the patient's baseline nutritional status and determine if he or she is at high risk (e.g., has had head and neck irradiation, glucocorticoid therapy).
- Obtain an oral and dental history; assess the patient's oral cavity.
- Determine whether and what types of complementary and alternative therapies and medications that can affect nutritional status may be in use.
- Measure the child's height, weight, and body mass index; plot these data at regular intervals on a standardized growth chart.
- Obtain a prospective, 3-day dietary history.
- Consult a dietitian regarding the patient's nutritional needs.
- Monitor the patient's bowel habits regularly.

Interventions:

- Educate the patient and the family regarding the nutrition-related side effects of therapy.
- Offer the patient frequent small meals and snacks.
- Encourage meticulous oral hygiene for the patient.
- Provide pain management for mucositis related to radiation or chemotherapy.
- Provide aggressive antiemetic therapy.
- Educate family members about enteral or parenteral feedings to ensure they are administering them properly, regularly assess their compliance with feeding schedules, and monitor the patient's weight.
- Refer the patient for psychosocial support, if necessary.

Expected Patient and Family Outcomes

- The patient maintains a positive nutritional status.
- The patient and the family understand the implications of poor nutrition on the patient's toleration of therapy, and on increasing the side effects or toxic effects of treatment.
- The patient and the family comply with recommended nutritional guidelines.

Growth and Development

Debbie Briseno-Toomey

Children frequently tolerate the immediate physical effects of cancer therapy better than do adults. However, growing children are more vulnerable to disruptions in their physical and psychological growth and development. Healthcare providers must be aware of this and must monitor children throughout their treatment to ensure the earliest possible intervention. Growth and development can be affected by any of the various treatment modalities used to treat childhood cancer. These side effects can be minimal, moderate, or severe, and can occur during treatment or years after all therapies are completed.

Risk factors: Risk factors are treatment at a young age (i.e., less than 6 years old); treatment after the onset of puberty; intensive combination chemotherapy; radiation higher than 2,400 cGy to the spine, long bones, hypothalamic-pituitary region, head, and neck; chemotherapy combined with radiation; suboptimal nutrition; and use of glucocorticoids.

Clinical presentation: A patient may have a developmental delay, delayed gross motor and/or fine motor development, and delays in personal or social skills or language development. Physical symptoms can include deficiencies in growth or thyroid hormone, malnutrition secondary to chronic illness, early onset of puberty, impaired spinal growth, failure of the vertebrae to develop, scoliosis, kyphosis, or dental and maxillofacial abnormalities. Neuroendrocrine dysfunction can be manifested by luteinizing hormone (LH), follicle stimulating hormone (FSH) deficiency, or both, demonstrated by failure to enter puberty and primary amenorrhea. A thyrotropin deficiency results in poor linear growth, excessive weight gain, lethargy, and delayed puberty. An adrenocorticotropic hormone deficiency can be accompanied by decreased stamina or lethargy. Hyperprolactinemia can result in pubertal delay or arrest, as well as amenorrhea with or without galactorrhea.

Medical management: Management includes measuring the patient's standing height every 3–6 months and plotting it on a standard growth curve. A sitting height measurement of patients who have received radiation to the spine, abdomen, or pelvis should be taken. Measurements of the ratio of the patient's weight to height and velocity of growth (i.e., cm/year) also should be made. Patients should be examined for scoliosis. Bone age and Tanner stage evaluation can be used to determine the child's physical age of development (**Table 5-10**).

Table 5-10. Secondary Sex Characteristics (Tanner Stages (Mean Age + SD)

	Breast Development (Female)	Genital Development (Male)	Pubic Hair (Male and Female)
Stage I	Preadolescent: elevation of papilla only Mean age: 11.2 years Range: 9.0–13.3 years	Preadolescent: testes, scrotum, and penis about the same size and proportion of early childhood	No pubic hair
Stage II	Breast bud: elevation of breast and papilla as small mound; enlargement of areolar diameter Mean age: 11.2 years Range: 9.0–13.3 years	Enlargement of the scrotum and testes; skin on the scrotum reddens and changes in texture; little or no enlargement of the penis Mean age: 11.6 years Range: 9.5–13.8 years	Sparse growth of long, slightly pigmented downy hair, straight or only slightly curled, chiefly at the base of the penis or along the labia **Females** Mean age: 11.7 years Range: 9.3–14.1 years **Males** Mean age: 13.4 years Range: 11.2–15.6 years
Stage III	Further enlargement and elevation of breast and areola; no separation of contours Mean age: 12.2 years Range: 10–14.3 years	Enlargement of the penis; first mainly in length; further growth of the testes and scrotum. Mean age: 12.9 years Range: 10.8–14.9 years	Considerably darker, coarser, and more curled; hair spreads sparsely over junction of pubes **Females** Mean age: 12.4 years Range: 10.2–14.6 years **Males** Mean age: 13.9 years Range: 11.9–16.0 years
Stage IV	Projection of the aerola and papilla to form a secondary mound above the level of the breast Mean age: 13.1 years Range: 10.8–15.3 years	Increased size of the penis with growth in breadth and development of the glans; further enlargement of the testes and scrotum and increased darkening of the scrotal skin. Mean age: 13.8 years Range: 11.7–15.8 years	Hair resembles an adult's in type; distribution is still considerably smaller than in adult; no spread to the medial surface of the thighs **Females** Mean age: 13 years Range: 10.8–15.1 years **Males** Mean age: 14.4 years Range: 12.2–16.5 years
Stage V	Mature stage: projection of the papilla is only due to recession of the areola to the general contour of the breast Mean age: 15.3 years Range: 11.9–18.8 years	Genitalia are adult in size and shape Mean age: 14.9 years Range: 12.7–17.1 years	Spread up the linea alba-"male escutcheon" **Females** Mean age: 14.4 years Range: 12.2–16.7 years **Males** Mean age: 15.2 years Range: 13.0–17.3 years

Because of the long-term effects of radiation to the thyroid gland or hypothalamus, thyroid functions should be assessed in patients who have received mantle, head and neck, spinal, or total body irradiation. The growth hormone status of patients who received radiation therapy to the hypothalamic-pituitary axis should be assessed in patients with documented growth delay (see Section X, "Late Effects of Childhood Cancer," for further details). In addition, a neuropsychological evaluation should be done and an early educational intervention provided, when appropriate.

Nursing Assessment and Interventions

Assessment:

- Assess the younger (birth to age 6 years) patient's developmental level with a standardized screening tool such as the Denver Developmental Screening Test.
- Assess cognitive and academic abilities routinely and compare with baseline measurements.
- Measure the patient's height and weight and plot the values on standard growth curves.
- Assess the child's Tanner stage of development.
- Assess the patient's menstrual history.
- Assess the impact of the illness on the patient's growth and development.

Interventions:

- Initiate age-appropriate activities that foster motor and cognitive development.
- Initiate activities that provide visual, auditory, verbal, and tactile stimulation.
- Collaborate with the patient's family and friends in stimulating the child's development.
- Communicate with the healthcare team, specifically through progress notes.
- Make appropriate referrals to neuropsychology and endocrinology, as indicated, to obtain baseline evaluations.
- Provide education, support, and reassurance to the patient and the family.
- Encourage and facilitate reintegration into the school system.

Expected Patient and Family Outcomes

- The patient continues to develop appropriately for his or her age.
- The patient is evaluated for developmental deficits or growth impairments.
- The patient and the family maintain ongoing contact with the healthcare team.
- The patient and the family demonstrate knowledge of, and participation in, appropriate interventions.

PAIN

Kathleen Jodarski and Karla Wilson

Pain is a devastating phenomenon that may be poorly managed because of lack of knowledge, inadequate assessment, and ineffective communication of the patient, family and healthcare team. Assessment and management of pain are complex issues for pediatric nurses because pain is interwoven with the emotions, perceptions, and previous experiences of the healthcare provider, the patient, and family members. In the last decade, there has been an increased awareness of, concern about, and improvement in pain management. The development of multidisciplinary pain management teams has driven much of this progress.

Acute and Chronic Pain

Definition: Pain is an unpleasant sensory and emotional experience associated with acute or potential tissue damage (see the discussion of procedure pain in Section VI, "Supportive Care," and of terminal pain in Section IX, "Care for the Terminally Ill Child and the Family").

Clinical presentation: Pain can be acute, chronic, or both. The signs and symptoms of acute pain can occur suddenly. The pain can be self-limiting and can result in restlessness, anxiety, hypertension, tachycardia, and tachypnea. The causes of acute pain in children with cancer are recent surgery, invasive medical procedures, and side effects of treatment, which can include infection, mucositis, myalgias, or peripheral neuropathies.

The signs and symptoms of chronic pain include persistent pain that usually lasts for more than 6 months. The pain can be constant or intermittent, accompanied by minimal alterations in the patient's vital signs, and result in depression. The causes of chronic pain in children with cancer can include disease progression, phantom-limb sensations, infection, and post-herpetic syndrome.

Myths about pain: Several myths surround the perception of pain:

- Children's nervous systems are immature; therefore, they have less pain.
- Active or sleeping children cannot be in pain.
- It is unsafe to administer opioids to children because of the possibility of respiratory depression or addiction.
- Children become accustomed to pain, so they no longer feel it.
- Children cannot tell you when they have pain.
- Neurologically impaired children do not feel pain.
- The best way to give an analgesic is intramuscularly.
- It is unsafe to give narcotics through central lines.
- Giving morphine means that a patient is dying.

Risk factors: Disease-related risk factors are infiltration or compression of soft tissue, bone, or nerves by tumor, and stimulation of pain receptors by effusions or edema.

Treatment-related risk factors include invasive diagnostic or treatment procedures as well as inflammation, mucositis, and infection.

Implications of pain: Therapy should address both the physiological and psychological components of pain.

Acute pain can be a major symptom that leads to a diagnosis of cancer or recurrent disease; however, a cause might not be readily identifiable.

Chronic pain can cause alterations in personality, lifestyle, and functional ability. It also can create a sense of hopelessness and a fear of impending death. In addition, it increases a patient's overall level of suffering.

Medical management: Clinicians should treat the underlying cause of the pain and provide definitive therapy.

Pharmacologic management using the World Health Organization's (WHO) stepladder provides a multisystem approach to pain management by providing a guide for instituting appropriate therapy based on the patient's reported level of pain (**Figure 5-6** and **Table 5-11**). Each step provides therapy based on the severity of reported pain. Therapy is not necessarily initiated at step one, but rather at the patient's current pain level. The ladder reminds caregivers to implement adjuvant therapies as part of the overall pain management program. Adjuvant therapies, such as palliative radiation and nonopioid medications, can enhance the analgesic effects of opioids, relieve contributing symptoms that enhance pain, and decrease the side effects of opioid drugs (**Table 5-12**).

Pain medications can be administered in many ways: through epidural or intraventricular agents, topical anesthetics, improved oral and rectal preparations, and transdermal and sublingual preparations. Some drugs are receptor-specific.

Potential complications include a build-up of physical tolerance to the medication, which requires increasing doses to achieve pain control. Physical dependence, particularly on narcotics, is another complication. Should such dependence occur, the patient must be weaned from medication, when appropriate, to prevent withdrawal symptoms such as anxiety, nausea, vomiting, diarrhea, and tremors. Psychological dependence involves drug-seeking behavior, which is extremely rare in cancer patients. The side effects of analgesics can be respiratory depression, urticaria, pruritis, constipation, urinary retention, nausea, vomiting, and sedation.

Nonpharmacological management includes preparing patients for procedures, behavioral therapy, hypnosis, guided imagery, distraction or relaxation techniques, transcutaneous electrical nerve stimulation (TENS), and physical therapy (see Section VI, "Supportive Care").

Palliative radiation is used to provide relief from pain associated with end-stage disease of some types of tumors.

Figure 5-6. Therapeutic Ladder

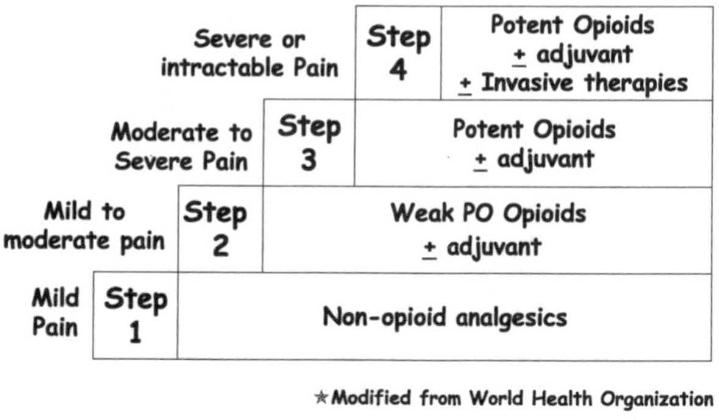

Severe or intractable Pain	Step 4	Potent Opioids ± adjuvant ± Invasive therapies
Moderate to Severe Pain	Step 3	Potent Opioids ± adjuvant
Mild to moderate pain	Step 2	Weak PO Opioids ± adjuvant
Mild Pain	Step 1	Non-opioid analgesics

*Modified from World Health Organization

Nursing Assessment and Interventions

Assessment:

- Assess pain on the basis of the patient's developmental stage.
  - Infant: An infant may cry intensely, be inconsolable, draw his or her knees to the chest, exhibit hypersensitivity or irritability, and be unable to eat or sleep.

Table 5-11. Starting Drug Doses of Commonly Used Opioids in Pediatrics

Drug	Usual IV Starting Dose (Patient < 50 kg)	Usual IV Starting Dose (Patient > 50 kg)	Usual Oral Starting Dose (Patient < 50 kg)	Usual Oral Starting Dose (Patient > 50 kg)
Morphine (MS Contin)	0.1 mg/kg q 3–4 hr[a]	5-10 mg q 3–4 hr	0.3 mg/kg q 3–4 hr	30 mg q 3–4 hr
Hydromorphone (Dilaudid)	0.015 mg/kg q 3–4 hr	1-1.5 mg q 3–4 hr	0.06 mg/kg q 3–4 hr	6 mg q 3–4 hr
Oxycodone (Roxicodone)	NA[b]	NA[b]	0.3 mg/kg q 3–4 hr[c]	10 mg q 3–4 hr
Meperidine (Demerol)[d]	0.75 mg/kg q 2–3 hr	75-100 mg q 3 hr	NR[e]	NR[e]
Fentanyl (Sublimaze)	0.5-1.5 µg/kg q 1–2 hr	25-75 µg q 1–2 hr	NA[b]	NA[b]

[a]Refers to intermittent opioid dosing.
[b]NA = not available as an oral agent.
[c]Smallest tablet size is 5 mg.
[d]Meperidine (Demerol) is not recommended for chronic use because of the accumulation of the toxic metabolite normeperidine.
[e]NR = not recommended.
Note: From Principles and Practice of Pediatric Oncology (3rd ed., p. 1189), by P.A. Pizzo and D.G. Poplack (Eds.), 1997, Philadelphia: Lippincott-Raven. Copyright 1997 Lippincott-Raven. Reprinted with permission.

Table 5-12. Coanalgesic Adjuvant Drugs

Category/Drug	Dosage	Indication	Comments
Antidepressants			
Amitriptyline	0.2–0.5 mg/kg PO hs Titrate upward by 0.25 mg/kg every 5–7 days as needed Available in 10 mg and 25 mg tablets Usual starting dose is 10–25 mg	Continuous neuropathic pain with burning, aching, dysthesia with insomnia	Provides anagesia by blocking re-uptake of serotonin and norepinephrine possibly slowing transmission of pain signals. Helps with pain related to insomnia and depression (use nortriptyline if patient is over-sedated) Analgesic effects seen earlier than antidepressant effects Side effects include dry mouth, constipation, urinary retention
Nortriptyline	0.2 to 1.0 mg/kg PO a.m. or bid Titrate up by 0.5mg q 5–7 days Max:25 mg/dose	Neuropathic pain as above without insomnia	
Anticonvulsants			
Gabapentin	5 mg/kg PO at bedtime Increase to bid on day 2, tid on day 3 Max: 300 mg/day	Neuropathic pain	Mechanism of action unknown. Side effects include sedation, ataxia, nystagmus, dizziness
Carbamzepine	<6 years 2.5 to 5 mg/kg PO bid initially Increase 20 mg/kg/24 hour divide bid q week prn Max: 100 mg bid 6–12 years 5 mg/kg PO bid initially Increase 10 mg/kg/24 hr divide bid q week prn to usual max: 100 mg bid >12 years 200 mg PO bid initially Increase 200 mg/24 hr divide bid q week prn to max: 1.6–2.4 gm/24 hr	Sharp, lancinating neuropathic pain Peripheral neuropathies Phantom limb pain	Similar analgesic effect as amitriptyline Monitor blood levels for toxicity only Side effects include decreased blood counts, ataxia, and GI irritation
Anxiolytics			
Lorazapam	0.03–0.1 mg/kg q 4–6 hr PO/IV; max: 2 mg/dose	Muscle spasm Anxiety	May increase sedation in combination with opiods Can cause depression with prolonged use
Diazapam	0.1 to 0.3 mg/kg q 4n to 6 hr PO/IV; max: 10 mg/dose	Muscle spasm Anxiety	May increase sedation in combination with opioids

(Continued)

Table 5-12. Coanalgesic Adjuvant Drugs *(Continued)*

Category/Drug	Dosage	Indication	Comments
Diazapam *(Continued)*			Can cause depression with prolonged use
Corticosteroids			
Dexamethasone	Dose dependent on clinical situation; higher bolus doses in cord compression, then lower daily dose. Try to wean to NSAIDS if pain allows Cerebral edema: 1–2 mg/kg load then 1–1.5 mg/kg/day divided every 6 hr; max: 4 mg/dose Anti-inflammatory: 0.08 to 0.3 mg/kg/day divided every 6–12 hr	Pain from increased intercranial pressure Bony metastasis Spinal/nerve compression	Side effects include edema, gastorintestinal irritation, increased weight, acne Use gastroprotectants such as H2 blockers (ranitidine) or proton pump inhibitors such as omeprazole for long-term administration of steroids or NSAIDS in end-stage cancer with bony pain
Others			
Clonidine	2 to 4 mcg/kg PO 4–6 hr May also use a 100 mcg transdermal patch q 7 days for patients >40 kg	Neuropathic pain Lancinating, sharp, electrical, shooting pain Phantom limb pain	Alpha 2 adenoreceptor agonist modulates ascending pain sensations Routes of administration include oral, transdermal and spinal Management of withdrawal symptoms Monitor for orthostatic hypertension, decreased HR Sedation common
Mexiletine	2 to 3 mg/kg/dose PO tid may titrate 0.5 mg/kg q 2–3 weeks as needed max 300: mg/dose	Neuropathic pain Lancinating, sharp, electrical, shooting pain Phantom limb pain	Similar to lidocaine, longer acting Stabilizes sodium conduction in nerve cells, reduces neuronal firing Can enhance action of opioids, antidepressants, anticonvulsants Side effects include dizziness, ataxia, nausea, vomiting May measure blood levels for toxicity

Note: From Pain management in children with cancer, pp. 36-37, by M. Hockenberry-Eaton, P. Barrera, M. Brown and J.B. O'Niell, 1999 Austin, TX: Texas Cancer Council. Reprinted with permission.

- Toddler: A toddler may be verbally aggressive, exhibit regressive behavior or withdraw, or guard the painful area.
- Preschooler: A preschooler may verbalize the intensity of the pain, may view the pain as punishment, and may understand that there can be a secondary gain associated with the pain.
- School-age child: A child at this age verbalizes pain, can use an objective measurement of pain, and resists movement. The child also can be influenced by cultural beliefs and can experience nightmares associated with pain.
- Adolescent: An adolescent can verbalize pain but may not request pain medications or may deny the pain in the presence of peers. An adolescent also can experience changes in sleep patterns and changes in appetite, or display regressive behavior in the presence of family members.

- Obtain the patient's pain history, including previous experience with analgesic medications.
- Use instruments to measure pain, but consider the child's developmental level and perspective; introduce the instruments before initiating painful procedures, when possible; and use the instrument consistently to assess the child's level of pain.
  - Numerical scale: This type of scale can be used with children 5 years of age and older. The most common range for numerical scale ratings is 0–10, but the high number should be no greater than the child's age.
  - Faces scale: This scale uses pictures of children's facial expressions to elicit information about the severity of a child's pain (**Figure 5-7**).

Interventions:

- Plan for managing pain by considering a patient's individual characteristics and cultural beliefs, considering the patient's pain threshold based on his or her current use of pain medications, assessing the patient's current or past use of illicit drugs or alcohol, addressing the patient's fears related to using drugs, and assessing the anxiety levels of the patient and the family.
- Educate the patient and the parents about pain management and the differences between acute and chronic pain.
- Discuss painful procedures honestly with the patient and the family and prepare them for the procedures (see Section VI, "Supportive Care").
- Document the patient's pain and evaluate interventions.

Expected Patient and Family Outcomes

- The patient and the family are active participants in the pain management process.
- The patient and the family understand the goals of pain management.
- The patient's medications are administered early in the pain cycle and on a regular schedule.
- The patient experiences pain control with minimal sedation or other side effects.
- The patient and the family recognize the need for changes in the pain management regimen when they are indicated by a change in the patient's pain level.
- The patient and the family understand how to appropriately manage the side effects of analgesics.
- The patient and the family are satisfied with pain control measures.

Figure 5-7. Wong-Baker Faces Pain Rating Scale

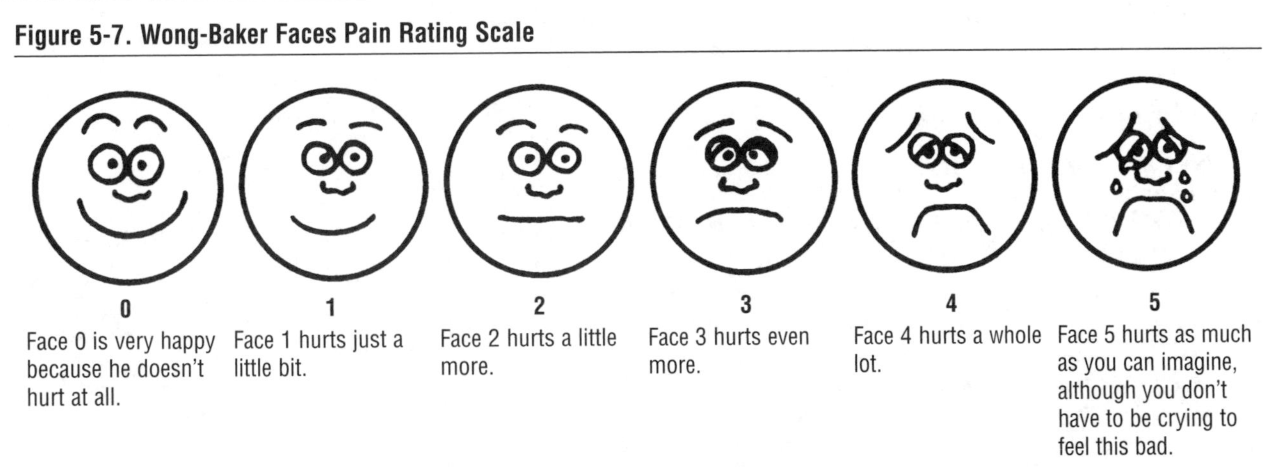

Note: Wong's essentials of pediatric nursing (6th ed., p. 1301), by D.L. Wong, M. Hockenberry-Eaton, D. Wilson, M.L. Winkelstein, and P. Schwartz, 2001, St. Louis: Mosby, Inc. Reprinted with permission.

Oncologic Emergencies

Karla Wilson, Rita Secola, and Debbie Reid

Oncologic emergencies are life-threatening events that can occur during a child's course of treatment for cancer. Some emergencies manifest at the time of diagnosis, as a direct result of cancer treatment, or when there is cancer recurrence.

Hyperleukocytosis

Definition: Hyperleukocytosis is a condition in which the peripheral white blood count is greater than $100{,}000/mm^3$, causing increased blood viscosity and blast cell aggregates and thrombi in the microcirculation.

Risk factors: The risk factors are acute lymphoblastic leukemia, seen in 10% of patients; acute nonlymphoblastic leukemia, seen in 20% of patients; and chronic myelogenous leukemia in the acute phase, seen in 100% of patients.

Clinical presentation: The signs can include shortness of breath, tachypnea, cyanosis, blurred vision, papilledema, agitation, ataxia, confusion, delirium, and stupor.

Medical management: Patients typically receive IV hyperhydration (approximately $3{,}000\ ml/m^2/day$), sodium bicarbonate, and allopurinol (Zyloprim). In addition, metabolic abnormalities are aggressively corrected. Other measures can include blood product support, leukopheresis, exchange transfusions, and chemotherapy.

Potential complications: Patients can experience hemorrhage, pulmonary leukostasis, metabolic alterations, and renal failure.

Nursing Assessment and Interventions

Assessment:

- Assess the patient's urine output and pH.
- Observe the patient's respiratory status for dyspnea, tachypnea, and pulmonary congestion.
- Assess the patient for signs or symptoms of bleeding.
- Evaluate the patient's neurological status and level of consciousness.
- Monitor dipstick urine for pH and presence of hematuria, and report a pH of less than 7 or greater than 8.5.
- Monitor the patient's weight closely.
- Perform a guaiac test on the patient's stools.

Interventions:

- Report critical changes in the patient's symptoms to his or her physician.
- Explain the purpose of the monitoring to the patient's family.

Expected Patient and Family Outcomes

- The patient and the family understand the implications of hyperleukocytosis and the potentially life-threatening situation.
- The patient and the family participate in making decisions about treatment and care.
- The patient and the family list the signs and symptoms that should be reported to the healthcare team.

Acute Tumor Lysis Syndrome

Definition: Acute tumor lysis syndrome (TLS) is a significant complication associated with initial chemotherapy for various subtypes of lymphomas and leukemias and other tumors with high growth fraction. TLS is defined as severe metabolic abnormalities that include hyperuricemia, hyperphosphatemia, hypocalcemia, and hyperkalemia. These metabolic abnormalities are a direct result of the death and degradation of tumor cells and the release of their contents into circulation. One abnormality or a combination of them may occur and lead to acute renal failure and potentially life-threatening cardiac dysfunction (**Figure 5-8**). Laboratory findings include: uric acid >8mg/dl; potassium >6meq/l; phosphorous >10mg/dl; calcium <8mg/dl; and elevated BUN and creatinine levels.

Risk factors: Patients who present with uric acid levels >8mg/dl, patients with high tumor burden and with aggressive histology of NHL (Burkitts, lymphoblastic), and children with leukemia (T-cell) and hyperleukocytosis are at high risk for TLS. These tumors are highly sensitive to chemotherapy and the extreme rapidity of tumor breakdown can quickly overwhelm the body's homeostasis. Additional risk factors for developing TLS are found in patients with a large tumor burden with lymphadenopathy, mediastinal mass, hepatosplenomegaly, large tumor, elevated LDH, and renal insufficiency. TLS also has been noted in neuroblastoma, small cell lung carcinoma, multiple myeloma, and other solid tumors.

Clinical presentation: TLS has a rapid onset and may manifest at prediagnosis, 6–48 hours after initial treatment, and up to 7 days thereafter. It is imperative to identify patients at risk and to complete a detailed history. Symptoms may include: abnormal laboratory findings (elevated

Figure 5-8. Cytoxic Therapy and/or Spontaneous Tumor Breakdown

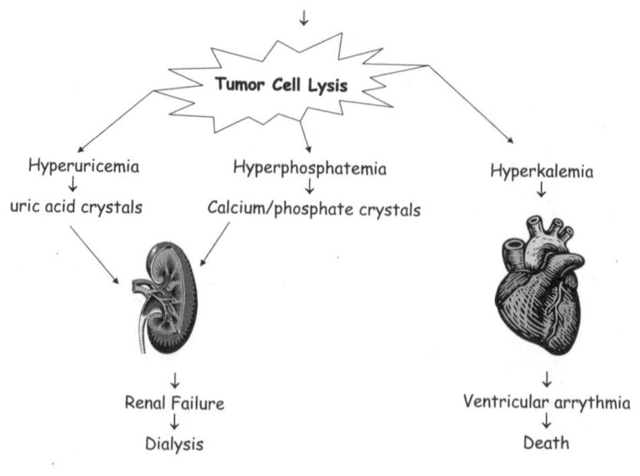

Tumor Cell Lysis
Hyperuricemia → uric acid crystals
Hyperphosphatemia → Calcium/phosphate crystals
Hyperkalemia
Renal Failure → Dialysis
Ventricular arrythmia → Death

WBC, phosphorous, uric acid, potassium, BUN, creatinine, LDH, and decreased calcium), flank pain, hematuria, decrease urine output, lethargy, nausea and/or vomiting, edema, muscle cramps and twitching, numbness and tingling, carpopedal spasms, seizures, diarrhea, respiratory distress, abdominal fullness or ascites, and irregular heartbeat.

Medical management: Early identification of high-risk patients with preexisting hyperuricemia, as well as taking prophylactic measures to prevent TLS, are critical in reducing the morbidity associated with it and in obtaining optimal patient outcomes. The single most important intervention is hydration.

- Administer intravenous hydration with D5 _ NS (no potassium) at 3L/m^2/day to attain a urine output of greater than 100cc/m^2/hr and a urine specific gravity of less than 1.010.
- Force diuresis (Lasix, mannitol).
- Manage hyperkalemia (remove sources of potassium, diuretics, Kayexalate, glucose/insulin IV infusion, IV calcium gluconate, sodium bicarbonate IV push, hemofiltration/dialysis).
- Manage hyperuricemia (alkalinization IV NaCCO3 40meq/L; Allopurinol PO 100mg/m^2/dose tid; maximum dose 800mg/day or IV 200mg/m^2/day in 1–3 doses; maximum 600mg/day; Rasburicase/Elitek 0.15 or 0.2mg/kg/dose IV Q day).
- Manage hyperphosphatemia (use oral phosphate binder, implement dietary phosphate restriction, remove phosphate-containing medications, peform IV glucose/insulin infusion).
- Manage hypocalcemia (treat hyperphosphatemia, keep serum bicarb <30, infuse calcium gluconate intravenously).
- Provide timely renal or ICU consults, as indicated.

Nursing Assessment and Interventions

- Give strict attention to fluid balance.
- Maintain strict input and output, maintain urine output at greater than 3–5cc/kg/hr.
- Monitor urine specific gravity (keep >1.010) and urine pH (keep 7.0–7.5) every 4 hours.
- Assess vital signs at least every 4 hours.
- Obtain "tumor lysis" laboratory specimens at least every 6–12 hours, as ordered, and evaluate values promptly.
- Perform ongoing respiratory assessments.
- Perform ongoing assessments for edema.
- Monitor weight bid.
- Provide ongoing neurological assessments (LOC, weakness, muscle twitching, numbness and tingling, seizures).
- Provide ongoing gastrointestinal assessment (nausea, vomiting, diarrhea).
- Provide ongoing assessment for Chvostek's (unilateral facial spasm) and Trouseau's (carpopedal spasms) signs.
- Maintain seizure precautions.
- Monitor for abnormal cardiac rate or rhythm (monitor for peaked T waves, QRS widening, ventricular arrhythmias).
- Administer IV hydration, as ordered, without potassium.
- Administer Alkalinization/Allopurinol and/or Rasburicase/Elitek, as ordered.

If these metabolic abnormalities cannot be controlled, more severe complications that can occur include the need for hemofiltration, dialysis, or both, heart block, and cardiac arrest.

Expected Patient and Family Outcomes

- The patient and family can verbalize their understanding of the seriousness of tumor lysis syndrome.
- The patient will have minimal symptoms of, or controlled tumor lysis syndrome.
- The patient will not experience any life-threatening events related to tumor lysis syndrome.

Septic Shock

Definition: Septic shock is a systemic response to pathogenic microorganisms and endotoxins in the blood that are usually gram-negative and arise from endogenous flora. Septic shock can lead to decreased tissue perfusion, cellular hypoxia, and death. Septic shock also is defined as sepsis with hypotension (systolic BP <90mm HG or a reduction of 40mm Hg from baseline) despite adequate fluid resuscitation, along with perfusion abnormalities that may include, but are not limited to, lactic acidosis, scant urination, or an acute alteration in mental status.

Risk factors: Risk factors include prolonged neutropenia (longer than 7 days), an ANC of less than 100mm^3, breaks in skin and mucus membrane integrity, invasive devices, malnutrition, and asplenia.

Clinical presentation: Not all children with sepsis will develop shock. Many times the febrile neutropenic patient will have the clinical symptoms of sepsis or shock until after antibiotics are initiated.

Sepsis should be considered a possibility whenever a patient presents with a known or suspected infection and with two or more of the following symptoms: fever or hypothermia, unexplained tachycardia and tachypnea, signs of peripheral vasodilation, leukocytosis or leukopenia, and reduced mental alertness. Severe sepsis is the diagnosis if any organ failure is confirmed.

If left untreated, or if the child is not responsive to treatment, then shock will progress. When shock is classified by etiology, the terms *hypovolemic*, *caridogenic*, and *distributive* are used. Hypovolemic shock is the most common manifestation of shock and is usually due to inadequate intravascular volume relative to vascular space (i.e., dehydration, hemorrhage, inflammatory condition [e.g., sepsis]). Distributive shock results from the inappropriate distribution of blood volume (i.e., sepsis, anaphylaxis). Cardiogenic shock is caused by myocardial dysfunction. Shock also is classified by its effects on blood pressure as compensated shock (i.e., early shock, tachycardia, and poor perfusion with normal blood pressure) or decompensated shock (i.e., late shock, weak central pulses, altered level of consciousness, oliguria, and hypotension). Septic shock is diagnosed when there is severe sepsis and hypotension despite fluid resuscitation, or when blood pressure is maintained with vasoactive drug support.

Medical management: Early recognition and prompt treatment of sepsis or septic shock are essential to the patient's survival.

Volume resuscitation is the most important treatment for patients with septic shock. Maintaining cardiovascular volume with isotonic or crystalloid boluses of 20cc/kg over 5–20 minutes to 60cc/kg or greater in the first hour often is required to help stabilize the child. However, when volume resuscitation is inadequate to restore blood pressure, vasoactive drugs are recommended. Along with volume replacements, the only other proven treatment for septic shock is the early administration of antimicrobials—preferably with broad spectrum antibiotics (see Section VI, "Supportive Care"), until the causitive pathogen is identified.

Potential complications: CNS complications include a decreased level of consciousness, anxiety, restlessness, confusion, disorientation, lethargy, and, in some cases, coma. Respiratory effects can include tacypnea, rales, wheezing, dyspnea, cyanosis, and pulmonary congestion. Cardiac difficulties comprise tachycardia, thready pulse, narrowing pulse pressure, decreased peripheral circulation, and cool, clammy skin. Renal complications are manifested by oliguria and anuria and can result in renal failure. Hematologic complications consist of bleeding or DIC or both. Complications result from the progression of shock and can lead to multiorgan failure and death if not treated promptly.

Nursing Assessment and Interventions

Assessment:

- Monitor the patient's physical status and vital signs continuously to assess for subtle changes in condition, and be aware that changes in a child's vital signs will lag behind deteriorations in physical status.
- Strictly monitor the patient's fluid intake and output.

Interventions:

- Obtain blood cultures immediately and administer IV antibiotics as soon as possible when a patient is febrile and neutropenic
- Provide support for the patient and the family

(See also Section VI, "Supportive Care".)

Expected Patient and Family Outcomes

- The patient and family understand the signs and symptoms of early infection and seek prompt medical attention
- The patient has minimal complications related to septic shock.

Disseminated Intravascular Coagulation

Definition: Disseminated intravascular coagulation (DIC) is the consumption of coagulation factors that is greater than the body's ability to replace them, thus inhibiting coagulation. Alterations in blood clotting mechanisms are manifested by decreased platelets, increased prothrombin, and decreased fibrinogen, which result in diffuse intravascular coagulation and tissue ischemia.

Risk factors: Risk factors are malignancy, infection, and trauma. Promyelocytic leukemia is the most common malignancy associated with DIC at initial diagnosis. The overall most common cause of DIC in children with cancer is gram-negative sepsis.

Clinical presentation: A patient can have petechiae, ecchymosis, and purpuric rash. There also can be diffuse uncontrolled bleeding, a platelet count of $<20{,}000/mm^3$, prolonged prothrombin (PT) time and partial thromboplastin (PTT) time, increased D-dimer assay, decreased antithrombin III levels, below-normal fibrinogen, and increased fibrin-degradation products.

Medical management: Treatment consists of symptom management and replacement of blood products (i.e., fresh-frozen plasma, cryoprecipitate, transfusions of platelet and packed red blood cells). Heparin, once a mainstay of DIC management, now is rarely used.

Potential complications: Complications include bleeding from puncture sites, GI bleeding, hematuria, oliguria, dyspnea, tachypnea, tachycardia, diminished peripheral circulation, restlessness, confusion, and lethargy.

Nursing Assessment and Interventions

Assessment:

- Monitor the patient for signs and symptoms of DIC.
- Assess the following for presence and amount of bleeding: urine, stool, emesis, and needle puncture sites.
- Assess changes in laboratory values.
- Assess tissue perfusion, including color, temperature, and peripheral pulses.

Interventions:

- Apply direct pressure to active bleeding sites.
- Administer pain medications, as needed.
- Elevate the sites of active bleeding when the patient can tolerate these measures.
- Administer blood products, as ordered.
- Provide support for the patient and the family
- Teach the patient and the family measures to prevent bleeding.

Expected Patient and Family Outcomes

- The patient and the family can identify risk factors for the development of DIC.
- The patient has minimal complications related to DIC.

Typhlitis

Definition: Typhlitis is a bacterial invasion of the cecum leading to necrotizing colitis. Tissue involvement ranges from inflammation to full-thickness infarction, perforation, or both. *Clostridium septicum* and *Pseudomonas aeruginosa* are the most common organisms associated with typhlitis.

Risk factors: Risk factors are severe neutropenia, high-risk acute leukemia, induction therapy for acute myelogenous leukemias, infection, and mucositis.

Clinical presentation: Symptoms can include profound neutropenia, fever, severe abdominal pain in the right lower quadrant, distended abdomen, high-pitched, diminished, or absent bowel sounds, nausea, vomiting, and diarrhea.

Medical management: Management consists of broad-spectrum antibiotic coverage, supportive management, and radiological evaluation. Surgical intervention may be indicated in the following situations: persistent GI bleeding despite resolution or correction of clotting abnormalities; evidence of free intraperitoneal perforation; clinical deterioration requiring support with vasopressors and hyperhydration, which suggests uncontrolled sepsis from infarction; and symptoms of an intra-abdominal process that would require surgical intervention in a nonneutropenic patient.

Potential complications: Complications can include sepsis, necrosis of the cecum, temporary or permanent ostomy, and death.

Nursing Assessment and Interventions

Assessment:

- Perform a physical assessment of the patient to evaluate bowel sounds and the degree of abdominal pain.
- Assess the patient's vital signs for signs of septic shock.
- Measure the patient's abdominal girth.
- Assess the patient for nausea, vomiting, and diarrhea.

Interventions:

- Provide pain management.
- Perform skin, oral, and perianal care for the patient.
- Provide support for the patient and the family

Expected Patient and Family Outcomes

- The patient and the family can identify the risk factors for typhlitis.
- The patient and the family seek early medical intervention for symptoms of severe abdominal pain, with or without fever.

Spinal Cord Compression

Definition: Spinal cord compression is a neurologic emergency that occurs in approximately 5% of patients with malignancies, either at the time of initial diagnosis or at recurrence. It is usually not life-threatening, but prompt assessment and intervention are needed to preserve neurological function. Compression can occur as a result of tumor invasion of the vertebrae, resulting in collapse of the spinal cord or increased pressure in the spinal canal. Some primary tumors also can invade the spinal cord.

Risk factors: Risk factors are primary CNS tumor of the spinal cord, neuroblastoma, lymphoma, and metastatic sarcoma.

Clinical presentation: Patients may exhibit local, referred, or diffuse pain; neck or back pain may occur. Other signs are motor deficits, including weakness, ataxia, hypotonic or hyporeflexic muscular reactions, paralysis, muscle atrophy, and sensory deficits such as bowel or bladder dysfunction, paresthesia, loss of pain sensation, and loss of temperature sensation. Specific symptoms depend upon the location and extent of tumor involvement.

Medical management: The patient should be given a diagnostic evaluation that includes a neurological examination and an MRI or CT scan of the spine, or both. The underlying disease may be treated with high doses of glucocorticoids, which are administered to reduce the edema and pain; emergent radiation therapy to the primary or metastatic lesion, which will result in a rapid decrease in the size of radiosensitive tumors; and surgical decompression involving a laminectomy.

Potential complications: Complications are temporary or permanent sensory or motor changes, or both, paralysis, muscle atrophy, a decrease in or loss of bowel or bladder function, and sexual impotence.

Nursing Assessment and Interventions

Assessment:

- Perform a comprehensive assessment of the patient.
- Observe the patient for early signs and symptoms, such as neck or back pain, motor weakness, and loss of sensation.
- Perform frequent neurological checks.
- Observe the patient for motor or sensory deficits.

Interventions:

- Help the patient with positioning and range of motion.
- Discuss safety issues related to altered mobility with the patient.
- Provide a regimen for skin care.
- Initiate consultation with a physical therapist and occupational therapist when the patient's condition has been stabilized.
- Educate the patient and the family about how to maintain some patient independence within the limitations caused by the compression.
- Provide supportive care for the patient and the family.

Expected Patient and Family Outcomes

- The patient and the family identify the symptoms associated with spinal cord compression and know the importance of seeking early medical intervention.
- The patient remains as independent as possible.
- The patient and the family participate in a rehabilitation program, as indicated.

- The patient and the family use available community resources.

Syndrome of Inappropriate Antidiuretic Hormone Secretion

Definition: The antidiuretic hormone acts on the distal renal tubules and collecting ducts to increase permeability, thus increasing water absorption. Excess production of antidiuretic hormone (ADH) from tumors that stimulate the posterior pituitary gland results in excessive water retention. The syndrome of inappropriate antidiuretic hormone secretion (SIADH) is caused by a continuous release of ADH without a relationship to plasma osmolality. SIADH is associated with a decrease in urine output and an increase in weight without edema, leading to hyponatremia and water intoxication.

Risk factors: Risk factors may be related to disease or treatment. The most common malignancies associated with SIADH are CNS tumors, Hodgkin's disease, and non-Hodgkin's lymphoma. Infectious causes are primarily pulmonary fungal or bacterial infections. Medications such as steroids, narcotics, thiazide diuretics, anesthetic agents, cisplatin, cyclophosphamide, and vincristine have been linked with SIADH. In addition, overhydration with hypotonic solutions may be a causative factor.

Clinical presentation: The signs of early SIADH (serum Na+ less than 130 mEq/l) are thirst, anorexia, headache, muscle cramps and lethargy, and weakness and lethargy.

The signs of midcourse SIADH (serum Na+ less than 125 mEq/l) are nausea, vomiting, hyporeflexia, and confusion.

The signs of late SIADH (serum Na+ less than 120 mEq/l) are seizures, coma, and death.

Medical management: The underlying disease is treated. Management of symptoms includes following the patient's serum chemistries as well as urine Na+ and urine osmolality and restricting fluids for patients with serum Na+ greater than 125 mEq/l. Corrections occur slowly over 7–10 days. Hypertonic saline solution may be administered for severe SIADH (i.e., serum Na+ less than 120 mEq/l).

Potential complications: Complications can include weakness, fatigue, altered mental status, nausea and vomiting, diarrhea, abdominal cramping, thirst, oliguria, weight gain, myalgias, muscle cramping, progressive lethargy, coma, and seizures.

Nursing Assessment and Interventions

Assessment:

- Determine if the patient is at risk for SIADH.
- Perform a comprehensive physical assessment of the patient.
- Monitor the patient's fluid intake and output strictly.
- Monitor laboratory values.
- Weigh the patient daily.

Interventions:

- Ensure that the orders for fluid restriction are followed.
- Educate the patient and the family about the importance of fluid restriction.

Expected Patient and Family Outcomes

- The patient and the family identify the risk factors associated with SIADH.
- The patient and the family report the signs and symptoms of SIADH in a timely manner.
- The patient has minimal complication related to SIADH.

Anaphylaxis

Definition: Anaphylaxis is an immediate hypersensitivity reaction to a foreign protein that can occur within seconds or minutes after exposure. An anaphylactic reaction is potentially life-threatening since it may result in respiratory or cardiac system dysfunction, or both. Generally, if the onset of a reaction is rapid, the more severe it will be.

Risk factors: Risk factors are IV administration of medications or chemotherapeutic agents, antibiotics (e.g., trimethoprim-sulfamethoxazole [TMP-SMZ, trade name Bactrim], penicillin [Pen-Vee-K], amphotericin B [Fungizone]), blood product infusions, intravenous immune globulin, chemotherapy agents (e.g., L-asparaginase [Elspar], etoposide [VP-16], teniposide [VM-26]), and radiological contrast media.

Clinical presentation: Symptoms of anaphylaxis can range from small urticarial lesions (hives) to a systemic response (**Table 5-13**).

Anaphylaxis manifests itself in the cutaneous system in the form of pruritis, erythema, urticaria, and angioedema; in the CNS by anxiety and agitation; in the respiratory system through hoarseness, coughing, sneezing, dyspnea, laryngeal edema, stridor, and cyanosis; in the cardiovascular system

Table 5-13. Grading Scale for Allergic Reactions

Grade 1:	Localized reaction at the injection site with hives measuring ≤6 cm and occurring ≤6 hours from time of administration
Grade 2a:	Generalized reaction with multiple widely spread hives each measuring ≤6 cm and occurring ≤6 hours from time of administration
Grade 2b:	Severe localized or generalized reaction with hives measuring >6 cm
Grade 3:	Serum sickness/severe bronchospasm, chest tightness, cough, chills, difficulty breathing, vomiting, tachycardia, cyanosis, agitation
Grade 4:	Anaphylaxis, severe hypotension, shock, and any of the above plus hypotension and shock (cardiorespiratory collapse)

Note: From *"Anaphylaxis to Asparaginase Preparations: Development of a Protocol,"* by E.C. Martingano and A. Ethier, 1997, Leukemia Nursing, 1, p. 5.

through tachycardia, hypotension, and decreased peripheral perfusion; and through the GI system through nausea, vomiting, and diarrhea.

Medical management: Test doses of high-risk medications should be administered to prevent anaphylaxis, and patients should be pretreated with diphenhydramine (Benadryl), hydrocortisone (Solu-Cortef), or both. Supportive management of anaphylactic reaction includes administering epinephrine and oxygen as well as intubation, when required. Commonly used secondary drugs in the management of allergic reactions and anaphylaxis are included in **Table 5-13**. The patients should be observed for a minimum of 4 hours after a mild anaphylactic reaction. A more severe reaction may require hospitalization. Patients receiving PEG-asparaginase are at risk for delayed or prolonged reactions.

Potential complications: Patients can have mild to moderate discomfort, experience respiratory arrest, or can develop cardiorespiratory arrest that results in death.

Nursing Assessment and Interventions

Assessment:

- Assess the patient's risk for anaphylaxis.
- Document in the patient's chart allergies and previous history of reactions.
- Ensure that an emergency cart and an oxygen delivery system are readily available.

Interventions:

- Educate the patient and family about the potential risk of allergic reactions.
- Stop IV infusion as soon as symptoms appear.
- Maintain intravenous access.
- Evaluate the patency of the patient's airway and assess vital signs.
- Notify a physician immediately.
- Administer emergency drugs, as ordered, or per institutional protocol.
- Remain calm.
- Instruct the patient of appropriate actions to take when at home if a suspected allergic reaction should occur.
- Inform patients about the risk of delayed reactions when given Peg-asparaginase.

Expected Patient and Family Outcomes

- The patient and the family know the patient's allergy history.
- The patient and the family recognize the symptoms of anaphylaxis (e.g., itching, hives, difficulty breathing, anxiety, restlessness).
- The patient maintains a patent airway and has minimal complications from anaphylaxis.

Bibliography

Impairment of the Immune System

American Academy of Pediatrics (2000). *Redbook 2000: Report of the committee of infectious diseases* (25th ed.). Elk Grove, IL: AAP.

Baggott, C.R., Kelly, K.P., Fochtman, D., & Foley, G.V. (Eds.). (2002). *Nursing care of children and adolescents with cancer*. Philadelphia: W.B. Saunders.

Bartlett, J. (2002). *Pocket book of infectious disease therapy* (11th ed.). Baltimore: Lippincott Williams & Wilkins.

Itano, J.K. & Taoka, K.N. (1998). *Core curriculum for oncology nursing* (3rd ed.). Philadelphia: W.B. Saunders.

Lehne, R. (2000). *Pharmacology for nursing care* (4th ed.). Philadelphia: W.B. Saunders.

Muskkowski, C., & Buchsel, P. (1999). *Oncology nursing*. St. Louis, MO: Mosby.

Pizzo, P., & Poplack, D. (Eds.) (2002). *Principles and practice of pediatric oncology* (4th ed.). Philadelphia: Lippincott Williams & Wilkins.

Central Nervous System Complications

Bates, B. (1999) *A guide to physical examination and history taking*, Philadelphia: Lippincott.

Cheetham, T., & Baylis, P.H. (2002). Diabetes insipidus in children: Pathophysiology, diagnosis and management. *Pediatric Drugs, 4*, 785–796.

Doxy, D., Bruce, D., Swift, D., & Shapiro, K. (1999). Posterior fossa syndrome: Identifiable risk factors and irreversible complications. *Pediatric Neurosurgery, 31*, 131–136.

Ettinger, A.G., Bond, D.M., & Sievers, T.D. (2002). Chemotherapy. In C. Rasco Baggott, K. Paterson Kelly, D. Fochtman, G. Foley. (Eds.). *Nursing care of children and adolescents with cancer.* (3rd ed., pp. 133–176). Philadelphia: W.B. Saunders.

Hussong, M.R. (2002). Non-Hodgkins lymphoma. In C. Baggott, K. Paterson Kelly, D. Fochtman, G.V. Foley. (Eds.). *Nursing care of children and adolescents with cancer.* (3rd ed., pp. 536–544). Philadelphia: W.B. Saunders.

Kirk, E.A., Howard, V.C., & Scott, C.A. (1995). Description of posterior fossa syndrome in children after posterior fossa brain tumor surgery. *Journal of Pediatric Oncology Nursing, 12*, 181–187.

Pollack, I.F., Polinko, P., Albright, A.L., Towbin, R., & Fitz, C. (1995). Mutism and pseudobulbar symptoms after resection of posterior fossa tumors in children: Incidence and pathophysiology. *Neurosurgery, 37*, 885–893.

Ryan Murray J., & Petriccione, M.M. (2002). Central nervous system tumors. In C. Rasco Baggott, K. Paterson Kelly, D. Fochtman, & G.V. Foley. (Eds.). *Nursing care of children and adolescents with cancer*, (3rd ed., pp. 503–523). Philadelphia: W.B. Saunders.

Saborio, P., Tipton, G., & Chan, J. (2000). Diabetes insipidus. *Pediatrics in Review, 21*, 122–129.

Shiminski-Maher, T. (1991). Diabetes insipidus and syndrome of inappropriate secretion of antidiuretic hormone in children with midline suprasellar brain tumors. *Journal of Pediatric Oncology Nursing, 8*, 106–111.

Shiminski-Maher, T., & Shields, M. (1995). Pediatric brain tumors: Diagnosis and management. *Journal of Pediatric Oncology Nursing, 12*, 188–198.

Strother, D.R., Pollack, I.F., Fischer, P.G., Hunter, J.V., Woo, S.Y., Pomeroy, S.L., et al. (2002). Tumors of the central nervous system. In P.A. Pizzo, & D.G. Poplack. (Eds). *Principles and practice of pediatric oncology* (4th ed.). Philadelphia: Lippincott Williams and Wilkins.

Thibodeau, G.A., & Patton K.T. (1992). *Anatomy and physiology*. (3rd ed.). St. Louis: Mosby.

Westlake, S.K., & Bertolone, K.L. (2002). Acute lymphoblastic leukemia. In C. Rasco Baggott, K. Paterson Kelly, D. Fochtman, G.V. Foley. (Eds.). *Nursing care of children and adolescents with cancer*. (3rd ed., pp. 503–523). Philadelphia: W.B. Saunders.

http://www.niddk.nih.gov/health/kidney/pubs/insipidus/insipidus.htm

http://diabetesinsipidus.maxinter.net/polydipsia_and_polyuria.htm

Ototoxicity

Bukowski, R. (1999). Cytoprotection in the treatment of pediatric cancer: Review of current strategies in adults and their application in children. *Medical and Pediatric Oncology, 32*, 124–134.

Fukunaga-Johnson, N., Sandler, H. M., Marsh, R.T.T., & Martel, M.K. (1998). The use of 3D conformal radiotherapy (3D CRT) to spare the cochlea in patients with medulloblastoma. *International Journal of Radiation Oncology Biology Physics, 41*, 77–82.

Huang, E., Teh, B.S., Strother, D.R., Davis, Q. G., Chiu, J.K., Lu, H. H., et al.(2002). Intensity-modulated radiation therapy for pediatric medulloblastoma: Early report on the reduction of ototoxicity. *International Journal of Radiation Oncology Biology Physics, 52*, 599–605.

Landier, W. (1998). Hearing loss related to ototoxicity in children with cancer. *Journal of Pediatric Oncology Nursing, 15*, 195–206.

Matz, G.J. (1993). Aminoglycoside cochlear ototoxicity. *Otolaryngology Clinics of North America, 26*, 705–712.

Rybak, L.P. (1993). Ototoxicity of loop diuretics. *Otolaryngology Clinics of North America, 26*, 829–844.

Endocrine Abnormalities

Balis, F.M., Holcenberg, J.S., & Blaney, S. (2002). General principles of chemotherapy. In P. Pizzo, & D. Poplack. (Eds.). *Principles and practice of pediatric oncology*. (4th ed., pp. 238–308). Philadelphia: Lippincott Williams & Wilkins.

Keene, N., Hobbie, W., & Ruccione, K. (2000). Hormone producing glands. In N. Keene, W. Hobbie, & K. Ruccione. (Eds.). *Childhood cancers survivors: A practical guide to your future*. (pp. 259–286) Sebastopol, California: O'Reilly & Associates, Inc.

Kenney, L.B., Laufer, M.R., Grant, F.D., Grier, H., & Diller, L. (2001). High risk of infertility and long term gonadal damage in males treated with high dose cyclophosphamide for sarcoma during childhood. *Cancer, 91*, 613–621.

Cardiac and Pulmonary Complications

Acuone, J.J., Steinhurz, L., Oblender, M.G., Barnard, D.R., & Ablin, A.R. (1997). Modification for toxicity. In A.R. Ablin (Ed.). *Supportive care of children with cancer: Current therapy and guidelines from the Children's Cancer Group* (pp. 79–111). Baltimore: The Johns Hopkins University Press.

Balis, F.M., Holcenberg, J.S., & Blaney, S.M. (2002). General principles of chemotherapy. In P.A. Pizzo, & D.G. Poplack. (Eds.). *Principles and practice of pediatric oncology*. (4th ed., pp. 237–308). Philadelphia: Lippincott Williams & Wilkins.

Loerzel, V.W. & Dow, K.H. (2003). Cardiac toxicity related to cancer treatment. *Clinical Journal of Oncology Nursing, 7*, 557–562.

Panzarella, C., Baggott, C.R., Comeau, M., Duncan, J.M., Groben, V., Woods, D.A., et al. (2002). Management of disease and treatment-related complications. In C.R. Baggott, K.P. Kelly, D. Fochtman, & G.V. Foley (Eds.). *Nursing care of children and adolescents with cancer* (3rd ed., pp. 279–318). Philadelphia: W. B. Saunders.

Gastrointestinal Complications

Baggott, C.R. (2002). *Nursing care of children and adolescents with cancer* (3rd ed., pp 285–297). Phildadelphia: W.B. Saunders.

DeVita, V.T., Hellman, S., & Rosenberg, S.A. (2001). *Cancer: Principles and practice of oncology*. (pp. 2854–2878). Philadelphia: Lippincott Williams & Wilkins.

Haskell, C.M. (2001). *Cancer treatment* (5th ed., pp. 327–340). Philadelphia: WB Saunders.

Miller, M. & Kearney, N. (2001). Oral care for patients with cancer: a review of the nursing literature. *Cancer Nursing, 24*, 241–254.

Pizzo, P.A. & Poplack, D.C. (2002). *Principles and practice of pediatric oncology* (4th ed., pp. 1317–1324). Philadelphia: Lippincott Williams & Wilkins.

Renal Complications

Balis, F.M., Holcenberg, J.S., & Blaney, S. (2002). General principles of chemotherapy. In P. Pizzo & D. Poplack (Eds.). *Principles and practice of pediatric oncology*. (4th ed., pp. 238–308). Philadelphia: Lippincott Williams & Wilkins.

Capizzi, R.L. (1999). Clinical status and optimal use of amifostine. *Oncology 13*, 47–59.

Keene, N., Hobbie, W., & Ruccione, K. (2000). Kidneys, bladders, and genitals. In N. Keene, W. Hobbie, & K. Ruccione (Eds.). *Childhood cancers survivors: a practical guide to your future*. (pp. 340–355) California: O'Reilly & Associates.

Kelly, K.M. (2003) Clinical emergencies in children with cancer. In M.A. Weiner & M.S. Cairo (Eds.). *Pediatric hematology/oncology secrets (The secrets series)*. (pp. 187–190). Philadelphia: Hanley & Belfus.

Lowenthal, R.M., & Eaton, K. (1996). *Toxicity of chemotherapy. Hematology Oncology Clinics of North America*, 10, 967–990.

Skin Changes

Altman, A.J., & Wolff, L.J. (1997). The prevention of infection. In A.R. Ablin (Ed.) *Supportive care of children with cancer: current therapy and guidelines from the Children's Cancer Group* (pp. 1–12). Baltimore: The Johns Hopkins University Press.

Panzarella, C., Baggott, C.R., Comeau, M., Duncan, J.M., Groben, V., Woods, D.A., et al. (2002). Management of disease and treatment-related complications. In C.R. Baggott, K.P. Kelly, D. Fochtman, & G.V. Foley (Eds.). *Nursing care of children and adolescents with cancer* (pp. 279–318). Philadelphia: W.B. Saunders.

Musculoskeletal Alterations

Dreyer, Z.E., Biait, J., & Bleyer, A. (2002). Late effects of childhood cancer and its treatment. In P. Pizzo & D. Poplack (Eds.). *Principles and practice of pediatric oncology*. (4th ed., pp. 1432–1452). Philadelphia: Lippincott Williams & Wilkins.

Granowether, L. (2002). Malignant bone sarcomas: Osteosarcoma and Ewing's sarcoma. In M.A. Weiner & M.S. Cairo (Eds.). *Pediatric hematology/oncology secrets (The secrets series)*. (pp. 177–185). Philadelphia: Hanley & Belfus.

Link, M.P., Gebhart, M., & Meyers, P. (2002). Osteosarcoma. In P. Pizzo & D. Poplack (Eds.). *Principles and practice of pediatric oncology*. (4th ed., pp. 1051–1080). Philadelphia: Lippincott Williams & Wilkins.

Nutritional Complications

Alexander, H.R., Rickard, K.A., & Godshall, B. (2002). Nutritional supportive care. In P.A. Pizzo & D.G. Poplack (Eds.). *Principles and practice of pediatric oncology* (3rd ed., pp. 1167–1181). Philadelphia: Lippincott-Raven.

Anderson, L., & Ward, D. (1997). Nutrition. In S.E. Otto (Ed.). *Oncology nursing* (pp. 728–745). St. Louis: Mosby.

Clark, J., McGee, R., & Preston, R. (1992). Nursing management of responses to the cancer experience: Nutrition. In J. Clark & R. McGee (Eds.). *Core curriculum for oncology nursing* (pp. 93–106). Philadelphia: W.B. Saunders.

Wilkes, G.M., & Yemma, T. (1997). Nutritional support. In C. Varricchio (Ed.). *A cancer source book for nurses* (pp. 200–213). Atlanta: American Cancer Society.

Growth and Development

Hobbie, W., Ruccione, K., Harvey, J., & Moore, I.M. (2002). Care of survivors. In C.R. Baggott, K.P. Kelly, D. Fochtman, & G.V. Foley (Eds.). *Nursing care of children and adolescents with cancer* (pp. 426–464). Philadelphia: W.B. Saunders.

Hockenberry, M., Wilson, D., Winkelstein, M.L., & Kline, N.E. (2003). *Wong's essentials of pediatric nursing*. (7th ed.). St. Louis: C.V. Mosby.

Pain

Hockenberry-Eaton, M., Barrera, P., Brown, M., Bottomley, S. J., & Brace-O'Neill, J. (1999). *Pain management in children with cancer*. Austin, TX: Texas Cancer Council.

SECTION VI

SUPPORTIVE CARE

Karla Wilson

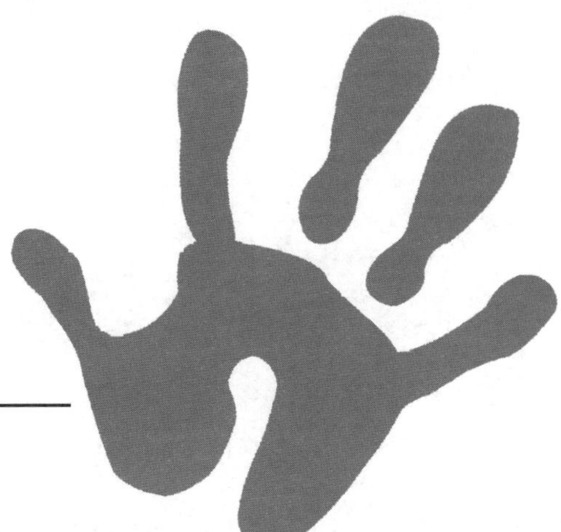

SECTION OUTLINE

Psychological Preparation and Support for Painful Procedures

Catherine Fiona Macpherson

Principles of Treatment

Preparing children psychologically to undergo an invasive procedure can decrease their anxiety and help them cope effectively with the event. Such preparation can give children a sense of security because they will have a more realistic picture of the event. If they are not given information, they will create in their minds what they believe will occur, and this creation may be more anxiety-producing than the actual event would have been. Psychological preparation also can create a foundation for developing positive coping skills children can use for future healthcare situations.

Role in Childhood Cancer

Invasive procedures occur frequently during cancer treatment, and require caregivers to help equip children to cope effectively with these situations. Furthermore, the protracted nature of most cancer therapies requires caregivers to be prepared to react to new types of anxieties as patients advance to higher cognitive levels during treatment.

Types of Preparation

- Provide age-appropriate information regarding the procedure the child will undergo.
- Provide information and support to parents who want to give the information to their child themselves.
- Teach coping strategies to be used during the procedure to give the child a sense of control and a focus.
- Show a videotape of how another child coped successfully with the procedure, thus allowing the child to perceive the event as manageable.
- Use medical play and dolls to teach the child about the procedure and to address any misconceptions he or she may express during the play session.
- Hold a one-to-one session between the child and the nurse prior to the procedure.
- Providing sensory information during the procedure as different aspects of it take place.
- Have the child meet with a child life specialist or other psychosocial support professionals, alone or with a nurse.

Nursing Assessment and Interventions

Assessment: Prior to the preparation session.

- Assess the child's chronological age and cognitive level (these may not correspond).
- Question the child and the caregiver about the child's past hospital experience, past procedures, reaction to pain, and coping techniques currently used during stressful situations.
- Determine the role the parent wants to assume, such as being present during the procedure, coaching, or coming into the room after the procedure. Support any role the parent can assume.

Assessment: During the preparation session.

- Ask the child what he or she expects will happen (e.g., how the procedure will be done), what he or she will feel, who will be present, where the procedure will take place, and how long it will last, thus allowing the child's misconceptions to be assessed.
- Continue to assess the child's understanding during the preparation session.
- Ask questions in different ways to determine if the child really understands and is not just repeating the words that have been said.
- Have the child reteach the staff person about the information conveyed during the preparation session as a way to assess the child's understanding.

Assessment: After the procedure.

- Assess the child's perception of the procedure.
- Assess with the child the effectiveness of his or her coping strategies.
- Reassess the child's understanding of the procedure over time, even for a procedure frequently experienced, since the child's needs and cognitive skills may change.

Interventions:

- Choose an environment free of distractions.
- Choose the most appropriate time for preparation (the younger the child, the closer to the event the preparation should be done).
- Prepare the child for all procedures, even those the staff considers routine and nonthreatening. Even when there is not time for formal preparation before a procedure, children still benefit from some type of preparation done either immediately before or during a procedure.
- Be aware that some children seek, and others avoid, information; attempt, but do not force preparation.
- Match preparation and support with the child's coping style.
- Present information at a developmentally appropriate level (**Table 6-1**).
- Give the child sensory information about the sequence of events.
- Explain how long the procedure will last as compared with the length of something with which the child is familiar, such as the length of a favorite TV show.
- Ensure that all information, including that regarding potential pain, is honest and accurate.
- Describe only what the child will see and feel. Avoid feeding the child's fears by describing potentially upsetting information, such as the size of a needle the child will not see when he or she has a lumbar puncture performed.
- Encourage the child to express all his or her feelings and concerns about the procedure.

Table 6-1. Developmental Considerations for the Psychological Preparation of Children

Stage	Developmental Characteristics	Concerns Related to Healthcare Experiences	Suggestions for Interaction
Infant	Is in the sensorimotor stage Is establishing a "self" versus others Forms attachments to favorite toys Attends to a variety of visual, auditory, tactile stimuli	Separation anxiety (8–24 months) Stranger anxiety	Include parents as often as possible. Prepare parents for tests and procedures. Encourage parents to support the child during the procedure. Maintain the crib as a safe place where no procedures are performed.
Toddler	Engages in preoperational thinking Is egocentric Can understand only concepts that he or she has experienced Mixes reality and fantasy Has a limited concept of time Has very little understanding of anatomy Has limited verbal skills Has limited self-expression skills Believes in imminent justice	Pain as "punishment" Fear of needles Separation Disruptive changes in familiar routines	Be truthful about pain. Be honest. Prepare the child for a procedure with tangible equipment and allow the child to manipulate safe equipment. Use dolls for preparation, not the child's transitional object (favorite toy). Provide simple explanations and information. Reassure the child that he or she is not being punished. Emphasize that there will be an end to the procedure. Clarify any misconceptions created by the child's fantasies. Provide only realistic choices. Maintain the bed as a place that is safe from invasive procedures.
Child of Preschool Age	Is in the preoperational stage Has better developed verbal skills than toddlers Uses play for self-expression Is egocentric Is acquiring a sense of initiative Engages in magical thinking Uses and repeats words that he or she does not understand	Fear of needles Magical thinking Fear of a new environment Fear of the unknown Fear of loss of control and body mutilation (a fear of older preschoolers)	Encourage questions. Address the child's fantasies. Reassure the child that the procedure is not being done to blame or punish. Use visual aids for teaching. Allow the child to manipulate safe equipment. Be honest. Allow the child to "play out" events. Maintain the bed as a place that is safe from invasive procedures.
Child of Primary School Age	Is at the stage of concrete operations Can think and reason logically but not abstractly Has a good concept of time Seeks autonomy and independence Understands cause and effect	Loss of control Bodily injury or mutilation Fear of death Fear of incompetency	Be honest. Offer help so the child can work through feelings and establish coping strategies early. Address the child's concerns about mutilation. Allow for realistic choices. Focus the child's preparation on sensory information and behavioral expectations. Use pictures, body outlines, dolls, or models for preparation.
Adolescent	Is at the stage of formal operations Thinks abstractly Engages in some magical thinking Is establishing his or her own identity Considers socialization with peers important Understands the body and bodily functions	Loss of control Privacy Loss of skills Body image Perception of peers Loss of independence	Allow for choices. Develop trust. Stress the importance of compliance. Promote peer contacts. Include the adolescent in decision making. Respect the adolescent's privacy. Begin the preparation with reason, then with concrete details. Maximize the adolescent's independence.

- Tell the child the reasons the procedure needs to be done to alleviate any misconceptions he or she might have.
- Tell the child about how he or she will be asked to behave during the procedure.
- Provide opportunities for hands-on learning by allowing the child to handle equipment, photos, videos, or dolls, or by encouraging medical play.
- Be extremely cautious about language; avoid using words with double meanings such as "shot" and "push."
- Choose words that convey a less frightening message, such as "gently slide the needle in" rather than "stick the needle in," or "warm" or "sting" rather than "burn."
- Use medical terms, but define them so the child can understand them.
- Teach coping skills.
  - Explain the rationale for using coping strategies.
  - Provide suggested techniques for procedures, such as distraction, imagery, relaxation, self-talk, and self-pacing.
  - Encourage the child to practice the techniques that have been chosen.
- Promote coping during the procedure.
  - Provide positive reinforcement during the procedure to enhance compliance and to help the child use coping strategies. Avoid saying "good girl" or "good boy," so that children do not equate compliance with being a good person; define the behavior that is being reinforced (e.g., "I really like the way you are holding so still").
- Allow for realistic choices (i.e., "Which arm should I use for the blood pressure cuff?", to give the child some control over the situation.
- Give the child a role during the procedure, such as holding the gauze or an adhesive bandage.
- Avoid using the child's bed for invasive procedures whenever possible to maintain the bed as a place of safety and security for the child.

Expected Patient and Family Outcomes

- The child has a developmentally appropriate understanding of the procedure, and misconceptions have been eliminated.
- The child has established coping strategies to employ during painful procedures.
- The child copes effectively during the procedure.

Sedation for Painful Procedures

Catherine Fiona Macpherson

Principles of Treatment

Pain during procedures such as bone marrow aspirations and lumbar punctures is often identified as the most distressing aspect of the entire experience for a child with cancer. Optimal management of pain associated with procedures through the use of sedation is likely to reduce the distress of dealing with cancer for the child and his or her family. Sedation ranges from minimal sedation/anxiolysis, to moderate sedation (formerly known as "conscious sedation"), to deep sedation and general anesthesia. Moderate ("conscious") sedation is defined as "a drug-induced depression of consciousness during which patients respond purposefully to verbal commands, either alone or accompanied by light tactile stimulation. No interventions are required to maintain a patent airway and spontaneous ventilation is adequate. Cardiovascular function is usually maintained" (American Society of Anesthesiologists, 2002, p. 1005).

Role in Childhood Cancer

The use of moderate ("conscious") sedation may reduce the pain and distress children with cancer associate with procedures such as bone marrow aspirations and lumbar punctures, and may prevent a child from developing negative expectations about pain and distress during procedures that must be repeated as part of the treatment protocol.

Types of Sedation Drugs

The combination of a benzodiazepine (e.g., midazolam [Versed]) and an opioid (e.g., morphine or fentanyl) is frequently recommended for intravenous (IV) sedation of children. Benzodiazepines have sedative, anxiolytic, and amnestic effects. Morphine and fentanyl, the opioids, have an analgesic effect (see **Table 6-2** for recommended drugs).

Method of Delivery

IV administration of a combination of benzodiazepines and opioids can provide both analgesia and sedation effectively and safely (**Table 6–3**). Unlike oral, intranasal, or intramuscular sedatives, this combination can be administered easily, has a predictable and rapid onset, short duration of action, can be titrated to individual patient response, and can be reversed with the appropriate antagonist (e.g., flumazenil [Romazicon] for midazolam [Versed], naloxone [Narcan] for morphine or fentanyl).

Potential Side Effects

Children with a known airway problem, apnea, hemodynamic instability, altered mental status, or who have experienced previous adverse events related to sedation or anesthesia are at increased risk for adverse cardiorespiratory effects. Also at increased risk are children younger than 6 years of age and those with developmental delays. These latter two groups of children may require more sedation to make them cooperate with the procedure team, but also they are more vulnerable to the effects of sedation on respiratory drive, airway patency, and protective reflexes. Research suggests, however, that patient characteristics are less important to adverse outcomes of sedation than are team reactions to rescue patients from such adverse events.

The American Academy of Pediatrics (AAP) has established comprehensive guidelines for monitoring pediatric patients during and after sedation (AAP, 1992, 2002) and has established recovery parameters for sedation of pediatric patients. The monitoring guidelines include continuous monitoring of oxygen saturation and assessment of respiratory rate, heart rate, and blood pressure at specific frequencies from baseline until the child has fully recovered from sedation. The recovery parameters include airway patency, stable cardiovascular function, and return of the child to his or her baseline level of alertness. These monitoring guidelines and recovery parameters are uniform and independent of specialty or care setting in which the sedation is administered (**Table 6-4**).

Adverse events related to sedation frequently are associated with drug overdoses or interactions. Respiratory depression resulting in hypoxemia is the most common serious adverse effect of sedation with a benzodiazepine-and-opioid

Table 6-2. Recommended Drugs and Dosages

Conscious Sedation Agents

Midazolam (Versed) 0.05 mg/kg IV initial dose. Additional doses of 0.05 mg/kg as necessary. Maximum total dose of 0.15 mg/kg. Dilute to a concentration of 1 mg/ml with 0.9% NaCl.

Fentanyl (Sublimaze) 0.5-1.0 mcg/kg IV undiluted. Note that because of small volume used, a toxic dose can be administered accidentally to young children; therefore, careful dosage calculation and volume measurement are mandatory.

Morphine 0.05-0.1 mg/kg IV. Dilute to a concentration of 1 mg/ml with 0.9% NaCl.

Reversal Agents

Naloxone (Narcan) 0.01 mg/kg IV repeated q 2-3 minutes as necessary for reversal of fentanyl and morphine.

Flumazenil (Romazicon) 0.2 mg/kg IV repeated q 1 minute as necessary to a maximum total dose of 3 mg/hour for reversal of midazolam.

Note: From "Conscious Sedation of Pediatric Oncology Patients for Painful Procedures: Development and Implementation of a Clinical Practice Protocol," by C.F. Macpherson and L.A. Lundblad, 1997, *Journal of Pediatric Oncology Nursing, 14*(1), p. 37. Copyright 1997 by W.B. Saunders. Adapted with permission.

Table 6-3. Protocol for Pediatric Conscious Sedation

Sedation Administration

1. Provide quiet environment, including parental presence for support of the child and use of relaxation techniques.
2. Follow the physician's order for conscious sedation agents. Midazolam (Versed) is used for sedation ± fentanyl (Sublimaze) or morphine for analgesia.
3. Verify patency of intravenous access prior to administration of conscious sedation agents.
4. Administer fentanyl (Sublimaze) or morphine by direct intravenous injection over 1-2 minutes followed by midazolam by direct intravenous injection over 1-2 minutes.
5. Wait 3-5 minutes following midazolam (Versed) administration to allow sedation to occur before beginning procedure. If sedation inadequate, administer additional dose of midazolam, wait 1-3 minutes and reassess adequacy of sedation.

Note. From "Conscious Sedation of Pediatric Oncology Patients for Painful Procedures: Development and Implementation of a Clinical Practice Protocol," by C.F. Macpherson and L.A. Lundblad, 1997, *Journal of Pediatric Oncology Nursing, 14*(1), p. 36. Copyright 1997 by W.B. Saunders. Adapted with permission.

Table 6-4. Pediatric Conscious Sedation Assessment and Interventions

Preprocedure Assessment

1. Assess indications and contraindications for conscious sedation.
2. Obtain informed consent from the child's parent/legal guardian.
3. Verify nothing-by-mouth (NPO) status:
   Child of 0-36 months: No milk or solids for 6 hours, no clear fluids for 2 hours prior to procedure
   Child of 36 months or older: No milk or solids for 8 hours, no clear fluids for 2 hours prior to procedure.
4. Make a clinical examination of the patient, including previous sedation/anesthesia, allergy, weight, respira-tory rate, heart rate, blood pressure, oxygen saturation, color of skin and nail beds.
5. Ensure the availability of
   a) emergency cart, oxygen, oral suction, naloxone (Narcan), flumazenil (Romazicon)
   b) at least one nursing or medical staff member trained in pediatric advanced life support
   c) consult PICU or pediatric anesthesia if patient has complex medical problem, abnormal airway, or if there are any questions regarding pediatric conscious sedation.

Nursing Interventions During and After the Procedure

1. Assess respiratory rate, heart rate, blood pressure, color of skin and nail beds, level of consciousness, responsiveness, and comfort level, and note any unusual responses to sedation q 5 minutes during procedure and q 15 minutes for a minimum of 60 minutes following the last dose of sedation administered or until the child returns to baseline level of consciousness and heart rate and respiratory rate ± 20% of baseline.
2. Provide continuous oxygen saturation and electrocardiographic monitoring during procedure and for a minimum of 30 minutes postprocedure. Continue intermittent oxygen saturation monitoring q 15 minutes for a minimum of 60 minutes following the last dose of sedation administered or until the child returns to baseline level of consciousness and heart rate and respiratory rate ± 20% of baseline.
3. Provide postconscious sedation discharge instructions as necessary.

Note: From "Conscious Sedation of Pediatric Oncology Patients for Painful Procedures: Development and Implementation of a Clinical Practice Protocol," by C.F. Macpherson and L.A. Lundblad, 1997, *Journal of Pediatric Oncology Nursing, 14*(1), p. 36. Copyright 1997 by W.B. Saunders. Adapted with permission.

combination (**Table 6-5**). Respiratory depression and hypoxemia may be prevented by careful calculation of the dose of each agent; and by titrating the doses until the desired effect is achieved. Continuous monitoring of the sedated patient for early indications of cardiorespiratory instability and rapid, effective response to such instability requires appropriate training and adequate numbers of personnel, monitors, resuscitation equipment, and medications appropriate to the child's age and size.

Nursing Assessment and Interventions

Nursing assessment and interventions for a child receiving sedation are most clearly and concisely presented in a clinical practice protocol.

Table 6-5. Respiratory Depression Protocol for Pediatric Conscious Sedation

Treatment of Respiratory Depression Occurring During or After the Procedure

1. Stop administration of drug immediately, reposition child to ensure adequate airway, stimulate child to breathe, administer 100% oxygen via mask. Notify physician stat.
2. If respiratory depression cannot be resolved with stimulation to breathe and administration of oxygen, administer reversal agent. For reversal of fentanyl (Sublimaze) or morphine, administer naloxone (Narcan) by direct intravenous injection. For reversal of midazolam (Versed), administer flumazenil (Romazicon) by direct intravenous injection. If both fentanyl or morphine and midazolam have been used, administer naloxone first, followed immediately by flumazenil. If respiratory rate < 10, or if there is no response to reversal agents, call for help, begin 100% oxygen by ambu bag and face mask, assist ventilation. If there still is no response, proceed to secure airway with appropriate size of endotracheal tube and assist ventilation.
3. Assess adequacy of response to reversal agents in resolving respiratory depression within 1 minute of administration. If respiratory depression fails to be resolved after administration of one dose of appropriate reversal agent or if there is persistent hypoxemia, obtain arterial blood gas and initiate airway management procedure.
4. Continue to assess oxygen saturation, heart rate, respiratory rate, blood pressure, color of skin and nail beds, and level of consciousness q 1-2 minutes until respiratory depression is resolved.
5. Once respiratory depression has been resolved, assess respiratory rate q 5 minutes, oxygen saturation, heart rate, blood pressure, color of skin and nail beds, and level of consciousness q 15 minutes for 2 hours.

Note: From "Conscious Sedation of Pediatric Oncology Patients for Painful Procedures: Development and Implementation of a Clinical Practice Protocol," by C.F. Macpherson and L.A. Lundblad, 1997, *Journal of Pediatric Oncology Nursing, 14*(1), p. 36. Copyright 1997 by W.B. Saunders. Adapted with permission.

Expected Patient and Family Outcomes

- The child experiences minimal pain and distress related to the procedure.
- The child receives effective sedation without incurring complications.

References

American Academy of Pediatrics Committee on Drugs (1992). Guidelines for monitoring and management of pediatric patients during and after sedation for diagnostic and therapeutic procedures. *Pediatrics, 89,* 1110–1115.

American Academy of Pediatrics (AAP) Committee on Drugs. (2002). Guidelines for monitoring and management of pediatric patients during and after sedation for diagnostic and therapeutic procedures: Addendum. *Pediatrics, 110,* 836–838.

American Society of Anesthesiologists, Task Force on Sedation and Analgesia by Non-Anesthesiologists. (2002). Practice guidelines for sedation and analgesia by non-anesthesiologists. *Anesthesiology, 96,* 1004–1017.

Central Venous Access

Joetta Deswarte Wallace

Principles of Treatment

To effectively treat children with cancer, clinicians frequently must have IV access to withdraw blood and to administer chemotherapy, supportive medications, fluids, and blood products.

Role in Childhood Cancer

Central venous devices (CVDs) minimize the need for venipunctures, thereby reducing patient discomfort. These devices minimize the emotional trauma associated with venipuncture and the placement of peripheral IV lines. Veins that are used frequently to administer chemotherapy are prone to scarring, thus, CVDs provide a safe route for administering vesicant chemotherapy.

Types of CVDs

Broviac, Hickman, and Quinton catheters: These external central venous catheters are threaded internally into a major blood vessel and advanced until the tip reaches the midportion of the superior vena cava (SVC), or at the junction of the SVC and right atrium. The catheter is tunneled from the entrance site through subcutaneous tissue or fascia and brought out through the skin (i.e., the exit site) on the chest (**Figure 6-1**).

The advantage of these catheters is that they are available as single-lumen or multiple-lumen catheters. Multiple-lumen catheters are recommended for patients who are on aggressive regimens and who may require simultaneous supportive therapies, such as parenteral nutrition, blood products, and antibiotics. External catheters make it possible for clinicians to draw blood without causing discomfort to patients.

Groshong catheter: This central venous catheter does not require heparinization (**Figure 6-2**). Its advantage is that it has a small self-sealing end that can be flushed with saline. However, it has had limited use in pediatrics because of its potential for valve failure

Permcath: This central venous access device is similar to a Vascath or Quinton catheter, and is used for dialysis. It is placed by a surgical technique similar to that used when placing Hickman and Broviac catheters. Its advantage is that it has a rigid wall that can withstand pheresis pressure. This catheter is appropriate for patients who will need pheresis for a peripheral blood stem-cell transplant.

Peripherally inserted central catheter (PICC): This is a threadlike, flexible catheter that is placed peripherally through a basilic or median cubital vein and advanced to the SVC. Its advantages are that it can be placed at the bedside by nurses trained in its placement and that it provides an economical and safe method of IV access for intermediate or long-term use. Nonetheless, placement of the PICC should be confirmed by a chest X ray.

Implanted venous access: These are surgically implanted central catheters whose placement is similar to that of a central venous line (CVL). The Port-a-Cath (PAC) catheter connects to a port, with a self-sealing silicone septum in the subcutaneous tissue of the patient's upper chest or abdomen (**Figure 6-3**). The PASport is similar to the PAC, except that it is placed in the inner part of the patient's arm and threaded to the SVC. The advantage of these catheters is that unless the ports are in use, no home maintenance is needed because they are implanted completely under the skin.

Potential Complications Associated with CVDs

Infection: Sepsis is the most common problem associated with CVDs.

Occlusion: Occlusion is the second most common complication associated with CVDs. The ease with which the CVD can be flushed depends upon whether the occlusion is partial or complete. Occlusions can be caused by a thrombus in the line or at the end of the catheter; by the fibrin sheath around the catheter tip, which allows fluids to flow through the CVD but inhibits blood withdrawal; or by precipitate caused by the administration of medications with incompatible fluids.

Malposition: A malposition can occur by pulling on the CVD or by improper placement of the catheter, causing withdrawal occlusion. The patient may experience chest pain or headache when the line is flushed.

Break in the CVD: An external break can result in blood loss, an air embolism, or sepsis. An internal break can cause the patient to experience edema at the site, or chest pain when the CVD is flushed.

Extravasation: Extravasation is caused by an infiltration of vesicants, evidenced by inflammation and pain at the exit site or withdrawal occlusion, or both, during or after administration of the vesicant.

Figure 6-1. Hickman® Dual-Lumen Catheter

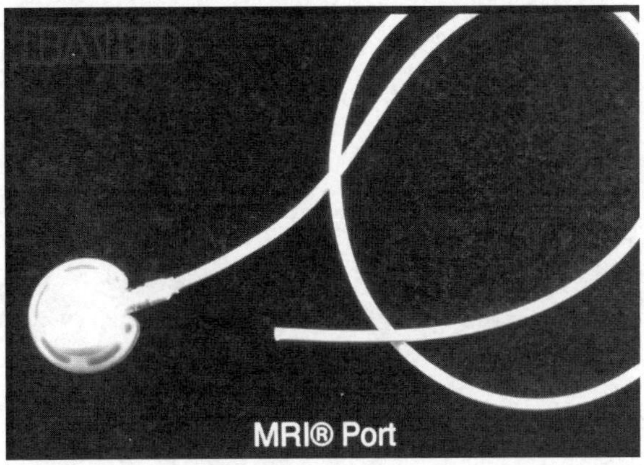

MRI® Port

Courtesy of Bard Access Systems

Figure 6-2. Groshong® OTG

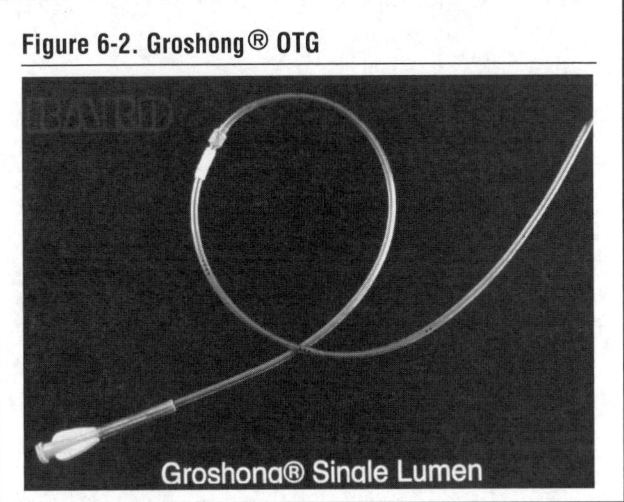

Courtesy of Bard Access Systems

Figure 6-3. Catheter with a Titanium Port

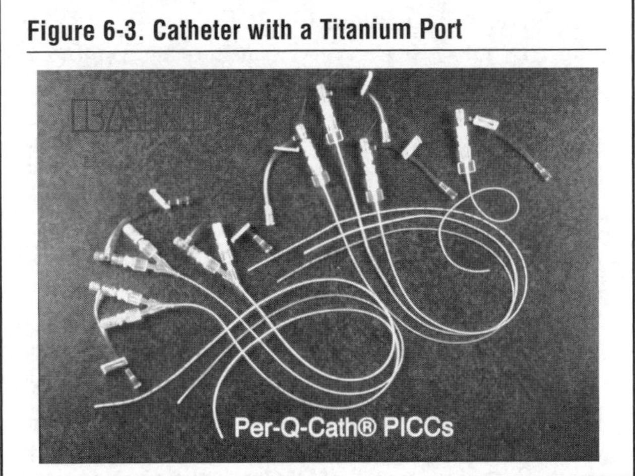

Courtesy of Bard Access Systems

Nursing Assessment and Interventions

Assessment:

- Determine which CVD is best for the patient by considering the family's ability to manage a catheter, the patient's body image, and the treatment protocol.
- Assess what the patient and the family know about the device and the care they will be expected to deliver.
- Assess the exit site for signs of infection (e.g., erythema, tenderness, swelling, drainage, foul odor).
- Evaluate the CVD for patency (i.e., it flushes without resistance or discomfort, has positive blood return).
- Observe the patient for facial swelling, distention of the neck vein, tachycardia, and shortness of breath—all of which could indicate SVC thrombosis.
- Ensure that the device is properly secured. To prevent dislodgment, a Hickman or a Broviac catheter should be coiled under the dressing, and the IV tubing connected to the CVD should be taped and pinned to the patient's clothing.
- Evaluate the integrity of the venous access device (i.e., monitor for kinking or twisting, or leaking fluid or blood).
- Ensure that the port needle is in the correct place to prevent infiltration or extravasation when vesicant chemotherapy is being infused.
- Assess the CVD dressing. Is it intact? When was it last changed?
- Evaluate the injection caps at the end of the line. Are they intact? Is there any leaking? Have blood clots formed? When were the caps last changed?

Interventions: Care of the CVL is one of the most controversial management issues in pediatric oncology. There are no national standards, but there are a multitude of institutional practices. Manufacturers of CVL products also provide guidelines for care. The following interventions are examples of guidelines for CVL care:

- Flush the lines with heparin (Liquaemin) regularly, according to institutional guidelines.
  - *Broviac and Hickman catheters:* Catheter flushes range from 10–100 units/ml of heparin, using 3–5 ml per flush, one to three times a day. It is important to exert positive pressure with the flush as the line is clamped to help decrease the potential for clot formation by minimizing backflow of blood into the catheter.
  - *Groshong catheter:* This type of catheter does not require daily heparin and can be flushed routinely with saline. However, the manufacturer recommends heparin flushes at least twice a month.
  - *Permcath:* Institutions use 100 or 1,000 units of heparin as a flush. When using 1,000 units, the clinician should withdraw the heparin from the line before flushing or administering medications so that the patient does not develop a systemic effect from the heparin. The line should be flushed by using a positive pressure technique.
  - *Ports:* To flush the device, use 10–100 units of heparin. If a port is to be deaccessed, 5 ml of 100 units/ml of heparin often is used. Ports can be deaccessed for a month.
- Change dressings according to institutional policy, or as determined by a patient assessment. Providine iodine (Betadine) can cause skin irritation at the catheter site.

One method of changing a dressing is to clean the site with alcohol and a solution of 2% aqueous chlorhexidine (Hibiclens) and then let it dry. A dressing can be placed around the line before it is coiled and covered with an occlusive dressing (e.g., Tegaderm, Bioclusive, Opsite). Dressings should be changed weekly if this method is used.

Another method is to cleanse the site with chlorhexidine (Hibiclens) and water and cover it with sterile gauze and tape. If this method is used, the dressing should be changed three times a week.

There are multiple methods for central line care:

- Change the injection caps at the end of the lumens while using a sterile technique, according to the institution's policy (caps usually are replaced weekly). Injection caps that are leaking or that contain clotted blood have the potential to become infected and should be changed promptly.
- Access the ports, as necessary, using aseptic technique.
  - Locate the port and cleanse the skin with providine iodine (Betadine) and alcohol or chlorhexidine; follow institutional guidelines.
  - Palpate and stabilize the port while inserting a noncoring needle (e.g., Gripper, Huber, or Whin) into its center.
  - Confirm the correct placement of the needle by aspirating blood from the port, then flushing the line without resistance.
  - Place an occlusive dressing over the accessed port, according to institutional policy.
  - Flush the port with heparin or connect it to IV fluid.
- Using a kit provided by the manufacturer, repair external breaks in a central venous line using sterile technique and according to institutional policy. Until the repair is made, clamp the line that is distal to the break and cover the end with sterile gauze to prevent an air embolism, excessive blood loss, or further contamination.
- Assess for internal breaks and occlusions. Signs of an internal displacement or a break can include a patient's complaint of chest or head discomfort, swelling around the exit site, or an inability to flush the CVD or to aspirate blood. It is important to make a prompt evaluation using a cathetergram (dye study). Signs of extravasation are erythema near the exit site or a patient's complaints about a burning sensation or pain in the chest or abdomen while a vesicant or irritant chemotherapy is being infused through the CVD. In this case, the infusion of chemotherapy should be stopped immediately and as much of the vesicant as possible should be aspirated from the CVD. If

an antidote for the extravasated chemotherapy is recommended, it should be administered into the surrounding tissue (see Section IV, "Childhood Cancer Treatment."). A plastic surgeon may need to be contacted to debride the wound.

- CVD occlusions: For blood clot and fibrin sheath occlusions, 1 mg (1 ml) Alteplase (tPA), could be put into the line and allowed to dwell for 1 hour. If the patency of the catheter is not resolved, a cathetergram should be done to document the clot. Based on the cathetergram results, a second dose of tPA may be instilled. If a thrombus is present, a continuous infusion of tPA over time may be necessary to dissolve the clot. When tPA is being continuously infused, the patient should be monitored for signs and symptoms of bleeding and pulmonary embolism. Clotting factors should be monitored and evaluated to prevent injury.
- An occlusion occasionally results from precipitate (i.e., from medications or parenteral nutrition) in a CVD. For a mineral precipitate, 0.2–1 ml of 0.1% hydrochloric acid (equal to the internal volume of the device) should be instilled and allowed to stand for 20 minutes to 1 hour. Many drugs are incompatable with heparin. For a medication precipitate, 1 mEq/ml of sodium bicarbonate should be instilled. For a lipid precipitate, 70%–95% ethyl alcohol or sodium hydroxide should be instilled. Many institutions use protocols with algorithms to manage clotted lines or lines that flush but do not have a blood return (**Figure 6-4**).

- Teach the patient and family about the care of a central venous line, the risks (i.e., infection, occlusion, displacement), and troubleshooting. Such instruction must be started early in the patient's hospitalization because it is a time-consuming task that requires reinforcement. The patient, the family, or both, must demonstrate the ability to provide competent catheter care. Ongoing education and evaluation are important whenever the patient returns to the hospital or clinic.
- Inform the patient that the external device must be covered with an occlusive dressing while he or she is showering and that the dressing must be changed after showering. Many institutions do not recommend that patients with external devices go swimming because of the risk of infection.
- Communicate with the appropriate home health agency (if necessary) about providing the patient with home supplies for line care and possible follow-up at his or her home.

Figure 6-4. Algorithm for "No Blood Return"

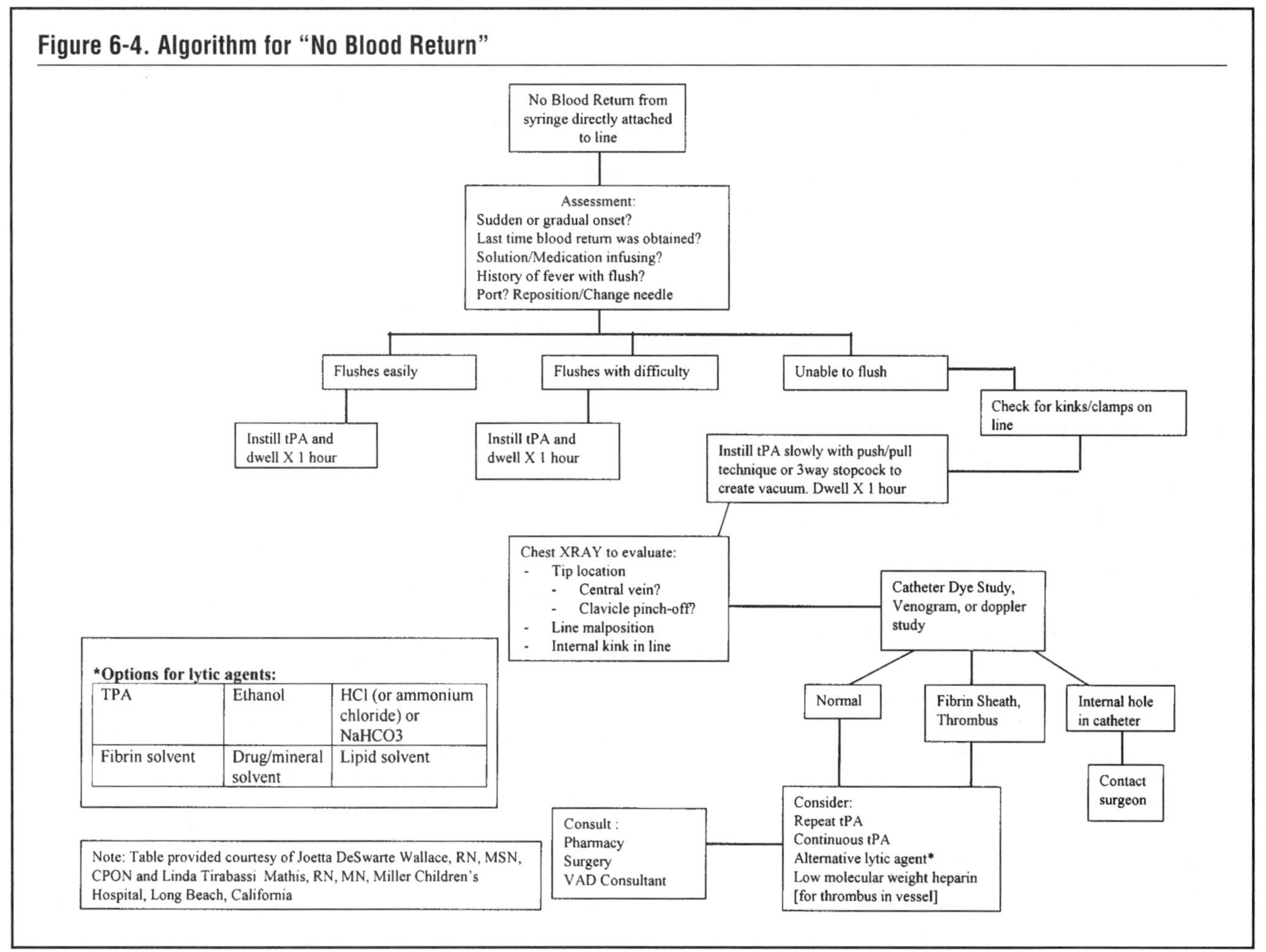

TPA	Ethanol	HCl (or ammonium chloride) or NaHCO3
Fibrin solvent	Drug/mineral solvent	Lipid solvent

Note: Table provided courtesy of Joetta DeSwarte Wallace, RN, MSN, CPON and Linda Tirabassi Mathis, RN, MN, Miller Children's Hospital, Long Beach, California

Expected Patient and Family Outcomes

- The patient and the family can competently perform line care (i.e., flushing, cap changes, dressing changes).
- The patient and the family know about the increased risk of infection with a CVL, a port, a Groshong catheter, or PICC line, and they understand why competent care of the line is essential.
- The family should demonstrate or explain the steps to take if the line breaks or becomes dislodged.
- The risks of having a CVD will be minimized as a result of proper care and prevention strategies.

Nutritional Support for Children with Cancer

Kenneth Lown

Principles of Treatment

The goals for nutritional intervention in children with cancer are to prevent or reverse nutritional deficits, promote normal growth and development, minimize morbidity, and optimize quality of life.

Role in Childhood Cancer

Nutritional assessment and support are essential for children with cancer to prevent malnutrition. Specific childhood cancers associated with the poorest prognoses (e.g., brain tumors, neuroblastoma, acute myelogenous leukemia [AML]), tend to have the most intense oncologic treatment regimens and the greatest association with malnutrition. Clinicians can anticipate that treatment (i.e., surgery, radiation, chemotherapy, and bone marrow transplantation) will cause sensory changes and prevent intake adequate to maintain or restore a child's nutritional status.

Recommended Calorie and Protein Intake

During illness, a child's protein needs increase, and children receiving chemotherapy may require more calories for tissue healing and energy. The recommended dietary allowances (RDA) (**Table 6-6**) are used to determine estimated calorie and protein needs. Because the RDAs were developed as recommendations for healthy populations, adjustments usually are necessary to maintain appropriate growth in sick children. The allowances may need to be increased 15%–50% to compensate for patients' previous weight losses, malnutrition, or metabolic changes. The estimation of resting energy expediture (REE) (**Table 6-7**) developed by the World Health Organization (WHO), along with appropriate activity and stress factors, may be more useful for accurately determining energy requirements for acutely ill patients.

Nutrition Assessment

Nutritional status should be assessed at the time of diagnosis and throughout therapy (**Table 6-8**).

Assessment of weight and height: A growth chart should be completed for inpatients and outpatients at the time of diagnosis and throughout therapy. When a child's weight or height percentile for his or her age has fallen two major percentile lines, he

Table 6-6. Recommended Dietary Allowances for Calories and Protein

Category	Age (in years)	g protein/ kg/day	kcal/ kg/day
Infants	0-0.5	2.2	108
	0.5-1.0	1.6	98
Children	1-3	1.2	102
	4-6	1.2	90
	7-10	1.0	70
Teen-aged	11-14	1.0	55
males	15-18	0.9	45
Teen-aged	11-14	1.0	47
females	15-18	0.8	49

Table 6-7. Estimating Daily Calorie Needs in Children 1 Year or Older

For children 1 year of age or younger, compute the estimated resting energy expenditure (REE) based on the World Health Organization (WHO) equations below. W = body weight in kilograms.

Age Range (Years)	Male	Female
1-3	60.9 W – 54	61 W – 51
3-10	22.7 W + 495	22.5 W + 499
10-18	17.5 W + 651	12.2 W + 746
18-30	15.3 W + 679	14.7 W + 496

REE = ______________________

Next, multiply REE by an activity/stress factor.

(REE) × (1.3) for a well-nourished child at bedrest with mild to moderate stress (mild surgery)

(REE) × (1.5) for a very active child with mild to moderate stress, an inactive child with severe stress (trauma, sepsis, cancer, extensive surgery), or a child with minimal activity requiring catch-up growth

(REE) × (1.7) for an active child requiring catch-up growth or an active child with severe stress

Note. From Energy and protein requirements (FAO/WHO/ UNV Expert Consultation Technical Report Series 724) (p. 71), by the World Health Organization (WHO), 1985, Geneva, Switzerland: Author. Copyright 1985 by WHO. Adapted with permission.

or she should be referred immediately for further nutritional evaluation. A weight loss of more than 5% from the onset of illness, or a weight loss of more than 5% over the previous month's weight, should be evaluated immediately. The percentage of weight lost should be derived from the patient's highest previous weight. Note that a weight is inaccurate when a child has edema, large tumor masses, and organs extensively infiltrated with tumor, effusions, or organ congestion, or has had an excess of fluids (i.e., twice the maintenance level) for chemotherapy. These guidelines apply to initially obese as well as lean patients.

Immediate referrals also need to be made for the following conditions:

- Weight is below the 5th percentile for the patient's age.
- Weight is below the 5th percentile for the patient's height.
- Weight is less than 90% of the ideal level for the patient's height.
- Height is below the 5th percentile for the patient's age.
- Nutrient intake is less than 80% of estimated needs.
- There is a physical change that crosses two major percentile lines on the growth chart.

The degree of malnutrition can be determined by using an ideal standard of body weight for height. The percentage of ideal body weight for height can be calculated with the following formula:

$$\frac{\text{actual weight}}{\text{weight at 50th percentile for current stature}} \times 100$$

Ideal body weight parameters are available in table format. Other, more sophisticated, means of evaluating nutritional status, including an assessment of muscle and subcutaneous fat stores, can be done by a registered dietitian.

Laboratory assessment: Laboratory values that can be monitored before and during repletion include biochemical studies that screen for organ function, including complete blood count, sodium, potassium, chloride, bicarbonate, glucose, creatinine, blood urea nitrogen (BUN), calcium, phosphorus, magnesium, total protein, albumin, triglycerides, cholesterol, alkaline phosphatase, alanine aminotransferase (ALT), g-glulamyltransferase (GGT), and total bilirubin. Serum albumin levels can be affected by hydration status and liver function. Serum albumin of less than 3.2 mg/dl may indicate depleted protein stores. Serum prealbumin below the normal level (normal value varies by a person's age) also may indicate depleted protein stores. The level can be increased because of impaired renal function and decreased as a result of altered hepatic function, but generally it is not affected by hydration status.

Types of Nutritional Interventions

Oral feeding: Early intervention should include a nutritionist at the time of diagnosis to provide nutritional assessment and counseling. This intervention includes providing guidelines for managing the complications of cancer treatment (e.g., anorexia, alterations in taste, mouth dryness, dysphagia, early satiety, nausea, vomiting, stomatitis, mucositis, diarrhea, or constipation) and for increasing protein intake or calories. Patients also may be given oral supplements, such as nutrition shakes and food bars (See **Table 6-9**). Another measure is to provide specific macronutrients as modular components (e.g., polycose powder, corn oil) to increase calorie intake. These macronutrients (protein, carbohydrate, and fat) can be added to a child's diet without increasing the volume of food needing to be consumed.

Table 6-8. Nutritional Monitoring Schedule for Children with Cancer

Parameter	Hospitalized patients on parenteral nutrition	Hospitalized patients on oral/tube feedings	Outpatients on parenteral nutrition	Outpatients on oral/tube feedings
Weight	Daily	Daily	Weekly	Monthly
Height	Monthly	Monthly	Monthly	Monthly
Head circumference	Weekly	Weekly	Monthly	Monthly
Arm anthropometrics	Monthly	As indicated	Monthly	As indicated
Intake/output	Daily	Daily	Daily to weekly	Weekly to monthly
Electrolytes/glucose	Daily	Weekly	Weekly	Monthly
Blood urea nitrogen, creatinine	Weekly	Weekly	Weekly	Monthly
Calcium, phosphorus, magnesium	Daily to weekly	Weekly	Weekly	Monthly
Triglyceride	Weekly	Monthly	Weekly	As indicated
Liver function tests	Weekly	Weekly	Monthly	Monthly
Trace elements	Monthly	As indicated	Biannually	As indicated
Carnitine	Monthly	As indicated	Biannually	As indicated
Vitamin levels	Monthly	As indicated	Biannually	As indicated

Adapted from Davis AM. Initiation, monitoring and complications of pediatric parenteral nutrition. In: Baker RD, Baker SS, Davis AM, eds. Pediatric parenteral nutrition. New York: Chapman & Hall, 1997:212.

Table 6-9. Enteral Products and Their Characteristics

	Children 1-10 Years of Age	Patients Above 10 Years of Age	
Type of Product	**Tube Feeding and Oral Feeding**	**Tube Feeding**	**Oral Feeding**
Standard or polymeric • Contain intact macronutrients intended as meal replacements • Require normal digestive and absorptive capacity • Are usually lactose-free unless otherwise indicated	Pediasure Nutren Junior Resource Just for Kids	Isocal Osmolite Nutren (unflavored) Compleat Modified Diet	Ensure NuBasic Nutrashake* Carnation Instant Breakfast* Scandishake* Sustacal pudding*
High-nitrogen • Contain intact macronutrients with >15% total calories as protein • Are useful in patients with increased protein needs (i.e., those whose wounds heal poorly or who have had radiation)		Isocal HN Osmolite HN Perative Replete	Ensure HN
Concentrated or high-calorie • Contain higher calories per cc than standard and generally are not well tolerated due to their high osmolality • May be used with fluid restriction		Nutren 1.5 (unflavored) Nutren 2.0 Two Cal HN Comply Magnacal	NuBasic Plus Ensure Plus Resource Plus
Predigested/elemental • Consist of predigested or partially hydrolyzed peptide-based diet that may be beneficial for child with impaired GI function (e.g., diarrhea, mucositis, atrophy of intestinal villi) • May contain medium-chain triglycerides to minimize fat intolerance • Can have high osmolality	Peptamen Junior (vanilla or unflavored) Neocate One Plus (flavored or unflavored) Vivonex Pediatric	Peptamen Peptamen VHP Reabilan Tolerex Vivonex TEN Vivonex Plus	Vital HN
Fiber-containing • Contain fiber from natural sources or added soy polysaccharides to aid in bowel function • Are disease-specific • Contain macro- and micronutrients modified for disease state	Kindercal Pediasure with fiber Nutren Jr. with fiber Liver: NutriHep Renal: Nepro, Suplena, Renalcal, Amin-Aid	Jevity Ultracal Nutren 1.0 with fiber Pulmonary: Pulmocare, Nutrivent	Nu Basics with fiber Ensure with fiber Altered fat absorption: Portagen, Lipisorb
Infant formulas	**Cow's Milk**	**Soy**	**Predigested**
Infant formulas (A variety of formulas are available for premature infants and for infants with poor feeding tolerance. Many infants are lactose-intolerant after chemotherapy and benefit from lactose-free formulas. Human breast milk should be used when possible; however, it contains lactose and may not be tolerated well after chemotherapy.)	Similac Enfamil Lactofree (lactose-free) Carnation Good Start Similac PM 60/40	Isomil Prosobee	Pregestimil Alimentum Nutramigen
Modular components	**Protein** Casec Pro-Mix ProMod NutriSource Protein Elementra	**Carbohydrate** Polycose Moducal Liquid Carbohydrate (LC) Sumacal NutriSource Carbohydrate	**Fat** Vegetable oil (long-chain triglycerides) Microlipid (long-chain triglycerides) Medium-chain triglycerides NutriSource (long- or medium-chain triglycerides)
Oral electrolyte solutions • Provide electrolytes, minimal calories, and water during periods of mild-to-moderate dehydration		Pedialyte Ricelyte Rehydralyte	

*Contain lactose

Enteral tube feeding: If oral feeding is not possible or is inadequate, tube feeding should be considered. It is important for a registered dietitian, physician, nurse, and social worker to provide support and suggest ways to improve the patient's acceptance of the feeding tube. Patients and families need to know that children receiving supplemental nutrition also can continue to eat. Tube feedings can be initiated when the patient has minimal mucositis, and an adequate platelet count to allow for insertion of a tube without the risk of excessive bleeding. The patient also needs to have a functional gastrointestinal (GI) tract, and any side effects of feedings (e.g., nausea, vomiting, and diarrhea) must be manageable. Tube feedings also are indicated when a patient meets the criteria for nutritional intervention, and oral intake is inadequate to meet his or her estimated needs for normal growth or repletion of nutritional losses.

Total parenteral nutrition (TPN)/hyperalimentation: Parenteral nutrition is indicated for patients when oral or tube feedings, or both, are unable to provide an adequate amount of nutrients, or when enteral feedings are contraindicated for a significant period of time. A nutritional assessment of the patient should be made before starting TPN. A central venous catheter is essential if total nutritional requirements are to be met for several weeks or months.

Enteral Feeding

The optimal access route for enteral nutrition is determined on the basis of the anticipated duration of the tube feeding, the risk of pulmonary aspiration, and indications for specific access routes.

Tube selection: The smallest possible tube should be used because it provides greater comfort (size 6 or 8 French nasogastric tubes will work in most patients). A larger tube is needed for delivering fiber-containing formulas or highly viscous formulas. Silicone and polyurethane nasoenteric tubes lessen physical irritation and have fewer associated risks of pulmonary aspiration. Weighted tubes are designed to assist with postpyloric tube placement and to maintain tube position. Placement is assessed by checking the pH level of aspirated contents or by X ray.

Types of tubes for enteral feedings: Nasoenteric tubes are designed for short-term use. They include silicone tubes and polyurethane tubes; tube lumen size range is 6 or 10 French. Tube choice should be based upon the age and size of the child and the viscosity of the formula. Orogastric tubes are used for infants whose gestational age is less than 34 weeks because they are obligatory nose breathers. Nasogastric tubes are easily intubated, but nasoduodenal or nasojejunal tubes can be easily dislodged and require radiographic proof of placement.

Enterostomy tubes are designed for long-term use. Gastrostomy tubes are made of silicone, polyurethane, rubber, or latex. Surgically or percutaneously placed gastrostomy tubes can be replaced with a button that is flush with the abdomen when a tract is formed. Jejunostomy tubes are made of rubber, latex, silicone, polyvinyl, silicone rubber, or polyethylene and are surgically placed. Complications with enterostomy tubes can include cellulitis and other infections (particularly when a patient is neutropenic), despite good hygiene practices.

Methods of administration: An enteral feeding pump provides a reliable, constant infusion rate, decreases the risk of gastric retention, and may prevent nausea, vomiting, abdominal cramping, bloating, and diarrhea. The flow rate with gravity-flow feeding can be adjusted with a clamp that applies pressure on the tubing.

Feeding schedules: There are two types of feeding schedules: bolus (intermittent or gravity), which closely mimics normal feeding; and continuous, which requires a feeding pump. A combination of continuous nocturnal feeding while the patient is sleeping and daytime bolus feedings works well. The feeding schedule will determine whether a portable or a standard pump is required and which pump is reimbursable by insurance.

Feeding formula: The formula is based upon the composition of required nutrients, the patient's GI function and age, and the cost and available resources (e.g., insurance coverage). Unflavored products are used for tube feeding. There are many products available for oral use and for tube feedings (**Table 6-9**). Oral products generally are not well accepted by children with cancer because of alterations in taste and smell, and because of mucositis. In addition, children with cancer generally are unable to gain weight with oral supplements and intake and therefore usually require supplemental tube feedings.

Initiation and progression of tube feeding: If a patient has had nothing by mouth for less than 3 days, full-strength formula at 1–2 cc/kg/hr may be started. Feedings may be increased by 1–2 cc/kg/hr per day, as tolerated, until the goal is achieved. If the patient has had nothing by mouth for more than 3 days, or if GI problems exist (e.g., mucositis, diarrhea, gut atrophy), half-strength formula at 1–2 cc/kg/hr can be started. The concentration should be advanced to full strength after 12–24 hours; the rate then should be increased by 1–2 cc/kg/hr per day to goal.

One option is to provide half of the patient's estimated needs continuously at night and the remaining half in 2–3 boluses during the day. The daily volume also can be divided into feedings every 2–4 hours, if desired. Most patients will tolerate continuous feedings better than bolus feedings, particularly if they are nauseated.

If the patient's fluid needs are not being met with oral intake and tube feeding, extra free water should be provided as flushes, or should be mixed with the feedings. The tube should be flushed frequently with water before and after all medications are administered. It should be flushed daily to maintain patency, even if no feedings are given.

Supplemental potassium, phosphorus, calcium, or magnesium should be given in divided doses throughout the day and mixed with feedings for better tolerance. Calcium and phosphorus should not be given at the same time, so that maximal absorption of both can be achieved. Medications can be very hyperosmolar and can cause GI irritation; therefore, the IV form of some medications (e.g., magnesium) can be given in tube feedings with less irritation.

Complications of Tube Feedings

Providing nutrition too rapidly to patients, particularly to those who are chronically deprived of adequate nutrition, can result in abnormalities. One such abnormality, called *refeeding syndrome*, is characterized by metabolic complications, severe fluid shifts, hypokalemia, and hypophosphatemia, and occurs in patients who are repleted both enterally and parenterally. Another abnormality is *tube-feeding syndrome*, which involves hypertonic dehydration, hypernatremia, and prerenal azotemia in patients receiving highly osmotic enteral feedings. Laboratory values, including sodium, potassium, chloride, bicarbonate, BUN, creatinine, calcium, magnesium, and phosphorus, should be monitored frequently.

A high gastric residual can be caused by delayed gastric emptying. Giving prokinetic medications (e.g., metoclopramide [Reglan]) and elevating the head of the patient's bed at least 30 degrees during and after feeding may help. Nasopharyngeal and nasolabial irritation can be lessened if small-bore tubes made of silicone or polyurethane are used and are taped securely to avoid pressure on the nares.

For patients with enterostomy tubes, skin irritation and excoriation at the ostomy site can be reduced through appropriate enterostomal therapy that uses topical or oral antibiotics during periods when the patient has severe or prolonged neutropenia.

To prevent obstruction of the feeding tube lumen, the tube should be adequately flushed before and after medications and boluses. During continuous tube feeding, the tube should be flushed every 4 hours. Liquid elixirs should be used when possible and diluted with water in a 1:1 ratio. If the tube is clogged, one crushed Viokase enzyme tablet should be mixed with one crushed tablet (324 mg) of sodium bicarbonate and 5 ml of tap water to prepare a pH 7.9 Viokase solution; 5 ml of this enzyme solution should be injected through a cartridge catheter inserted into the feeding tube and left to sit for 5 minutes. The feeding tube should be reirrigated with 20 to 30 ml water. To maintain the tube's patency, the tube can be flushed with 1 tablespoon of seltzer mixed with 1/8 teaspoon of baking soda once a day. Enteral tubes can stay in place 4–6 weeks before needing to be replaced. Older adolescents may choose to place the tube daily for nocturnal feedings.

Patient monitoring during tube feeding includes checking body weight, fluid intake and output, and GI function on a daily basis, or as needed. Biochemical indices, such as fluid balance, calcium, phosphorus, and magnesium, should be assessed. If refeeding syndrome or depleted stores are suspected, laboratory studies should be monitored on a daily basis and calories should be increased slowly.

Initiating Total Parenteral Nutrition

Parenteral nutrition should be provided when oral feeding, tube feeding, or both provide inadequate nutrients or when enteral feedings over a significant period of time are contraindicated.

Determine the patient's fluid needs: Fluid needs are determined according to body weight as follows:

- 1–10 kg: 100 cc/kg/day
- 11 to 20 kg: 1,000 cc + 50 cc for each kg > 10 kg/day
- 20 to 30 kg: 1,500 cc + 20 cc for each kg > 20 kg/day
- > 30 kg: 35 cc/kg/day.

Compute the patient's calorie needs: The patient's parenteral calorie needs are computed as follows.

- Preterm infant, 90–100 kcals/kg/day; full-term infant, 90–100 kcals/kg/day; and infant younger than 1 year old, 80–100 kcals/kg/day.
- For older children, use RDAs (**Table 6-6**) or WHO's equations (**Table 6-7**) for calculating estimated needs.

Determine the patient's protein needs: Protein provides 4.0 kcal of energy per gram. The patient's protein needs can be determined as follows:

- Preterm infant, 2.5– 3.5 g/kg/day; full-term infant, 2.5– 3.0 g/kg/day; infant less than 1 year old, 1.5–2.5 g/kg/day.
- Child 1–10 years old, 1.0–2.0 g/kg/day.
- Child 11–18 years old, 0.8–2.0 g/kg/day.

Administer amino acids: Amino acids are given routinely in parenteral fluids as follows:

- TrophAmine, for children 6 months old or younger.
- Novamine, for children 6 months of age or older.

Determine the appropriate lipid dose (g/kg/day): Lipids are provided in a solution available in 10% (1.1 kcal/ml) or 20% (2 kcal/ml) concentrations. To prevent essential fatty acid deficiency, 0.5–1.0 g/kg/day of fat or lipids must be provided. Parenteral fat intake should not exceed 4g/kg/day, or 60% of total calories.

Determine carbohydrate and glucose needs: Dextrose nutrient provides 3.4 kcal/g. Normal glucose infusion rates are as follows:

- Infants up to 1 year of age, 5–12 mg/kg/min.
- Children 1–18 years old, 5–8 mg/kg/min.
- Adults, 2–5 mg/kg/min.

Determine electrolyte needs: A patient's electrolyte needs can be altered due to chemotherapy, medications, or both (e.g., cisplatin [Platinol] causes an increased loss of potassium, calcium, magnesium, and phosphorus; amphotericin [Fungizone] can cause increased losses of potassium and renal tubular acidosis, requiring acetate replacement in TPN).

Guidelines for advancing peripheral-line TPN: On day 1, administer 10% dextrose; protein, as required; lipids at 1–2 g/kg/day. On day 2, lipids should be increased by 1 g/kg/day until the goal level is achieved.

Guidelines for advancing central-line TPN: On day 1, administer 10% dextrose; protein, as required; lipids at 1–2 g/kg/day. On day 2, dextrose solution and lipids should be increased to goal.

Monitoring TPN: A laboratory baseline screening panel (see the earlier section titled "Nutrition Assessment") should be done, then checked weekly. If the patient is at risk for refeeding syndrome, calories should be increased more slowly (i.e., 10%–15% per day), regardless of the type of IV access. The patient's weight should be checked every day.

Intake and output: Intake and output should be monitored daily.

Cycling: Many patients benefit from having TPN cycled over 10–12 hours to allow more time off for normal activity. A portable pump can be used to increase the patient's mobility during TPN administration. The infusion rate of TPN solutions with more than 10% dextrose should be decreased by 50% during the last hour of the infusion to prevent rebound hypoglycemia.

Complications of Total Parenteral Nutrition

Complications of TPN can include hypoglycemia; therefore, sudden discontinuation of TPN should be avoided (i.e., the rate should be decreased gradually). If hyperglycemia is a problem, the dextrose concentration can be decreased or insulin can be administered with TPN or provided subcutaneously. To prevent occurrence of a fatty liver, excessive infusion of carbohydrates should be avoided, and an appropriate balance of dextrose, protein, and lipids should be provided. To avoid cholestatic jaundice, TPN should be cycled as soon as possible, and enteral feeding should be provided.

Expected Patient and Family Outcomes

- The patient will have appropriate nutritional supplementation throughout treatment.
- The patient and the family are knowledgeable about the nutritional options available during treatment.
- The patient will have minimal complications associated with nutritional supplementation.

Treatment of Infections

Asako Komiya

Principles of Treatment

Complications of infectious diseases commonly occur in an immunocompromised host. Now that intensive treatment regimens for childhood cancer include high-dose chemotherapy, radiation therapy, and bone marrow transplantation, the percentage of pediatric cancer patients becoming immunocompromised has increased. Antibiotics are essential components of supportive care.

Risk Factors Associated with Infection

Certain malignancies are associated with immune deficits. Children with leukemia are more prone to develop severe gram-negative infections as a result of granulocytopenia associated with the disease. Children with Hodgkin's disease or lymphomas are at greater risk for viral and fungal infections because of abnormalities in their cellular immune systems. Granulocytopenia, induced by high-dose chemotherapy or radiation therapy, causes patients to be at increased risk for bacterial infection. Corticosteroid therapy affects immune system functioning and decreases a host's defenses. Patients with disrupted skin or mucous membrane integrity are more likely to develop infections. Patients with poor nutritional status are at increased risk for infections.

Clinical Presentation

Fever and neutropenia: Symptoms are fever ≥ 101° F and absolute neutrophil count (ANC) <500. Fever may be the first sign of infection; other signs of inflammation can either be subtle or absent.

Bacteremia: Fever, chills, and other symptoms depend on the site of origin (e.g., the respiratory, perianal, perioral, GI tract, or the genitourinary system).

Pneumonia: Fever, productive or nonproductive cough, malaise, anorexia, chest pain, and rales may or may not be detectable on auscultation.

Otitis media: Symptoms are fever, earache, otalgia, hearing loss, irritability.

Esophagitis: Symptoms are retrosternal burning chest pain, odynophagia, anorexia, dehydration, and fever.

Oral mucositis: Symptoms are fever, ulceration, vesicles, lesion, pain, burning, anorexia, dehydration.

Cutaneous infections: Symptoms are fever, pain, burning, tingling, pruritus, erythema, vesicles, pustules, inflammation, warmth, drainage, bleeding.

Sinusitis: Symptoms are fever; nasal drainage; tenderness in frontal, maxillary, and ethmoid area; cough; sore throat.

Typhlitis: Symptoms are subacute or acute onset of right lower quadrant pain, fever, diarrhea, and prostration.

Pseudomembranous (antibiotic-associated) colitis: Symptoms are fever, abdominal pain, diarrhea (may contain blood or mucus), nausea, vomiting.

Urinary tract infection (UTI): Symptoms are fever, abdominal pain or distention, urgency or frequency urination, dysuria, hematuria, malodorous urine.

Perirectal cellulitis: Symptoms are perirectal tenderness or pain, erythema, induration, and fever.

Ventricular peritoneal (VP) shunt infection:. Some patients have no symptoms, whereas others may have a wide range of symptoms, including fever, headache, vomiting, neurological changes, and meningeal signs (i.e., central nervous system irritability, neck rigidity).

Diagnostic Workup

The diagnostic workup depends upon a patient's presenting signs and symptoms, but commonly includes one or more of the following:

- A blood culture and sensitivity (for bacteremia).
- Chest X ray (for pneumonia).
- Urine analysis and culture (for UTI).
- Stool culture, computed tomography of the abdomen (for typhlitis).
- Cerebrospinal fluid culture (for a VP shunt infection).

Medical Treatment

Fever and neutropenia: Treatment for these includes broad-spectrum antibiotic therapy until the causative pathogens are identified or cultures return a negative result (**Table 6-10**).

Table 6-10. Antibiotic Therapy

Aminoglycosides

Aminoglycosides are bactericidal antibiotics active against many aerobic gram-negative and some aerobic gram-positive bacteria. Anaerobic bacteria are resistant because transport of aminoglycosides into cells is oxygen-dependent. Aminoglycosides are also inactive against fungi and viruses. In combination with penicillins or vancomycin (Vancocin), aminoglycosides often act synergistically to kill gram-positive bacteria. Aminoglycosides have a postantibiotic effect against gram-negative bacteria that allows for less frequent dosing.

	Indications	Potential Side Effects	Dosage and Administration
Gentamicin sulfate (Garamycin) **(Warnings: Ototoxicity may be directly proportional to the amount of drug given and the duration of treatment. Dosing adjustment is required for patients with renal impairment.)**	*P. aeruginosa, Enterobacter* spp, *Enterococcus*	Hearing loss, tinnitus, loss of balance, high-frequency deafness, peripheral neuritis, numbness, tingling of skin, granulocytopenia, anemia, thrombocytopenic purpura, proteinuria, changes in BUN, oliguria	**Infants and children** *IM, IV:* 2-2.5 mg/ kg/dose every 8 hours up to a maximum of 300 mg/day **Adults** *IM, IV:* 1-1.7 mg/ kg/dose every 8-12 hours
Tobramycin sulfate (Tobrex) **(Warnings: Ototoxicity may be directly proportional to the amount of drug given and the duration of treatment. Dosing adjustment is required for patients with renal impairment.)**	Similar to gentamicin (Garamycin) except not as active against *Enterococcus*	Changes in SGOT (AST), SGPT (ALT), and LDH, pancytopenia, nausea, vomiting, headache, fever, lethargy	**Infants and children** *IM, IV:* 2.5 mg/kg/ dose every 8 hours up to a maximum of 300 mg/day **Adults** *IM, IV:* 1-1.8 mg/kg/dose every 8-12 hours
Amikacin sulfate (Amikin) **(Warning: Dosing adjustment is required for patients with renal impairment.)**	*Serratia, Proteus, Pseudomonas, Enterobacter* spp, *Providencia*	Drowsiness, headache, unsteady gait, paresthesias, tremors, hypotension, tachycardia, oliguria, hematuria, thirst, tinnitus, high-frequency hearing loss, bleeding reactions	**Children and Adults** 10 mg/kg/dose every 8 hours; dosage should be based on an estimate of ideal body weight; maximum dose is 15 g/day

Extended-spectrum penicillins

Extended-spectrum penicillins are bactericidal. They are more active against enteric gram-negative bacilli than natural penicillins, penicillinase-resistant penicillins, and aminopenicillins because they are more resistant to inactivation by β-lactamase-producing gram-negative bacteria. These drugs may also penetrate the outer membrane of gram-negative organisms more readily than their penicillin precursors. Extended-spectrum penicillins are active in vitro against most gram-positive and gram-negative aerobic cocci (except penicillinase-producing strains), some gram-positive aerobic and anaerobic bacilli, and many gram-negative aerobic and anaerobic bacilli. They are inactive against mycobacteria, *Mycoplasma, Rickettsia,* fungi, and viruses.

	Indications	Potential Side Effects	Dosage and Administration
Penicillin G (Bicillin) **(Warning: Dosing adjustment is required for patients with renal impairment.)**	*S. pneumoniae, S. pyogenes, S. viridens, S. bovis, Neis-seria,* most anaerobes	Dizziness, neuromuscular hyperirritability, seizures, decreased sense of taste and smell, stomatitis, flatulence, diarrhea, pancytopenia, hypokalemia, and changes in liver and kidney function	**Infants and children** 100,000-300,000 units/kg/day divided every 4 hours up to a maximum of 24 million units/day **Adults** 2-24 million units/ day in divided doses given every 4 hours
Nafcillin sodium (Nafcil) **(Warnings: This drug is a vesicant. Dosing adjustment is required for patients with severe hepatic impairment.)**			**Children** 150-200 mg/kg/day divided every 6 hours up to a maximum of 12 g/day **Adults** 500 mg-2 g every 4-6 hours

Table 6-10. Antibiotic Therapy *(continued)*

	Indications	Potential Side Effects	Dosage and Administration
Ampicillin (Omnipen) **(Warning: Dosing adjustment is required for patients with renal impairment.)**	*S. fecalis, Listeria monocytogenes, Haemophilus, E. coli, Salmonella, Proteus*	Nausea and vomiting, hypokalemia	Serious infections (meningitis [higher end of dosing range preferred], sepsis): **Children** *IM, IV:* 150-300 mg/kg/day divided every 6 hours up to a maximum of 12 g/day **Adults** *IM, IV:* 1-2 g/dose every 4-6 hours Mild to moderate infections: **Children < 20 kg** *Oral:* 50-100 mg/kg/day divided every 6 hours to a maximum of 2-3 g/day *IM, IV:* 100-200 mg/kg/ day divided every 6 hours **Children > 20 kg** *Oral:* 250-500 mg every 6 hours *IM, IV:* 100-200 mg/kg/day divided every 6 hours
Ticarcillin disodium (Ticar) **(Warning: Dosing adjustment is required for patients with renal impairment.)**	*P. aeruginosa, E. coli, P. mirabilis,* anaerobes		**Infants and children** *IV:* 200-300 mg/kg/day in divided doses every 4-6 hours; maximum of 24 g/day **Adults** *IM, IV:* 2-4 g every 4-6 hours
Piperacillin sodium (Pipracil) **(Warning: Dosing adjustment is required for patients with renal impairment.)**	*Proteus, Enterobacter, Serratia* spp, *Acinetobacter, Providencia, Klebsiella* spp, plus increased activity against *P. aeruginosa*	Prolonged bleeding	**Infants and children** 200-300 mg/kg/ day in divided doses every 4-6 hours up to a maximum of 24 g/day **Adults** 3-4 g every 4-6 hours to a maximum of 24 g/day

Cephalosporins

Cephalosporins are usually bactericidal in action. They are classified as first, second, third, or fourth generation based on their spectrum of activity. First-generation cephalosporins are active in vitro against gram-positive aerobic cocci. They have limited activity against gram-negative bacteria. Second-generation cephalosporins are active in vitro against organisms susceptible to first-generation cephalosporins and have more activity against gram-negative organisms. Third-generation cephalosporins are less active in vitro against gram-positive organisms than first-generation cephalosporins but have an extended spectrum against gram-negative organisms.

First-Generation

	Indications	Potential Side Effects	Dosage and Administration
Cefazolin sodium (Ancef) **(Warning: Dosing adjustment is required for patients with renal impairment.)**	*E. coli, Klebsiella, Proteus, Haemophilus, S. aureus, S. epidermis, Streptococcus*	Dizziness, vertigo, headache, nausea, vomiting, diarrhea, anorexia, abdominal cramping, pancytopenia, changes in liver and renal function studies, oliguria	**Infants > 1 month and children** 50-100 mg/kg/ day in three divided doses; maximum dosage is 6 g/day **Adults** 1-1.5 g every 8 hours; maximum dosage is 12 g/day

(continued on the next page)

Table 6-10. Antibiotic Therapy *(continued)*

	Indications	Potential Side Effects	Dosage and Administration
Second-generation Cefoxitin sodium (Mefoxin) **(Warning: Dosing adjustment is required for patients with renal impairment.)**	*E. coli, Klebsiella, Proteus, Haemophilus, S. aureus, S. epidermis, Streptococcus*, anaerobes	Hypersensitivity reactions, eosinophilia, superinfection	**Children ≥ 3 months** *IM, IV:* 80-160 mg/kg/day divided every 6-8 hours; may dose every 4 hours for severe infections, maximum dosage is 12 g/day **Adults** *IM, IV:* 1-2 g every 6-8 hours (IM injection is painful); for severe infections, may dose 2 g every 4 hours or 3 g every 6 hours; maximum dosage is 12 g/day
Third-generation Cefotaxime sodium (Claforan) **(Warning: Dosing adjustment is required for patients with renal impairment.)**	*E. coli, Klebsiella, Proteus, Haemophilus, S. aureus, S. epidermis, Streptococcus, Enterobacter* spp, *Proteus, H. influenzae, Citrobacter* spp, *Serratia* spp, and some *P. aeruginosa, Bacteroides* spp	Transient leukopenia, thrombocytopenia, and phlebitis	**Infants and children 1 month-12 years (< 50 kg)** 100-200 mg/kg/day divided every 8 hours (for meningitis, 300 mg/kg/ day divided every 8 hours) to a maximum of 12 g/day **Children > 12 years (≥ 50 kg) and adults** Moderate-to-severe infection, 1-2 g every 8 hours; for life-threatening infection, 2.5 g every 8 hours
Other Antibiotics Chloramphenicol (Chloromycetin) **(Warnings: Serious and fatal blood dyscrasias have occurred after both short-term and prolonged therapy; should not be used when less potentially toxic agents are effective. Use with caution in patients with impaired hepatic or renal function.)**	*Haemophilus, B. fragilis, S. pneumonia, Neisseria, Salmonella, Klebsiella, Rickettsia,* most anaerobes	Headache, depression, confusion, nausea, vomiting, diarrhea, perianal irritation, stomatitis, xerostomia, abdominal distention, blotching skin, cyanosis, hypothermia, bone marrow depression, and aplastic anemia	**Infants and children** 50-75 mg/kg/day divided every 6 hours (for meningitis, 75-100 mg/kg/day divided every 6 hours) to a maximum of 4 g/day **Adults** 50-100 mg/kg/day divided every 6 hours to a maximum of 4 g/day
Erythromycin (EES)	*Legionella, Mycoplasma, S. pyogenes*	Abdominal cramping and distention, diarrhea, and phlebitis	**Children** *Oral:* 30-50 mg/kg/day in four divided doses every 6 hours to a maximum of 2 g/day *IV:* 20-40 mg/kg/day as a continuous IV infusion (every 6 hours in divided doses by intermittent IV infusion) to a maximum of 2-4 g/day **Adults** *Oral:* 250 mg to 1 g every 6 hours to a maximum of 4 g/day (for severe infections) *IV:* 15-20 mg/kg/day to a maximum of 4 g/day (for very severe infections) by continuous infusion or in divided doses at intervals no greater than 6 hours

Table 6-10. Antibiotic Therapy *(continued)*

	Indications	Potential Side Effects	Dosage and Administration
Sulfisoxazole and erythromycin (Pediazole)	*H. influenzae, S. pyogenes*	Diarrhea, abdominal pain	**Children** *Oral:* 40-50 mg/kg/day (based on erythromycin content) in four divided doses for 10 days to a maximum of 2 g/day For severe infections, it is recommended that children be given no less than 300 mg/day regardless of body weight
Clindamycin (Cleocin) **(Warning: Can cause severe and possibly fatal colitis. Contraindicated in patients with previous pseudomembranous colitis or hepatic impairment.)**	*B. fragilis, clostridium* spp, *S. pneumoniae, S. viridans, S. pyrogenes, S. aureus*	Diarrhea, abdominal pain, bloating, nausea, vomiting, decreased taste, neutropenia, thrombophlebitis, jaundice, abnormal liver function studies, and severe colitis	**Infants > 1 month and children** *Oral:* 10-30 mg/kg/day divided every 6-8 hours *IM, IV:* 30-40 mg/ kg/day divided every 6-8 hours to a maximum of 4 g/day **Adults** *Oral:* 150-600 mg/dose every 6-8 hours to a maximum of 1.8 g/day *IM, IV:* 1.2-1.8 g/day in three to four divided doses to a maximum of 4.8 g/day *Topical:* Apply a thin film to affected area twice daily
Vancomycin (Vancocin) **(Warnings: Rapid infusion is associated with erythematous reaction including hypotension and rash involving the face, neck, upper trunk, back, and upper arms. Dosing adjustment is required for patients with renal impairment.)**	*C. difficile, S. aureus, S. epidermis, S. fecalis, corynebacterium* spp, and *S. bovis*	Vertigo, dizziness, phlebitis, tinnitus, ototoxicity, increased BUN and creatinine, and superinfection	**Infants > 1 month and children** For meningitis, 60 mg/kg/day divided every 6 hours to a maximum of 2 g/day; for staphylococcal central nervous system infection, 60 mg/kg/day in divided doses every 6 hours to a maximum of 1 g/dose **Children** *Oral:* 40 mg/kg/day in divided doses every 8 hours, not to exceed 2 g/day *IV:* 40 mg/kg/day divided every 6 hours **Adults** *Oral:* 1 g/day in divided doses every 12 hours (for those with normal renal function, 1 g every 12 hours)
Trimethoprim-sulfamethoxazole (Bactrim) **(Warning: Dosing adjustment is required for patients with renal impairment.)**	*P. carinii, S. aureus, S. pneumoniae, S. pyogenes, Salmonella, Listeria, E. coli, Proteus, Serratia, Haemophilus, Neisseria*	Myelosuppression, aplastic anemia, Stevens-Johnson syndrome, and hepatic necrosis	Dosage is based on trimethoprim (TMP) content. **Children > 2 months** For a minor infection, 6-12 mg TMP/kg/day divided every12 hours For a serious infection (e.g., *Pneumocystis*), 15-20 mg TMP/kg/day divided every 6-8 hours For *Pneumocystis* prophylaxis, 10 mg TMP/kg/day or 150 mg TMP/m^2/day divided every 12 hours For prophylaxis of urinary tract infections (UTI), 2-4 mg TMP/kg/day once daily **Adults** For UTI or chronic bronchitis, one double-strength tablet every 12 hours for 10-14 days

(continued on the next page)

Table 6-10. Antibiotic Therapy *(continued)*

	Indications	Potential Side Effects	Dosage and Administration
Antiviral Agents Acyclovir (Zovirax) **(Warnings: Rapid IV infusion can cause acute renal failure. Dosing adjustment is required for patients with renal impairment.)**	Herpes simplex virus (HSV) and varicella zoster virus	Renal toxicity and neurotoxicity	**Children and adults** *Oral:* For mucocutaneous HSV, 10 mg/kg/day (maximum: 2 g/day) divided every 6 hours for 5 days For chicken pox, 20 mg/kg (maximum: 4 g/day) four times a day for 5 days; start therapy at the earliest sign or symptom *IV:* For mucocutaneous HSV, 5-10 mg/kg/dose every 8 hours for 5-7 days For HSV encephalitis, 10-15 mg/kg/dose every 8 hours for 14-21 days For disseminated zoster, 10 mg/kg/day divided every 8 hours for 7 days For varicella zoster in immunocompromised patients, 30 mg/ kg/day (1,500 mg/m^2/day) divided every 8 hours for 7 days *Topical:* 1/2-in. ribbon of ointment every 3 hours (six times/day) for 7 days
Antifungals Amphotericin B (Fungizone) **(Warnings: This drug is a vesicant. Dosing adjustments are *not* necessary for patients with renal impairment. If decreased renal function is due to amphotericin, the daily dose can be decreased by 50%, or the total dose can be given every other day.)**	*Candida, Aspergillus,* Zygomycetes, *Cryptococcus, Histoplasma*	Fever, headache, sedation, weakness, paresthesia, flushing, arrhythmias, hypotension/ hypertension, tinnitus, hearing loss, vertigo, nausea, vomiting, diarrhea, coagulation deficits, electrolyte imbalances (decreased potassium, magnesium, sodium), pancytopenia, and hepatic dysfunction	**Children and adults** *Maintenance:* Initial 0.25 mg/kg/day over 2-4 hours and increase by increments of 0.25 mg/kg/day to 0.5-1.5 mg/kg/day; the maximum daily dosage is 1.5 mg/kg/ day *Intrathecal or intraventricular:* 0.025-1 mg/dose every day or every other day
Flucytosine (Ancobon) **(Warning: Do not administer to infants due to possible hepatic damage. Dosing adjustment is required for patients with renal impairment.)**	*Cryptococcus, Candida,* chromomycosis		**Children and adults** *Oral:* 75-150 mg/kg/day in divided doses every 6 hours
Clotrimazole (Lotrimin)	*Candida* spp	Erythema, stinging, blistering, peeling, edema, and pruritus with topical application	**Children > 3 years and adults** *Oral:* 10-mg troche dissolved slowly five times/day for 14 days *Topical:* Apply twice daily and massage gently
Miconazole nitrate (Monistat) **(Warning: Avoid contact with eyes.)**	*Candida* spp, *Aspergillus* spp, Zygomycetes, *Cryptococcus, Blastomyces, Histoplasma, Coccidioides, Sporothrix*	Dizziness, anxiety, drowsiness, arrythmias, nausea, vomiting, diarrhea, anemia, hyponatremia, phlebitis, fever, allergic reaction, anaphylaxis	**Children < 1 year** *Intrathecal:* 20 mg/dose every 3-7 days **Children > 1 year** *IV:* 20-40 mg/kg/day divided every 8 hours to a maximum of 15 mg/kg/dose *Topical:* Apply twice daily for 2-4 weeks *Vaginal:* Insert 100-mg suppository at bedtime for 7 days

Table 6-10. Antibiotic Therapy *(continued)*

	Indications	Potential Side Effects	Dosage and Administration
Miconazole nitrate (Monistat) *(continued)*			**Adults** *Intrathecal:* 20 mg every 1-2 days *IV:* Initial dose of 200 mg, then 1.2-3.6 g/day divided every 8 hours for up to 20 weeks *Topical:* Apply twice daily for 2-4 weeks *Vaginal:* Insert 100-mg suppository at bedtime for 7 days
Ketoconazole (Nizoral) **(Warning: Hepatic toxicity can be fatal.)**	Similar to miconazole (Monistat)	Gynecomastia, adrenal insufficiency, hepatic toxicity	**Children > 2 years** *Oral:* 5-10 mg/kg/day divided every 12-24 hours for 2-4 weeks, not to exceed 800 mg/day **Adults** *Oral:* 200-400 mg/day divided every 12-24 hours

Bacteremia: Treatment includes antibiotic therapy directed at specific causative pathogen(s).

Pneumonia: Treatment includes antibiotic therapy directed at specific causative pathogen(s).

Otitis media: Treatment includes broad-spectrum antibiotic therapy. Supportive measures include antipyretic and pain control.

Esophagitis: Treatment includes antacids; histamine antagonists; antifungal, antibacterial, or antiviral therapy; pain control; and IV hydration.

Oral mucositis: Treatment includes antibiotic therapy specific for anaerobes and Candida, as well as antifungal therapy. Supportive measures include an alcohol-free mouthcare regimen, pain control, IV hydration, and nutritional support.

Cutaneous infections: Treatment of these includes broad-spectrum antibiotic, antifungal, or antiviral therapy. Supportive measures include medications to control pain or pruritus.

Sinusitis: Treatment includes broad-spectrum antibiotic therapy, antifugal therapy if a fungal infection is suspected, topical nasal steroids, and decongestants. Supportive measures include pain control and IV hydration, if needed.

Typhlitis: Treatment includes antimicrobial therapy. Supportive measures include nasogastric suction, IV hydration, and pain control. Surgical resection of a necrotic bowel can be performed, but it is a rare procedure.

Pseudomembranous (antibiotic-associated) colitis: Treatment includes antibiotic therapy (metronidazole) and pain control.

UTI: Treatment includes pathogen-specific antibiotic therapy.

Perirectal cellulitis: Treatment includes broad-spectrum anaerobic coverage, as well as administration of an antianaerobic agent. Supportive measures include sitz baths, stool softeners, a low-bulk diet, and pain control.

VP shunt infection: Treatment includes appropriate antimicrobial therapy and surgical intervention (e.g., externalization of the VP shunt, removal of the shunt).

Nursing Assessment and Interventions

Assessment:

- Perform a detailed patient history, including information such as temperature range; presence of chills or rigors; pain (including its intensity, duration, and quality); appetite level; urinary and bowel habits; GI disturbances; and neurological changes.
- Complete a comprehensive physical examination, including an assessment for abnormalities or changes in vital signs, assessment of chills (especially during IV boluses or infusions); assessment of skin and mucous membrane integrity; an evaluation for signs of shock (e.g., delayed capillary refill, tachycardia, hypotension, confusion); and neurological, GI, and respiratory assessments.

Interventions:

- Encourage the patient's compliance with prophylactic antibiotic therapy (postsplenectomy and prophylactic *Pneumocystis carinii* regimens) so that the risk of infection is decreased.
- Educate the patient and the family regarding care of the central line to decrease the patient's risk of infection.
- Ensure that appropriate diagnostic tests are ordered, and the results are obtained.
- Administer antibiotics to a neutropenic patient as soon as possible.
- Perform patient assessments on an ongoing basis to ensure that any associated complications will be identified as early as possible.
- Provide developmentally appropriate education to patients and families regarding the early diagnosis and treatment of cancer-related infections.

Expected Patient and Family Outcomes

- The patient and the family adhere to prophylactic antibiotic regimens.

- The patient and the family learn about and appropriately care for the central line.
- Parents of the patient recognize the signs of infection and know when to seek medical intervention.

Blood Product Support

Kathleen Adlard

Definition

Blood components are products derived from human whole blood, which, when broken down, forms red blood cells (RBCs), platelets, white blood cells (WBCs), and plasma. Plasma can be further processed to obtain cryoprecipitate. Many children with cancer require infusions of one or more blood components during the course of their cancer therapy due to specific hematological deficiencies. These deficiencies can result from an increased loss, increased destruction, or a decreased production of a blood component.

Indications for Blood Product Infusions

Indications for infusions of blood products are to restore blood volume, improve oxygen-carrying capacity, minimize bleeding, correct coagulopathies, and/or replace plasma proteins.

Pathophysiology of Blood Component Deficits

Tumor cells can replace normal cells within the bone marrow space. Bone marrow production becomes suppressed because of chemotherapy, radiation therapy, or both. Kidney damage, a side effect of several chemotherapeutic agents such as cisplatin (Platinol), cyclophosphamide (Cytoxan), or ifosphamide (Ifex), also may result in reduced production of erythropoietin.

Sources of Blood Components

There are two sources of blood components, donor and autologous. Donor blood components are collected from volunteer donors for transfusion to another person and may be donated for a specific recipient (designated donors). Autologous blood is collected from the patient and stored for later reinfusion.

Types of Blood Components

Whole blood: Whole blood contains RBCs, WBCs, platelets, and plasma. Whole blood is rarely administered but may be used to restore RBCs and volume when massive blood loss has occurred. It occasionally may be used for exchange transfusions.

Volume guide. Volume is 20 ml/kg initially to replace massive blood loss.

Crossmatching. Donor and recipient blood must be ABO-identical and Rh-compatible.

Packed RBCs: These cells are used to improve tissue oxygenation and correct anemia without causing a significant increase in blood volume, and generally are administered when a patient's hemoglobin is > 7 g/dl. They are prepared by removing the plasma portion of whole blood. The shelf life of pRBCs is 21–42 days. Their life span after they have been transfused is approximately 30 days.

Volume guide. The volume guide for pediatric patients shows that 10 ml/kg will increase Hgb 3 g/dl; 15 ml/kg is the maximum amount given in a single transfusion.

Crossmatching. Crossmatching is done within 72 hours prior to transfusion. The donor's and patient's blood must be ABO-identical and Rh-compatible.

Transfusion time. Transfusion normally takes 3–4 hours. A transfusion must be completed within 4 hours of the blood's removal from a blood bank.

Filter. A 40-micron microaggregate (leukopore) filter must be used for all pRBC transfusions.

Platelets: One unit of platelets is obtained from 500 ml of fresh whole blood. An apheresis unit is equal to 6–8 random donor units.

Platelets are suspended in a small amount of plasma and stored at room temperature on an agitator for up to 5 days. The types of platelet preparations are:

- Random-donor platelets, which combine aliquots of platelets from different donors and expose the recipient to multiple foreign antigens.
- Single-donor platelets, which minimize a recipient's exposure to foreign antigens.
- Human lymphocyte antigen (HLA)-matched platelets, which are obtained by apheresing an HLA-identical donor to further minimize a recipient's exposure to foreign antigens

One unit of platelets should increase a patient's peripheral blood level by 10,000 cells/mm^3. Platelets are administered when a patient is actively bleeding and/or when the platelet count is less than 10,000 cells/mm^3. Platelet infusions may be given prophylactically in children with vascular brain tumors prior to invasive procedures or surgery, sepsis, or other infections if the count is less than 50,000 cells/mm^3.

Platelet counts can be drawn 60 minutes after an infusion. Failure to achieve adequate increases in circulating platelet counts often is due to infection, fever, disseminated intravascular coagulation (DIC), splenomegaly, or formation of antibodies to antigens in the donated blood. Exposure to multiple tissue antigens leads to formation of antibodies to the antigens, which results in patients' inability to experience a platelet rise after platelet transfusions.

Volume guide. Pediatric volume is 10 ml/kg or 1 random unit per year of age. Adult volume is 6–10 units.

Crossmatching. Crossmatching is not required, but ABO-identical and Rh-compatible platelets are preferred.

Transfusion time. The transfusion time should be as fast as a patient can tolerate but should be within 4 hours after the platelets are released from a blood bank.

During transfusion, it is recommended that the bag and volume control chamber (burretrol) be gently agitated every 30 minutes to prevent platelets from clumping and/or sticking to the bag and tubing.

Granulocytes: Granulocytes may be used to treat patients who are severely neutropenic and have absolute neutrophil counts of >500 x 10^9 with documented infections, especially those caused by gram-negative organisms that are not responding to antibiotics. Granulocytes are not recommended for patients whose bone marrow functions are not likely to recover.

Granulocytes are collected from a single donor and stored at room temperature. They contain large numbers of leukocytes, many platelets, and some RBCs.

Febrile and allergic reactions are common as the recipients' antibodies react to the antigens on the donor leukocytes. Diphenhydramine (Benadryl), acetaminophen (Tylenol), or hydrocortisone (Solu-Cortef) may be ordered before a transfusion to prevent these reactions. Infusions can lead to pulmonary sequestrations, especially if the recipient is receiving amphotericin (Fungizone). Due to their low survival time after infusion, high degree of toxicity, and limited clinical evidence of benefit, granulocytes are rarely used.

Volume guide. The volume usually is 1 unit per day until the patient's condition improves, and there are signs of neutrophil recovery.

Crossmatching. Crossmatching is required because there are many RBCs contained within the volume of granulocytes to be transfused. The donor and the recipient must be ABO-identical and Rh-compatible.

Transfusion time. Granulocytes are transfused over 2–4 hours (5 ml/kg/hr). A standard-size filter (170 microns) should be used for administering granulocytes. **A 40 micron microaggregate filter should not be used because it will filter out the granulocytes.**

Fresh-frozen plasma: Plasma is the clear-fluid portion of blood that remains when RBCs are removed from whole blood. Fresh-frozen plasma (FFP) is separated and frozen less than 6 hours after its collection. FFP contains plasma proteins and stable coagulation factors (fibrinogen and factor IX) and unstable coagulation factors (factor V and factor VIII). FFP contains approximately 1 unit/ml of each coagulation factor. FFP is used to replace coagulation factors in bleeding patients with multiple coagulation factor deficiencies as a result of liver disease, DIC, or dilutional coagulopathy (i.e., because of massive blood replacement). The FDA recently approved frozen plasma (FP) as a new option for patients. The new product is plasma frozen within 24 hours of its collection. The main difference between FFP and FP is that FP has a lower amount of factor VIII.

Volume guide. The volume is 10–30 ml/kg.

Crossmatching. Crossmatching is not required. However, the patient and the donor must be ABO-identical. Rh compatibility is not required because the product does not contain RBCs.

Transfusion time. FFP is transfused over 2–4 hours. It must be infused within 6 hours of the time it has been thawed.

Albumin (5% or 25% solution) and plasma protein fraction (PPF) (5% solution): Albumin contains 96% albumin and 4% globulins, and plasma protein fraction contains 83% albumin and 17% globulins. Both are treated with heat to destroy viruses. Albumin and PPF are used to treat patients who are both hypovolemic and hypoproteinemic. Both treatments must be used with caution in patients susceptible to fluid overload.

Volume guide. The volume is 0.5–1 g/kg = 10 ml/kg of 5% solution; 1 g/kg = 4 ml/kg of 25% solution.

Crossmatching. Crossmatching is not required.

Transfusion time. The transfusion rate for a 5% solution is 1–2 ml/minute (60–120 ml/hr) or more rapidly if the patient is in shock. The transfusion rate for a 25% solution is 0.2–0.4 ml/minute (12–24 ml/hr).

Cryoprecipitate: Cryoprecipitate is prepared by thawing FFP. The cryoprecipitate is used to replace fibrinogen and clotting factor deficiencies. It contains clotting factors VIII and XIII, fibrinogen, and von Willebrand factor.

Volume guide. The dosage varies depending upon a patient's disease and condition. Doses are usually repeated every 8–12 hours until bleeding is stopped or the desired factor VIII level is attained.

Crossmatching. Crossmatching is not required. ABO compatibility is suggested, not required.

Transfusion time. The transfusion time is 1–2 hours, but it must be transfused within 6 hours of the time the frozen plasma has been thawed.

Clotting concentrates: Factor VIII and factor IX clotting concentrates are used to treat specific clotting deficiencies. They provide a known dosage in a small volume. One unit provides the amount of factor activity that is normally present in 1 ml of normal plasma.

Volume guide. One unit/kg of factor VIII should increase a patient's plasma level by 2%; 1 unit/kg of factor IX should increase a patient's plasma level by 1%.

Crossmatching. Crossmatching is not required.

Transfusion time. The transfusion time is 5–15 minutes. The factor is withdrawn from a vial using a filter needle.

Special Component Preparations

Irradiated blood products: T lymphocytes that are present in the blood of a donor can cause graft-versus-host disease (GVHD) in an immunocompromised recipient. Immunocompromised recipients include patients with malignancies, chemotherapy recipients, candidates for bone marrow transplant, and/or neonates. The lymphocytes in the donor's blood attack the recipient's tissue, which is unable to reject incompatible foreign cells, resulting in GVHD. Irradiation of a donor's blood makes the WBC lymphocytes nonviable. All donor blood components are irradiated by a blood bank just before transfusion.

Leukocyte-reduced blood products: Leukocyte-reduced RBCs and platelets are indicated for all patients receiving chemotherapy and for individuals who have repeated febrile reactions associated with RBC transfusions, platelet transfusions, or both. Patients who receive frequent transfusions may become alloimmunized to leukocyte antigens and sometimes to platelet antigens. This sensitization can manifest itself as febrile transfusion reactions and/or refractoriness to a transfusion of platelets. Leukocyte reduction also decreases the risk of transmitting cytomegalovirus (CMV) to the recipient.

Leukocytes can be removed from the blood products by centrifugation, filtration, or washing the RBCs in saline solution. Washed RBCs are preferred for patients with severeallergic reactions to transfusions.

Cytomegalovirus negative components: CMV is an easily transmitted virus that can cause serious infections and possibly even death in immunosuppressed individuals or premature infants. The virus can persist in a carrier state in the blood of a previously infected person even though antibodies are present. It is generally accepted that leukocyte reduction during the collection process is an effective method of reducing CMV transmission to a CMV-negative recipient. Candidates for a bone marrow transplant who are CMV-negative and neonates weighing less than 1,250 grams at birth usually receive CMV-negative blood components.

Potential Complications

Febrile response: Symptoms include fever, chills, muscle pain, chest pain, flushing, and headache.

Allergic reaction: Symptoms include itching, hives, dyspnea, wheezing, respiratory arrest, and cardiac arrest.

Circulatory overload: Symptoms include hypertension, hypotension, bradycardia, tachycardia, cyanosis of the extremities, and clammy skin.

Sepsis: Symptoms include fever, chills, bleeding, DIC, nausea and vomiting, diarrhea, and abdominal cramping.

Nursing Assessment and Interventions

Assessment:

- Assess the child's pretransfusion status, including weight, clinical condition, laboratory values, indications for component therapy, previous transfusion history, and indications for premedication.
- Assess the child's and the family's understanding of the transfusion process.
- Assess the child's intravenous access and patency of the child's veins.
- Verify the physician's orders, including the type of component, special requirements (e.g., irradiated blood products, leukocyte-reduced blood products); the number of millimeters or units to be given, the date and time they are to be administered; and the length of the infusion.
- Monitor the patient for acute hemolytic reactions to the transfusion (most are a result of clerical error either by the nurse or blood bank technician).
- Verify with a second healthcare provider the following things, according to institutional policy:
  - The type of product, blood group, and Rh type.
  - That the patient's identification band containing patient's name and medical record is worn by the patient at all times.
  - That the transfusion service record and/or labels on the bag matches pertinent identification, compatibility, crossmatching (if required), ABO group, unit number, expiration date of the product, lot numbers (if given), and any other information on or attached to the product.
- Perform a baseline assessment and check the patient's vital signs before beginning the infusion.
- Monitor the patient according to institutional policy; at a minimum, this includes observing the patient for the first 15 minutes and reassessing or taking the patient's vital signs every hour.

Interventions:

- Obtain a crossmatch and label the specimen according to institutional policy.
- Administer premedications, when indicated.
- Do the following when there is a suspected transfusion reaction:
  - Stop the transfusion.
  - Draw 3–5 ml and discard the blood specimen, flush the IV line with saline, and maintain venous patency.
  - Notify the physician and the blood bank.
  - Assess the patient's condition and vital signs.
  - Check the blood bag for a compatibility label and the patient identification label for clerical errors.
  - Return the untransfused portion with tubing set to the blood bank.
  - Obtain blood and urine samples from the patient.
  - Document the reaction in the patient's medical record. Include the date and time the transfusion was begun, venipuncture sites, venous access device, the unit number of the blood component, type of product and filter used, times of any filter and/or tubing changes, the volume infused, vital signs, observations of the patient's tolerance, education the patient and family had received, and any medications that had been omitted or given to the patient.

Expected Patient and Family Outcomes

- The child and the family understand the purpose of the infusion of the blood product.
- The child and the family understand the signs and symptoms of a transfusion reaction.
- The blood component is infused safely.

Bibliography

Psychological Preparation and Support for Painful Procedures

Chen, E., Joseph, N.H., & Zeltzer, L.K. (2000). Behaviorial and cognitive interventions in the treatment of pain in children. *Pediatric Clinics of North America, 47,* 513–525.

Christensen, J., & Fatchett, D. (2002). Promoting parental use of distraction and relaxation in pediatric oncology patients during invasive procedures. *Journal of Pediatric Oncology Nursing, 19,* 124–132.

Walker, C.L., Wells, D., Heiney, S.P., & Hymovich, D.P. (2003). Family-centered psychosocial care. In C.R. Baggott, K.P. Kelly, D. Fochtman, & G.V. Foley (Eds.), *Nursing care of children and adolescents with cancer* (3rd ed., pp. 365–390). Philadelphia: W.B. Saunders.

Sedation for Painful Procedures

Collins, J.J., & Weisman, S.J. (2003). Management of pain in childhood cancer. In N.L. Schechter, C.B. Berde, & M. Yaster (Eds.), *Pain in infants, children, and adolescents* (2nd ed., pp. 517–538). Philadelphia: Lippincott Williams & Wilkins.

Cote, C.J., Karl, H.W., Notterman, D.A., Weinberg, J.A., & McCloskey, C. (2000). Adverse sedation events in pediatrics: Analysis of medications used for sedation. *Pediatrics, 106,* 633–644.

Cote, C.J., Notterrman, D.A., Karl, H.W., Weinberg, J.A., & McCloskey, C. (2000). Adverse sedation events in pediatrics: A critical incident analysis of contributing factors. *Pediatrics, 105,* 805–814.

Finley, G.A., & Schechter, N.L. (2003). Sedation. In N.L. Schechter, C.B. Berde, & M. Yaster (Eds.), *Pain in infants, children, and adolescents* (2nd ed., pp. 563–577). Philadelphia: Lippincott Williams & Wilkins.

Central Venous Access

Anton, M. & Massicotte, M.P. (2001). Venous thromboembolism in pediatrics. *Seminars in Vascular Medicine, 1,* 111–122.

Maki, D.G., Stolz, S.M., Wheeler, S., & Mermel, L.A. (1997). Prevention of central venous catheter-related bloodstream infection by use of an antiseptic-impregnated catheter: A randomized, controlled trial. *Annals of Internal Medicine, 127,* 257–266.

Pearson, M.L., & Abrutyn, E. (1997). Reducing the risk for catheter-related infections: A new strategy. *Annals of Internal Medicine, 127,* 304–306.

Zaoutis, T.E., Greeves, H.M., Lautenbach, E., Bilker, W.B., & Coffin, S.E. (2004). Risk factors for disseminated candidiasis in children with candidiasis. *Pediatric Infectious Disease Journal, 23,* 635–641.

Nutritional Support for Children with Cancer

American Cancer Society. (2003, February 4). In ACS introduction to childrens' nutrition [on-line]. Available: www.cancer.org.

Bechard, L.J., Adviv, O.E., Jaksic, T., & Duggan, C. (2002). Nutritional supportive care. In P.A. Pizzo & D.G. Poplack (Eds.), *Principles and practice of pediatric oncology* (4th ed., pp. 1285–1301). Philadelphia: Lippincott Williams & Wilkins.

Capra, S., Bauer, J., Davidson, W., & Ash, S. (2002). Nutritional therapy for cancer-induced weight loss. *Nutrition in Clinical Practice, 17,* 210–213.

Novy, M.A., & Saavedra, J.M. (1997). Pediatric nurtrition therapy. Nutrition therapy for the pediatric cancer patient. *Topics in Clinical Nutrition, 12*(4), 16–25.

Skolin, I., Hernell, O., Larrson, M.V., Wahlgren, C., & Wahlin, Y.B. (2002). Percutaneous endoscopic gastrostomy in children with malignant disease. *Journal of Pediatric Oncology Nursing, 19,* 154–163.

Skolin, I., Hutsti, U.K., & Wahlin, Y.B. (2001). Parents' perception of the child's food intake after the start of chemotherapy. *Journal of Pediatric Oncology Nursing, 18,* 124–136.

Treatment of Infections

American Academy of Pediatrics. (2000). *2000 Red Book: Report of the Committee on Infectious Diseases* (25th ed.). Elk Grove Village, IL: Author.

Groll, A.H., Irwin, R.S., Lee, J.W., et al. (2001). Management of specific infectious complications in children with leukemias and lymphomas. In C.C. Patrick (Ed.), *Clinical management of infections in immunocompromised infants and children* (pp. 111–143). Philadelphia: Lippincott Williams & Wilkins.

Mitchell, D.K., & Pickering, L.K. (2001). Enteric infections. In C.C. Patrick (Ed.), *Clinical management of infections in immunocompromised infants and children* (pp. 413–449). Philadelphia: Lippincott Williams & Wilkins.

Soloway-Simon, D., & Levy, M. (2001). Dermatologic findings with infection. In C.C. Patrick (Ed.), *Clinical management of infections in immunocompromised infants and children* (pp. 470–508). Philadelphia: Lippincott Williams & Wilkins.

Blood Product Support

American Association of Blood Banks (AABB). (2000). Facts about blood. www.aabb.org.

Brown, M., & Whalen, P.K. (2000). Red blood cell transfusion in critically ill patients. *Critical Care Nurse.*

Fitzpatrick, L. (2002). Blood products. *Nursing, 32*(5), 36–42.

Herberg, A., (2003). Blood product administration. In V.R. Bowden, & C. Smith Greenberg (Eds.) *Pediatric nursing procedures.* Philadelphia: Lippincott Williams & Wilkins, 122–132.

Miller, R.L.S. (2002). Blood component therapy. *Urologic nursing, 22*(5), 331–342.

Norville, R. & B (2002). Blood component deficencies. In C. Rasco-Baggott, K. Patterson-Kelly, D. Fochtman, & G.V. Foley (Eds.), *Nursing care of children and adolescents with cancer* (3rd ed., pp. 347–364).

Rossetto, C.L., & McMahon, J.E. (2000). Current and future trends in transfusion therapy. *Journal of Pediatric Oncology Nursing, 17,* 160–173.

SECTION VII

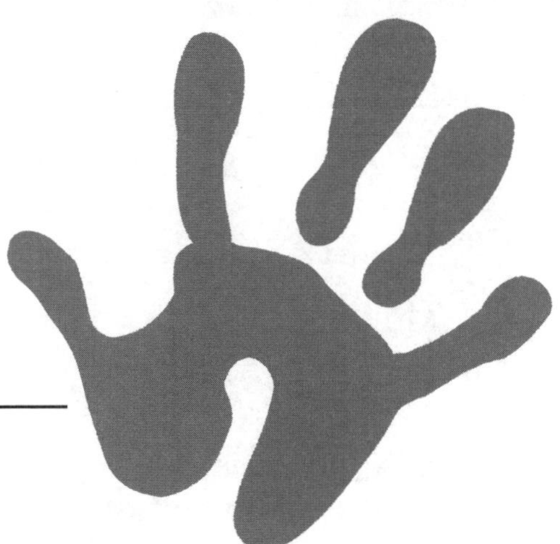

Psychosocial Issues

Mary C. Hooke

Section Outline

Development of Infants (Birth to 1 Year)

Mary C. Hooke

Normal Development

Psychosocial stage of trust versus mistrust: Infants work to develop a sense of trust while overcoming a sense of mistrust. Infants trust that their needs for food, comfort, stimulation, and caring will be met. Mistrust develops in response to a lack of trusting experiences.

Cognitive stage: This is the sensorimotor stage during which simple learning takes place through sensory experiences and exploration. Infants progress from reflex behaviors to simple repetitive acts and imitative activities. Infants work toward developing a sense of object permanence.

Emotional and social characteristics: Infants' temperaments or behavioral styles influence their human interactions.

Body image and sense of self: Infants' sensorimotor experiences provide the first perceptions of their own body, and the mouth is an infant's primary area of pleasure. Infants develop an awareness of their hands and feet, which they suck or play with. They acquire a sense of object permanence through sensorimotor development. Infants then recognize themselves as distinct from their parents.

Fears: Infants' fear of strangers and of separation from their parents are important to the development of healthy parent-child attachments. Infants also may have fears related to loud noises, bright lights, sudden movements, animals, and heights.

Significant relationships: An infant's attachment to a mothering figure is of primary importance. By 6 months, an infant shows a distinct preference for his or her mother and shows attachment to the father by 7 months.

Risks to infants with cancer: Hospitalization often causes infants to be separated from their parents for significant periods of time. Cancer therapy can cause side effects such as fatigue, pain, mucositis, central nervous system toxicities, and immobility, which can interfere with sensorimotor experiences and the infant's development. Hospitalization and cancer treatment also bring about changes in routines and patterns that provide security to an infant. Furthermore, cancer treatment involves experiences that infants fear, such as those involving separation, strangers, loud noises, bright lights, and sudden movements.

Nursing Assessment and Interventions

Assessment:

- Assess the relationship between the infant and the parent (i.e., bonding behaviors, responsiveness, and interplay between the parent and the child).
- Assess the infant's level of development by using assessment tools or developmental milestones.
- Assess the infant's sensorimotor experiences.
  - Have oral-motor experiences and pleasure been affected by the disease or treatment?
  - Is the infant able to roll and move his or her hands and feet to the mouth?
  - Has the infant received neurotoxic therapies that can affect neurological function (e.g., intrathecal [IT] medications, therapies that cross the blood-brain barrier, radiation therapy)?

Interventions:

- Encourage the development of trust.
- Encourage the parents to visit and room in with the infant.
- Allow the parents to hold the infant as much as possible.
- Encourage comforting touch.
- Perform examinations as quickly as possible.
- Provide sensorimotor experiences for the infant.
- Provide pleasurable visual, auditory, tactile, taste, and movement mechanisms for the infant's stimulation.
- Encourage the development of the infant's oral-motor pleasure through such actions as sucking and oral intake.
- Consult with an occupational therapist or a speech therapist if the infant's oral functioning is impaired.
- Consult with a physical therapist and an occupational therapist if the infant has developmental delays or is receiving neurotoxic therapies.
- Encourage age-appropriate developmental skills.

Expected Patient and Family Outcomes

- The outcomes of nursing interventions have been evaluated, and the plan of care has been adjusted accordingly.
- A comprehensive developmental assessment is completed every 2 months and as needed for infants who have developmental delays or impairments.

Development of Toddlers (1–3 Years)

Mary C. Hooke

Normal Development

Psychosocial stage of autonomy versus shame and doubt: Toddlers develop a sense of independence and self-mastery. They discover that their behavior is their own and has predictable effects on others. They learn that gratification must sometimes be delayed, and limits on their behavior will be set. Continued dependence at this stage can cause a sense of doubt about their ability to control their own actions.

Cognitive stage: Toddlers continue to develop in the sensorimotor phase of cognitive development (12–24 months), during which they increase their understanding of object permanence and sense of cause and effect through trial and error. Toddlers develop their language skills (i.e., they develop mental symbolism); they show curiosity and engage in experimentation, exploration, and mimicry. They are egocentric in their thinking. During their later preoperational phase, toddlers become preconceptual thinkers. They increase their ability to use speech, but they continue to be egocentric in thought, play, and behavior. Toddlers do not think logically, but rather can be magical in their thinking based on their perception of an event.

Emotional and social characteristics: Toddlers may express their frustration through temper tantrums as they are striving for autonomy. They respond with negativism to requests and questions. They are vulnerable to stress due to their limited ability to cope.

Body image and sense of self: Toilet training is the major task of toddlers. During this stage in their development, they learn the names of body parts and their purposes, and they learn to recognize differences between the sexes. They are unable to understand the concepts of body integrity and internal organs. They find intrusive experiences and procedures very threatening. Toddlers are able to separate from their parents for brief periods but are fearful of strangers when their parents are not present. They learn that they are individuals separate from others, but they see the world as revolving around themselves.

Fears: Toddlers fear separation from their parents. They fear strangers, especially when their parents are not present. They also may fear sleep, animals, and loud noises.

Significant relationships: Parents are the primary people of importance in a toddler's life. Interactions with other people, however, start to become more important for toddlers. They demonstrate parallel play with other children.

Risks to toddlers with cancer: Hospitalization may cause separation from parents and the introduction of strangers, both of which are major sources of fear and stress for toddlers. Cancer therapy can cause side effects, such as fatigue, pain, isolation, central nervous system toxicities, and immobility, which can interfere with a toddler's normal needs for exploration, experimentation, and development of autonomy. A toddler's normal negativism and temper tantrums can be exacerbated by a sense of loss of control, pain, and the side effects of medications such as steroids.

Toddlers are unable to understand what cancer is and how treatment works. They have limited verbal skills with which to explain their perceptions and sensations to others. Cancer treatment and hospitalization also cause changes in discipline and routines that normally provide toddlers with a sense of security. A toddler can fail to achieve success in toilet training due to regression, illness, bladder abnormalities, and high levels of IV hydration. The duration of a toddler's cancer treatment can range from 6 months to 3 years, encompassing this entire developmental stage.

Nursing Assessment and Interventions

Assessment:

- Use developmental tools and milestones to assess the toddler's developmental level.
- Interview the family about the toddler's normal behavior, routines, sleep patterns, fears, security objects, toilet training, ability to communicate and use language, responses to limits and discipline, and effective comfort measures.
- Assess the toddler's responsiveness to interactions with his or her parents.
- Assess for the impact of disease and treatment on the toddler's current developmental level (e.g., regression in achievement of milestones, language, toilet training).
- Assess whether the toddler received neurotoxic therapies (IT medications, therapies that cross the blood-brain barrier, radiation therapy).

Interventions:

- Use assessment data from an interview with the toddler's parents to individualize the patient's care plan to maintain consistency; address topics,such as the toddler's normal behavior, routines, fears, toilet training, limits, and discipline.
- Encourage independence by providing opportunities for the toddler to participate in care and by offering appropriate choices.
- Encourage mobility and independence by allowing the toddler to engage in physical activity or to move around using a wagon or stroller.
- Encourage the toddler's need to explore, play, and experiment with the environment while, at the same time, providing safe boundaries.
- Arrange for rehabilitation services for toddlers who have developmental delays or who are receiving neurotoxic therapies.
- Use consistent caregivers for the toddler to promote the development of trusting relationships.
- Provide opportunities for play to help the toddler work through fears; consult child-life resources about the use of therapeutic play.
- Support the parents in their toilet-training efforts with the toddler by providing frequent opportunities for toileting and the use of training pants instead of diapers.
- Provide simple explanations describing sensations and desired behavior, because a toddler does not understand causal relationships.
- Teach parents about the toddler's response to illness and ways to promote the toddler's development during the illness; use resources for education such as child-life specialists and child psychologists.
- Discuss the toddler's need for socialization with the parents and develop creative ways to meet these needs when the toddler is at home.

Expected Patient and Family Outcomes

- The outcomes of nursing interventions are evaluated, and the plan of care has been adjusted accordingly.
- A comprehensive assessment of development is completed every 6 months, and as needed, for toddlers who have developmental delays or impairments.

Development of Preschoolers (4–6 Years)

Mary C. Hooke

Normal Development

Psychosocial stage of initiative versus guilt: Preschoolers develop mastery over their physical skills and are energetic learners. They feel satisfaction in their play and work. If they overstep the limits of appropriate behavior, they feel guilty.

Cognitive stage: Preschoolers move from preconceptual thought processes that are egocentric and symbolic to intuitive thought that enables them to think and verbalize their mental processes. They are beginning to consider other viewpoints during this stage. Preschoolers use magical thinking when relating one event to another and believe that thoughts are all-powerful. Preschoolers have only a limited understanding of time and relate it to a specific event (e.g., lunch time). They also attribute lifelike qualities to inanimate objects and believe that everyone thinks as they do.

Emotional and social characteristics: Preschoolers have increased mastery over their fear of strangers and separation; however, they find prolonged separation stressful and need their parents' support. They are more social and willing to please than toddlers. They have internalized the standards of their culture. They find support in security objects and can work through fears and anxieties through play.

Body image and sense of self: During this stage, children are beginning to understand the concepts of desirable and undesirable appearances. They are at risk for developing their own prejudices or experiencing the prejudices of others. They develop their sexual identity through identification with the parent of their sex and will imitate roles (e.g., what mothers and fathers do) through play. Preschoolers continue to have a poor sense of their internal anatomy and its functions and find intrusive procedures to be frightening.

Fears: Preschoolers may be afraid of the dark, of being left alone, and of having their body mutilated. They are fearful of pain as well as the objects and people associated with pain. They also are afraid of witnessing others who are in pain.

Significant relationships: Their parents and family continue to be of primary importance to preschoolers. They may attend an early childhood program and kindergarten, which provide opportunities for social development with their peers and significant adults other than their parents.

Risks to preschoolers with cancer: The experience of having cancer and undergoing treatment separates a preschooler from social relationships that are important for the development of social skills. Cancer therapy can cause side effects, such as fatigue, pain, isolation, and immobility, which can interfere with a preschooler's energetic play and work and deprive him or her of developmental experiences and a sense of accomplishment. Central nervous system toxicities also can interfere with a preschooler's cognitive development.

Hospitalization can cause prolonged, stressful periods of separation from parents. Furthermore, preschoolers with cancer may have decreased opportunities to be with both parents, especially if one parent takes on the role of primary caregiver. This circumstance can affect the development of the child's sexual identity. Preschoolers also may develop a poor sense of body integrity if they have experienced physical impairments. In addition, their tendency to engage in magical thinking places them at risk for increased fears. If they witness someone else's pain or injury, they may develop fears about experiencing that pain or wound as well because of their ability to imagine an event without having experienced it.

Nursing Assessment and Interventions

Assessment:

- Use parental history and developmental milestones to assess the preschooler's current developmental level.
- Assess the impact of disease and treatment on the preschooler's current developmental level.
- Assess whether the preschooler received neurotoxic therapies (IT medications, therapies that cross the blood-brain barrier, radiation therapy).
- Interview family members about the preschooler's normal behavior, routines, sleep patterns, fears, coping skills, security objects, toileting and hygiene skills, concerns about himself or herself, limits and discipline, and comfort measures.
- Assess the responsiveness of the interaction between the parents and the preschooler.
- Listen to the preschooler's conversations and observe his or her play; assess for the child's understanding of his or her disease and its treatment.
- Observe for fearful or anxious behavior and try to determine the source of the child's fear.

Interventions:

- Individualize the patient's care plan to include information from the interview with the parents; address information about the preschooler's normal routines, self-care skills, fears, coping, comfort measures, bathroom routines, security objects, as well as limits and discipline.
- Encourage the child's mastery of self-care skills and promote independence in activities of daily living.
- Provide opportunities for stimulating play and success while providing safe boundaries.
- Arrange for neuropsychology consultation and rehabilitation services for the preschooler who has developmental delays or is receiving neurotoxic therapies.
- Consult child-life resources when using therapeutic play to learn about illness and promote the child's adaptive skills.
- Provide simple, brief explanations about treatments and experiences while keeping in mind the limits of a preschooler's understanding of time.
- Maintain the child's bed and room as safe areas; protect the child from witnessing pain in other children.

- Discuss with the parents their child's need for socialization and devise creative ways to meet them.
- Use a school reentry program for a child who is returning to a preschool group or kindergarten (see the discussion of school reentry in this section); provide guidance and assistance as the child makes the transition and help with appearance and adjustment issues.
- Teach the parents about preschoolers' responses to illness and ways to promote their child's development during illness; use resources for education such as child-life specialists and child psychologists.

Expected Patient and Family Outcomes

- The outcomes of nursing interventions are evaluated, and the plan of care is adjusted accordingly.
- A comprehensive developmental assessment is completed every 6 months, and as needed, for preschoolers who have developmental delays or impairments.

Development of School-Age Children (7–12 Years)

Linda Madsen

Normal Development

Psychosocial stage of industry versus inferiority: The challenge for children at this stage is to become proficient at accomplishing tasks as they become increasingly independent from their parents. At this time, the peer group is a source of feedback for socially acceptable behavior, and conformity to the group is valued. If a child is unable to perform tasks in the social, physical, and academic realms, he or she can develop feelings of inadequacy that lead to a sense of inferiority. A sense of industry is developed if competence at these skills is adequate. The overall goal for children at this stage is to answer the question, "What can I do?"

Cognitive stage: This is the stage of concrete thinking or concrete operations. Children at this stage are able to conceptualize and think through concepts without having had a similar experience to rely upon. They are able to classify, sort, and order things; perform inductive reasoning; and understand the concepts of reversibility and object conservation. Children of this age also see things in absolute terms and consider rules as being inflexible. Their primary focus is on mastery of school subjects and productive development of skills.

Emotional and social characteristics: Children of this age are beginning to place importance on peer relationships and approval. Their peers give them feedback about acceptable behavior. They value conformity; physical differences may be threatening to the group. They wish to please and try to be cooperative. Confidence often exceeds a child's true capabilities at this age. They need privacy and strenuous physical activity. Their self-esteem is linked to their competence at performing tasks.

Fears: Children at this age have fears about losing control, being faced with the physical aspects of illness, failing to accomplish tasks, and being isolated from their peers.

Significant relationships: Children at this stage of development have significant relationships with their parents and other family members, school staff, and peers.

Risks to children with cancer:

Lost productivity. This risk is associated with being absent from school, weakness, fatigue, decreased endurance, or disability that interferes with normative functions, and the lowered expectations placed on them by the significant adults in their lives. Central nervous system toxicities also can interfere with the school-age child's cognitive development.

Poor peer relationships due to isolation from the group. Sick children may fail to interact with the group because of frequent absences from school and inability to participate in social activities. Poor self-esteem because of physical changes can lead children to isolate themselves and perceive themselves as being different from the group. The peer group also might reject these children because they are perceived as being different.

A sense of loss of control. Children may feel that they have lost control over their emotions because of having to undergo painful procedures and stressful situations. Children who have experienced a loss of physical function or endurance or who have experienced weakness may feel a loss of body integrity. They also may sense that they are incapable of functioning independently if they have experienced a loss of function or weakness or if their parents overprotect them.

A sense of inferiority resulting from unrealistic expectations. Parents and teachers may have unrealistically high or low expectations that are inconsistent with the child's true abilities.

Information deficit. Children may feel responsible for the diagnosis. As they grow older, children may need new information to successfully deal with the new challenges related to their illness.

Nursing Assessment and Interventions

Assessment:

- Assess current growth and development.
- Determine level of success in interpersonal relationships, and evaluate these key relationships through questioning and observation:
  - the extent of contact with peers in school and during outside activities
  - the level of involvement in school and extracurricular activities
  - the quality of peer relationships
  - the level of inclusion in the peer group.
- Assess the parents' and the teachers' ability to normalize and adapt their expectations.
- Assess the effect of changes on self-image by using verbal and nonverbal cues:
  - the extent of physical limitations

- the perception of these limitations
- the effects of the limitations on activities of daily living.

- Assess for signs that the child is using healthy strategies for coping, and assess his or her level of adjustment by observing and questioning the child and the family about
  - the child's ability to incorporate the changes imposed by the disease and its treatment into the activities of daily living
  - the child's level of involvement with his or her own care
  - the child's personal affect
  - the child's ability to establish normalcy in relationships and activities
- Determine if there are school-related issues, such as attendance and the child's ability to maintain his or her previous academic performance.
- Assess whether the school-age child has received neurotoxic therapies (IT medications, therapies that cross the blood-brain barrier, radiation therapy).
- Assess level of knowledge and information needs about the disease and its treatment through discussions with the child and the family; consider the child's previous experiences and any past illnesses.

Interventions:

- Foster the child's sense of mastery and development of self-esteem.
  - Give the child tasks and actively involve the child in his or her own care.
  - Encourage play so the child can master skills and overcome fears related to the diagnosis and treatment.
  - Encourage the child to share knowledge about the condition so that he or she can feel powerful in the eyes of peers.
  - Encourage the child to participate in hobbies, sports, social events, and schoolwork that highlight his or her strengths.
  - Encourage activities that draw upon fine and gross motor skills to develop physical skills.
- Foster normalcy whenever possible.
  - Encourage the child to maintain routines and usual activities.
  - Be flexible, within reason, with the timing of treatments and tests.
  - Encourage the parents to maintain discipline and consistency in their approach to parenting.
  - Encourage parents to maintain their expectations about academic achievements in school and at home.
  - Encourage the child to maintain relationships with peers and family members.
  - Encourage the child to maintain his or her usual level of responsibility within the family.
- Foster positive peer relationships.
  - Encourage the child to maintain contact with peers through visits, involvement with social activities, phone calls, videotapes, videophone, and letters.
  - Encourage socialization with peers, including those with cancer (e.g., camps, playroom, shared social activities).
  - Teach the child how to cope with teasing and name-calling.
- Foster the development of healthy coping.
  - Encourage play that will help the child maintain control during invasive procedures.
  - Prepare the child for procedures by explaining the sensations the child will feel, the reasons for them, and how they will occur; use visual aids and strategies the child can use to maintain self-control.
  - Help the child save face when the child loses his or her composure.
  - Praise the child for any signs of helpful behavior or positive coping.
  - Explain the cause of the disease and alleviate any feelings of responsibility and guilt the child might have.
  - Encourage open and honest communication and serve as a role model for this behavior.
- Facilitate the child's educational endeavors.
  - Use games to teach concepts.
  - Explain new information while building upon past experiences.
  - Educate teachers and school officials about the importance of normalizing their expectations and of providing tutors when they are needed.
  - Facilitate prompt reentry into school.
  - Encourage daily attendance at school.
  - Educate classmates about the child's condition and needs, dispel any myths they might have, and elicit their support.
  - Arrange for neuropsychology consultation and interventions if the child has developmental delays or is receiving neurotoxic therapies.
- Foster the child's independent functioning.
  - Avoid unnecessary restrictions.
  - Encourage involvement in tasks related to the treatment and reporting of side effects.
  - Encourage the parents to give the child freedom and responsibility to learn about his or her illness and its management.
  - Allow the child to have some control over some aspects of care.
  - Offer choices about tasks that must be accomplished, such as receiving medication, whenever possible.
  - Encourage self-care activities, such as dressing and brushing teeth.
  - Encourage the child to do as much for himself or herself as possible.

- Have a physical therapist and an occupational therapist work on the child's muscle strength, mobility, and ability to perform activities of daily living, as appropriate.
- Ensure that the child maintains a balance between rest and play.
- Help maintain privacy.

Expected Patient and Family Outcomes

- The outcomes of the nursing interventions are evaluated, and the plan of care is adjusted.
- The assessment is comprehensive, and reassessments are made on an ongoing basis.

Development of Adolescents (13–18 Years)

Linda Madsen

Normal Development

Psychosocial stage of identity versus identity confusion: The challenge for adolescents is to establish their own identity by examining and integrating their values and beliefs with those of society. Physical changes are rapid during this time; society's reactions to these changes acutely influence the self-concepts that adolescents have. The peer group is instrumental in helping an adolescent shape and try out future roles. The goals during this stage are to be able to make choices about an occupation and to form meaningful relationships outside the family. The framework is to develop values and ideologies that further the individual's future. An adolescent's overall goal is to answer the question, "Who am I?"

Cognitive stage: Adolescents are capable of abstract thought. They are also at the stage of formal operations, or the ability to reason and make predictions about things beyond their actual experience or knowledge. They can engage in introspection and are able to enhance the development of their values and beliefs. During this new intellectual stage in their development, they question theories and generate hypotheses.

Emotional and social characteristics: Teenagers' developing independence is their key characteristic. They vacillate between dependent and independent functioning. They believe that people around them are aware of all of their flaws—social, emotional, intellectual, and physical—leading them to feel embarrassed over small issues. Egocentrism and idealistic thinking are two of their characteristics. They are careful critics of the world and people around them, and see the world primarily from their own perspective.

The dominant focus of adolescents is to be accepted by and included in their peer group, which provides feedback about normative behavior. Their position in the peer group structure has a great influence on their sense of self-esteem. They value conformity. Physical differences may be threatening to the group.

Adolescents need privacy. Body image issues are acutely important; teens are extremely self-conscious about changes in their bodies and feel that others are acutely aware of these changes. Body image and how a person feels about body functioning and effectiveness are linked to a sense of worth; adolescents' self-esteem is linked to peer acceptance. A person's positive self-esteem is linked to recognition and approval by others of his or her accomplishments. Teenagers, however, have a tendency to feel personally inadequate. On the other hand, teens can have difficulty admitting a need for information or assistance.

Teenagers tend to focus on immediate or short-range goals and are interested in immediate gratification. They are emotionally labile because the hormonal changes they are undergoing lead to extreme fluctuations in emotions. Engaging in risk-taking behavior is common among adolescent, who tend to believe that bad things "won't happen to me" (i.e., the concept of the "personal fable"). This attitude also can lead to noncompliant behaviors.

Fears: Teenagers fear rejection by their peers, loss of self-control, loss of identity, loss of their ability to attain future goals, and loss of previously acquired independence.

Significant relationships: The most significant relationships teenagers have are with their peers, adult role models, and their families.

Risks to teenagers with cancer:

Loss of control and of independent functioning. Teenagers with cancer have an imposed dependence upon their caregivers, which can be exacerbated should their parents tend to overprotect them.

Devastating impact of alterations in body image or the ability to identify with peers. Teenagers' inability to identify with their peers and be accepted as part of the group can be detrimental to their self-esteem. Among the physical changes that can occur in teens with cancer are hair loss, moon face, acne, weight gain or loss, surgical incisions, and amputation, as well as their dependence on central lines and feeding tubes. They also can experience functional limitations, such as hemiparesis and weakness.

Poor peer relationships due to isolation from the group. Because of frequent absences from school and social events, teens might have too little interaction with their peers. In addition, poor self-esteem because of alterations in body image may lead a teen to avoid his or her peer group.

Rebellion and lack of compliance with treatment or supportive care. In their desire to be like their peers, teens may rebel and refuse to comply with their treatment or supportive care. Other factors associated with treatment noncompliance include a teenager's normal short-range focus and risk-taking behavior.

Loss of or change in the teen's goals for the future. Because of the rigors of therapy or a permanent disability or change in body functioning as a complication of disease or treatment, teens may have altered goals for their future. Goals also may change because they have shifted their priorities after facing a life-threatening disease.

Information deficits. Information deficits can occur because of teens' characteristic inability to admit to their knowledge gaps. A large volume of information is needed for patients to successfully manage their treatment.

Nursing Assessment and Interventions

Assessment:

- Assess current growth and developmental level.
- Determine the patient's level of success in interpersonal relationships and evaluate key relationships by questioning and observation.
- Assess the teen's ability to speak for himself or herself and participate significantly in decision-making, as well as the parent's ability to respect their teen's decisions.
- Identify key support people within the family, community, healthcare, and school settings.
- Interpret verbal and nonverbal cues about the effect of body image changes on the patient's self-concept. Take into account the extent of the changes to the body, the patient's perspective on these changes, and the amount of interest the patient has in his or her appearance.
- Assess the patient and family for healthy coping strategies and their level of adjustment by observing and questioning the following areas:
  - the ability to incorporate changes imposed by the disease and treatment into daily life
  - the level of the family's involvement in the teen's care and the teen's level of independence
  - the quality of the teen's relationships and level of involvement in his or her peer group
  - the ability to establish normalcy in relationships and activities
  - the level of participation in high-risk activities
  - the teen's personal affect and level of interest and involvement in life.
- Assess through discussion with the patient, family, and school staff the teen's ability to maintain academic performance and attendance, and whether he or she has taken an interest in planning for the future.
- Assess the impact of cancer and cancer therapies (including side effects and late effects) on the teen's future goals and aspirations.
- Assess the teen's level of sexual involvement and functioning to determine educational needs regarding sexuality, which should include
  - the use and importance of birth control measures during treatment
  - the use and importance of taking precautions against sexually transmitted diseases (STDs), including HIV
  - the potential effects of cancer treatment on fertility and sexual functioning.
- Assess the teen's ability to adhere to the treatment plan through ongoing dialogue about treatment and lifestyle considerations.
- Assess the patient's level of knowledge and desire for information about the disease and its treatment by having a discussion with the patient about his or her previous experience.

Interventions:

- Support the adolescent's autonomy.
  - Encourage the teen to take an active role in managing the disease.
  - Encourage caregivers to allow the teen the freedom and responsibility to learn and manage as many aspects of the illness as possible.
  - Encourage collaborative decision-making with the healthcare team.
  - Allow the teen control over as many aspects of his or her care as possible.
  - Respect the teen as an individual separate from parents by addressing questions to him or her and by discussing the teen's concerns without a parent present.
- Encourage self-care and maintenance of independence.
  - Through education, facilitate early recognition and careful, proactive management of side effects, such as pain and nausea, to minimize their effect on well-being.
  - Encourage the teen to do as much as possible for himself or herself.
  - Help the patient accept help when it is truly needed. Emphasize that such acceptance is a sign of strength and maturity, and that there are times when a problem is too difficult to solve alone.
  - Facilitate physical and occupational therapy referrals, if needed, to maintain or improve muscle strength, mobility, and the ability to perform activities of daily living.
  - Encourage the teen to break out of his or her role as "the sick one" and be as involved in life as feasible.
  - Respect the teen's wishes concerning the amount of assistance he or she needs.
- Encourage normalcy whenever possible.
  - Facilitate the teen's maintenance of routines and usual activities.
  - Be flexible with the timing of treatments and testing, when possible.
  - Encourage parents and teachers to maintain reasonably normal performance expectations of the teen.
  - Encourage parents to maintain discipline and be consistent in their approach to parenting.
  - Encourage the teen to maintain relationships with important people in his or her life.
- Encourage socialization and social support.

- Foster positive peer relationships (e.g., match patients on a one-to-one basis with peers who are off therapy).
- Provide information about online chat rooms for cancer patients.
- Provide opportunities for socialization with other patients such as retreats, camp, common in- and outpatient meeting places, and social events.
- Encourage contact with peers at home and school through phone calls, visits, letters, the Internet, and attendance at social activities.

• Foster the development of healthy self-esteem by promoting a positive body image.
  - Maintain privacy.
  - Encourage activities that enhance personal hygiene and appearance.
  - Encourage the teen to get up and dressed every day, even when hospitalized.
  - Encourage the patient to plan for hair loss by selecting attractive head coverings (e.g., wigs, hats, scarves).
  - Facilitate control of acne.
  - Encourage dress and cosmetics that minimize attention to scars, pigment changes, and weight changes.
  - Emphasize the temporary nature of the changes to the body.
  - Encourage activities that focus and build on strengths.

• Support adolescent hoping and coping.
  - Provide nursing care using a calm, competent approach. Facilitate the open expression of feelings, anxieties, beliefs, goals, and needs. Listen and respond honestly and be nonjudgmental. Alleviate symptoms promptly and anticipate needs.
  - Use humor and have a light-hearted approach. Let the patient tease you, if appropriate.
  - Maintain a positive, optimistic attitude.
  - Provide hopeful stories of others in similar situations.
  - Convey genuine concern for the individual's well-being.
  - Provide opportunities for spiritual support. Honor the patient's beliefs and values.
  - Teach the teen to put cancer in its place by accepting what is uncontrollable, and focusing instead on what he or she can control.
  - Help the teen develop a realistic focus and plan for the future using a goal-oriented approach. Help the teen see his or her strengths and how they can contribute to a healthy future. Give honest, positive feedback.
  - Provide psychological preparation for invasive and disfiguring procedures.
  - Model and encourage open and honest communication.
  - Normalize fears and concerns. Emphasize that a diminished sense of physical well-being is normal during treatment.
  - Allow the teen time alone for self-reflection, introspection, and thought.
  - Help the teen realize that he or she already possesses the strength to cope.
  - Approach teaching and the provision of support by explaining the common concerns and feelings of people in similar situations.
  - Facilitate the use of relaxation and imagery techniques for coping with side effects, pain, and anxiety.
  - Suggest hand-holding and other strategies that minimize anxiety and help maintain control during painful procedures. Offer your own hand to the patient to hold.

• Focus on wellness in the areas of adequate nutrition, rest and activity patterns, responsible sexual behavior, and avoidance of smoking, alcohol, and illicit drug use.
  - Explain how the individual can take control in all of these areas in order to be as well as possible.
  - Teach teens to pace activities and rest to lessen the effects of fatigue.
  - Teach the importance of birth control and precautions against STDs. Educate the teen about fertility and sexual functioning as they relate to therapy and the potential short-term and late effects of therapy.

• Facilitate a focus on education and career issues. Show how to adapt these goals, when necessary.

• Encourage attendance at school or facilitate tutoring when attendance is not feasible.
  - Assist with school accommodations as needed for disabilities or treatment.
  - Provide programming for school reentry if the teen wishes it.

• Educate the teen about the disease and treatment, including areas the individual can affect.
  - Provide multiple opportunities over the course of treatment for the teen to learn with staff.
  - Reinforce the importance of taking oral medications at home and adhering to the treatment plan. Partner with the adolescent to strategize ways to do this.
  - Suggest books, articles, videos, and computer resources for independent learning.
  - Look for signs that additional information may be needed. Clarify misinformation, dispel myths, and provide more in-depth information for those who seek it.
  - Encourage the teen to discuss with the healthcare team any information he or she finds independently. Some sources may be inaccurate or incomplete, or may be misunderstood.
  - Provide resources for learning about and writing advance directives (e.g., living will).

Expected Patient and Family Outcomes

- The outcomes of the interventions are evaluated, and the plan of care is adjusted.
- Comprehensive ongoing assessments are made.

Development of Young Adults (18–25 Years)

Linda Madsen and Mary C. Hooke

Normal Development

Psychosocial stage of intimacy versus isolation: The goals of young adulthood focus on committing oneself to concrete affiliations and partnerships. This stage builds on the identity established in adolescence. The egocentrism of adolescence is replaced by reciprocity in relationships. A young adult learns to develop an intimate, interpersonal relationship in which it is possible merge his or her identity with someone else without fear of losing the sense of self. The adolescent who does not have a secure identity will have difficulty developing intimacy in young adulthood. Relationships will remain shallow, and the young adult will experience a sense of isolation and loneliness.

Cognitive development: Piaget describes formal operational thought as the ability to reason about what is possible as well as what is real. Formal operational thought includes the ability to reason about hypotheses related to objects and problems, both present and future, and to reflect on the uniqueness of one's own thoughts and perspective. Adolescents should develop to this level, but typically reason in egocentric and narrow ways. They may reason that the best solutions to global problems (e.g., overpopulation, pollution) are the logical ones and be unable to appreciate mitigating factors, such as world politics and culture differences. As the adolescent becomes a young adult, the quality of thought may not change, but the quantity of what is reasoned will increase.

Emotional and social characteristics: Young adults are focused on developing adult identities. They are beginning to realize their potentials and to set and work on goals. They are transitioning from the relatively egocentric focus of adolescence to a more outward focus as they realize their interdependence on society. They begin to explore their place in society and how their individuality relates to relationships with other people. Significant others—partners, spouses, friends, family—may include their own children, coworkers, or members of the community. The ability to form intimate and caring relationships with others is key. Relationships are more mature and based on independent individuals finding connectedness, which is the foundation for deeper commitments. Initial exploration toward career goals lays the groundwork for a career.

The individual begins to strive toward financial, psychological, and physical independence and autonomous living. He or she is becoming accountable for his or her choices and the consequences of those choices. The young adult must deal with life's challenges and problems largely independently. The individual gets help only when necessary, when self-determination and resources are overwhelmed by the complexity of the challenges he or she faces.

The young adult begins to internalize morals and ideals. The goal is to be socially, physically, and intellectually competent to accomplish tasks. The well-adjusted young adult is able to maintain individuality and independence while remaining connected to the family. He or she has a sense of self-confidence and competence, character, connection to the larger world, and caring or compassion toward others. To successfully complete development, the healthy, productive adult must

- find a valued place in a constructive group
- learn how to form close, durable human relationships
- feel worthwhile as an individual
- achieve a reliable basis for making informed choices
- know how and when to use support systems
- express constructive curiosity and exploratory behavior
- find ways to be useful to others
- believe in a promising future with real opportunities

Fears: The young adult facing a diagnosis or relapse of cancer may fear isolation, loneliness, and loss of independence (both physical and psychological), self-determination, usefulness, and future goals and aspirations. The patient may fear becoming less physically attractive or a burden to a spouse or romantic partner. The patient may worry about his or her future fertility or about children he or she already has. Educational or career plans may need to be put on hold. The necessity of maintaining employer-provided health insurance can limit career options. However, treatment can make it difficult for the patient to continue working. Treatment expenses or the loss of his or her job or supportive relationships can force the young adult to depend on his or her parents financially. Mortality comes into the young adult's reality at a time when planning for the future normally is the primary focus.

Risks:

Altered body image. Altered physical appearance or body image can have a devastating impact on the young adult's ability to pursue or maintain intimate relationships. Physical attractiveness can be affected by acne, hair loss, moon face, weight changes, surgical incisions, loss of limb functioning, and so on, potentially inhibiting the individual's perceived or real ability to pursue romantic relationships.

Isolation from school/work/community. Such isolation may mean the loss of opportunities to develop relationships with others and pursue and explore career goals.

Loss of ability to maintain or develop intimacy with significant others. Real or perceived changes may lead to isolation. The patient may be deprived of opportunities to explore social relationships or lack the energy to do so.

Change of goals or timeline for achieving goals. The complications of living with cancer can cause a change in the timeline for goal achievement or a complete inability to attain previously planned goals. Goals also might change because facing a life-threatening disease may cause a young adult to realign his or her priorities.

Loss of independent functioning. Perceived or necessary financial, social, or physical dependence on others. Dependence may be overemphasized because some families tend toward overprotection.

Nursing Assessment and Interventions

Assessment:

- Assess the patient's current growth and developmental level.
- Determine the patient's level of success in interpersonal relationships, and evaluate key relationships by questioning and observation.
- Assess the extent of the patient's peer contacts and involvement in work, school, community, and outside activities.
- Assess the patient's ability to make independent decisions and the ability of the patient's parents and significant others to respect those decisions.
- Identify key support persons within the family, community, healthcare, school, and work settings.
- Interpret verbal and nonverbal cues about the effect of body image changes on the patient's self-concept. Take into account the extent of the changes to the body, the patient's perspective on these changes, and the amount of interest the young adult has in his or her appearance.
- Assess the patient, family, and, if applicable, the significant other for healthy coping strategies and their level of adjustment by observing and questioning the following areas:
  - the ability to incorporate changes imposed by the disease and treatment into daily life
  - the level of the family's involvement in the patient's care
  - the patient's level of independence
  - the ability to establish normalcy in relationships and activities
  - the level of participation in high-risk activities
  - the young adult's personal affect and level of interest and involvement in life
- Assess the young adult's ability to maintain work and/or academic performance and attendance and level of interest in planning for the future.
- Assess the impact of cancer and cancer therapies (including side effects and late effects) on the young adult's future goals and aspirations.
- Assess caregiving resources for patients who are responsible for own children.
- Assess the young adult's level of sexual involvement and functioning to determine educational needs regarding sexuality, which should include
  - the use and importance of birth control measures during treatment
  - the use and importance of taking precautions against STDs, including HIV
  - the potential effects of cancer treatment on fertility and sexual functioning.
- Assess the young adult's ability to adhere to the treatment plan through ongoing dialogue about treatment information and lifestyle considerations.
- Assess the patient's level of knowledge and desire for information about the disease and its treatment by having a discussion with the patient about his or her previous experience.
- Assess the patient's knowledge of advance directives.
- Assess the patient's ability to act as his or her own advocate in the healthcare system.

Interventions:

- Support the young adult's autonomy.
  - Encourage the young adult to take an active role in managing the disease.
  - Encourage self-advocacy and collaborative decision-making with the healthcare team.
  - Allow the young adult control over as many aspects of care as possible.
  - Respect the patient's privacy, keeping discussions with him or her confidential, and sharing information with support persons only after the patient has given permission to do so.
- Encourage self-care and maintenance of independence.
  - Through education, facilitate early recognition and careful, proactive management of side effects, such as pain and nausea, to minimize their effect on well-being.
  - Encourage the young adult to do as much for himself or herself as possible.
  - Help the patient accept help when it is truly needed. Emphasize that such acceptance is a sign of strength and maturity, and that there are times when a problem is too difficult to solve alone.
  - Facilitate physical and occupational therapy referral, if needed, to maintain or improve muscle strength, mobility, and the ability to perform activities of daily living.
  - Encourage the young adult to break out of his or her role as "the sick one" and to be as involved in life as possible.
  - Respect the individual's wishes concerning the amount of assistance he or she needs.
- Encourage normalcy whenever possible.
  - Facilitate the maintenance of the patient's routines and usual activities.
  - Be flexible, when possible, with the timing of treatments and testing.

- Encourage family, teachers, and colleagues to maintain reasonably normal school and work expectations.
- Encourage the patient to maintain important relationships.
- Encourage the patient to fulfill his or her responsibilities.
- Encourage the young adult to care for his or her children and to obtain child care, when needed.

• Encourage socialization and social support.
- Foster positive peer relationships (e.g., match patients on a one-to-one basis with peers who are off therapy).
- Provide information about online chat rooms for cancer patients.
- Provide opportunities for socialization with other patients, such as retreats, young adult conferences, common inpatient and outpatient meeting places, and social events.
- Encourage contact with peers at home, work, and/or school through phone calls, visits, letters, the Internet, and attendance at social activities.
- Facilitate the patient's ability to have time alone with his or her significant other.

• Foster the development of a healthy self-esteem through a positive body image.
- Maintain privacy.
- Encourage activities that enhance hygiene and personal appearance.
- Encourage the patient to get up and dressed every day, even when hospitalized.
- Encourage the patient to plan for hair loss by selecting attractive head coverings (e.g., wigs, hats, scarves).
- Facilitate control of acne.
- Encourage dress and cosmetics that minimize attention to scars, pigment changes, and changes in weight.
- Emphasize the temporary nature of the changes to the body.
- Encourage activities that focus on and build strengths.

• Support the young adult's hope and coping skills.
- Provide nursing care using a calm, competent approach. Facilitate the open expression of feelings, anxieties, beliefs, goals, and needs. Listen and respond honestly, and be nonjudgmental. Alleviate symptoms promptly and anticipate needs.
- Use humor and have a lighthearted approach. Let the patient tease you, if appropriate.
- Maintain a positive, optimistic attitude.
- Provide hopeful stories of others in similar situations.

Resources for Patients, Families, Health Professionals, and Educators

Web Sites

American Association for Cancer Education
http://www.aaceonline.com/index.asp

American Cancer Society
http://www.cancer.org

Association of Pediatric Oncology Nurses
http://www.apon.org

Bandaids & Blackboards
http://www.faculty.fairfield.edu/fleitas/contents.html

CancerSourceKids
http://www.cancersourcekids.com/

Cancervive
http://www.cancervive.org

CaringBridge
http://www.caringbridge.org/

Children's Oncology Group
http://www.childrensoncologygroup.org/

Leukemia & Lymphoma Society
http://www.leukemia.org

National Childhood Cancer Foundation
http://www.conquerkidscancer.org/

National Cancer Institute Cancer Information
http://www.nci.nih.gov/cancerinfo

National Cancer Institute Clinical Trials
http://www.nci.nih.gov/clinicaltrials

KidsHealth
http://www.kidshealth.org

Starbright Pediatric Network
http://www.starbright.org

Teens Living with Cancer
http://www.teenslivingwithcancer.org

Publications

Fighting Chance: Journeys through Childhood Cancer
Harry Connolly, Woodholme House Publishers, 800/488-0051

I Will Sing Life: Voices from the Hole in the Wall Gang Camp,
Larry Berger and Dahlia Lithwick, Little, Brown & Co., 800/759-0180

The Alphabet About Kids with Cancer
Rita Berglund, The Children's Legacy, 303/830-7595

In addition to the publications listed here, numerous cancer publications are available through organizations whose Web sites are listed here.

- Convey genuine concern for the individual's well-being.
- Provide opportunities for spiritual support. Honor the patient's beliefs and values.
- Teach the young adult to put cancer in its place by accepting what is uncontrollable. Encourage the patient to focus on what he or she can control.
- Help the individual develop a realistic focus and plan for the future using a goal-oriented approach. Help the individual to see their own strengths and how they can contribute to a healthy future. Give honest, positive feedback.
- Provide psychological preparation for invasive and disfiguring procedures.
- Model and encourage open and honest communication.
- Normalize fears and concerns. Stress that a diminished sense of physical well-being is normal during treatment.
- Facilitate the patient taking time alone for self-reflection, introspection, and thought.
- Help the young adult realize that perhaps without realizing it, he or she already possesses the strength to cope.
- Approach teaching and the provision of support by explaining the common concerns and feelings of people in similar situations.
- Facilitate the use of relaxation and imagery techniques for coping with side effects, pain, and anxiety.
- Suggest hand-holding and other strategies that minimize anxiety and help the patient maintain control during painful procedures. Offer your own hand to the patient to hold.

• Focus on wellness, such as adequate nutrition, rest and activity patterns, responsible sexual behavior, and avoidance of smoking, alcohol, and illicit drug use.
  - Explain how the individual can take control in all of these areas to remain as healthy as possible.
  - Teach the patient to pace activities and rest to help alleviate and compensate for feelings of fatigue.
  - Teach the importance of birth control and precautions against STDs. Educate the young adult about fertility and sexual functioning as they relate to therapy and the potential short-term and late effects of therapy.
  - Facilitate a focus on education and career issues. Show how to adapt goals, when necessary.
• Encourage the patient to attend school, or facilitate tutoring when attendance is not feasible.
  - Assist the patient to obtain the necessary documentation for work or school if medical treatment or assistance with disabilities is needed.
  - Educate the young adult about the disease and treatment, including areas he or she can affect.
  - Provide multiple opportunities over the course of treatment for the patient to learn with staff.
  - Reinforce the importance of taking oral medications at home and adhering to the treatment plan. Partner with the patient to strategize ways to do this.
  - Suggest books, articles, videos, and computer resources for independent learning.
  - Look for signs that additional information may be needed. Clarify misinformation, dispel myths, and provide more in-depth information for those who seek it.
  - Encourage the young adult to discuss with the healthcare team any information he or she finds independently. Some sources may be inaccurate or incomplete, or may be misunderstood.
  - Provide resources for learning about and writing advance directives.

Expected Patient and Family Outcomes

• The outcomes of the interventions are evaluated, and the plan of care is adjusted.
• Comprehensive ongoing assessments are made.

Family Systems

Lona Roll

Definition

The diagnosis of cancer in a child is a critical life event for the entire family. A complete assessment of such a family requires a multidisciplinary approach that involves all members of the healthcare team and their evaluations of different aspects of the family's dynamics. Collaboration among team members is essential.

The Institute for Family-Centered Care (2003) recognizes that a family-centered approach empowers the healthcare team and families, fosters independence, supports family caregiving and decision-making, respects patient and family choices, respects their cultural background, builds on individual and family strengths, and involves patients and families when delivery and evaluation of heathcare services are being planned.

The definition of family in this era has become complex. The basic definition of the family resides with the family itself. Identifying key members of the family, how they interact, and who ultimately will be responsible for the care of the child permits the nurse to plan interventions tailored to that family's particular needs and level of comprehension. Family approaches to the crisis of cancer in a child vary depending upon a cancer's stage of development and the degree of support that is available. Parents of a young toddler who are not yet comfortable in their parenting role will deal with issues that are different from those of the parents of a teenager who are dealing with the adolescent stage of their child's development.

Understanding the coping strategies that family members have used in previous crises can help a nurse support them through the many challenges of cancer therapy. Coping is a response to a stressful event that can be viewed as a process that leads to a desirable outcome. Coping strategies will change over time. There is no objective definition of "good" or "bad" coping; instead, these strategies should be appraised in light of their outcomes.

People will use coping strategies based upon their appraisal of a stressful situation. For example, some parents will seek information when faced with the unknown challenge of childhood cancer as a way of taking control of the situation. Others may find that some form of denial or avoidance will help them through the initial trauma caused by a cancer diagnosis. Problems may arise when one parent uses a coping strategy that is at odds with that of the other parent.

Being aware of various coping styles, and identifying those that are being used by family members, can help clinicians develop intervention strategies, such as identifying which parent to educate about the home care needs of the patient, or determining how to support the family through the difficult days after a diagnosis. Clarke-Steffen (1993) presented a model showing the transition of a family from its state before a child's diagnosis to a "new normal" state (**Figure 7-1**), which the author says is "characterized by a new daily routine that incorporates the medical regimen, uncertainty, and a new world view" (p. 290). All families move through this transition at their own pace and require varying degrees of support from their treatment team.

Because the family system is a dynamic, changing system, the nursing process in relation to family assessment should be used for each stage of cancer therapy, including diagnosis, treatment, end of treatment, relapse, and terminal care.

Nursing Assessment and Interventions

Assessment: Assessment of a family of a child diagnosed with cancer is an ongoing process in which all members of the multidisciplinary team (medical, nursing, psychology, social work, and child-life staff) participate.

At the time of diagnosis. The initial assessment at the time of diagnosis unfortunately must occur at a time when the family is undergoing a major crisis.

- Assess the following characteristics of the family:
  - family composition (i.e., who are the members of the family)
  - occupation and educational levels of family members
  - cultural and religious traditions

Figure 7-1. Model of Family Transition to Living with Childhood Cancer

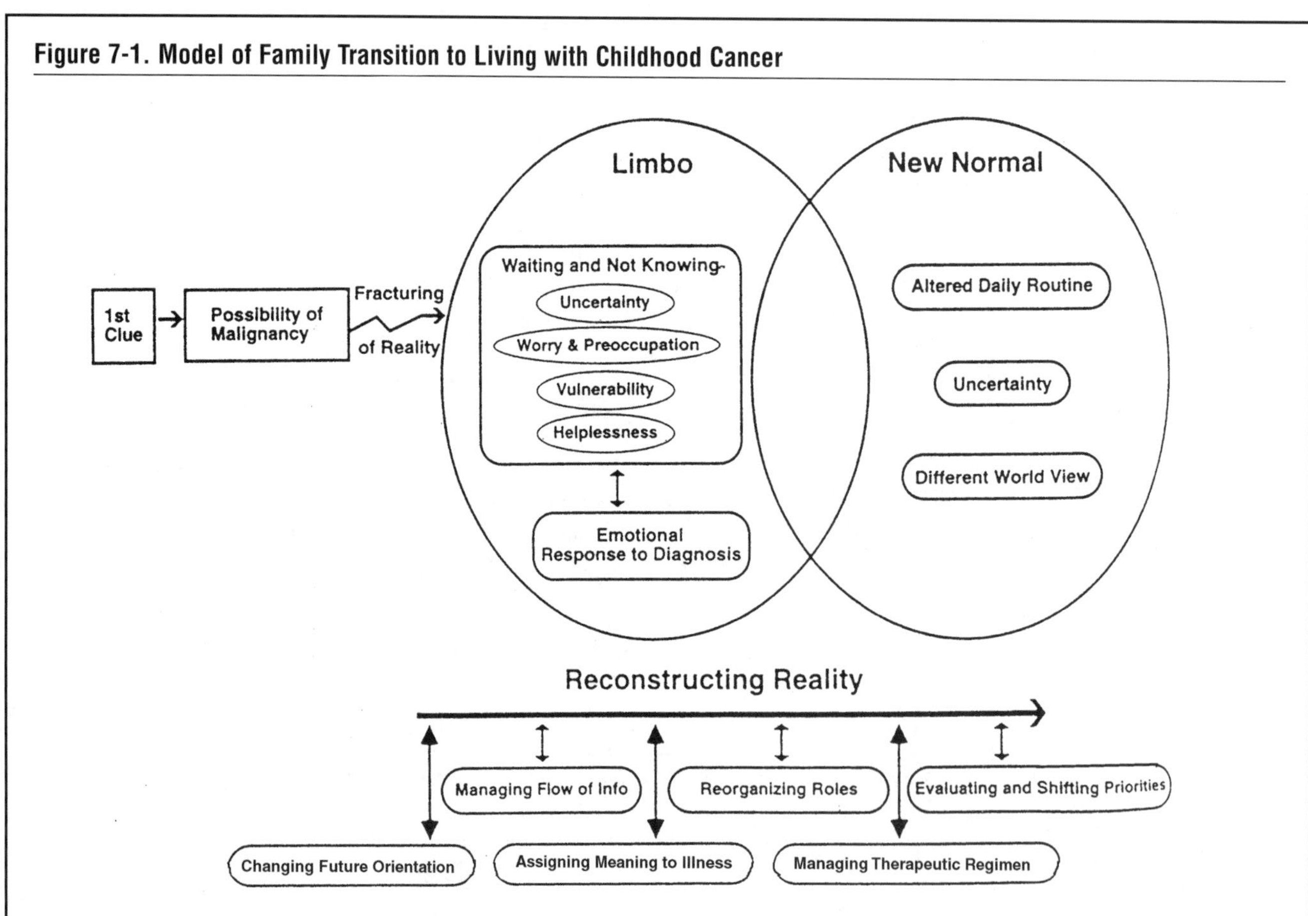

Note: From "A Model of the Family Transition to Living with Childhood Cancer," by L. Clarke-Steffen, 1993, Cancer Practice, 1, p. 288. Copyright 1993 by Lippincott-Raven. Adapted with permission.

- communication and interaction patterns (i.e., how members relate to each other and express their emotions)
- decision-making and problem-solving dynamics (i.e., who makes and enforces family rules and follows through on family members' problems).

- Perform an emotional assessment of the varied responses of family members.
- Assess for shock, disbelief, and fear:
  - Do family members ask for second or third opinions?
  - Do they seek medical information?
  - Do they use protective mechanisms to soften the reality of the cancer diagnosis?
- Assess for expressions of guilt and anger:
  - Family members may direct their anger at the treatment team or, many times, at those who initially informed them of the diagnosis.
  - Parents may express feelings of guilt and ask why their child has cancer, what they could have done to have caused it, and why they did not detect it earlier.
- Assess for factors that may make it very difficult for families to cope, such as having a single-parent or stepfamily structure, preexisting physical or mental health problems, economic problems, language differences, or isolation from cultural supports.

During treatment. The assessment of the family's adaptation to living with illness should continue during the child's treatment. The assessment should include

- the family's adjustment to having the child live at home after inpatient care, caring for the child, and sharing the burden of care
- the family's return to "routine"
- the family's compliance with maintaining the child's medical regimens
- the ability of the patient's siblings to adapt to and cope with their new lifestyle.

After treatment ends. This assessment should include the family's reaction to the end of the child's treatment routine and the family's fears about relapse in the absence of active treatment. Continue the ongoing assessment and follow-up with the patient to monitor for potential long-term effects of the cancer therapy.

During a relapse. This period is viewed as the most difficult time for many families because they are aware of the struggles ahead and the decreased likelihood of a patient's long-term survival. This assessment should include

- the family's need for further preparation regarding their child's possible need for more intensive chemotherapy
- the family's support system (i.e., who has proven to be a strong support for the family and can continue to help it during this very trying time).

During the period of terminal care.

- Assess the family's coping abilities and whether they need and desire further, possibly unconventional treatment or have accepted that all further care will be terminal care.
- Determine what the family's desires are concerning where the child should die (i.e., at home or in a hospital) when such a choice is possible (see Section IX, "Care for the Terminally Ill Child and the Family").
- Assess the needs of the patient's siblings and extended family. For further details, see the discussion of terminal care in Section VIII, "Patient and Family Education."

Interventions: Psychosocial interventions for the family of a child diagnosed with cancer require planning and support from the entire treatment team, including professionals from the areas of medicine, nursing, psychology, social work, and child-life, who must work together to develop coordinated approaches for each family.

At the time of diagnosis. (**Table 7-1** lists the family's coping tasks and interventions at the time of diagnosis.) Healthcare professionals need to perform the following interventions:

- Help the family meet its basic needs, including those involving sleeping arrangements, food, clothes, and care of the patient's siblings.
- Help the family interpret medical information; ideally, the primary nurse should be present at the initial discussion with the family to clarify the information that is being presented.
- Explain and review hospital routines and the care being given to the child.
- Encourage the parents to maintain their parenting role by comforting the child, explaining the diagnosis to the child, and setting limits on the child's behavior, as needed.
- Prepare the family for the child's transition to the home:
  - Begin early in the child's hospitalization to provide information related to the patient's eventual discharge.
  - Reassure the parents that they still are the best caregivers for their child.
  - Reassure the parents that someone from the treatment team always will be available to them when they are at home.

During treatment. (**Table 7-1** lists the family's coping tasks and interventions during treatment.)

- Continue to help the family understand the treatment protocol.
- Help the family identify the side effects of the treatment and appropriate interventions.
- Reassure the family that it is doing well in interpreting events that occur in relation to the sick child (i.e., do some hand-holding with the family).
- Help the parents reestablish their protective, nurturing role.

At the end of treatment. (**Table 7-2** lists the family's coping tasks and interventions at the time treatment ends.)

- Prepare the parents for the transition from treatment to survival and the task of "getting on with life."
- Encourage the parents to view their child as normal.

Table 7-1. Family Coping Tasks and Nursing Interventions During Diagnosis and Treatment

Essential Coping Tasks	Interventions
At the time of diagnosis	
Gaining control of emotions	Allow time for parents to be alone to grieve.
Alleviating acute anxiety	Maintain hope for the child no matter how serious the situation is. Allow family members to express their feelings and fears.
Understanding the diagnosis	Spend time discussing the diagnosis and its meaning before presenting a plan for treatment.
Explaining cancer to the child	Use terms the child can understand; tell the child about cancer and the need for treatment.
Establishing the treatment regimen	Begin discussions with the parents and the child about the treatment regimen and its side effects.
Preventing anxiety regarding discharge and home care	Begin early to discuss care for the child at home. Identify key individuals who will assist the family at home.
Allowing for participation of family members	Discuss with siblings and other family members the child's diagnosis and treatment. Encourage siblings to visit the child.
During treatment	
Accepting the diagnosis	Allow for ongoing discussion of the diagnosis with parents and family members. Reinforce with the parents that it is normal to have continued fears and doubts.
Understanding the treatment and its side effects	Throughout the treatment, continue discussions of the treatment and its side effects to increase the family's understanding.
Identifying support systems	Help the family to identify individuals and groups who will support the family during times of crisis.
Establishing alternative routines, lifestyle	Provide opportunities for the family to begin reestablishing its lifestyle to meet each family member's needs. Encourage activities the family participated in before the diagnosis. Stress the importance of the child's return to school.
Providing support for the child	Allow the child to express his or her own thoughts and feelings, separate from those of the parents. Provide opportunities for age-appropriate play therapy, especially for invasive procedures. Provide the child with explanations for body changes occurring as a result of the disease or treatment.
Encouraging siblings' participation	Stress the importance of including siblings in conversations and care. Allow siblings to accompany the child to the hospital when possible. Stress that the parents need to provide time alone with their other children at home.

Note: From *Pediatric Oncology and Hematology: Perspectives on Care* (pp. 436, 440), M.J. Hockenberry and D.K. Coody (Eds.), 1986, St. Louis: C.V. Mosby. Copyright 1986 by C.V. Mosby. Adapted with permission.

- Review the follow-up plan and reassure the parents that the child still will be followed closely by the treatment team for signs of relapse or late effects of therapy.

At the time of a relapse. (**Table 7-3** lists the family's coping tasks and interventions when the child has a relapse.)

- Provide empathy and support to family members as they adjust to the initial shock of the child's relapse.
- Provide information to the family about new treatment plans.
- Arrange assistance for family members if they must travel to another treatment center with the child for specialized care.
- Explain the meaning of relapse and new treatment options to the extended family and to other support systems.

During the period of terminal care. (See section IX, "Care for the Terminally Ill Child and the Family," for a discussion of interventions.)

Expected Patient and Family Outcomes

- A multidisciplinary team approach is used to assess family coping and use of resources at each stage of care.
- Families are able to move through all stages of the diagnosis and treatment of childhood cancer with their psychological care needs being met by a multidisciplinary team.

Table 7-2. Family Coping Tasks and Nursing Interventions at the Time of Discontinuation of Therapy

Essential Coping Tasks	Interventions
Adapting to discontinuing treatment	Begin discussions several months before therapy is discontinued. Allow time for the parents and the child to ask questions and verbalize their concerns.
Recognizing the fear of a relapse	Discuss openly the possibility of relapse. Review the concerns of the parents and the child regarding what to expect if a relapse should occur.
Realizing the impact of a parent's attitude	Discuss the importance of the parents' attitudes and how they affect the child. Stress the importance of verbalizing fears while recognizing the positive situation of discontinuing therapy.
Supporting the child's needs and preventing fears	Reassure the child that therapy would not be discontinued unless he or she was doing well. Allow the child to express fears separately from the parents (provide support and stress the need for courage and trust).

Note: From Pediatric Oncology and Hematology: Perspectives on Care (p. 443), M.J. Hockenberry and D.K. Coody (Eds.), 1986, St. Louis: C.V. Mosby. Copyright 1986 by C.V. Mosby. Adapted with permission.

Table 7-3. Family Coping Tasks and Nursing Interventions at the Time of a Relapse

Essential Coping Tasks	Interventions
Alleviating the initial shock of the relapse	Allow the parents to express their shock and disbelief. Provide time for grieving before initiating discussion of a treatment plan.
Understanding the impact of a relapse	Discuss the seriousness of the relapse, yet provide hope in the situation. Offer facts regarding the possible outcome of the disease.
Discussing the relapse with the child	Express the importance of being truthful with the child. Discuss the relapse with the child and the need to begin therapy again (realize the child will perceive the seriousness of the situation by observing his or her parents and the staff).
Expressing appropriate feelings of grief	Encourage an expression of feelings and the need for the family to maintain a realistic outlook toward the situation. Identify key support individuals to maintain a close follow-up with all family members.

Note: From *Pediatric Oncology and Hematology: Perspectives on Care* (p. 446), M.J. Hockenberry and D.K. Coody (Eds.), 1986, St. Louis: C.V. Mosby. Copyright 1986 by C.V. Mosby. Adapted with permission.

References

Clarke-Steffen, L. (1993). A model of the family transition to living with childhood cancer. *Cancer Practice, 1,* 285–292.

Institute for Family Centered Care (2003). *What is Family Centered Care?* Retrieved August 29, 2003, from: http://www.familycenteredcare.org/

Family Resources

Suzanne Nuss

Many childhood malignancies that were once considered fatal now are curable. Because of this fact, pediatric oncology patients today require nursing interventions that were not needed in the past. Prevention of acute and late toxic effects of therapy, maintenance of wellness in the child during and after therapy, and support of the efforts of patients' families as they cope with a chronic, life-threatening illness, are major functions of nursing.

Nursing strategies to promote the family's role as primary caregivers for the child include recognizing and accepting diverse styles of family coping, helping families recognize their strengths and methods of coping, reassuring parents that their roles are important and essential, promoting family-centered care and communicating with local healthcare teams to offer continuity of care (Scoti-Findlay & Chalmers, 2001; Walker, Wells, Heiney, & Hymovich, 2002).

It is important to stress that the patient's entire family is affected by a cancer diagnosis. Preexisting factors, such as cultural influences, employment situations, family dynamics, home environment, finances, socioeconomic situations, or support systems, affect how a family functions or copes. If any of these factors are unstable when a cancer diagnosis is made, the entire family system can break down. Nurses have a responsibility to perform a thorough assessment to determine the types of resources that a family may require to cope with the cancer experience of one of its members.

Nursing Assessment

The home environment: All children with cancer have special needs; however, those from rural areas must deal with adverse circumstances not encountered by children from urban areas, where the university-based tertiary medical centers that provide the majority of pediatric oncology care are located. These circumstances include lack of tertiary health care and the need to travel long distances for treatment, necessitating the family to take on more responsibility for the child's care (Scoti-Findlay & Chalmers, 2001). As a result of the special needs of these children, the National Association of Children's Hospitals and Related Institutions (NACHRI) has developed recommendations for caring for children with cancer in the home setting (NACHRI Patient Care Oncology FOCUS Group, 2000).

- Assess the accessibility of the child's home in relation to the child's special needs.
  - Is the home easy to enter and exit?
  - Does the home have stairs? Is the child capable of climbing stairs? Is the caregiver capable of carrying the child if the child is unable to climb stairs?
- Assess the level of cleanliness of the child's home.
  - How clean is the environment? Are there infestations or rodents?
  - Is there an area where Hickman catheter care can be performed or IV medication can be given?
  - Does the home have running water?
- Determine the proximity of the child's home to the treatment center and assess the family's plan for their child in an emergency situation, such as high fever or neutropenia.
- Assess the family's transportation needs.
  - Does the family have access to a car? Is the car reliable?
  - Does the family have access to public transportation if it is needed?
  - If the patient should have to be taken to the hospital by ambulance, is the treatment center the closest hospital, or would advance arrangements need to be made with an ambulance company?
- Does the family have a telephone? If not, is there a nearby phone that can be used in an emergency?

Finances and medical coverage: According to Scoti-Findlay and Chalmers (2001), rural families who lived long distances from the medical center experienced "great financial hardship" (p. 215) because of excessive travel to and from the tertiary care center (including fuel and car maintenance), lodging, and meals. In addition, patients from rural areas often are from farm families. Consequently, time away from the farm for treatments adds to the financial burdens of these families. Often, there is little or no financial assistance to help families defray these additional expenses.

- Determine whether the family has medical insurance; if not, determine whether the family should be referred to a financial counselor.
- Make an assessment of possible incidental expenses the family could incur (e.g., buying meals, paying for housing near the medical center). Does the family have the funds to cover these incidental expenses?
- If the family has medical insurance, determine whether the policy covers home care; if so, determine what is covered, including how many hours of nursing care.
  - How much must the family pay on its own before the insurance will pay 100% of the child's medical expenses? Does the family have the funds to cover these out-of-pocket expenses?
  - Does the family's insurance program include a prescription plan?
  - Does the insurance company require precertification for all hospital admissions? If so, who will ensure that precertification is done?

Family dynamics: In American society, individualism, competition, nuclear families, and a future orientation are highly valued. Despite these values of the dominant culture, many diverse groups continue to maintain their ethnic self-identity, values, norms, behaviors, and language. People from diverse ethnic groups may place a higher value on the needs and traditions of the group, such as conformity, extended family, and mutual empathy. A thorough assessment of the family dynamics must be made so that the family can be supported appropriately.

- Assess the family's primary cultural influences.
  - Are there any types of restrictions?
  - Does the family's culture prevent family members from asking questions?
- Determine the parents' employment status.
  - Do the parents work?
  - Must they work for financial reasons?

FAMILY RESOURCES: A CASE STUDY

Delilah is an 18-year-old female who received an unrelated bone marrow transplant (BMT) more than 2 years ago as treatment for acute mylogenous leukemia (AML). Although her actual BMT course was fairly uneventful, Delilah developed chronic graft-versus-host disease (cGVHD) of the skin (scleraderma). The cGVHD was treated with steroids and photopheresis. Due to prolonged immunosuppression, Delilah developed pulmonary *aspergillus* and atypical mycobacterium, which was diagnosed with bronchcoscopy. Despite treatment, her chest X ray and chest CT scan remained abnormal. It was decided that a lung biopsy was necessary to determine if the treatment was appropriate. A needle biopsy was inconclusive, so an open-lung biopsy was performed that indicated *Bronchiolitis obliterans* (a pulmonary manifestation of cGVHD). During her postoperative period, Delilah developed a pneumothorax and pericardial effusion. She required mechanical ventilation for approximately 5 weeks and, eventually, a tracheostomy.

Family history revealed that Delilah lived with her mother, father, sister, and brother in a small town approximately 120 miles from a tertiary care center. Her mother worked in the business office of a nursing home and carried the family medical insurance. Her father was a truck driver, but was presently out of work. Delilah's sister was attending college, but quit to be with Delilah when she became ill. Her brother worked full-time.

The mother had a tendency to become overly anxious with even slight changes in Delilah's condition. Delilah and mother had similar personalities, so when the mother became anxious, Delilah's anxiety also escalated, and she usually required an antianxiety medication. Her sister and father stayed fairly calm during these high anxiety situations. The brother had minimal involvement with Delilah or with her care. Delilah's home care needs included total parenteral nutrition (TPN), tracheostomy care, physical therapy, and speech therapy.

Delilah's home was at least 7 miles from the local hospital—a small, rural hospital with limited resources. Three home care companies were contacted before one agreed to provide services for Delilah in her small town.

Below are the issues that arose as discharge planning for Delilah was initiated, and the nursing interventions that were made for each of these issues.

Assessment:
There is a need to care for Delilah and her new tracheostomy, but without a healthcare facility nearby.

Interventions:

- All aspects of tracheostomy teaching were initiated 7–10 days prior to discharge.
- Delilah was transferred to a cooperative care inpatient unit (unit where family provides major care, with nurses available to answer questions) as a transition to home.
- Tracheostomy supplies were delivered to the family at the tertiary care center instead of home, and Delilah was discharged to the campus hotel so that the family was responsible for all care, using home supplies, but was only an elevator ride away from healthcare personnel.

Assessment:
There is a need to deal with the baseline anxiety of family members.

Interventions:

- Delilah's sister was trained as primary caregiver, her father as secondary caregiver, and her mother as tertiary care giver.
- Teaching was reinforced as often as possible.

Assessment:
Concern was expressed regarding what to do in an emergency once home.

Interventions:

- A plan to drive to the ER, instead of calling an ambulance, was discussed.
- The plan was put into written form so the family could read it in case of an emergency (to decrease anxiety level).
- A local physician was notified of Delilah's return to the community.

Assessment:
The distance of Delilah's hometown to tertiary care center and home health agencies was a barrier to care.

Interventions:

- Numerous calls were made until a home care company could be found that would accept Delilah as a home care patient.
- Availability by phone of tertiary care center staff to local healthcare professionals was offered to local agencies.

Assessment:
There existed a potential for multiple medical referrals to be made by various caregivers.

Interventions:

- Tracheostomy care and supplies were provided by one company only; TPN and central line supplies were provided exclusively by a second company; and physical therapy and speech therapy were provided only by home health.
- For consistency, the pediatric oncology clinical nurse specialist made all referrals.
- A listing of all of these companies, the contact person, and the phone numbers, as well as the contact personnel from the tertiary care center, was compiled and placed in Delilah's chart .

Assessment:
There was an urgent need for continued medical insurance.

Interventions:

- Attempts were made to schedule all follow-up care (oncology, surgery, ENT) for the same day to minimize trips to the tertiary care center as much as possible.
- Delilah's father was encouraged to bring Delilah to appointments so that her mother's absences from work were minimized.

- Will the parent(s) continue to work?
- Do they have flexible work hours?
- Will the parents be able to leave work for emergencies?

- Assess the composition of the family constellation.
  - Who lives in the household?
  - What is the developmental stage of the family?
- Determine whether there are other children in the family and whether there are other family members who are also receiving medical care.
- Determine the level of the parents' involvement in their children's care.
  - Are there two parents living with the family, or is the child from a single-parent household?
  - If this is a single-parent family, does the parent have to work for financial reasons and medical benefits?
  - When the patient is hospitalized, who will provide care for the patient's siblings, if there are any?
- Assess various members' roles within the family structure.
  - What roles did the family members play before the cancer diagnosis?
  - Will family members' roles change as a consequence of the child's illness?
  - How will those role changes need to be renegotiated when treatment has been completed?
- Find out whether the family has any spiritual concerns.
  - Does the family rely on religion, spirituality, or both?
  - Does the family have the support of the religious community to which it belongs?
- Assess the stability of the family.
  - Does the family have any preexisting, ongoing concerns (e.g., marital difficulties, financial concerns)?

Resources: The coping strategies and available support systems for the patient and the family vary. The way in which patients or families accept assistance also varies. The major strategies that parents use to cope with their children's illnesses include reading books about different aspects of childhood cancer, talking with a counselor during times of stress, talking with another parent whose child has cancer, and attending group meetings. Many parents also obtain information from the Internet. (Caution must be advised, however, as not all of the information that is found on the Internet is accurate.) Although there are many community-based resources available to help patients and families with treatment, rehabilitation, and financing, patients and their families frequently are unaware of the services that are offered. Assess the family's resources.

- Determine the family's availability (i.e., is it available to learn about the child's illness and treatment).
- Assess the family's emotional capabilities (i.e., are members emotionally capable of absorbing the information).
- Establish whether there are existing support systems for the family (e.g., friends, other family members, clergy, teachers).
- Determine how much the family understands about the child's illness and treatment.
- Determine whether the family has communication barriers.
  - Do the members of the healthcare team and the family speak the same language? If not, is an interpreter readily available?
- Ascertain whether family members have any learning disabilities that might prevent them from learning about the child's disease and its treatment.
- Determine whether the family perceives a need for support; if so, is it willing to accept support?
- Find out whether any other family members have illnesses or physical limitations.
  - Does the primary caregiver have any medical conditions or physical limitations that might prevent him or her from caring for the patient?
- Assess the family's coping skills.
  - Has the family ever had a stressor of this magnitude?
  - Do family members have similar or different coping skills?

Nursing Interventions

The home environment:

- Refer the family to a social worker as needed (e.g., to arrange for new housing or to arrange for a telephone).
- Be prepared to anticipate situations beforehand (e.g., make arrangements with a local ambulance service to take the child to the treatment center and not to the closest hospital, as some are required to do).
- Offer suggestions (e.g., if the house is not clean, suggest keeping one area clean for use when changing the dressing for a patient with a Hickman catheter).

Finances and medical coverage:

- Refer the family to a social worker as needed (e.g., if the family is medically indigent or needs assistance with housing and meals to be with a child hospitalized far from home).
- Provide information about organizations that offer financial assistance (e.g., Leukemia Society of America, pharmaceutical companies that may offer free medication for children in hardship situations).
- Determine who will be responsible for precertification (i.e., a family member or nurse).

Family dynamics:

- Learn about the family's specific culture, including restrictions that might have an impact on health care.
- Include siblings as much as possible in teaching sessions, family meetings, and support groups.
- Be as flexible as possible, especially in accommodating to the parents' work schedules.

- Offer anticipatory guidance with respect to role changes that may occur within the family.
- Include the family's religious community in providing support to the family.
- Refer the family to a social worker, as needed.

Resources:

- Include the family's existing support systems to the extent possible.
- Use interpreters, as necessary, when there is a language barrier.
- Offer information about support groups.
- Introduce parents new to the experience of having a child with cancer to parents who have already undergone a similar experience.
- Individualize plans of care to take advantage of family members' effective coping skills and to minimize any detrimental strategies.
- Offer teaching sessions as often as necessary and in different formats (e.g., group sessions, one-on-one sessions, teaching packets).
- Offer information on outside resources (e.g., American Cancer Society, Candlelighters, Leukemia Society of America, National Children's Cancer Society).

Expected Patient and Family Outcomes

The home environment:

- The home will be accessible and clean.
- The family will have access to a telephone, either in the home or nearby.
- A plan will be in place for ambulance transportation in case of an emergency, if the child's home is not near a treatment center.
- The family will have access to a car or to public transportation if the treatment center is nearby.

Finances and medical coverage:

- Social services staff will be involved if the family does not have medical insurance or is not eligible for Medicaid benefits.
- The family will experience minimal out-of-pocket expenses.
- The family will not become overburdened financially.

Family dynamics:

- The plan of care will be tailored to the family's culture.
- The parents and siblings will verbalize their support.
- The parents will have minimal absences from work.
- All family members will adjust to their role changes with minimal anxiety.
- The family's religious community will be included in the plan of care.
- Social services staff will be included in the plan of care, as necessary.

Resources:

- The family will make use of its available resources.
- The family will demonstrate an understanding of the illness and its treatment.
- The family will exhibit effective coping skills and strategies.

References

National Association of Children's Hospitals and Related Institutions (NACHRI) Patient Care Oncology FOCUS Group. (2000). Home care requirements for children and adolescents with cancer. *Journal of Pediatric Oncology Nursing, 17*, 45–49.

Scott-Findlay, S., & Chalmers, K. (2001). Rural families' perspectives on having a child with cancer. *Journal of Pediatric Oncology Nursing, 18*, 205–216.

Walker, C. L., Wells, L. M., Heiney, S. P., & Hymovich, D. P. (2002). Family-centered psychosocial care. In C. R. Baggott, K. P. Kelly, D. Fochtman, & G. V. Foley (Eds.). *Nursing care of children and adolescents with cancer* (3rd ed., pp. 365–390). Philadelphia: W. B. Saunders.

Wells, L.M., Heiney, S.P., Swygert, E., Troficanto, G., Stokes, C., & Ettinger, R.S. (1990). Psychosocial stressors, coping resources, and information needs of parents of adolescent cancer patients. *Journal of Pediatric Oncology Nursing, 7*, 145–148.

Cultural Care

Jane Hennessy

Definition

The rapidly increasing diversity of client populations is challenging healthcare professionals to develop a better understanding of the role culture plays in clients' beliefs, responses, and behaviors regarding health and illness. Many misunderstandings between clients and professional healthcare providers can be attributed to the fact that each uses different culturally based concepts and reasoning processes to determine and manage health and illness states. By understanding and appreciating the impact of culture on health behavior, healthcare professionals are able to explore ways of identifying and incorporating patients' and families' belief systems about health into the plan of care in a culturally sensitive, yet clinically effective, manner.

The literature demonstrates the tremendous controversy that exists regarding the exact definitions of *culture*, *ethnicity*, *minority status*, and *ancestry*. *Culture* can be defined as "the sum total of socially inherited characteristics of a human group that comprises everything which one generation can tell, convey, or hand down to the next" (Fejos, 1959, p. 44). Endelman and Mandel (1986) define culture as learned patterns of living, including health beliefs and behaviors, that have been handed down from generation to generation. Culture also has been described as patterned ways in which humans have learned to think about and act in their world.

Ethnicity focuses on the cultural characteristics of a particular group and the norms, values, attitudes, and behaviors that are typical of an ethnic group and that stem from a common culture of origin transmitted across generations. Ethnicity is closely tied to culture, ethnic identity, and minority status. A person's ethnic identity is that aspect of self that includes a sense of membership in an ethnic group and the attitudes and feelings associated with that membership.

Minority status refers to the status of the ethnic group within the larger society. It implies less power, disproportionately low representation of group members in positions of authority and leadership, unequal social and economic position, and a greater experience with prejudice and discrimination than the majority population.

Ancestry is defined as an individual's specific nationality, group, or country from which the person or his or her parents or ancestors resided before emigrating to the United States. It is important to recognize that although many culturally diverse groups share the characteristics of a dominant culture, they may continue to maintain their own ethnic identification, values, language, and behaviors. For example, Hispanics are commonly considered to be one ethnic group but, in fact, they represent many different countries, dialects, religions, and cultural identities.

Culture encompasses not only the concept of ethnic background, but also the many subcultures to which an individual is exposed (e.g., rural, urban, immigrant, native, laborer, professional). Likewise, cultural background cannot be viewed as being mutually exclusive of personal, familial, and social experiences when considering the framework of an individual patient's perception of health and illness.

Demographics of Ethnic Populations

Since 1970, diversity in the racial and ethnic makeup of the U.S. population has been increasing. The 2000 census shows that the Caucasian race group remains the largest, but accounts for a smaller portion of the total population than it once did (80.3% of the population in 1990; 75.1% in 2000). The African American population remained relatively stable; it constituted 12.1% of the population in 1990 and 12.3% in 2000. The proportion of Asians and Pacific Islanders has increased from 2.9% of the total population in 1990 to 3.8% in 2000. Alaska Native and American Indians accounted for 0.8% of the population in 1990 and 0.9% in 2000, and those claiming some other race accounted for 3.9% of the population in 1990 and 5.5% in 2000. People who declared that their ancestry includes two or more races accounted for 2.4% of the population in 2000. In 1980, the U.S. census asked people for the first time if they had Hispanic ancestry, and included individuals of any racial background. Since 1980, this population has almost doubled in size—in 2000, it comprised 12.5% of the U.S. population, or 35.3 million people (Hobbs & Stoops, 2002)

Cancer Survival and Diversity

Healthy People 2010: Understanding and Improving Health described a statistical disparity in cancer deaths (U.S. Department of Health and Human Services [HHS], 2000). African Americans are more than twice as likely to die from cancer as are Pacific Islanders, Asians, Hispanics, or American Indians; they are approximately 34% more likely to die of cancer than Caucasian Americans (HHS, 2000).

It has been suggested that preventive measures such as changes in dietary habits and quitting smoking can decrease cancers by 50%. Cancer survival rates also may be improved by improving access to healthcare resources. This access can be improved by making certain that information given is appropriate linguistically and culturally, and that all groups have access to both prevention and treatment options (HHS, 2000).

In December 2000, the HHS's Office of Minority Health issued standards for delivering appropriate health care to people who belong to racial, cultural, linguistic, or ethnic minorities. These standards are guidelines meant to help healthcare agencies set up programs that will meet the needs of the minority populations they serve. These guidelines address the need for competent interpreter services and for health agencies to monitor the changing cultural composition of the communities they serve (Shaw-Taylor, 2002).

According to *Healthy People 2010,* a higher income, health insurance, and ongoing health care are predictive of the ability to obtain quality health care. Eleven million children in the United States are not covered by health insurance (HHS, 2000).

Cancer Clinical Trials and Minority Groups

Minority and economically disadvantaged populations are underrepresented in national cancer clinical trials. Information and an understanding of the ethnic and cultural environment of these populations, as well as the barriers they face with regard to participation in clinical trials are required if recruitment and minority inclusion levels are to be improved.

Barriers to participation include physical access and affordability (e.g., lost work time, transportation costs), patient and family perceptions of health, and specific attitudes toward research trials. Other barriers are fear and mistrust, insufficient recruitment efforts, consent information that has not been translated into the language used by the patient, and insufficient availability of valid and culturally appropriate questionnaires and sampling tools.

Attention to these factors could facilitate participation: adequate information and education about the risks, benefits, costs, and required time commitment; peer group norms that are supportive of the goals of the trials; endorsement of the goals of the clinical trials by church, cultural, or social groups and by employers; improved access to the healthcare system and specific locations where trials are being conducted; a perceived benefit to the individuals from their participation; and minimal actual cost to individuals or families in terms of time lost from work or because of associated transportation and child care needs.

Culture and the Family

The family is the basic unit of every society and the basic unit for the transmission of culture. In some cultures, the family is central; in others, it is peripheral to a greater governing body. Depending upon its cultural norms, a family can act as the primary decision-making body for all of its members, or it can defer to the individual the right to decide. In American society, decision-making does not rest with a single authority—sometimes it is in the hands of the individual, sometimes the family makes the decision, and sometimes neither the individual or the family has the final say. In many other societies in which the rules clearly state that the family makes the decision for the individual, there may be a designated decision maker or consensus may be reached through family discussions. In these societies, it is rare for an outside authority to interfere in family matters.

American society is a composite of many, often conflicting, cultures with different values and beliefs. When different values clash in a way that may be important to society as a whole (e.g., parents who are Jehovah's Witnesses who object to a healthcare professional's decision to provide their child with a blood transfusion), the state may become the decision maker, determining which value is correct. Thus, decision-making regarding children can be taken away from parents.

Healthcare professionals who work primarily with children and adolescents must assess the strengths, culture, and structure of each family and must be aware of the role these will play in decision-making about health care. A compromise must be achieved when potentially conflicting cultural beliefs exist, especially when dealing with issues of informed consent, treatment planning, and end-of-life decisions.

Culturally Sensitive Cancer Care

Communication is the basis of any relationship between a healthcare professional and a patient and his or her family. Language can be a critical barrier to effective communication, but issues related to educational level, income, and socioeconomic status also figure prominently.

Professionals in healthcare settings must

- educate themselves regarding the cultural characteristics of their targeted populations
- identify the points of access and key leaders in the targeted ethnic communities
- develop institution-based programs targeted at overcoming economic and logistical barriers in these specific ethnic groups
- provide professional translation services that incorporate training in medical translation.

Assessment of Culture and Perceptions of Health and Illness

Culture influences illness and health behaviors. Illness behaviors can be influenced by a culture's definition of the appropriate steps to take in seeking health care. Culture also can affect beliefs about the cause of illness, symptom presentation and interpretation, and expectations and decision-making regarding treatment.

At the time of assessment a nurse must keep in mind the beliefs and assumptions that healthcare providers bring to the workplace. Assessment can be made easier by remembering that in all cultures, parents communicate with their children and respond to a child's distress. How parents communicate or answer a cry varies from culture to culture (Trawick-Smith, 2000).

Nursing Assessment and Interventions

A cultural assessment and related interventions at the time of an initial diagnosis, treatment planning and intervention, at relapse, and/or at the terminal phases of illness will enhance overall compliance with the treatment plan and contribute to comprehensive, high-quality care.

Assessment:

At the time of the initial diagnosis.

- Assess the patient's and the family's preferred pattern of communication (i.e., verbal or nonverbal) as well as their language preferences.
- Learn about the parenting and child-rearing practices of the family, and assess what impact these may have on the patient's future compliance with and adherence to the treatment plan.
- Identify potential culturally driven barriers to communication, compliance, acceptance of the diagnosis, and adherence to the treatment plan.
- Explore the family's ethnic beliefs regarding cancer and its causes and treatments.
- Assess the focus of control (e.g., is it in the hands of the individual, the medical professional, a healer, or God?).
- Identify potential financial, transportation, or other logistical barriers that may impede care.

During treatment planning and intervention.

- Identify the primary caretaker(s) as well as the primary decision maker(s) within the family structure.

At the time of relapse or during the terminal phases of illness.

- Assess the child's interpretation of the pain experience in the context of cultural norms and beliefs.
- Reevaluate and document the family's beliefs and wishes regarding the rights of the child to information and inclusion in the decision-making process.
- Become familiar with ethnic-specific mourning and grieving practices, as well as with dying and burial traditions and beliefs.
- Consider the following when assessing a child's pain, evaluating its intensity, or developing treatment strategies:
  - cultural beliefs regarding demonstrating pain (i.e., emotionally or stoically)
  - cultural acceptance of medications via oral, IV, or invasive routes
  - the use of alternative methodologies to manage the child's pain.

Interventions:

At the time of the initial diagnosis.

- Provide culturally appropriate and language-appropriate information, patient education, treatment-related information, and informed-consent materials.

- Respect the parenting and child-rearing practices of the family as much as possible.
- Discuss in detail the family's diet and nutritional practices, paying particular attention to herbal or other medicinal practices, views regarding nutrition for infants and toddlers, and beliefs regarding the relationship between diet and the causes of illnesses.

During treatment planning and intervention.

- Use the influential members of the family unit or ethnic community (e.g., religious leaders, community gatekeepers, healers) to assist the family in decision-making. Arrange to have these key people at the informed-consent and treatment-planning conferences whenever it is appropriate and desired by the family.
- Discuss the family's cultural beliefs regarding the rights of children, including their right to assent and consent and to be included in making day-to-day decisions.
- Discuss with the child and the family the comfort measures and remedies they used to manage the illness prior to the diagnosis, and incorporate these practices into the treatment plan whenever possible.
- Avoid using family members as interpreters during sensitive conversations (i.e., those regarding treatment options, informed consent, end-of-life decisions). Relatives or close friends may have an unknown level of competency, violate the family's confidentiality and privacy, tend to take a protective role, or omit, change, or add valuable information.
- Encourage patients and their families to share their cultural beliefs regarding intrusive or invasive procedures.
- Recognize that patients from some ethnic groups mistrust their healthcare institutions or services for a variety of reasons (e.g., they see them as too invasive, they are unable to recognize the metaphysical or natural causes for diseases, they have fears related to the status of their U.S. residency).

At the time of relapse or during the terminal phases of illness.

- Recognize that some patients and families may have a religiously based belief that suffering is a necessary or inevitable part of life, and they may not wish curative or palliative therapy to be administered.
- Discuss with the child and the family their beliefs regarding the use of alternative therapies; help the family to distinguish between a palliative and curative intent.
- Help patients die in a manner that is consistent with their values and the way they have lived.

Expected Patient and Family Outcomes

- The patient and the family receive culturally sensitive cancer care that incorporates their cultural beliefs and values into the management plan, minimizes barriers to prompt and effective intervention, and facilitates access to state-of-the-art and research-based treatment.

References

Endelman, C., & Mandel, C. (1986). *Health promotion throughout the lifespan.* St. Louis: Mosby.

Fejos, P. (1959). Man, magic, and medicine. In I. Goldstein (Ed.), *Medicine and anthropology* (pp. 46–53). New York: International University Press.

Hobbs, F., & Stoops, N. (2002). *Demographic trends in the 20th century* (Census 2000 Special Reports, Series CENSR-4). Washington, DC: U.S. Government Printing Office.

Shaw-Taylor, Y. (2002).Culturally and linguistically appropriate health care for racial or ethnic minorities: Analysis of the U.S. Office of Minority Health's recommended standards [Electronic version]. *Health Policy, 62,* 211–221.

Trawick-Smith, J. (2000). *Early childhood development: A multicultural perspective* (2nd ed.). Upper Saddle River, NJ: Prentice-Hall.

U.S. Department of Health and Human Services. (2000). *Healthy People 2010: Understanding and improving health* (2nd ed.). Washington, DC: U.S. Government Printing Office.

Spirituality

Brian Brooks

Definition

Spirituality is the deepest core of our being, the essence of who we are as human beings. Spirituality is the dimension of ourselves that seeks to understand and connect with God or the divine, with other persons, and with the world around us. It is an awareness of something beyond our senses, telling us our perception of reality is limited. Assigning meaning to the experiences of life also is a part of being a spiritual person. Spirituality is the source of hope, peace, strength, resiliency, connection, and purpose.

Spirituality and religion are similar, but distinct, concepts. Religion is a set of beliefs, language, and rituals that are used to express spirituality in a structured format. These elements often are shared by a religious community—a group of individuals who have a common understanding or approach to spiritual life and practice. Adherents come together in the religious community to worship, learn about the tenets of their religion, and share spiritual life together. Religions have encoded sets of beliefs or doctrines that are shared by adherents. Many religions have sacred writings or scriptures from which people find direction for their faith and practice or which adherents believe reveals the nature of God. Many religions also include formalized forms of worship or spiritual discipline, such as prayer, fasting, or meditation.

The diagnosis of an oncologic disease is a time of crisis, distress, and uncertainty for children, adolescents, and their families. A traumatic event can threaten one's worldview or spiritual or religious understanding and cause patients and families to face difficult emotions, such as hopelessness, fear, loneliness, anger, guilt, depression, and separation from God or their religious community. Families or patients facing a cancer diagnosis may find themselves questioning the understanding of God and the way the world works. Many times, families will reevaluate their priorities in life, their relationships, their relationship with God, and the spiritual practices that have brought them hope and meaning.

In general, patients and families will move from spiritual crisis to a new place of spiritual understanding or equilibrium during their cancer journey. Some families and patients will experience changes in their beliefs and practice as a result of a cancer diagnosis. Others will find that the experience reinforces or strengthens their existing spiritual practices and beliefs. Another way to look at the spiritual journey of cancer patients is to view it as a movement from chaos (at diagnosis) to the development or integration of a new or modified approach to experiencing spirituality.

Nursing Assessment and Interventions

Assessment: Barnes, Plotnikoff, Fox, and Pendleton (2000) have proposed "Seven Questions for Learning About Connections Families and Children Make Among Spirituality, Religion, Sickness, and Healing." These seven questions are helpful in assessing the understanding and meaning families attach to illness. The questions are

1. How is ultimate health understood?
2. How are affliction and suffering explained?
3. What are the different parts of a person?
4. How is the child's illness/sickness/disease understood and explained?
5. What intervention and/or care is seen as necessary?
6. Who is seen as qualified to address the different parts that need healing?
7. What do the child and family mean by efficacy or healing? (Barnes, p. 904)

Additional issues to consider.

- Observe the patient's surroundings for spiritual or religious articles, symbols, or copies of sacred scriptures.
- Observe the patient and family for use of religious or spiritual language, literature, or music.
- Observe whether the patient or family engages in religious rituals (e.g., prayer) within the healthcare setting.
- Observe whether the family receives visits from clergy or other spiritual leaders.
- Observe for behaviors and expressions of emotions that might indicate spiritual distress (e.g., hopelessness, fear, loneliness, anger, guilt, depression, regressive behavior).
- Consider the impact of the family's cultural heritage upon their spiritual and religious beliefs and practices.

Interventions:

- Communicate respect for the individual's religious beliefs and practices.
- Encourage visitation and contact from family members, friends, and clergy or spiritual leaders.
- Use books and other written materials to provide comfort and encourage the expression of emotions. Appropriate books, poetry, and storytelling enable children to identify their feelings and reflect upon their own experiences.
- Listen carefully to the concerns of the patient and family.
- Use age-appropriate language when talking with children about spiritual concerns.
- Refer patients and families who exhibit symptoms of spiritual distress or ask for religious or spiritual rituals to the institution's chaplaincy department.
- Facilitate communication between the family, chaplains, community faith leaders, and healthcare providers.

Expected Patient and Family Outcomes

- The patient's symptoms of spiritual distress improve.
- The patient and family are able to identify and claim sources of hope and strength.
- The patient and family maintain or develop spiritual or religious practices.
- The patient and family move from spiritual distress to spiritual equilibrium.
- A trusting relationship between the nurse, the patient, and the family develops.

Reference

Barnes, L.L., Plotnikoff, G.A., Fox, K., & Pendleton, S. (2000). Spirituality, religion, and pediatrics: Intersecting worlds of healing. *Pediatrics, 106,* 899–908.

School Reentry

Diane Dingley

Long-term survival and the potential to cure cancer both open possibilities and pose challenges to the child with cancer, his or her family, and healthcare professionals. From the moment of diagnosis, the child's future should be given just as much consideration as the current situation. Patients and their parents must learn the terminology, procedures, and issues of their particular cancer diagnosis and treatment. Healthcare professionals must anticipate the social, emotional, and cognitive needs of these patients, who will most likely grow into adulthood and become productive citizens.

School attendance is an important factor in preparing children for a productive future. A child with cancer has as much need for and draws as much benefit from school as his or her healthy peers do. School not only is a place for academic learning, but also a place for social growth and personal development. The continuation of attendance at school sends a strong message to children that life goes on, that there is hope, and that there are expectations for the future. School provides young people with the opportunities and resources to develop the intellectual and interpersonal skills they will need to cope successfully with their illness and to function in the world.

Pediatric oncology nurses have an opportunity and a responsibility to help patients maneuver through their treatments with an outlook toward the future by promoting school attendance and participation. Given the intensity of treatment protocols, some people may suggest that it would be easier for the child not to attend school or keep up with his or her studies. However, the child, who already has the burden of a disease, is then at risk of being additionally burdened with falling behind in required classroom studies, underachievement, and lower self-esteem. Part-time attendance may be a reasonable goal, particularly during the initial phases of treatment. Katz, Varni, Rubenstein, Blew, and Hubert (1992) state

> *The child who is denied continued school participation is, in effect, being denied a major opportunity to engage in age-appropriate, goal-oriented behavior. Such interference with normal activities of daily living may lead to a sense of learned helplessness, reinforcing feelings of hopelessness and despair, thus obstructing the child's ability to cope with his/her illness and rehabilitative process. (p. 69)*

School reentry is a collaborative effort. Many treatment centers have developed school reentry programs to ease a patient's transition from a hospital or the home back to school. Even if such programs do not exist in a patient's particular setting, nurses can take a number of measures to facilitate a child's return to school.

Nurses first must identify other members of the child's treatment team who are involved or should be involved in this endeavor. These can include professionals in the fields of child-life, psychology, social work, rehabilitation, and neuropsychology, as well as physicians and nurses. The patient and his or her parents are vital members of this reentry team; the child's teachers and other school staff (e.g., the school nurse, counselor, principal) also are members.

Nursing Assessment and Interventions

Assessment: In assessing a child's readiness for and needs related to school, nurses must consider various factors.

- Assess the child's previous school history.
  - Has the child attended school regularly?
  - Has the child been absent recently due to illness?
  - How do the child and family view the importance and benefits of school?
  - Is the child home-schooled?
- Anticipate the child's treatment schedule.
  - How long will the treatment last?
  - Does it require frequent or extended hospitalizations, or both?
  - How often might the child reasonably be expected to attend or miss school?
- Assess the child for any special learning needs.
  - Assess the child's anticipated learning needs related to treatment.
  - Is there a likelihood that treatment, such as radiation or surgery, could cause the child immediate or future learning problems?
  - Could the child benefit from baseline neuropsychological testing in anticipation of changes in cognitive abilities (and therefore learning abilities)?

Interventions: Successful planning for a child's reentry to school depends upon both medical and developmental issues. For children under age 11, a large part of school involves learning to make friends and developing physical skills. Preteens and adolescents have made friends and are at the stage of seeking their ongoing approval and support. The plan for the child's return to school must include preparing the patient and the patient's classmates and friends. The planning and implementation can be done as a collaborative effort by a nurse or a member of the psychosocial team, or both.

Implementation of the plan for a child's return to school is the next step in this collaborative process. A visit to the classroom provides opportunities to present accurate information and to clarify misconceptions classmates may have about the impact of treatment on their affected classmate and on themselves. This preparatory step is particularly effective when the child with cancer is personally present because it reinforces in children and adults alike the message of hope and the expectation of a future for the sick child. An approach that combines some education about the child's cancer along with students' participation in brainstorming, problem-solving, and role-playing will promote the development of empathy on the part of the child's peers and will help dispel the negative stigma and fear that often accompany a cancer diagnosis.

In addition, concrete materials can be sent prior to the visit for students and teachers to review, or they can be used at the time of the visit or left for use later to reinforce the content of the visit. Photos of the child, the treatment center, and the child with healthcare providers provide a meaningful connection between the information presented and the classmates. The Internet is another source of information and is a means of communication between the ill child, classmates and teachers, parents, and school personnel. Still other resources are available through national and local health departments and associations (**Table 7-4**).

An instruction sheet for the teacher and other school staff can be helpful in easing a child's transition to school. Such a form can outline the child's treatment plan and identify special considerations, such as physical limitations, as well as instructions for handling fever, nausea, fatigue, and exposure to chicken pox, for example. It also can help to ensure that an appropriate follow-up is done during the school year by building in a process of ongoing communication between the school and the treatment facility. There should be a clearly identified coordinator at each setting. Parents should be included in this structure as well. The benefit of such a plan is that it increases the opportunities for early intervention if a problem should arise. It also presents timely opportunities for further assessments of the child and referrals to developmental, educational, or mental health services.

Communicating with the classroom teacher.

- Clarify the child's diagnosis and treatment.
- Identify the child's need for a tutor if or when the child is homebound or hospitalized, and assist in securing a tutor. Check state law and school district policy regarding the timeframe of absences and provision of tutor services. These laws and policies vary from state to state and district to district.
- Determine whether a visit to the class by representatives from the child's treatment facility is possible.
- Identify the child's daily or weekly school schedule so that medical appointments can be planned with the least amount of interruption in school attendance.

Coordinating the classroom visit.

- Identify representatives from the healthcare institution who can visit the patient's class, and schedule a visit.
- Communicate with the school nurse, social worker, or both about any particular medical or psychosocial issues the child might have to identify and solve potential problems associated with school reentry.
- Notify the child's family about the scheduled date and time of the visit.

Preparing the child and the family.

- Solicit the child's input into the content of the school visit and the extent to which he or she wishes to participate.
- Help the child identify current and potential concerns related to being at school.
- Consider having the patient role-play the actual entrance into the classroom on the first day back to help promote the child's sense of readiness and confidence.
- Identify the concerns of the child's siblings and the possible need for a visit to their classrooms.
- Acknowledge the parents' fears and concerns about their child's attendance at school.

Expected Patient and Family Outcomes

- The nurse coordinates a plan with other caregivers, the patient, the patient's parents, and school staff for assessing the effectiveness of the intervention.
- The patient and the family provide anecdotal reports during routine medical visits, reporting not only their response to the child's initial reentry to school, but also their perceptions of the ongoing adjustment of the child and his or her peers.
- The child's caregivers inquire specifically about whether the child has been the object of ridicule or teasing and about how involved and welcome the child feels at school.
- The child's caregivers answer any question that may arise from peers about the chronic nature of the child's condition or the extended period of a child's changed physical appearance or stamina—even if the child has been back at school for a long time.
- The child's healthcare team helps the parents if they report new anxieties or if the child's medical condition changes and affects school performance and peer relationships.
- The child's parents note positive outcomes of the child's regular attendance at school.
- The child's teachers and classmates provide feedback, which is equally important to that of the child and the parents. This can be elicited by means of a written evaluation tool with some basic questions about their level of understanding of childhood cancer before and after the patient's return, their comfort level with the student, and classmates' willingness to maintain normal peer relationships with the child.
- The child, the child's peers, and the child's teachers feel able to engage in what they consider to be a normal way of functioning within the school setting; this is a likely indicator of the effectiveness of the school reentry intervention.

Reference

Katz, E., Varni, J., Rubenstein, C., Blew, A., & Hubert, N. (1992). Teacher, parent and child evaluative ratings of a school reintegration intervention for children with newly diagnosed cancer. *Children's Health Care, 21*(2), 69–74.

Table 7-4. Educational Resources for Families

Resources	Title	Availability
Videos	"Please Stand By"	Available through the American Cancer Society
	"Why, Charlie Brown, Why?"	Available through most large pediatric cancer centers
Puppet Program	"Kids on the Block"	Available through Kids on the Block, Inc., 9385-C Gerwig Lane, Columbia, MD 21046, 800/368-KIDS (5437)
Publications	*Students with Cancer*	National Cancer Institute
	When Your Student Has Cancer	American Cancer Society
	School Reentry Resource Manual	The Candlelighters Childhood Cancer Foundation Canada, 10 Alcorn Avenue, Suite 200, Toronto, ON M4V 3B1, Canada
	An Alphabet About Kids with Cancer	Rita Berglund, The Children's Legacy, Denver, CO 80203, 303/830-7595

Nurse-Patient Relationships

Jill Brace O'Neill

Definitions

Nurse-patient relationship: According to the National Council of State Boards of Nursing (2002), nursing is both an art and a scientific process founded on a professional body of knowledge. It is a learned profession based on an understanding of the human condition across the lifespan and the relationship of a client with others and within the practice environment. Nursing is a dynamic discipline that is continually evolving to include more sophisticated knowledge, technologies, and client-care activities. Florence Nightingale saw the work of nursing as more of an art than a science and felt that the role of the nurse was not to heal, but rather to create an environment to facilitate healing (1860). Caring is a human science, the ethical and philosophical core of oncology nursing. Caring itself is not a behavior. It is a way of being that has meaning and motivates action (Watson, 1994). The nurse-patient relationship also is characterized by availability, nurturance, and advocacy on the part of the nurse and a sense of mutual trust between the patient, family, and nurse. This relationship is a professional one rather than a social one. It is, however, goal-oriented, theory-based, and open to supervision. Many definitions and descriptions exist describing the "ideal" nurse-patient relationship. Examples of some of these descriptions include the following:

- The nurse assesses the patient's needs and creates individualized interventions based on those needs.
- Caregivers develop and maintain caring, clear, well-defined relationships with children and families. These relationships are positive and professional (McKlindon & Barnsteiner, 1999).

As these definitions demonstrate, there continues to be no consensus in the literature regarding the "ideal" nurse-patient relationship, as exemplified by the lack of consistent terminology used to identify and refer to this professional relationship. Terms used include the therapeutic relationship, the authentic relationship, a guarded alliance, and a relationship with maintenance of professional boundaries.

Oncology nurses are known for caring and compassion, and for alleviating the suffering of others. They have the privilege of being intimate with patients and their families, often at the most stressful moments of their lives. Nurses have always had to contend with the dichotomy of the desire to care for others and the ability to control and define the act of caring. The dilemma for nurses is how to be caring in a professional manner (Murphy & Gosselin, 2001). Furthermore, circumstances exist in the specialty of pediatric nursing that confound the setting of boundaries between nurses and their patients. The care of pediatric patients often includes dealing with the patient's family, which is in crisis and which also receives care from the nurse. Care of the child is important to the family, but care of the family is central to the care of the child.

Four types of nurse-patient relationships: Morse (1991) has identified four types of nurse-patient relationships.

Clinical relationship. A clinical relationship occurs when the patient is treated for a minor concern and has brief contact with the nurse. During this interaction, the nurse makes an assessment and applies a treatment, and the patient is satisfied with the provided care. The patient has no expectations of the nurse beyond the care that was required and given.

Therapeutic relationship. Most nurse-patient relationships fall into the category of a therapeutic relationship—this is a relationship considered ideal by administrators and educators. Usually of short duration, this relationship occurs when the patient's needs are not complex, care is given quickly and effectively, and the diagnostic evaluations or treatments given are not medically complicated. The nurse views the care recipient first, as a patient and second, as a person with a life outside the treatment center.

Connected relationship. In this relationship, the nurse, while maintaining a professional perspective, views the patient first, as a person and second, as a patient. The patient and the nurse have been together long enough for the relationship to have evolved beyond a clinical and therapeutic relationship (unless the process is accelerated because of the patient's extreme need). The nurse also serves as the patient's advocate. Moreover, the patient will consult the nurse about recommendations regarding proposed changes in treatment modalities. The patient in this type of relationship believes that the nurse has "gone the extra mile," respects the nurse's judgment, and feels grateful; the nurse believes that his or her care has made a difference to the patient.

Overly involved relationship. A nurse in this type of relationship also may be described as having crossed or violated boundaries. This relationship involves the care of a patient who has extraordinary needs by a nurse who chooses to meet those needs. Such a relationship also can develop when a patient and a nurse have spent an extended amount of time together and mutually respect, trust, and care for each other. The nurse becomes committed to the patient as a person, and this commitment overrides the nurse's commitment to the treatment regimen, the multidisciplinary team, the institution, and his or her nursing responsibilities for other patients. If the patient is discharged or the nurse is transferred to another unit or institution, the nurse in this type of relationship will remain a key figure and advocate for the patient. The nurse views the patient as a person with a life outside the treatment center. The patient relinquishes the patient role, and the nurse relinquishes the professional relationship. This type of relationship between a patient and a nurse is considered dysfunctional (refer to case studies).

A Nurse's Self-Assessment and Interventions

Self-assessment: A nurse and a patient or the patient's family achieve a "connectedness" within their relationship. They are separate and autonomous, yet actively and meaningfully related to each other. Morse's (1991) research found that oncology nurses reported a greater attachment and affection for their patients than did nurses working in other specialties.

Self-assessment for indicators of connectedness.

- Assess one's ability to develop one's advocacy role and ability to facilitate the patient's care.
- Ascertain whether the patient, the family, or both feel empowered.
- Determine whether there can be disagreement and differences without causing a threat to the relationship with the patient.

Self-assessment for indicators of overinvolvement. Overinvolvement results in a loss of objectivity, which can destroy the team approach to nursing.

- Determine whether there is a lack of empowerment in the relationship.
- Assess whether one has become dependent upon the patient or the family, serves a parental role, or has become enmeshed with either the patient or the family.
- Note whether one has become territorial about providing care.
- Ascertain whether one has become secretive and reluctant to share information with other staff about the relationship with the patient or the patient's family.
- Note whether one shows favoritism to the patient or the patient's family.
- Look for a pervading sense of discomfort or confusion related to feelings toward a patient or the patient's family or both.
- Note whether the patient's care is becoming destructive to the patient and the family or to oneself.
- Ascertain whether one's own needs supersede the needs of those who are receiving the care.

Burnout: Burnout describes the end result of stress in a nurse's professional relationship and may be the result of a combination of emotional exhaustion, depersonalization, and limited personal accomplishment. This problem is common among healthcare workers in every specialty and not only may affect personal satisfaction but also the quality of care delivered to patients. Burnout is especially prevalent in oncology, where caregivers work closely with patients with life-threatening illnesses and therapies sometimes have limited impact. The Peak and Nadir Study (Hinds, 2000) further demonstrated that pediatric oncology nurses experienced moderate to high role-related stressors, but also reported positive consequences, including high job satisfaction, high group cohesion, and low intent to leave the specialty. High levels of role-related meaning seem to sustain the commitment of pediatric oncology nurses in their efforts to deal with role-related stressors.

Members of the International Society of Paediatric Oncology (SIOP) formed a working committee on psychosocial issues in pediatric oncology and specifically addressed the issue of burnout in pediatric oncology staff (Spinetta et al., 2000). The first stage of burnout is mental and physical exhaustion characterized by feelings of emptiness and lack of energy. The next stage is indifference; affected individuals seem cynical and disinterested. Individuals go on to experience a sense of failure as a professional, which may be accompanied by a fear of committing serious errors. The next stage is a sense of failure as a person. The individual feels isolated and hopeless. The final stage is feeling "dead inside." This is when the individual lacks affect and may leave the profession altogether.

Causes of burnout in pediatric oncology nursing are the nature of the work (i.e., dealing with life-threatening illness daily), the work environment (lack of support from peers, the institution, or both), and characteristics of the individual nurse.

Self-assessment for risks that may lead to burnout. Characteristics that can predispose a nurse to burnout include

- poor preparation for this type of work
- high demands of oneself
- expecting too much from one's work
- difficulty asking for help
- difficulty taking time off
- difficulty seeking counseling
- not sharing thoughts
- not using peers as support
- feelings of fear, guilt, or helplessness; feeling that one did not do all that should be been done
- becoming too involved with particular patients or families
- difficulty in sharing work issues at home
- not getting enough rest
- wanting to change jobs, but feeling financially trapped
- being unable to say "no" to families or staff
- not having a healthy balance between work and one's personal life.

Self-assessment for indicators of burnout. Symptoms of burnout for the nurse can include, but are not limited to

- withdrawal
- inappropriate anger or irritability
- inability to enjoy life
- a sense of being overwhelmed by endless tasks
- chronic fatigue
- rigidity
- a sense that one's work has become routine
- shortened attention span
- headaches and nonspecific gastrointestinal symptoms.

Interventions: One nurse's boundary is not necessarily equal to another nurse's. The ability to find comfortable boundaries in nursing practice is not an innate skill. Time and experience teach nurses the margins of their practice. It is only through experience that nurses can learn the boundaries of their care. Crossing the line can be a powerful teacher, and its lesson can be empowering. Yet it is not caring, but the loss of caring, that causes burnout, and the cure is to return to caring.

One study found that from the patient's perspective, excellent care was characterized by professional knowledge, continuity, attentiveness, coordination, partnership, individualization, rapport, and caring (Radwin, 2000). Both the nurse and the patient have control over factors that will increase or decrease the level of involvement in the developing relationship. Empowerment is central to the development of these therapeutic partnerships. The less dependent a child or family is upon a caregiver, the more successful that caregiver will feel. Caregivers should encourage children and families to acquire control over their situation.

Ways for the nurse to empower the patient and his or her family include

- using a family-centered care model for working with patients and families
- interviewing patients and families to ascertain their strengths and weaknesses
- working with patients and families to decrease dependence upon the nurse or healthcare institution, including helping them to separate their needs from that of caregivers and encouraging them to solve family problems among themselves, without undue interference
- being aware of the "power disequilibrium" that places nurses in a powerful position in relation to the patient and family
- providing education for patients and families to support their knowledge of and success in managing healthcare issues
- developing systems of care that meet both patient and family needs as well as the needs of the staff
- providing private, quiet, family-friendly areas for gathering, as well as places designated for education
- implementing systems that enhance communications, including interpreter services, educational resources for patients and parents with disabilities, and other educational resources
- formulating systems that enhance the continuum of care from one aspect of care to the next, such as care managers who plan transitions between inpatient, outpatient, and home care (McKlindon & Barnsteiner, 1999).

Benner (1984) stated that it is through experience that nurses learn the boundaries of their care. She described the boundaries of professional practice as narrow paths traversed by nurses. She stated that this path was best negotiated through the support of others who understand the nurse-patient relationship. Building personal coping strategies and supportive collaborative relationships within the work environment is essential to the enhancement of self-esteem and professional effectiveness.

Ways to support the healthy nurse-patient relationship:

Refresh and update communication skills. Nurses should be as attentive to developing communication skills as they are to developing therapeutic or clinical skills. Nurses often share intimate and personal moments with patients and families. Nurses disclosing information about their personal lives should consider

- whose needs the disclosure meets (staff versus patient or family)
- how the information being shared by the nurse will be perceived
- the purpose or intended impact of the disclosure
- whether the disclosure could potentially shift focus off the family to the nurse
- the impact the disclosure will have on the nurse-patient relationship.

Identify family strengths. By shifting the focus from a family's limitations to its strengths, emphasis is placed on the supports that exist. Nurses have numerous opportunities to reinforce this fact—during shift report, in transfer summaries, or during interdisciplinary team meetings.

Develop neutrality. Neutrality is the ability to connect with all individuals in an equally caring and professional manner. In nurse-patient relationships, aim to meet each individual where he or she is. Recognize strengths in an effort to empower each family member and the family as a whole.

Think before acting. Thinking through the larger implications of an action, such as giving or receiving gifts, is a necessary and important component of establishing and maintaining therapeutic relationships.

Methods of self-care for the nurse:

Set life priorities. When others define your success, your self-esteem suffers. Decide what *you* think is important in your life.

Be your own best friend. Do things that nurture your feelings of self-acceptance. That little voice in your head that gives you feedback can either be a cheerleader or your worst critic.

Find time to be alone. In a profession that is defined by doing for others, it is not uncommon to be "othered" out. Schedule a solitary activity.

Take a real vacation. Vacations are designed for rest, relaxation, revitalization, and exploration. When you plan a vacation, leave anything work-related behind.

Build loving personal relationships. Learn to talk about and meet your personal relationship needs outside the work setting and seek professional help if you are feeling particularly vulnerable. Nurses who seek a balance between their personal priorities and their professional obligations find their work more satisfying and are more effective on the job.

Acknowledge your feelings. Feelings of grief, failure, and disappointment are inevitable in the practice of nursing. Denying these normal human reactions can lead to problems. Find a safe, comfortable way to share your feelings. Professionals who reach out to their colleagues strengthen their own sense of humanness, which in turn improves their connection to patients' needs.

Learn to say "no" and still feel good. The tendency to want to please everyone by saying "yes" ultimately leads to taking on the impossible. Also, when you say "yes" and really mean "no," anger and resentment can build to self-destructive levels. Go back to your life priorities and values and see if saying "yes" really fits. If it doesn't, saying "no" will build your sense of self-esteem and sense of personal freedom.

Avoid overworking and leave your work at the office, hospital, or clinic. The nurse's other roles—father, mother, neighbor, community member, spouse, daughter, son, and so on—enhance his or her personal growth and effectiveness. Letting the work role overshadow the others leads to one-dimensional relationships and ultimately to becoming an isolated, lonely, incomplete human being. Nurses find great rewards when they learn to delegate appropriately and set limits with patients.

Providing terminal care to a dying child: As an oncology nurse, knowing what to do or say to meet the changing needs of the terminally ill comes from knowledge of the patient, the family, their experience with cancer, and their needs while approaching death. It involves being fully present as a source of validation, education, comfort, and support during life's most difficult transition. The more threatening the situation, the greater the patient's dependence on the nurse.

The death of a child not only affects the nurse's heart, but also can transform a nurse's practice. Nurses who work with children who die need to find meaning in their work that helps resolve their grief. Self-care on the nurse's part is vital during times when he or she is caring for a dying child.

Strategies for the nurse dealing with grief issues:

- Recognize that symbols and rituals surrounding a death are important to an understanding and acceptance of death as a part of the life cycle.
- Seek meaning in the circumstance of the death (e.g., freeing the child from suffering).
- Apply knowledge, particularly knowledge gained through past positive experiences in dealing with death; knowledge of human responses to stressful circumstances also is empowering.
- Recognize personal limits and the need for breaks.
- Be honest with both the patient and his or her family.
- Spend time with the patient by sitting, listening, providing company, and accompanying him or her during vulnerable moments (e.g., painful procedures).
- Separate work and family life or feel comfortable sharing one's experience with friends and family.
- Share feelings surrounding grief with other nurses and healthcare providers.
- Withdraw temporarily. This can be a useful strategy if it enables the nurse to carry out necessary tasks; however, it can be destructive and not allow a nurse to deal with grief if it is the primary coping method utilized.
- Follow through. Stay with the child until the moment of death, talk with and support the family, and attend the patient's funeral.

Expected Patient and Family Outcomes

- The patient and the family feel empowered when engaged in making healthcare decisions.
- The patient and the family develop a mutually agreed-upon relationship with the nurse that meets their needs, but the relationship is not a dependent one.
- The family maintains or builds a connection with the community to further foster its independence, accountability, and overall support and to help to meet its long-term needs.

Expected Nursing Outcomes

- The nurse has increased confidence in his or her competence specifically in relation to communication skills and interpersonal relationships.
- The nurse experiences job satisfaction and shows a decreased tendency to burn out.
- The nurse feels empowered.

Examples of Nurse-Patient Relationships

A Crossed Boundary

Chris, a recent nursing school graduate, has been working on a pediatric medical unit for 6 months. The patient population she most enjoys working with is children with cancer. She cared for one newborn patient with acute lymphoblastic leukemia for 2 months. Unfortunately, the infant began to do poorly and did not respond to any therapy he received. Chris found herself doing more and more for this patient and his family. She brought in clothes and toys for the infant routinely, she sometimes stayed late into the next shift to spend time with the family, and she attended the infant's baptism. Chris was not always comfortable doing these types of activities with the patient and family, but she thought to herself, "I can't always stop and sort it all out; I just have to keep going and doing whatever this family needs of me. I don't want to talk to other staff because they will know that I need help, and they'll see me as weak. I can do this without help!" Other patients and families notice the unusual attention Chris is paying to this patient and his family and comment to the staff and administrators.

Chris is a new nurse who needs the support and guidance of her more experienced mentors during this difficult case. She seems to know there are alternatives to how she is managing this patient and family, but is not sure exactly what these are or how to put them into practice. Chris's reluctance to discuss her actions and review her nursing practice with peers or mentors is a red flag. Some helpful activities for this nurse may be role-playing with more senior nurses (e.g., how to handle an invitation from a patient's family), discussing her feelings and confusion related to this case with her peers, and reviewing institutional policies regarding giving and receiving gifts. As a new nurse, Chris needs assistance defining the boundaries of her practice.

Handling Inappropriate Gift-Giving

Dan, an experienced pediatric oncology nurse for a number of years, was hired by a palliative care service. He had had positive experiences with a number of patient deaths and was ready to pursue a more permanent role supporting patients and families through the most difficult experience anyone will face—the death of a child. He was put in charge of caring for a young boy who had received treatment in another country. The boy and his family came to the United States for Phase I treatment. Unfortunately, but not unexpectedly, the treatment did not cure the young boy's cancer. The family decided to remain at Dan's institution because they were very impressed with the care and the pain control that their son received. This family was very appreciative and grateful for all the staff had done for them in their routine professional activities.

One morning, when Dan arrived for work, he was greeted by the sight of a large wrapped package. Dan was very embarrassed. He immediately sat down with the family and asked that they keep their gift. An alternative, he offered, might be to make a donation to the unit. Such a donation would help nurses with educational or travel expenses to attend national meetings. The boy's family was quite persistent and talked with Dan extensively about their wishes for the gift. This was the only way they knew to express their gratitude. Dan continued, with caring perseverance, to explain to this family why he believed supporting the nursing staff as a whole was better for their relationship. Eventually the family relented and made a donation to the unit nursing staff to support their attendance at an upcoming conference. Periodically, as their son became more ill and more dependent upon the expertise of the staff, they would revisit giving Dan gifts as expressions of their gratitude. But, in a caring manner, he persisted too.

Dan had experience being able to provide expert nursing care in a caring manner, which made a difference in the lives of this patient and his family. Dan also knew that accepting a gift from this family would convey to fellow staff that he was somehow valued more. Furthermore, this acceptance would say to other patients and families that they needed to give gifts or money to receive a certain standard of care. This is untrue, but assumptions would abound. By directing families to established ways of giving to the institution and staff, he empowered this family. Furthermore, Dan recognized the good work of his fellow nurses and did not send a misleading message to other patients.

An Unintended Dependent Relationship.

Paula was a clinical nurse specialist who worked in a clinic. She had the most experience of all her peers working with patients with solid tumors, particularly neuroblastoma (NB) patients. When Holly, a 10-year-old girl diagnosed with NB, arrived in the clinic, Paula quickly became the expert in her care. Holly was being treated on a new vaccine protocol with which only Paula had had experience. Holly had multiple reactions to this treatment, but Paula knew what to watch for and how to act quickly to avert a crisis. Paula taught Holly's parents and family how to respond to these reactions and how to work with the medical team efficiently, but their impression was that Paula was the only nurse who could safely care for their daughter. Furthermore, Paula fostered this misperception by failing to introduce other nurses or providers to the family. As time went on, Paula became resentful of the demands this family put on her during clinic visits. She felt them to be very needy, something she had not noticed during the early months of working with them.

Although Paula did not verbally reinforce the family's perception of her as the only staff member who could care for Holly, her actions did (e.g., not including other nurses in this patient's care, not teaching other staff about this patient's protocol). Paula became resentful of the demands this case put on her during the family's clinic visits, yet she had fostered a dependent relationship with this patient and family. Ways to rectify this nurse-patient situation are to include other staff in this patient's care, teach other nurses about the new protocol and give them hands-on experience working with it, and teach and support this family in utilizing all parts of the multidisciplinary team.

References

Benner, P.E. (1984). *From novice to expert: Excellence and power in clinical nursing practice.* Menlo Park, CA: Addison-Wesley.

Hinds, P.S. (2000). Testing the stress-response sequence in pediatric oncology nursing. *Journal of Pediatric Oncology Nursing, 17,* 59–68.

McKlindon, D., & Barnsteiner, J.H. (1999). Therapeutic relationships: Evolution of the Children's Hospital of Philadelphia model. *The American Journal of Maternal/Child Nursing, 24,* 237–243.

Morse, J. (1991). Negotiating commitment and involvement in the nurse-patient relationship. *Journal of Advanced Nursing, 16,* 455–468.

Murphy, M.C., & Gosselin, T. (2001). A vision of unity: Nurses must seek professional unity and respect through education. *American Journal of Nursing,* April Supplement, 44–46.

National Council of State Boards of Nursing. (2002). Model Nursing Practice Act. Retrieved March 26, 2004, from http://www.ncsbn.org/regulation/nursingpractice_nursing_practice_model_practice_act.asp

Nightingale, F. (1860). *Notes on nursing.* New York: Appleton.

Radwin, L. (2000). Oncology patients' perceptions of quality nursing care. *Research Nursing Health, 23,* 179–190.

Spinetta, J.J., Jankovic, M., Ben Arush, M.W., Eden, T., Epelman, C., & Greenberg, M.L., et al. (2000). Guidelines for the recognition, prevention, and remediation of burnout in health care professionals participating in the care of children with cancer: Report of the SIOP working committee on psychosocial issues in pediatric oncology. *Medical and Pediatric Oncology, 35,* 122–125.

Watson, J. (1994). *Applying the art and science of human caring.* New York: National League for Nursing Press.

Bibliography

Growth and Development

Haluska, H.B., Jessee, P.O., & Nagy, M.C. (2002). Sources of social support: Adolescents with cancer. *Oncology Nursing Forum, 29,* 1317–1324.

Hendricks-Ferguson, V.L. (1997). An analysis of the concept of hope in the adolescent with cancer. *Journal of Pediatric Oncology Nursing, 14,* 73–80.

Ishibashi, A. (2000). The needs of children and adolescents with cancer for information and social support. *Cancer Nursing, 24,* 61–67.

Kusch, M., Labouvie, H., Ladisch, V., Fleischhack, G., & Bode, U. (2000). Structuring psychosocial care in pediatric oncology. *Patient Education and Counseling, 40,* 231–245.

Lahteenmaki, P.M., Huostila, J., Hinkka, S., & Salmi, T.T. (2002). Childhood cancer patients at school. *European Journal of Cancer, 38,* 1227–1240.

Leondari, A., & Kiosseoglou, G. (2000). The relationship of parental attachment and psychological separation to the psychological functioning of young adults. *The Journal of Social Psychology, 140,* 451–464.

Lerner, R.M., & Thompson, L.S. (2002). Promoting healthy adolescent behavior and development: Issues in the design and evaluation of effective youth programs. *Journal of Pediatric Nursing, 17,* 338–344.

McDonald, J.T. (2001). Helping adolescents cope with cancer. *Journal of Pediatric Oncology Nursing, 18,* 138–139.

Richie, M. (2001). Sources of emotional support for adolescents with cancer. *Journal of Pediatric Oncology Nursing, 18,* 105–110.

Richie, M.A. (2001). Self-esteem and hopefulness in adolescents with cancer. *Journal of Pediatric Nursing, 16,* 35–42.

Vance, Y.H., & Eiser, C. (2002). The school experience of the child with cancer. *Child Care, Health & Development, 28,* 5–19.

Walker, C.L., Wells, L.M., Heiney, S.P., & Hymovich, D.P. (2002). Family-centered psychosocial care. In C.R. Baggott, K.P. Kelly, D. Fochtman, & G.V. Foley (Eds.), *Nursing care of children and adolescents with cancer* (3rd ed., pp. 365–390). Philadelphia: W.B. Saunders.

Family Systems

Hersh, S., & Weimer, L. (2002). Psychiatric and psychological support for the child and family. In P.A. Pizzo & D. G. Poplack (Eds.), *Principles and practice of pediatric oncology* (4th ed., pp. 1365–1391). Philadelphia: Lippincott.

Hockenberry, M., & Kline, N.E. (2002). Nursing support of the child with cancer. In P.A. Pizzo & D.G. Poplack (Eds.), *Principles and practice of pediatric oncology* (4th ed., pp. 1333–1349). Philadelphia: Lippincott.

Lazarus, R., & Folkman, S. (1984). *Stress, appraisal and coping.* New York: Springer Publishing Company.

Walker, C.L., Wells, L.M., Heiney, S.P., & Hymovich, D.P. (2002). Family-centered psychosocial care. In C.R. Baggott, K.P. Kelly, D. Fochtman, & G.V. Foley (Eds.). *Nursing care of children and adolescents with cancer* (3rd ed., pp. 365–390). Philadelphia: W.B. Saunders.

Family Resources

Aitken, T.J., & Hathaway, G. (1993). Long distance-related stressors and coping behaviors in parents of children with cancer. *Journal of Pediatric Oncology Nursing, 10,* 3–12.

Association of Pediatric Oncology Nurses. (2000). *Scope and standards of pediatric oncology nursing practice.* Washington, DC: American Nurses Publishing.

Enskär, K., & von Essen, L. (2000). Important aspects of care and assistance for children with cancer. *Journal of Pediatric Oncology Nursing, 17*(4), 239-249.

Hendricks-Ferguson, V. L. (2000). Crisis intervention strategies when caring for families of children with cancer. *Journal of Pediatric Oncology Nursing, 17*(1), 3-11.

Hicks, M.D., & Lavender, R. (2001). Psychosocial practice trends in pediatric oncology. *Journal of Pediatric Oncology Nursing, 18*(4), 143-153.

Murray, J.S. (2001). Social support for school-aged siblings of children with cancer: A comparison between parent and sibling perceptions. *Journal of Pediatric Oncology Nursing, 18*(3), 90-104.

Ritchie, M.A. (2001). Sources of emotional support for adolescents with cancer. *Journal of Pediatric Oncology Nursing, 18*(3), 105-110.

Cultural Care

Spector, R. (2000). *Cultural diversity in health and illness.* Norwalk, CT: Prentice Hall Health.

Spirituality

Carpenito, R.J. (2001). *Nursing diagnosis: Application to clinical practice* (9th ed.). Philadelphia: Lippincott Williams & Wilkins.

McEvoy, M. (2003). Culture and spirituality as an integrated concept in pediatric care. *The American Journal of Maternal/Child Nursing, 28,* 39–43.

Pfund, R. (2000). Nurturing a child's spirituality. *Journal of Child Health Care, 4,* 143–148.

Steen, S.E., & Anderson, B.A. (2002). Caring for children of other faiths. *Journal of Christian Nursing, 19*(1), 14–21.

School Reentry

Cabat, T., & Shafer, K. (2002). Resources for facilitating back to school programs. *Cancer Practice, 10,* 105–108.

Eiser, C., & Vance, Y. (2002). Implications of cancer for school attendance and behavior. *Medical and Pediatric Oncology, 38,* 317–319.

Heffer, R., & Lowe, P. (2000). A review of school reintegration programs for children with cancer. *Journal of School Psychology, 38,* 447–467.

Kliebenstein, M., & Broome, M. (2000). School re-entry for the child with chronic illness: Parent and school personnel perceptions. *Pediatric Nursing, 26,* 579–582.

Nurse-Patient Relationships

Baake, A., & King, D. (2000). A fundamental aspect of supportive care delivery: The nurse's opportunity to shape the caring encounter. *Journal of Pediatric Oncology Nursing, 17,* 182–187.

Benner, P.E. (2000). The wisdom of our practice: Thoughts on the art and intangibility of caring practice. *American Journal of Nursing, 100*(10), 99–105.

Brace-O'Neill, J. (1998). Professional boundaries in pediatric nursing. *Journal of Pediatric Healthcare, 12,* 225–227.

Lev, E. (2003). Issues for the nurse caring for dying patients. *Oncology Nursing Updates, 1*(1). Retrieved, March 26, 2004 from http://www.ons.org/xp6/ONS/Library.xml/ONS_Publications.xml/Oncology_Nursing_Updates.xml/Volume_One_Number_One.xml

Lillibridge, J., Axford, R., & Rowley, G. (2000). The contribution of nurses' perceptions and actions in defining scope and stabilizing professional boundaries of nursing practice. *Collegian, 7*(4), 35–39.

Ljungman, G., McGrath, P.J., Cooper, E., Widger, K., Ceccolini, J., & Fernandez, C.V., et al. (2003). Psychosocial needs of families with a child with cancer. *Journal of Pediatric Hematology/Oncology, 25,* 223–231.

Penson, R.T., Dignan, F.L., Canellos, G.P., Picard, C.L., & Lynch, T.J., Jr. (2000). *Burnout: Caring for the caregivers. Oncologist, 5,* 425–434.

SECTION VIII

Patient and Family Education

Nancy E. Kline

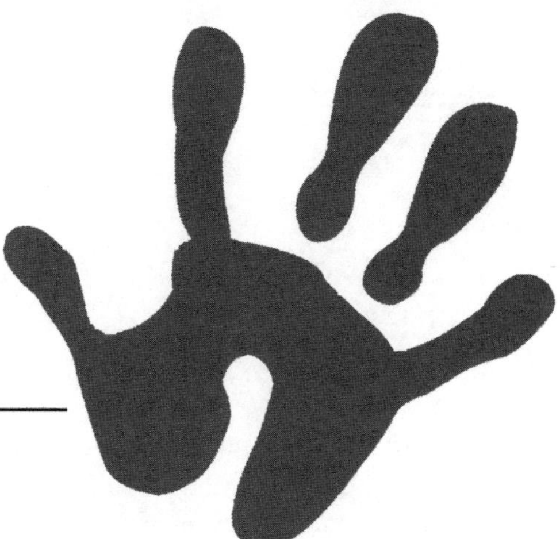

Section Outline

Teaching by Developmental Level

Wendy Landier

Children's ability to understand a diagnosis of cancer and a required treatment regimen are dependent upon their developmental levels. Nurses therefore must use developmentally appropriate teaching strategies to optimize patients' learning experiences (**Table 8-1**). Education about the disease and its treatment should begin during the diagnostic phase and continue through treatment and follow-up. As children grow and enter new developmental phases, more detailed explanations regarding cancer and its treatment are necessary. Siblings also require age-appropriate education regarding a cancer diagnosis and cancer treatment.

Developmental Differences According to Age

Infants:

- rely on sensory input and body movement to form concepts (sensorimotor stage)
- require the maintenance of a consistent relationship with a primary caregiver (usually the mother), which is important in establishing a sense of trust

Table 8-1. Teaching According to a Pediatric Patient's Developmental Level

Developmental Level	Cognitive Level	Psychosocial Level	Key Teaching Strategies
Infant	Sensorimotor	Trust versus mistrust	Teach parents the importance of having consistent caregivers and maintaining an infant's normal routine within the limits of medical constraints. Encourage parents to use sensory measures, such as cuddling, giving a pacifier, and talking in a soothing voice, to comfort an infant.
Toddler	Preoperational-preconceptual	Autonomy versus shame and doubt	Give explanations in terms of the senses—what a toddler will hear, smell, feel, or see. Teach only about external body parts because toddlers cannot conceptualize internal body parts. Limit teaching sessions to 10 minutes or less. Choose words carefully because toddlers interpret words literally. Implement procedural teaching just prior to a procedure.
Preschooler	Preoperational-intuitive	Initiative versus guilt	Use simple terms to explain procedures and treatments. Engage in supervised medical play with dolls. Use picture books and body outlines because preschoolers can understand simple explanations about internal body parts. Keep teaching sessions about 10-15 minutes in length. Implement procedural teaching shortly before a procedure.
Child of school age	Concrete operations	Industry versus inferiority	Use correct medical terminology when teaching. Use concrete terms when giving explanations. Allow children to have hands-on practice with equipment by using a doll and body outline for younger children and a body outline alone for an older child. Prepare the child for procedures several hours prior to or the day before the procedures are scheduled to occur. Limit teaching sessions to about 20 minutes in length.
Adolescent	Formal operations	Identity versus role confusion	Provide explanations using correct medical terminology and detail. Include patients in family conferences and decisions regarding the plan of care. Teach about how treatment will affect body image; describe possible interventions (e.g., wigs and scarves for alopecia). Provide opportunities for teaching patients when their parents are not present. Keep in mind that teaching children with their peer group is effective.

- communicate nonverbally (e.g., cry, smile, coo, laugh)
- develop stranger anxiety between 8 and 12 months of age.

Toddlers:

- use words in a general fashion, but are unable to form true concepts (preconceptual phase of the preoperational stage)
- often exhibit negativism and ritualistic behavior
- engage in animistic thinking (i.e., a belief that objects can think, feel, and come alive)
- imitate adult
- display a strong desire for independence and mastery of their environment.

Preschoolers:

- use words to represent objects, feelings, and actions (the intuitive phase of the preoperational stage)
- engage in egocentric and magical thinking (may have difficulty distinguishing between reality and fantasy at times)
- often have imaginary playmates
- may view illness and treatment as punishment for perceived misdeeds
- show extreme concern regarding bodily integrity
- typically are full of enthusiasm (i.e., show initiative) and are eager to learn.

Children of school age:

- are capable of logical, concrete thought
- are able to comprehend physical causes for phenomena
- invest much energy in mastering cognitive, motor, and social skills and build self-esteem with the mastery of new skills.

Adolescents:

- are capable of abstract, formal operational thought
- are able to imagine possibilities and to think introspectively
- lack breadth of experience; may make unwise choices
- want to establish their own identity and uniqueness.

Nursing Assessment and Interventions

Assessment:

- Determine the child's developmental and cognitive levels, psychosocial level, language ability, degree of apprehension, and illness state (i.e., his or her physical and emotional readiness to learn).
- Identify appropriate interventions and teaching methods to use with the child.

Interventions:

- Consider a variety of teaching methods, including individual or group instruction, medical play, books and other written materials, audiotapes, videotapes, and computerized instruction.
- Document teaching or other interventions and their outcomes.
- Select an appropriate teaching method on the basis of the child's developmental level (**Table 8-2**).

Infant.

- Focus most instructions on the parents.
- Inform the parents of the infant's need to maintain a close relationship with the primary caregivers.
- Encourage parents to room-in (parents may require assistance when planning for the care of their other children).
- Allow parents to stay with their infant during procedures.
- Provide comfort measures involving the senses of touch (e.g., cuddling, stroking), motion (e.g., rocking, pacifier), sight (e.g., mirrors, brightly colored toys), and sound (e.g., soft voice, music, audiotapes).
- For older infants, begin basic teaching by allowing them to explore medical equipment; model the use of the equipment (e.g., stethoscope) first on a doll, then on their parents, and finally on the child.

Toddler.

- Approach the child at eye level.
- Use simple words and short sentences.
- Do not use words that can be misinterpreted by the literal-thinking toddler (e.g., "a stick in the finger" may be interpreted literally as a tree branch coming out of a finger).
- Keep explanations brief.
- Focus on the sensory aspects of experiences, such as what the toddler will feel, hear, taste, or see.
- Do the teaching in the presence of a parent to prevent toddlers from experiencing separation anxiety.
- Use transition objects, such as dolls, puppets, and play equipment, for teaching.
- Do not use body outlines because toddlers are not capable of conceptualizing internal body parts.
- Emphasize aspects that allow the toddler to preserve his or her autonomy, and allow choices whenever possible (e.g., ask questions, such as "Would you like juice or milk to drink with your medicine?").

Preschooler.

- Emphasize that the child did not do anything to cause the illness and that illness is no one's fault.
- Use dolls and medical play (e.g., a body outline can be used in conjunction with dolls because a preschooler is capable of understanding simple explanations regarding the internal body).
- Use picture books and videotapes designed for preschoolers. Discuss issues related to bodily integrity and emphasize placement of Band-Aids after a needle stick or surgical procedures.
- Avoid words that could be misinterpreted by literal-thinking preschoolers.
- Encourage the child's questions and interactions during teaching sessions.

Child of school age.

- Use concrete explanations that emphasize the physical aspects of the disease and treatment.

Table 8-2. Examples of Teaching According to a Pediatric Patient's Developmental Level: Explaining the Diagnosis and Treatment of Leukemia

Developmental Level	Concept	Explanation
Infant	Diagnosis Treatment	Explanations using adult learning concepts should be given to the infant's parents or other caregivers.
Toddler	Diagnosis	"Your blood is sick."
	Treatment	"This medicine is to help your blood get better."
Preschooler	Diagnosis	"Do you remember how you have been very tired and your nose has been bleeding? You came to the hospital to find out why you were having these troubles. We checked your blood and your bone marrow—the place where your blood is made—and found out what was causing the trouble. Your blood is sick. This sickness is called leukemia."
	Treatment	"We will give you some special medicine, called 'chemo,' to help fix your blood."
Child of school age	Diagnosis	"You know that since you came to the hospital, we have been checking your blood and bone marrow to find out why you have been so tired and pale and have been having nosebleeds. It is important to find out what is causing these troubles so that we can help you to get well again. We found out that there is a problem in your bone marrow. Your bone marrow is a factory that makes your blood. Your blood is made of cells. Cells are the very smallest parts of you. When you look at blood, it looks red, but there are really three kinds of cells in your blood—red blood cells, white blood cells, and platelets. The red blood cells give your body oxygen for energy. The white blood cells are like soldiers—they fight infection and keep you from getting sick. And the platelets stop the bleeding when you get a cut or nosebleed. Right now there are too many white blood cells in your bone marrow. There are so many white blood cells that they are crowding out your red blood cells and platelets. And all those white blood cells aren't even doing their job of being soldiers to fight infection—they are just causing trouble. This trouble is called leukemia—it is a cancer of the white blood cells."
	Treatment	"We need to give you special medicines, called chemotherapy, to help you get well again. The chemotherapy will get rid of the leukemia cells and let your healthy bone marrow cells get back to work. Some of the medicine can be taken by mouth either in pills or liquid, whichever way is easiest for you. Some of the medicine will be given in shots; we will tell you when you will be getting these shots. Some of the medicine will be given in your lower back; we call this a spinal tap. And some of the medicine needs to go right into your blood, into a vein. The blue lines on your hands and arms are called veins—they are like highways that carry your blood around your body. We will put a tube, called an IV (or a central line [if applicable]) in one of your veins to give you some of your chemotherapy."
Adolescent	Diagnosis	Explanations of disease using concepts presented for a child of school age should be given to an adolescent, but scientific terminology should be used.
	Treatment	The names, routes of administration, potential side effects, and dosage regimens of chemotherapeutic drugs should be given. The patient should be involved in the consent process. The prognosis and possibility of a fatal outcome should be discussed with patients in their upper teens.

- Describe the treatment from the child's experiential viewpoint (e.g., provide information about whether the medication will be given as a pill or a shot; whether the child will receive treatment in the hospital or the clinic; and when the child will be able to return to school).
- Use analogies to explain complex topics (e.g., "Your white blood cells are like soldiers—they fight the invading germs").
- If the child is deemed to be too old for dolls, refer to a teaching doll as a "dummy," or use a body outline.
- Provide the child with written materials at his or her reading level, and allow the child to have hands-on experiences to increase understanding of the disease and treatment (e.g., arrange for the child to view his or her blood smears under the microscope).
- Use developmentally appropriate audiotapes, videotapes, and computerized instruction.
- Reassure the child that nothing he or she did was the cause of the illness and that illness is not anyone's fault.

Adolescent.

- Give a detailed, scientific explanation of the disease and its treatment.

- Offer to include the adolescent in medical conferences and treatment decisions, if the patient so desires.
- Arrange for teaching sessions with the adolescent, either individually or with his or her peers.
- Use body outlines to clarify information.
- Use developmentally appropriate written materials, audiotapes, videotapes, and computerized instruction.
- Assure the adolescent that he or she did nothing to cause the illness.
- Anticipate concerns regarding the adolescent's changing body image (e.g., give the patient an opening to express concerns by saying, "Many teens your age are concerned about losing their hair while on chemotherapy. Are you worried about that?").

Expected Patient and Family Outcomes

Infant:
- The parents verbalize an understanding of the infant's disease and treatment plan.
- The infant maintains a trusting relationship with the parents.
- The infant begins to adjust to medical equipment that will be used frequently, such as a stethoscope and a sphygmomanometer.

Toddler:
- The toddler is able to verbalize a simple explanation of the illness and treatment (e.g., "I go to the hospital because my blood is sick").
- The toddler is able to cooperate for routine aspects of treatment, accepting the elements of autonomy that are offered (e.g., the toddler takes medicine well when allowed to choose between juice or milk to drink with the medicine).

Preschooler:
- The preschooler is able to describe the basic concepts of the illness (e.g., "I have leukemia; my bone marrow makes blood, and my blood got sick").
- The preschooler is able to describe the basic aspects of treatment (e.g., "I have to take chemo and come to the clinic so my blood can get better").
- The preschooler is able to verbalize that illness is not his or her fault and that treatment is not a punishment for anything that he or she did.

Child of school age:
- The child is able to describe the illness in simple detail (e.g., the child can describe how blood is produced in the bone marrow, the functions of red blood cells, white blood cells, and platelets and how leukemia affects healthy blood cells).
- The child is able to name and explain the various modalities of treatment that he or she is receiving.
- The child is able to verbalize that he or she did not do anything to cause the illness.

Adolescent:
- The adolescent is able to use scientific terminology to describe the disease in detail.
- The adolescent participates in treatment conferences and consent decisions.
- The adolescent is able to verbalize that he or she did not do anything to cause the illness.
- The adolescent is able to describe treatment modalities and to verbalize an understanding of the treatment schedule and overall plan.

Family Education

Amanda Carnes

Family education is a process by which a child's primary caregivers (usually the parents) learn about the child's cancer, the treatment plan, and how to deal with expected and potential treatment-related effects, complications, and stressors (**Table 8-3**). This process, based upon adult learning and teaching principles, consists of a variety of informal and structured learning activities and experiences designed to promote active involvement, application, and learning.

Table 8-3. Benefits of Family Education

Education helps the family of a patient with cancer deal with the following stressors:
- coping with the crisis of a cancer diagnosis
- coping with the stress of assimilating a vast amount of extensive and detailed information
- participating in informed decision making about the child's treatment
- coping with the anxiety related to caring for the child with cancer
- learning how to deal with treatment-related conditions, side effects, and emergency situations
- coping with disruptions in normal individual and family functioning and the psychological distress the patient or other family members may be experiencing
- learning how to use available resources
- learning about possible delayed consequences of the original cancer or its treatment or both

Principles of Adult Learning

Principles of adult learning furnish the nurse with a series of actions to begin, maintain, and enhance the effectiveness of an educational event (**Table 8-4**). These principles not only highlight the nurse's roles as clarifier, coach, and transmitter of information, but also enhance the potential for learning across the care continuum by families of children with cancer, as well as nurses. These are the general principles related to how adults learn:

Table 8-4. Guidelines for Adult Education

1. Conduct a comprehensive assessment to determine the adult's learning needs.
2. Create a safe environment conducive to adult learning.
3. Cultivate a positive teacher-learner relationship and dialogue based on mutual trust and respect.
4. Formulate objectives (i.e., the directions of the learning).
5. Incorporate cognitive, psychomotor, and affective aspects of learning in the design and enactment of learning activities and experiences.
6. Determine the proper sequencing of content and effective reinforcement methods.
7. Promote inductive and deductive learning through practice and reflection.
8. Respect the learners as decision makers and subjects of their own learning.
9. Establish learning activities and experiences that allow the learners to see the immediate usefulness of what they have just learned.
10. Measure progress and reassess learning needs (i.e., evaluate the educational process).

- They decide for themselves what is important to be learned and are generally self-directed.
- They attach more meaning to learning gaine by experience and may have fixed viewpoints.
- They become ready to learn when they feel the learning situation is of interest or if they have to cope with an unfamiliar situation.
- They have a problem-centered learning orientation and seek learning opportunities that focus on solutions and increase competence.
- They must apply what they have learned immediately and expect that their new knowledge will be useful immediately.

Nursing Assessment of a Family's Learning Needs

Preassessment: A preassessment includes

- investigating the child's medical history, diagnosis, treatment plan, and prognosis
- discovering what information the family and child have already been given
- obtaining a general sense of what the family and the child currently understand through a dialogue with the primary physician and other healthcare providers on the team
- recognizing that the parental response to a diagnosis and anticipated management of their child with cancer may interfere with their ability to concentrate on and comprehend what has been taught.

Assessment: An assessment involves

- determining the family's current knowledge base and validating their understanding (e.g., by asking them to describe, in their own words, the child's disease, treatment plan, and what the child already knows about the disease)
- assessing the child's current health maintenance routines (e.g., hygiene, nutrition)
- discovering what issues and topics are of immediate concern to the family
- determining the family's preferred learning styles (e.g., discussion, reading, practice)
- identifying situations and conditions that can present barriers to effective learning (e.g., inability to read and comprehend English; physical impairments, such as deafness or blindness; financial constraints, such as unemployment or lack of health insurance; psychosocial stressors, such as a divorce, a recent death in the family, a sibling with a physical or mental disability, or chronic illness; the family's current health status; a limited support system; the family's culture and religious beliefs)
- ascertaining the family's current coping style(s).

Planning and Intervention

The following are the planning and intervention measures that should be taken:

- Determine the outcomes of family education.
  - Family members will possess accurate current information about the child's cancer and treatment plan.
  - Family members will know when to watch the child closely, how to deal with problems, and when to be more protective.
  - Family members will continue to perceive the child with cancer in a developmentally appropriate way.
- Identify and agree on learning objectives with the family.
- Formulate a teaching plan that includes the characteristics of adult learning and teaching principles (**Table 8-5**), prioritizes the information the family needs to know rather than the information that is nice to know, and bases the content, teaching methods, sequencing, and resources on identified learning objectives, the family's perceptions, concerns, current knowledge base, and learning styles, as well as the child's diagnosis and treatment plan.
- Select appropriate teaching and learning strategies.
- Teach in an environment conducive to learning; minimize distractions.
- Use clear explanations; avoid medical jargon.
- Explain and reinforce complex concepts by using analogies and definitions.
- Introduce educational materials and resources to promote and reinforce learning (e.g., books, pamphlets, written guidelines, handbooks, computerized instruction programs, videotapes, as well as medication and follow-up calendars to reinforce the cognitive component of learning). Puppets

Table 8-5. Characteristics of Adult Learners and Their Educational Implications

Characteristics	Implications for Teachers
Learn by their own and others' experiences	Teach by providing actual experiences. Use simple definitions, analogies, and storytelling.
Have mixed motives for learning	Provide support, guidance, feedback, and resources.
May need more time to learn	Give learners some control over their pace. Prioritize content from general to specific. Use resources for reinforcement.
Are problem-centered learners	Address perceived problems and issues first.

or dolls may be used with parents and children to explain medical procedures. To ensure readability of health education materials, it is recommended the materials be presented at the fifth-grade level.

- Give parents opportunities to practice with equipment and to demonstrate what has been taught to reinforce the psychomotor component of learning.
- Use individual and group discussions and support groups as educational opportunities.
- Encourage parents and children to keep a journal to reinforce the affective component of learning.
- Focus on the actions and outcomes the family needs to know.
- Clarify and expand on the information that already has been conveyed.
- Consider alternative approaches, such as using interpreters, foreign-language cards and pamphlets, and assistive equipment, to overcome physical and linguistic barriers to learning.
- Select the appropriate content focus, which may include, but is not limited to, cancer pathophysiology, diagnostic tests and procedures, cancer treatments (e.g. chemotherapy, radiation therapy), basic healthcare habits, bone marrow suppression, management of general physical side effects (e.g., nausea, vomiting, alopecia), psychosocial care, oncologic emergencies, central venous access devices, discharge planning, home care, and delayed consequences of cancer therapy.
- Document the content that has been taught, the learning level the family has attained, remaining learning gaps, and a recommended plan to address the child's and the family's other learning needs.
- Use accepted methods to standardize and enhance learing (**Table 8-6**).

Table 8-6. Family Education Checklist: What the Family Should Know

Treatment plan

The type of chemotherapy the child is receiving and its side effects
The date, time, and location of the next appointment
Important telephone numbers
The days on which blood counts should be done

Important signs to report

Signs of infection
- fever (temperatures of 101°F/38.3°C and above)
- cough or rapid breathing
- earache
- sore throat
- the child's inability to bend his or her neck
- stomach pain
- red or irritated skin around the child's bottom
- blisters, rashes, ulcers on the skin
- redness, swelling, pus around the central line

Change in behavior or level of consciousness
Break in the central line
Leaking around or from the central line
Bleeding, increased bruising, or petechiae
Difficulty or pain when eating, drinking, or swallowing
Changes in bowel habits (e.g., constipation, diarrhea)
Uncontrolled nausea and vomiting
Paleness, increased fatigue
Inability to drink or eat
Exposure to chicken pox

Important precautions

Do not give the patient aspirin (Ecotrin) or products containing aspirin.
Do not take the child's temperatures rectally or otherwise manipulate that area, and do not give the patient suppositories.

Healthcare habits and infection precautions

Good handwashing
Proper nutrition
Proper mouth care
Avoidance of crowds and contagious persons
Daily bath or shower
Sufficient rest
Knowing the proper way to take a temperature
Proper central line care

Supportive medications (including the reason for their use and information about dosage and administration)

Pneumocystis carinii prophylaxis (TMP-SMZ [Bactrim])
Colony-stimulating factor therapy (G-CSF [Neupogen])
Supplemental or adjuvant medications (e.g., allopurinol [Zyloprim], magnesium, calcium)
Antiemetic, bowel, and/or pain medication regimens

Miscellaneous

Nutritional support (e.g., total parenteral nutrition, lipids, supplements)

Evaluating the Outcomes of Family Education

- Measure family outcomes by assessing if family members can do the following:
  - Describe the type of cancer the child has and its treatment plan.
  - Verbalize an understanding of expected and potential immediate and delayed treatment-related effects, procedures, and follow-up care.
  - Demonstrate the skills needed to care for the child at home.
  - Verbalize how and when to contact appropriate healthcare team members about problems encountered at home.
  - Discuss the preventive and precautionary measures and symptoms associated with treatment-related effects that can pose an immediate threat to the child's well-being.
- Use the following evaluation strategies:
  - verbalization
  - demonstrations and opportunities for family members to demonstrate what has been taught
  - identification of learning gaps
  - reconsideration of learning objectives, content focus, and sequencing
  - modification of teaching plan.

Critical Learning Periods

Angela Ethier

Critical learning periods for children with cancer and their families are characterized by uncertainty, change, and the need to gain knowledge. Common critical learning periods in the care of children with cancer and their families include diagnosis, beginning treatment, receiving ongoing treatment, relapse or recurrence, relocation to a different healthcare center, completion of treatment, and palliative care.

Educational Priorities for the Newly Diagnosed Patient and Family

An overview of the common concerns about childhood cancer: An overview for patients and their families should include information about the pathophysiology of cancer, the development of cancer, its diagnosis and prognosis, diagnostic test results, misconceptions about cancer, remission and relapse, as well as stable, progressive, and recurrent disease.

Definition of childhood cancer treatment: Defining childhood cancer treatment includes providing facts about how different therapies work, how treatment is administered, what supportive care measures the patient needs, and what the risks and long-term implications of treatment modalities are.

A review of investigational protocol issues: The investigational protocol issues that should be addressed are the patient's rights, informed consent, and how to read a roadmap (i.e., the outline describing the patient's treatment schedule).

A description of the general side effects of treatment: Patients and families should be informed about bone marrow suppression, nausea and vomiting, diarrhea, constipation, mucositis, alopecia, the risks of exposure to sun, altered nutrition, chemotherapy-related precautions, pain, and behavioral changes (see Section V, "Side Effects of Treatment," for more information on side effects).

Information on bone marrow suppression: The aspects of bone marrow suppression that patients and families should be informed of are blood cell function; normal blood cell values; absolute neutrophil count and neutropenia; and risk and treatment of infection, including the symptoms of infection, correct assessment of temperature, fever reporting and management, chicken pox precautions, and immunization restrictions. Parents should be taught when to call the healthcare provider. Other areas that should be discussed are the risk of bleeding, including information about the symptoms of thrombocytopenia, nosebleed management, and medications that should be avoided (e.g., aspirin [Ecotrin], ibuprofen [Advil]); the risk of anemia; the symptoms of anemia; and blood product administration (see Section V, "Side Effects of Treatment," for more information).

Description of venous access devices for children: This description should include the reasons for venous access, a description and model of the catheter that will be used, information on maintenance of the catheter, the need and schedule for dressing changes and flushing, and signs of catheter-related infection. Other issues to be addressed are care of the catheter after completion of therapy and how to obtain supplies (see Section VI, "Supportive Care," for further discussion on venous access devices).

Discussion of the impact of treatment on the child's activities: The topics for this discussion are restrictions, maintaining a normal lifestyle, educational services that can be provided while the child is in the hospital, when to return to school, a school reentry program, obtaining access to school district services, and locating teachers for homebound students (see Section VII, "Psychosocial Issues," for more information).

Discussion of family issues: This discussion should focus on the family's existing support systems, coping issues, availability of community and financial resources, applications for assistance, the names of support services and groups, the needs of the patient's siblings, concerns about discipline, child care concerns, issues related to disclosure of information to the child with cancer and to the child's siblings, and issues related to the parents' employment (see Section VII, "Psychosocial Issues," for more information).

Educational Priorities for the Patient and Family During Treatment

During treatment, informed consent should be reviewed as the treatment phases change. New chemotherapy agents and their side effects must be discussed. In addition, the patient and the family must learn to plan ahead for anticipated hospital and clinic visits. They also might need help with issues related to day-to-day living, such as maintaining a normal lifestyle, school versus at-home education for the patient, sibling considerations, discipline, coping, community and financial resources, and issues related to the parents' employment.

Educational Priorities for the Relapsed Patient and Family

Reinforcement of treatment-related information: The issues for these patients and their families include investigational therapies, new chemotherapy agents and their side effects, new treatment modalities and their side effects, the addition of biologic response modifiers and their side effects, as well as anticipated hospital and clinic appointments. Families also must be briefed on the need to sign new informed-consent documents.

Facilitation of coping strategies and communication: The goals are to promote honesty within the family, use age-appropriate information with the child and his or her siblings, listen to the entire family's concerns, and explore community and financial resources.

Educational Priorities for the Patient and Family Who Move to a New Geographic Area

Information that will provide a smooth transition to the new cancer center: The patient and the family may need help establishing a relationship with a new oncologist and staff, and obtaining addresses, locations, and telephone numbers of physicians and treatment centers in the city to which they are moving. Other issues that may arise include establishing a date for the patient's next clinic or hospital visit and treatment, review of the treatment protocol and determination of the patient's and family's level of understanding of the treatment protocol, and review of the anticipated side effects of ongoing treatment.

Educational Priorities for the Patient and Family Who Have Completed Therapy

Help with a smooth transition at the completion of therapy: This assistance includes acknowledging the positive and negative aspects of completing treatment, reviewing the possible late effects of treatment, describing the importance of attending a clinic for long-term survivors and reviewing the location of the follow-up clinic, and providing a schedule for follow-up care and a follow-up routine.

Discussion of the family's and the patient's fears regarding a recurrence: The patient and the family should have opportunities to discuss their concerns about a recurrence and should be given referrals to support groups. Test results should be reported to the patient and family on a timely basis.

Discussion of the importance of returning to a normal life: Assistance in this area includes reviewing the signs that a family is returning to normalcy, discussing school-related concerns, assessing family relationship issues, and fostering the child's needs for increasing independence.

Discussion about changes in healthcare providers after therapy has been concluded: This discussion involves the changing relationship with the oncology staff and the role of the primary care physician.

Educational Priorities for the Patient and Family During Palliative Care

Information about the palliative care phase of illness: The concept of palliative care is discussed. This includes a review of the options for care: hospice, home care, and hospital. The parents' ability to provide interventions also must be considered. In addition, healthcare providers should address changes in care, such as a decreased need for blood work and clinic visits, and provide information about the child's anticipated disease progression.

Discussion of children's concept of death: When talking with parents about their children's understanding of death, discussion should center on the developmental age of the child and sibling(s) and how that developmental age affects their ability to relate to or conceptualize death. Encourage the parents to explain death to the child and sibling(s) in a developmentally appropriate honest, caring, and open way.

Discussion of the need for comfort measures: A discussion of comfort measures includes changes in the child's physical condition and a review of the child's need for supportive measures, such as oxygen, pain medications, and other interventions.

Discussion of the importance of having parents communicate with their terminally ill child and with the child's siblings: The goal of this discussion is to promote honesty within the family by teaching the parents about the common responses that children in similar situations give so that they can provide age-appropriate information to their terminally ill child and the child's siblings.

The family's need to be aware of grieving: The family needs assistance with understanding the grieving process as well as with referrals to support groups and to available community resources (see Section IX, "Care for the Terminally Ill Child and the Family").

Nursing Assessment and Interventions Related to the Patient's and the Family's Learning Needs

Assessment:

- Identify specific learning goals for the patient and the family for their identified critical learning period.
- Assess the patient's and the family's needs to understand the disease and its treatment, their developmental and educational levels, language barriers, literacy barriers, emotional and physical barriers, cultural and religious beliefs, and the availability of resources or support.

Interventions:

- Select individualized methods and resources for teaching the patient and the family.

- Define methods for evaluating the patient's and the family's achievements, such as direct observation of their behavior, oral questioning, written tests, and self-reports.
- Prioritize goals in collaboration with the patient, the family, and the healthcare team.
- Include the patient and the family in planning and teaching sessions.
- Develop a teaching plan for the patient's and the family's critical learning period.
- Document educational strategies or other interventions and their outcomes.

Expected Patient and Family Outcomes

- The patient, the family, or both are able to verbalize the information that has been taught.
- The patient, the family, or both are able to satisfactorily demonstrate the skills they have been taught.

The Pediatric Oncology Nurse as Educator

Karen A. Conley

Pediatric oncology nurses are responsible not only for patient and family education, but also for providing information to other healthcare professionals regarding the care of children with cancer. Teaching strategies should be tailored to each audience based upon individual learning needs. Pediatric oncology nurses also are responsible for their own continuing education.

Educating New Oncology Nurses

Information on disease, treatment, and symptom management should be presented to new oncology nurses. This information can be presented through inservice sessions, one-on-one teaching segments, self-paced modules, and electronic or Internet offerings. Orientation and mentoring should be provided for all new oncology nurses. A comprehensive orientation program includes skill validation, review of institutional policies and standards, introduction to available resources, and identification of a preceptor or mentor.

Educating Nurses from Other Specialties

Nurses from other specialties, such as emergency medicine, intensive care, and community health, often are required to care for children with cancer. The pediatric oncology nurse should serve as a resource to nurses in other specialties by providing information on disease, treatment, and symptom management and by being available for ongoing consultation. Nursing education should be directed to specific patient-identified outcomes (e.g., getting access to implanted central venous catheters, administering chemotherapy, monitoring for side effects, interpreting lab values, and recognizing the signs and symptoms of neutropenia).

Educating School Nurses and Other School Staff

Issues related to a patient's reentry to school should be addressed with family, school nurses, and other school staff members (see the discussion on school reentry in Section VII, "Psychosocial Issues"). This information should include input about possible limitations on the patient's physical activities as well as background on the patient's potential or actual learning problems. A well-organized reentry plan helps the child, family, teacher, classmates, and school personnel deal realistically with the special needs of children with cancer.

Educating Multidisciplinary Team Members

Multidisciplinary team members should receive basic information on disease, treatment, and symptom management. They also should know about how the side effects of treatment can affect the delivery of discipline-specific care. Their general and specific concerns about patients should also be addressed.

Individual Continuing Education and Professional Development

Nurses working in the area of pediatric oncology should be responsible for their own ongoing education. The field is changing rapidly, and pediatric oncology nurses should have the knowledge necessary to maintain state-of-the-art and state-of-the-science nursing care.

Professional practice and patient care may be enhanced by becoming a certified pediatric oncology nurse (CPON®). This certification is offered by the Oncology Nursing Certification Corporation (see www.oncc.org for further information). Pursuing a graduate degree in the specialty is another way to obtain clinical and professional advancement. Finally, joining professional organizations such as the Association of Pediatric Oncology Nurses (APON) and the Oncology Nursing Society (ONS) provides pediatric oncology nurses with peer support as well as clinical and professional advancement opportunities.

Nursing Assessment and Interventions

Assessment:

- Review the learner's past experiences.
- Consider the value of the information to be taught.
- Determine the learner's readiness and ability to learn.
- Identify barriers to learning.
- Identify educational outcomes.

Interventions:

- Review the principles of adult education.
- Schedule a specific time for disseminating information.
- Provide an outline or an overview of the material that is to be presented.
- Identify available resources.
- Document the teaching that has been done.

Expected Educational Outcomes

- The learner is able to verbalize the information that has been taught.
- Various evaluation methods have been used; they include demonstrations, informal observations, tests, structured observations, discussions, and checklists.
- The learner is able to demonstrate satisfactorily the skills that have been taught.
- The patient and the family receive optimal care from members of the multidisciplinary healthcare team.

Bibliography

Teaching by Developmental Level

Bukatko, D., & Daehler, M.W. (2001). *Child development: a thematic approach* (4th ed.). Boston: Houghton Mifflin.

Hockenberry, M.J., Wilson, D., Winkelstein, M.L., & Kline, N.E. (2003). *Wong's nursing care of infants and children* (7th ed.). St. Louis: Mosby.

Jackson, P.L., & Vessey, J.A. (2000). *Primary care of the child with a chronic condition* (3rd ed.). St Louis: Mosby.

Redman, B.K. (2001). *The practice of patient education* (9th ed.). St. Louis: Mosby.

Family Education

Baggott, C.R., Kelly, K.P., Fochtman, D., & Foley, G.V. (2002). *Nursing care of children and adolescents with cancer* (3rd ed.). Philadelphia: W.B. Saunders.

Chelf, J.H., Agre, P., Axelrod, A., Cheney, L., Cole, D.D., Conrad, K., et al. (2001). Cancer-related patient education: An overview of the last decade of evaluation and research. *Oncology Nursing Forum, 28,* 1139–1147.

Friesen, P., Pepler, C., & Hunter, P. (2002). Interactive family learning following a cancer diagnosis. *Oncology Nursing Forum, 29,* 981–987.

Critical Learning Periods

Baggott, C.R., Kelly, K.P., Fochtman, D., & Foley, G.V. (2002). *Nursing care of children and adolescents with cancer* (3rd ed.). Philadelphia: W.B. Saunders.

Cagen, D., Franco, M., & Vasquez, D. (2002). The ABCs of low blood cell count. *Clinical Journal of Oncology Nursing, 6,* 34–35.

Freeman, K., O'Dell, C., & Meola, C. (2000). Issues in families of children with brain tumors. *Oncology Nursing Forum, 27,* 843–848.

Hicks, M.D., & Lavender, R. (2001). Psychosocial practice trends in pediatric oncology. *Journal of Pediatric Oncology Nursing, 18,* 143–153.

Landier, W. (2001). Childhood acute lymphoblastic leukemia: Current perspectives. *Oncology Nursing Forum, 28,* 823–833.

The Pediatric Oncology Nurse as Educator

Agre, P., Dougherty, J., & Pirone, J. (2002). Creating a CD-ROM program for cancer-related patient education. *Oncology Nursing Forum, 29,* 573–580.

Gomez, E., & Clark, P. (2001). The Internet in oncology nursing. *Seminars in Oncology Nursing, 17,* 7–17.

Mooney, K. (2000). Oncology nursing education: Peril and opportunities in the new century. *Seminars in Oncology Nursing, 16,* 25–34.

http://www.apon.org (Association of Pediatric Oncology Nurses)

http://www.ons.org (Oncology Nursing Society)

SECTION IX

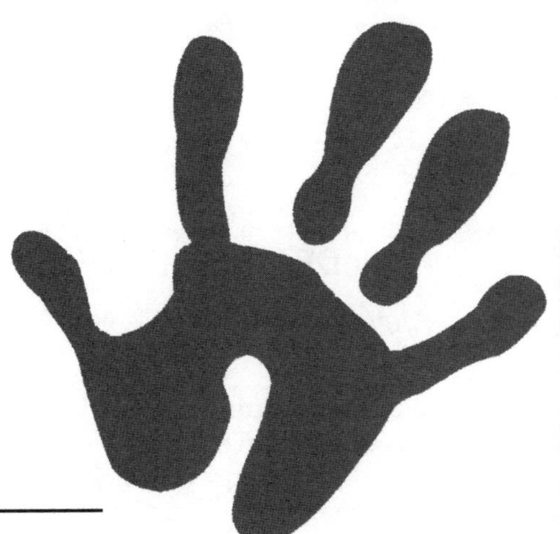

Care for the Terminally Ill Child and the Family

Nancy E. Kline

Section Outline

Children and Death

Angela Ethier

General Principles

A diagnosis of cancer is the prelude to the question asked by most children with cancer, "Am I going to die?" Other members of their family ask, "Is my brother or sister going to die?" or "Is my child going to die?" These questions are not always verbalized. When children's questions about dying and death are avoided, their fears are magnified. Nurses and other healthcare providers should acknowledge and address the possibility or reality of dying and death and provide emotional support and education on an ongoing basis.

The process of understanding death begins when one is a child and continues throughout one's life. One's concept of death matures as one ages. A child's concept of death is influenced by his or her personal experiences with it and by the explanations and attitudes of others. Nurses can help parents relate to children's age-specific understanding of death. A family's ability to cope can be supported by others' attitudes and expressions of acceptance, patience, and respect.

It is imperative that professionals achieve their own self-awareness regarding death and grief. They also should be mindful of the need for continuous reflection and self-care.

Ages and Stages in Understanding Death

Infants and toddlers (0–2 years): We do not know how preverbal children view death. It is believed that they have no concept of death.

Some toddlers may perceive death as temporary. They are affected by their mothers' and fathers' emotional and physical state and respond to the emotions of others. They react to separation from caregivers and alterations in their routine and surroundings. Behavioral responses can include crying, fussiness, clinging, biting, hitting, turning away, withdrawal, regression in speech, regression in toileting, and changes in eating patterns.

Preschool children (3–5 years): Preschoolers have a limited understanding of the concept of death. They perceive death as a state of being less alive (similar to the state of someone who is sleeping or who is away on a trip). They view death as reversible and temporary. Their magical thinking can lead them to believe that their misdeeds or thoughts have caused their illness. In addition, preschoolers might feel guilty and responsible for having caused someone's illness or death. Preschoolers understand words literally, so euphemisms regarding death should be avoided. For example, children at this age who hear of a pet being "put to sleep" may fear going to sleep. Preschoolers' greatest fear about death is being separated from their parents.

Children of this age often hear, see, and understand more than adults are aware they do. Their ideas and feelings about death are strongly influenced by the reactions of their parents. Due to their limited coping strategies for dealing with loss, they may appear to be indifferent or be unable to tolerate feelings of grief for long. Playing can provide them with relief and an alternative method of coping. Behavioral responses can include repetitive questioning, disturbed eating and sleeping, physical symptoms (e.g., a stomach ache, headaches), intensification of normal fears, emotional outbursts and irritability, and regression.

School-age children (6–11 years): School-age children have a deeper understanding of death, although children 6–9 years old may continue to believe their own thoughts or misdeeds can cause death and feel guilt and responsibility for death. They frequently personify death as a bogeyman. By the age of 9 or 10, children typically understand death in a realistic sense (e.g., they understand that death is final and universal). They ask more questions about life and death than younger children do, including questions about what happens to the body after death. They know they can die and they fear death.

Dying is a threat to the school-age child's sense of security. Behavioral responses can include repetitive questioning, disturbed eating and sleeping, physical symptoms (e.g., a stomach ache, headaches), intensification of normal fears, emotional outbursts and irritability, and regression.

Adolescents (11–20 years): Adolescents and young adults understand death in a way that is much like that of adults. They ask about dying and death, search for the spiritual meaning of death, and ponder what happens to the soul after death. Their immediate concerns may relate to their physical appearance and being different from their peers rather than the possibility of death. At this stage in life, they are separating from the family, yet holding on at the same time. As death draws near, adolescents may find it difficult to cope with increased isolation from their peers and dependence on their family. Adolescents often display intense emotional reactions toward dying and death. Their behavioral responses can include anger, withdrawal, an intensified fear of death, and risk-taking behaviors (e.g., reckless driving, drug use, and sexual activity).

Grief in Children Who Have Lost a Sibling or Friend

Four tasks of grief work: Children and adolescents who are grieving should be allowed to complete the process, which includes these tasks:

- Telling the story of their loved one.
- Identifying their emotions and expressing them.
- Finding meaning in the experience and the loss.
- Making the transition from their relationship with the physical presence of the deceased person to a relationship based on the history, memories, and the notion of who the person would have been.

Facilitating the grieving process: Children and adolescents can be supported as they undergo the grief process; this support includes providing a safe and predictable environment with supportive and trusted individuals. Children and adolescents work through their grief through play and art activities, as well as through conversation and introspection. Typical grief responses include denial, sadness, anxiety, guilt, bodily distress, anger, blame, depression, and acting-out behaviors.

Children and adolescents may experience complicated grief. It is the intensity and duration of the behaviors that may be the deciding factors in determining whether referral to a mental healthcare provider is indicated. Warning signs of an intense, possibly destructive response include an absence of grief; persistent blaming or feelings of guilt; aggressive, antisocial, or destructive acts; suicidal thoughts or actions; an unwillingness to speak about the deceased or an expression of only positive or only negative feelings about the deceased; prolonged dysfunction in school; accident proneness; and addictive behavior (e.g., drug use, overeating).

Nursing Assessment and Interventions

Assessment:

- Realize that children and adolescents rework their loss and grief as they mature and will achieve developmental milestones in a normal manner.
- Recognize that children and adolescents should be provided with a safe and nonjudgmental environment in which they can express their grief.
- Consider the child's developmental level, the developmental stage of the family, and the family's history prior to any intervention.
- Recognize that young children learn best through the medium of play.
- Become knowledgeable about issues related to normal childhood developmental patterns; the patterns of physical, intellectual, psychological, emotional, and social development; the child's personal history and issues regarding death; the family's dynamics; as well as the characteristics of the grief process and complicated grief.
- Assess the family's structure and dynamics, coping mechanisms, cognitive and emotional functioning, previous history with loss, family support system, and spiritual and religious beliefs on a continual basis.
- Recognize that children and families will be affected, whether positively or negatively, by the actions, attitudes, and skills of healthcare professionals.

Interventions:

- Use art supplies, musical instruments, puppets, and toy figures to help the child express what he or she is experiencing and feeling.
- Use interventions such as identifying the child's and the family's current understandings or beliefs; promoting honesty in all communications by avoiding euphemisms or trite expressions; providing facts related to the child; educating the family about the grief process; answering questions; avoiding unnecessary or unwarranted information; modeling appropriate behaviors; sharing personal feelings of grief to demonstrate that sadness, tears, anger, disbelief, or guilt are acceptable; finding healthy ways for the family to remember the deceased child, such as storytelling, developing rituals, and creating memory books; and avoiding idealization of the ill or deceased child.
- Contact school, religious, and community-based youth groups as a helpful way to address the grief and bereavement needs of children and adults in these settings.
- Make referrals to other healthcare providers, such as social workers, psychologists, psychiatrists, counselors, marriage and family therapists, pastoral counselors, and school-based guidance counselors.
- Use resources that include support groups, bereavement camps, literature, and individual, marital, or group counseling.

Physical Care of the Terminally Ill Child

Nancy E. Kline

General Principles

Research related to symptom management in children with terminal illnesses is limited. Formal assessment tools for symptoms other than pain in children are not available. The assessment of symptoms is often a synthesis of the child's own description and the parents' observations and opinions.

Approaches to symptom management should include pharmacologic and nonpharmacologic therapy, practical nursing care, and holistic support for the child and the family.

Dimensions of Terminal Illness

The concepts discussed in this section are described in **Table 9-1**.

Terminal phase: The terminal phase is usually the last 2–3 months of life, though it can have a longer or shorter duration. Conventional or experimental methods are no longer feasible for a cure or remission at this stage of the illness.

Terminal period: This period comprises the actual dying process. It usually involves the last 2–3 weeks of life.

Terminal event: The terminal event includes the actual physical dying process, which spans the last days or hours during which death is imminent.

Bereavement: Bereavement encompasses an indefinite period of mourning the death of the child. In the face of progressive life-threatening illness, this phase can begin before the death and extend up to several years after a child's death (see a more detailed discussion titled "Bereavement" later in this section).

Symptom Management for Children Dying of Cancer

Pain: The majority of children with solid tumors who are terminally ill will require pain control. These tumors commonly have metastases to the spine and major nerves. Effective pain relief may require aggressive measures.

A minority of children with hematological malignancies experience disease-related pain. The onset of their pain is rapid, so pain management is most significant during the terminal period.

Table 9-1. Signs of Approaching Death

	Weeks to 1–3 months preceding death	Days to 1–2 weeks preceding death	Minutes to hours preceding death
Physical changes	*Central nervous system:* Patients need more sleep. *Gastrointestinal:* Patients lower their intake.	*Central nervous system:* Patients have a heightened sensitivity to sight, sound, smell, and activity; increased pain, confusion, and weakness; and varied sleep-and-wake patterns. Patients have decreased awareness or a surge of energy. *Respiratory:* There are respiratory irregularities. *Circulatory:* Patients have temperature fluctuations and color changes. *Gastrointestinal:* Patients have decreased intake. *Genitourinary:* Patients have decreased bladder control and a decreased amount of urine.	*Respiratory:* Breathing will gradually slow and cease. *Circulatory:* Heartbeat and pulse are not present; skin color changes to gray. *Genitourinary:* The patient may have an involuntary loss of stool and urine.
Possible support measures related to physical changes	Provide food and fluids if the patient desires them. Plan periods of rest and activity according to the patient's ability to tolerate these measures.	Give medications to relieve the patient's pain, symptoms, and discomfort. Provide familiar comfort measures (see Table 9-2). Provide assistance with the patient's physical care needs at night. Dress the patient in light cotton clothing; provide light bedcovers. Anticipate the patient's bowel and bladder control needs.	
Emotional and spiritual changes	The patient "cocoons."	The patient is afraid of being alone, especially at night. There is a diminishing circle of visitors that consists of family only. The patient is restless, agitated, and/or anxious. The patient shows anger or impatience with loved ones. The patient talks with the unseen or unheard and has out-of-body experiences. The patient finishes "unfinished" business.	
Possible support measures related to emotional and spiritual changes	Accept and allow the child to set the pace.	Listen quietly. Keep the child in touch with time and place. Touch the child gently if it is appropriate. Continue to laugh and play with the child. Respect the child's privacy. Use soft, indirect lighting in the child's room. Have someone stay with the child at night. Acknowledge the child's experiences.	Say good-bye in whatever way is possible. Honor the child's dignity. Touch the child gently when cleansing the body.

Pain is a complex sensation influenced not only by the degree of physical damage to tissues but also by the psychological, social, and cultural factors that are unique to each person. Pain management requires an approach that is family- centered, interdisciplinary, and collaborative. Clinicians must have knowledge of the principles of childhood development to enable them to use appropriate tools when measuring children's pain. Consistent use of a pain assessment tool is critical. Healthcare providers must have a sound understanding of the anatomical and physiological basis of pain perception. Knowledge of the underlying pathophysiology of the disease process also is essential (see the discussion of pain in Section V, "Side Effects of Treatment").

Principles of terminal pain management. Certain actions must be taken to provide the most effective system for managing the pain of children with terminal illnesses:

- At regular intervals, conduct a thorough, but rapid, assessment of the child's pain.

- Avoid unnecessary delays in pain treatment.
- Educate the child and the family about pain and pain control and include them in devising and implementing the treatment plan.
- Set these goals:
  - The child can sleep undisturbed by pain.
  - The child at rest experiences complete relief from pain.
  - The child is pain-free when moving around or being handled.
- Follow a stepwise approach to analgesia that considers the severity of the pain. This model of analgesic prescription, firmly established by the World Health Organization, includes stepwise progression from a nonopioid analgesic (e.g., acetaminophen [Tylenol]) to a weak opioid (e.g., codeine) and, finally, to a strong opioid (e.g., morphine) (see the discussion of pain in Section V, "Side Effects of Treatment").
- Consider adjuvant therapy. These drugs have little or no intrinsic analgesic effects but produce useful pain relief as an adjunct to standard analgesic drugs. They include nonsteroidal anti-inflammatory drugs, corticosteroids, antidepressants, anticonvulsants, muscle relaxants, and anxiolytics (see the discussion of pain in Section V, "Side Effects of Treatment").
- Give drugs orally, when possible.
- Constant pain requires regular administration of analgesics. Schedule medications to be given around the clock to maintain adequate drug levels.
- Develop a plan for treating breakthrough pain.
- Try to prevent the side effects associated with analgesic drug therapy, when possible, and when they occur, treat them aggressively to promote comfort.

Anemia and bleeding: Patients may develop anemia and thrombocytopenia during the terminal phase of the disease. These sequelae also may occur in patients who have solid tumors with metastases to the bone marrow. Ongoing discussions with the patient's family should be conducted regarding how to handle the symptoms associated with underlying bone marrow failure.

The ambulatory status of the patient can be used as a guide for recommending a transfusion of packed red blood cells. For example, if the patient is up and about and demonstrating symptoms of anemia (e.g., decreased strength, dizziness, shortness of breath, tachycardia) or showing signs of continued blood loss, periodic transfusions of red blood cells could be an appropriate course of action. There should be no assumption that transfusions will continue once they have been started because the patient's clinical situation could change and, eventually, transfusions will be unlikely to provide any clinical benefits.

A patient's clinical status should be considered when determining his or her need for platelet transfusions. If a child manifests symptoms of bleeding (e.g., nosebleeds, hematuria, bloody stools), then a platelet transfusion should be considered. Massive external bleeding is an unusual event in terminally ill pediatric patients. However, as a precaution in the event an overwhelming hematemesis or hemoptysis should occur, a bleeding kit along with an appropriate analgesic and sedative should be readily available.

Seizures: Seizures are most common in patients with brain tumors or brain metastases. Seizures can occur spontaneously when central nervous system bleeding caused by thrombocytopenia occurs, or when the child develops hypocoagulability. Seizures also can occur due to tumor growth that causes increased intracranial pressure.

Medical treatment for seizures is given to prevent or control their occurrence or severity. When seizures occur in a patient who is already on anticonvulsant therapy, the seizures usually can be controlled by increasing the doses of the medications that have already been prescribed. A short-acting benzodiazepine can be used to quickly suppress the seizures. Diazepam (Valium) per rectum (PR) or IV is the usual first line of treatment. A variety of anticonvulsants are available, and each agency or institution may have a particular treatment preference. When seizures are a strong possibility, families caring for a child at home should have a supply of diazepam (an IV formulation or a compounded suppository) or lorazepam (Ativan), in either tablet or intensol liquid form, and they should be taught how to administer the drug.

A frequent side effect of anticonvulsant therapy is sedation. An acceptable balance between seizure control and lethargy should be achieved.

Dyspnea: The development of air hunger and respiratory distress can be one of the most disturbing and difficult symptoms to treat. The etiology of the respiratory distress must be established to determine the most appropriate treatment. Respiratory distress is caused by pulmonary disease or damage, infection, malignant infiltration, pleural effusion, cardiac failure, obstruction of the superior vena cava, or extrathoracic problems, such as anemia, ascites, or pain in the chest wall.

Although palliative measures, such as radiation or drainage of ascites or effusions, provide only temporary relief, they still may be worthwhile. Each episode should be considered individually to determine the goal of an invasive procedure. If the underlying cause of dyspnea is not amenable to treatment, the best possible relief may be achieved by combining a variety of pharmacologic methods with supportive measures. Simple, practical measures to relieve respiratory distress, such as using a fan, keeping the windows in the patient's room open, finding the optimal position for the patient, and using progressive relaxation techniques, may be useful.

The sensation of air hunger also can be decreased with opioid drugs. Opiates reduce anxiety and alleviate pain, which itself can lead to dyspnea. In addition, opiates have a specific effect on the respiratory center by reducing its sensitivity to changes in blood oxygen and carbon dioxide tensions. They can, therefore, produce significant improvement in dyspnea, regardless of the cause. Nebulized opioids provide an additional route for administering site-specific dosing to treat dyspnea. Recent reports about the success of this method have been encouraging (Cohen & Dawson, 2002).

Oxygen can give some short-term relief to patients suffering from dyspnea; however, some children may have a claustrophobic reaction to the oxygen cannula or mask. Anxiolytic agents (e.g., alprazolam, diazepam) also can be helpful in relieving the anxiety associated with dyspnea.

Children with pulmonary metastases are more likely to have increased oxygen requirements. Preparation for meeting the oxygen requirements of a patient being cared for at home usually includes liquid oxygen. Malignancies with no pulmonary involvement usually are managed effectively with either a regular oxygen tank or an oxygen concentrator.

Excessive secretions can be problematic for some children as their disease progresses. This is a chronic problem for some children, whereas for others, excessive secretions are associated with the terminal event. Scopolamine hydrobromide (Isopto-Hyoscine) administered subcutaneously or by patch is an effective agent for reducing secretions.

Fever and infections: Families of children with cancer are reminded repeatedly that fever can signal a life-threatening complication if a child is neutropenic. The shift from curative to palliative care may be a difficult concept for them to assimilate as they observe their child develop a fever without emergent action being taken. Families should be informed that fever in terminally ill children might not necessarily be indicative of infection, but could instead be related to the disease process.

The decision to treat the fever with antibiotics or antifungals should be made jointly by the family and members of the child's healthcare team. Issues that should be considered are how responsive to treatment the infection might be, whether medications could be administered in the patient's setting of choice, whether either the drugs or their administration could result in significant toxicity, and how uncomfortable the child might be if antibiotics were withheld. Treatment of fever in a child in the terminal stage of disease could include simple measures, such as sponging with tepid water, and/or administering acetaminophen (Tylenol) at regular intervals.

Nausea and vomiting: The neurophysiology and control of nausea and vomiting are complex and not fully understood. The act of vomiting appears to be coordinated by the vomiting center in the medulla and can be induced by a variety of stimuli. Antiemetic agents may work either at one or a number of sites (e.g., vomiting center, neurotransmitter receptors in the gut wall, vestibular pathways) and can be selected rationally according to the presumed cause.

Persistent nausea and vomiting can be exhausting symptoms to control. The etiology of a patient's nausea should be established in order to determine appropriate treatment. The cause of vomiting often can be deduced from a knowledge of the disease process, inquiry about the nature of vomiting and the circumstances in which it occurs, and the presence of associated symptoms, such as headache or constipation. Nausea and vomiting also can be the result of tumor invasion or as a consequence of opioid therapy.

There are many pharmacological approaches to the treatment of nausea and vomiting, and clinicians must make their decisions on the basis of each patient's previous experience with antiemetic agents and their evaluation of the current problem. Persistent vomiting may require a combination of several drugs that have different mechanisms of action.

Constipation: Constipation is a common problem that can cause anorexia, nausea, discomfort, and overflow diarrhea. Contributing factors include lack of GI motility, a poor or low-fiber diet, low fluid intake, decreased physical activity, weakness and muscle wasting, and medications (i.e., opioids, phenothiazines, anticholinergics). At least one, and often many, of these factors contribute to constipation in terminally ill children.

Prevention is the best course of treatment. Docusate sodium, lactulose, senna, and bisacodyl are common agents used in combination for the treatment and prevention of constipation. Adequate doses and a combination of oral drugs should be tried before resorting to suppositories (bisacodyl) or enemas (sodium citrate or docusate sodium).

Anorexia: Treatable causes of anorexia should be considered and include nausea, vomiting, constipation, mucositis, depression, or excessive portions of food. It is natural, however, for children near death to become less interested in food. Severely ill children, who have a minimal level of activity, can survive comfortably for extended periods with little nutrition. However, a child's failure to eat often is a problem for parents and other family members because for many families, eating is equated with nurturing and maintaining the child's strength.

Support should be focused on the family. Family members should be helped to accept the child's natural loss of appetite. The family may wish to offer frequent small portions of the child's favorite foods. Intravenous hydration or total parenteral nutrition usually is inappropriate for a child during the terminal period. However, if the family has had previous experiences with IV nutrition for the child, they may insist on this intervention (see the discussion of ethical dilemmas later in this section).

Restlessness and anxiety: A patient's restlessness can be the result of pain, anxiety, or sleeplessness. Restlessness in a child should be evaluated promptly, or the child's narcotic regimen should be reevaluated. Restlessness and anxiety also can be signs that a child needs communication, reassurance, and emotional support. Pharmacological agents cannot and should not replace time spent listening and talking with a child about his or her fears and anxieties.

Medications such as benzodiazepines may be indicated when a child is very close to death, a time when agitation and confusion occur as a result of irreversible organ failure.

Nursing Assessment and Interventions

Assessment:

- Recognize that management of terminal symptoms is not standardized.

Table 9-2. Measures that Enhance the Patient's Sense of Comfort and Security

Measure	Description
Quiet presence	Sit calmly and quietly, not necessarily touching.
Massage	Use oils or lotions that will not irritate the patient's skin; play music quietly to help the patient relax.
Therapeutic touch	This is done only by a person trained in therapeutic touch, a method that works with a person's energy field to bring comfort and relief from physical and emotional pain.
Music, videos, toys, blankets	Help to maintain a link with what is familiar from the child's home; children may come to the hospital or hospice with their favorites.
Family gatherings	Explore ways to create lasting memories, treasures, and rituals that will keep the child's presence felt after his or her death.
Picture board	Have family members and friends gather pictures of times shared together; place them on a bulletin board near the bed where everyone can see them.
Room environment	Encourage the family to bring items that will provide comfort from home; modify the patient's room according to his or her developmental age and preferences.
Books	Engage the child in choosing an appropriate book (many children enjoy having someone read to them).
Family, friends, a spiritual support person, pets	Respect and enable the dying child to see people and pets. At times, the child's requests may seem very spontaneous and not practical, but to the child it may be part of finishing unfinished business.

- Explore the child's and the family's fears related to the onset of certain symptoms or the inability to control them.
- Consult with the family and help them care for their child in a manner that is compatible with their wishes.
- Recognize that physiological signs and symptoms tend to develop more quickly in children.
- Recognize that symptoms are rarely simple physical events; it is more likely that they are complex experiences with physical, emotional, social, and spiritual components (see the discussion on the psychosocial care of a terminally ill child in this section).

Interventions:

- Prioritize the patient's comfort as the primary goal. Remember that families vary in their ability and willingness to tolerate symptoms, so the meaning of comfort for individuals and families also varies (**Table 9-2**).
- Determine the family's preferences for treatment and intervention; a compromise between the family's wishes and the physician's orders may be required.
- Emphasize symptom management that focuses on the uses of noninvasive, palliative approaches.
- Provide a cohesive team approach to determining the strategy of care for the child; team members should contribute their own personal and professional skills.
- Ensure ongoing, direct, and honest communication between team members and the family.
- Provide anticipatory guidance for the child and the family regarding the course of the child's illness and appropriate teaching to ease their fears and anxiety.
- Understand that the satisfaction of having coped with difficulty and provided the best possible care for their child often is a source of comfort for parents.

Reference

Cohen, S. P. & Dawson, T. C. (2002). Nebulized morphine as a treatment for dyspnea in a child with cystic fibrosis. *Pediatrics, 110,* e38.

Psychosocial Care of the Terminally Ill Child

Nancy E. Kline

General Principles

Initiating a plan of care for a terminally ill child requires a multifaceted approach. The healthcare team, along with the child and family, must work together as partners to guide decisions for future interventions. The team can best actuate the goals of care after a complete assessment of the child's and family's values, beliefs, and wishes.

Nurses work with professionals from other healthcare disciplines to facilitate psychosocial care. Nurses play a primary role in helping to present and explain care options, the side effects of interventions, and patients' expected physical changes. These conversations usually raise numerous psychosocial issues for a child and a family. It is during these critical moments that children and families benefit from the therapeutic psychosocial support that nurses have to offer.

Goals of Family-Centered Care

Questions that should guide the care of terminally ill patients and their families include the following:

- What are the current roles of the family members?

- How will the child's death alter the roles of other family members?
- What is the family's previous history with death or other loss?
- What are the family's coping patterns?
- Are there situations that can cause added stress and loss for the family?

Attend to the needs of the family: The death of a child causes trauma and disconnection within a family. Family members can become isolated from each other and their friends. Family members may disagree about the approach to care. Friends may be unable to tolerate the intense pain of the loss.

In addition, communication between family members may be strained due to the difficulty they may have in coping with the loss. The child and the family may pretend that everything is all right while knowing that the reality is much different; this protective denial among family members only serves to isolate them more.

The family's feelings of loss of control may have started at the time of the child's diagnosis. Facing the terminal aspects of the disease can worsen the sense of being out of control. The family's need for normalcy may be impossible to achieve during this stage of the child's disease.

Financial concerns may increase. Often, one or both parents need to consider a leave of absence from their place of employment. In addition, insurance coverage often is limited. Pediatric hospice benefits frequently often do not cover what is considered routine pediatric terminal care (e.g., private-duty nursing, at-home blood transfusions). Requests for exceptions or an acknowledgment of necessity must be obtained to provide this essential care.

Actuate care goals: The values and wishes of the child and the family about care at the end stage of the disease should guide medical interventions (e.g., home versus hospital; high-tech versus low-tech interventions). When possible, the child and family should be given options. The family then can weigh carefully the risks and benefits of each option and make an informed decision. The child and family should be informed about current and anticipated physical changes. Most families can cope better if they know what to expect. It is not necessary to go into great detail, however, until the changes are likely to occur.

Attend to the needs of the dying child: Comfort for a dying child should be the primary concern. Other goals include pain control, expert symptom management, and emotional peace. Dying patients often have a fear of being alone, so loved ones should be encouraged to remain nearby. Terminally ill children also are concerned about the future of their families. The child should be reassured that the family will survive the loss.

Communication is critical. A dying child may need "permission" to talk about the dying process. This permission can be given by providing simple, honest, age-appropriate information about what is happening. Family members, nurses, and other healthcare providers should talk about what the child needs to discuss, answer questions, and update information as the need arises. Explanations may need to be given more than once. The child also may want to talk, not just listen.

The dying child should remain connected with the people in his or her lives. This connection can be maintained by having the child spend time with or be involved in activities with siblings, parents, and other people who are important to him or her. Having safe and familiar surroundings helps to alleviate unnecessary anxieties (see the discussion of children and death in this section).

Attend to the needs of siblings: Emotional comfort for siblings is important. A change in the family's routine patterns and the parents' inability to parent are usual occurrences during the terminal stages of a child's illness. These children may witness inconsolable distress in their parents; the anguish this can bring to the dying child's siblings may be difficult to bear.

Siblings should receive information about what is happening to their dying brother or sister. They should be given simple, honest, age-appropriate information about the situation. They should be allowed to talk about whatever they need to discuss, and their questions should be answered and updated when the need arises. Siblings often struggle emotionally when contradictory information is disclosed. What they have overheard and what has been told to them may be very different.

Siblings need to spend special time and to be involved in activities with the dying child. Participation, no matter how minor, in the care of the dying child can be crucial to the sibling's ability to cope.

Saying good-bye is very important for siblings. They should be encouraged to view their sibling after he or she has died. Young children usually benefit by actually witnessing that their brother or sister is no longer breathing or moving.

Siblings may fear that life will never be the same after their brother's or sister's death. They also recognize that the parent they view as powerful cannot fix the situation. Furthermore, siblings often are the last family members whose loss is acknowledged. As a result of their brother's or sister's death, siblings may have lost their companion, playmate, rival, idol, or parent substitute. They may fear that they will be expected to fill the dying child's role (see the discussion of children and death in this section).

Attend to the needs of the parents: Parents need information about how to care for themselves, their dying child, and their other children. They should be encouraged to spend time with all of their children and to maintain as much normal activity as possible (see the discussion of children and death in this section).

Support from a spouse may be difficult at this time. Feelings of helplessness or fear of burdening a spouse may make mutual support impossible. Spouses should be encouraged to maintain a united approach to care, and family members should be encouraged to share their feelings clearly and honestly. Open communication and compromise are the goals.

The dying child's parents may need assistance with crucial decisions, such as those involving palliative management of pain and other symptoms, hospice and hospital admissions, home-based care, support groups, disclosure of information, and planning a funeral.

Attend to the needs of the grandparents: Grandparents can experience physical and emotional isolation from the terminally ill child and other family members. This isolation can be self-imposed due to their own intense feelings of grief and loss. Coping with the death of a grandchild is a double loss because the grandparents not only are experiencing the loss of a grandchild, but also are witnessing their own child suffer the worst loss imaginable for a parent.

Respect the individual's and the family's spiritual beliefs: It is important to determine families' religious preferences and to respect individual customs. A terminally ill child and the child's family should be encouraged to talk about their beliefs. The child and the family may need to find meaning in the child's suffering. Feelings of guilt and a need for forgiveness and reconciliation should be acknowledged as being normal.

The family should be assured that rituals and traditions (i.e., those related to holidays and celebrations) that normally create special memories and meaning should be continued in the absence of the child. If a family finds solace in prayer, they should be supported. Spiritual beliefs are often challenged during a crisis involving a dying child. Family members' perceptions of the meaning of life can change; they may even question their faith.

Facilitate pediatric-focused hospice care: The parents are the primary caregivers and decision makers, and they may request palliative care measures for their child (e.g., IV fluids, antibiotics). Children with cancer are familiar with and may expect a high-tech approach to care. Making the transition to a philosophy of care that offers a number of options for symptom management may be difficult for the child to understand and require significant flexibility (see the discussion of ethical dilemmas in this section).

Each family may have different reimbursement considerations related to the child's care; therefore, a discussion with the family's insurance case manager may be beneficial for determining the most appropriate payment source. Hospice insurance may not be the most cost-effective option because a 6-month prognosis is required by many hospice programs. This determination can be difficult to make for children because they often can withstand the excessive stress and strain of progressive tumor growth and live longer than expected. In addition, a prognosis is not always an appropriate guide for making a referral to a hospice. Many children with a prognosis of more than 6 months should be referred to hospices, especially if their disease is incurable. Nurses and other healthcare professionals should check with their local pediatric hospice program for guidance.

Parents may not be able to sign a do-not-resuscitate order, but they might agree to nonaggressive treatment for their child. This fact does not necessarily mean that hospice care is inappropriate. Until the moment of their child's death, many parents sustain the hope that their child will be cured or will not die.

Nursing Assessment and Interventions

Assessment:

- Evaluate the wishes, beliefs, and values of the child and family for direction concerning the child's terminal care.
- Assess the family members' feelings and concerns.
- Recognize that nurses in this situation share an intimate, personal experience with the child and family.
- Acknowledge that age is not necessarily an accurate predictor of sophistication regarding how children face death. Differences in children's concepts depend upon their life experiences, developmental level, intellect, and level of precocity. Their cultural and ethnic backgrounds also are influential. Each child is unique and demands careful understanding, consideration, and compassion.

Interventions:

- Allow the child and the family to maintain control over the direction of care.
- Respect and support the child's and the family's decisions.
- Develop a multidisciplinary plan of care that addresses the physical, emotional, and spiritual comfort of the child and the family.
- Refer the child and the family to a pediatric hospice program, if they so desire.
- Promote honest, open communication among all family members.
- Share the dying experience with the child and the family.
  - Validate all feelings as normal.
  - Explain to the family that the grief process is very individualized.
  - Provide emotional support for each issue or crisis as it occurs.
  - Promote a trusting relationship with all healthcare providers.
  - Respond promptly to requests for information.
- Recognize that palliative care includes expert pain and symptom control, recognition of the futility of life-saving treatment, an emphasis on open communication within the family and between the family and the healthcare team, and support for the bereaved.
- Work with the family to balance their hopes and fears, and help them face death realistically; emphasize that the parents have done all that could be done to save their child.
- Recognize the healing power of listening, touch, books, art, and music.
- Remember that professionals have chosen their roles in this field, but parents of dying children have not chosen this experience.

Bereavement

Marci Klein Gross

General Principles

Bereavement is the state of having suffered a loss; grief is the emotional reaction to the loss. The type of grief and bereavement experience depends upon many factors, including the significance of the survivors' relationship with the deceased person and the circumstances of the death. Bereaved parents have the difficult task of discovering a new life without the physical presence of their child.

The death of a child is perhaps the most difficult loss to endure because the loss of a child is unnatural. The event represents not only a physical loss but also a loss of the past and an end to parents' future hopes and dreams. Parents lose a part of themselves when their child dies.

Stages of Bereavement

Elisabeth Kübler-Ross (1993) identified five stages of grief and bereavement a person goes through when coping with the death of a loved one. The stages are denial, anger, bargaining, depression, and acceptance.

Tasks of Bereavement

The tasks of bereavement comprise accepting the loss, experiencing the pain, and adjusting to an environment without the deceased person.

Parental Bereavement Tasks

The bereavement tasks of parents are

- facing the finality of loss
- remembering past events and experiences with their child
- processing the feelings of failure as a parent and of personal diminishment
- building a family life without the child
- discovering healthy ways to continue the relationship with the deceased child on a spiritual and an emotional level.

Unique Features of Parental Bereavement

The death of a child is out of sequence with the natural order of events in a family's life. Fathers' and mothers' grieving styles may be different and may even conflict, so they may be unable to support each other or their surviving children. Parents may even feel they are "going crazy." Parents will experience grief throughout their lifetime, and significant events may trigger acute grief reactions.

The death of a child is an assault on the parents' sense of identity as parents, protectors, and providers. Feelings of guilt may be related to their perceived failure to protect the child, their past transgressions, and the mere fact of their survival beyond the lifetime of their child.

The second year of grieving may be more difficult than the first. Often, parents recall the first year as "feeling numb." Between the second and third years of bereavement, family members may realize they are forever changed, may feel their grief declining, may feel renewed energy, and may be ready to reinvest themselves in their work and the important relationships in their lives.

Nursing Assessment and Interventions

Assessment:

- Assess the factors that are unique to parents' bereavement.
- Determine the relationship or role each family member had with the child (e.g., Was the child an only child? If not, what was his or her birth order? Were siblings of the same sex? Did the siblings have a "soul mate" relationship? Did the family member share similar interests?).
- Determine the family's history of previous losses, and ascertain if they have any other concurrent stresses.
- Evaluate the existing support systems available to each family member.
- Assess the family's anticipatory grieving and involvement with the child prior to the child's death, including their ability to communicate openly about the death, the quality and quantity of the time they spent with the child, and the opportunity they had to say good-bye and to make memories.
- Recognize that grief and bereavement experiences are individual and unique to each person and that the family's culture, community, faith, and support system will influence this process significantly.
- Recognize that the degree to which each family member will grieve and successfully work through bereavement is related to the extent they allow themselves to grieve.

Interventions:

Interventions prior to the child's death.

- Establish a primary care team for inpatient, outpatient, and home care of the child.
- Encourage the family's mutual participation in caring for the child.
- Facilitate communication between the family and the team regarding all healthcare decisions.
- Encourage the family to use its own support systems, but also offer others (e.g., a social worker, counselor, chaplain).
- Assist the child and family with good-byes, last wishes, and making memories.
- Reinforce the family's positive role in the child's life.
- Prepare the child and the family for the physical changes and emotions that might occur near death.

Interventions at the time of the child's death.

- Be sensitive to the family's cultural and religious preferences.
- Assist with notification of death and funeral or memorial arrangements, if assistance is requested.
- Prepare the child's body with or without the family's assistance–some parents will want to bathe and dress the child.
- Provide compassionate postmortem care.

Resources for Families

National Organizations

The Candlelighters Childhood Cancer Foundation
7910 Woodmont Avenue, Suite 240
Bethesda, MD 20814
800/366-2223

Center for Loss and Grief Therapy
10400 Connecticut Avenue, Suite 514
Kensington, MD 20985
301/942-6440

Centering Corporation
1531 N. Saddle Creek Road
Omaha, NE 68104-5064
402/553-1200

Children's Hospice International
2202 Mt. Vernon Avenue, Suite 3C
Alexandria, VA 22301
800/24-CHILD (242-4453) or 703/684-0300

Compassionate Friends
PO Box 3696
Oak Brook, IL 60522-3696
630/990-0010

Rainbow Connection
479 Hannah Branch Road
Burnsville, NC 28714
704/675-9670

Rainbow, Inc.
1111 Tower Road
Schaumburg, IL 60173-4305
800/266-3206

- Include the child's siblings in the after-death experience; even very young children should be included.

Interventions after the death of the child.

- Provide active listening statements; "I'm sorry" or "I care" can be comforting.
- Comfort with physical touch, if appropriate (e.g., hugging, hand-holding).
- Use the words "death" and "died," because children can be confused by substitute words such as "lost" or "taken."
- Contact the family to extend sympathy, send a card with a written memory, call the family, or make a visit.
- Refer the family to other sources of support (see the list of resources for families at the end of this section).
- Speak about the child; most parents appreciate that their child has been remembered and welcome an opportunity to talk about their grief or to share their memories.
- Educate the family about grief and bereavement experiences.
- Effective interventions for families can be simple, or they can be part of a structured bereavement program.
- Implement bereavement rounds during which the care team can discuss the death and identify areas of concern that can be addressed during bereavement follow-up.
- Implement a structured bereavement program and arrange for bereavement materials to be sent to families at certain intervals (e.g., on the anniversary of the child's death, birthdays, holidays).
- Develop rituals of remembrance at the institution (e.g., a memorial service).

Reference

Kübler-Ross, E. (1993). *On death and dying.* New York: Maxwell Macmillan International.

Professionals' Grief, Distress, and Bereavement

Cynthia A. Stutzer

General Principles

Grief is a normal, healthy process. It is the "affective and cognitive component of bereavement, involving a wide array of emotions (e.g., sadness, despair, numbness,...anger, fear, relief)....and cognitive responses (e.g., shock, indecision, denial search for meaning)" (Valente & Saunders, 2002, p. 9). Grief may begin well before a child dies. It can start at the time of the diagnosis, at relapse, or at any time during the treatment or palliative care phases. Distress occurs when people do not allow themselves to express grief.

Bereavement is an individual's physical, psychosocial, spiritual, and cultural response to the death of a significant person.

Factors and Situations that Influence Professionals' Grief

Factors and situations at the time of a child's death: A number of factors and situations can affect a healthcare professional's experience of grief, including

- the immediate circumstances of the death
- the decision making before, during, and after the death
- a perception that the death was preventable
- a perception that the child suffered
- the suddenness of the death
- the nurse's conception of a "good" death; and the family's reaction to the death.

Environmental factors: Environmental factors also affect the level of grief professionals' are able to express. These factors include

- the workplace culture (i.e., "being professional means you don't cry")
- the level of support offered by the healthcare facility (including education support)
- presence or absence of supportive colleagues and friends
- workplace stress
- the number of concurrent stresses or crises in the nurse's life at the time of the child's death, include other losses (bereavement overload)
- the nurse's level of satisfaction with his or her job
- time available for emotional support and debriefings
- policies that may conflict with the nurse's values and beliefs
- fear of legal action
- stigma of the death, especially if it was iatrogenic.

Intrapersonal factors: Intrapersonal factors that affect the grief experience include the nurse's

- values and beliefs
- work and life experiences
- social, cultural, ethnic, religious, or spiritual background
- previous experiences of grief and loss (including whether he or she is regrieving past losses)
- coping patterns and skills
- perception of unfinished business with the deceased child and the child's family
- personal expectations within the situation
- assigned meaning to the death
- need to feel in control of a situation
- level of self-esteem
- self-blame
- experience as a nurse
- professional identity
- ability to deal with his or her own emotions and openly express grief.

Interpersonal factors: Interpersonal factors include

- the nature of the relationship with the child and the child's family (including the nurse's perception of his or her place in, and contribution to, the child's life)
- the nurse's relationships with other team members, the patient, and the family
- conflict and communication problems among team members and with the family
- fear or criticism
- level of ability to provide input into the decision-making process regarding the child's care
- the extent to which the nurse incorporates the emotions of the child, the family, and colleagues into his or her own grieving process.

Responses to Grief

Physical symptoms: The physical responses professionals can experience include insomnia or increased desire to sleep, nausea, stomach pain, weight loss or gain, fatigue, lack of strength, hyperactivity, restlessness, heart palpitations, sighing, loss of or increase in sexual desire, hair loss, diarrhea, constipation, shortness of breath, crying, nervousness, tension, feelings of emptiness or heaviness, impatience, irritability, and a tightness in the throat.

Emotional or psychological symptoms: Professionals can experience symptoms such as sadness, depression, anger, inability to concentrate, feeling out of control, vulnerability related to their own or their loved ones' mortality, frustration, feelings of inadequacy, a sense of powerlessness over their inability to change the outcome, doubt about their professional competence, lower self-esteem, loneliness or isolation, feeling overwhelmed by the unfairness of the situation, and guilt.

Professionals might feel some emotional numbness, which is a self-protective reaction that can be beneficial in helping them do what needs to be done to care for a dying child and the child's family. However, this reaction can be harmful if it continues to the point where individuals are unable to find an appropriate outlet for grief. These professionals also might undergo a physical or an emotional withdrawal from patients and families whose uncertain futures could eventually cause them pain and grief.

Other reactions include feeling valued or, sometimes, devalued by the child, the family, and other members of the healthcare team. Some professionals feel grateful that they have done everything possible for the patient, that they have been able to facilitate a peaceful and dignified death, that the child has taught them so much, and that they have shared a part of life with the patient and family. In addition, professionals may acquire a renewed appreciation of life, a feeling of relief that suffering has ended, and a sense of peace.

Strategies for Professionals Dealing with Grief

- Recognize the inevitability of the death, and revise goals from focusing on cure to ensuring a comfortable and dignified death for the child.
- Find some kind of meaning in the child's death (i.e., What does this child's life and death mean to others? How has life been changed positively by knowing this child and his or her family? What has the experience taught about life and humanity?).
- Discover or develop a personal sense of spirituality.
- Develop and apply increased personal knowledge about the physical and psychosocial aspects of care during the period of dying, death, and grief to deliver the best possible care to other patients and their families.
- Realize that some situations cannot be changed, no matter how good the care delivered was. Reflect upon the interventions that worked, and discuss with colleague those that did not go well. Learn from every experience, both positive and negative; acknowledge feelings about them;

and then let those feelings go. Self-blame for situations a caregiver has no power over or experience with should be avoided. Sometimes the best legacy a child who has died can bequeath is the increased skill, knowledge, and understanding that the child's caregivers can bring to similar situations in the future.

- Strive to separate work and personal life by developing a ritual or process for leaving work behind when off duty. This should become easier as experience in coping with grief increases.
- Use briefing and debriefing sessions to share experiences with colleagues, and seek support from colleagues, friends, and professional grief counselors. Letting others know what is happening at the time it is happening often helps one anticipate and prepare for a patient's death.
- Maintain good health by continuing to exercise and eat properly, rest, and get enough sleep. Create a routine that will promote health and prevent illness. Develop a balance between the demands of work, family life, and other individual needs.
- Draw on internal resources.
- Use the expertise of colleagues, and ask questions when trying to find ways to cope with grief. Use others as role models for grieving.
- Plan ahead, anticipate grief, and focus actions and interventions to influence it. For example, being honest and being with the child and family may help to avoid regrets later when looking back on the experience. Conversely, physical or emotional withdrawal might help professionals avoid pain and grief in the short term, but withdrawal could result in feelings of regret at a later time.
- Complete unfinished business by finding a way to say good-bye, whether by attending the patient's funeral or creating a memorial of some type in the child's honor. Some facilities have memorial services or "remembrance teas," for example. Many nurses have created their own rituals (e.g., lighting a candle, walking on the beach, reading a special poem, or listening to a piece of music) to honor dead patients who have touched their lives. Writing a note to a bereaved family can mean a great deal to them and can help bring closure to the relationship.
- Learn about the normal grief process. Distinguish between grief reactions and depression—manage each appropriately.
- Develop an awareness of personal grief reactions and triggers, and identify the characteristics that trigger a more intense grief reaction. For example, a child who is the same age as a nurse's own child or who reminds the nurse of another patient who has died may trigger a grief reaction. Children with certain physical or personality characteristics might also stimulate a more intense grief response.
- Take time to create joy and peace and to affirm life. Learn to self-nurture. Recognize the need to laugh and have fun even in the midst of sorrow.
- Seek professional help, if necessary, to work through personal feelings of grief.

Management has a role to play in helping professionals deal with grief. Managers need to identify the ways in which the workplace affects grief. For example, if a nurse wants to be informed when a child has died, provisions should be made to provide the notification and give the nurse the option of remaining home from work to avoid facing the patient's empty bed.

Facilitating or providing educational opportunities for staff to learn about grief and bereavement, developing policies that acknowledge and support professionals' grief, changing assignments, giving professionals time off, changing their work schedules, providing mentoring opportunities, forming stress management teams for critical incidents, instituting "bereavement rounds," and holding multidisciplinary team debriefings are ways in which an institution can play a role in helping professionals deal with grief. Debriefing can consist of an individual or a group meeting, but it is important to have a skilled facilitator who will not be caught up in the emotions of the situation. Skilled facilitators can lead a discussion as participants discuss the death, its meaning, their feelings and emotions, and the impact of the death on themselves, the work group, and others.

Proposed Models for Professionals' Grief and Bereavement

Most traditional models that describe the experience of those who have lost a loved one do not accurately describe the grief and bereavement experienced by healthcare professionals. Although there are no well-tested models for professionals' grief and bereavement, reviewing the following models may help nurses explore their own grief reactions and lead to self-understanding.

Kaplan (2000) proposed a model with three interactive and integrated components. These dynamic, nonlinear components are

- "emotional tension," that is, managing strong feelings while maintaining professional caregiving
- personal grief
- physical and emotional symptoms.

Influencing factors may help or inhibit this process. Papadatou (2000) describes factors that affect the grieving process and its outcomes. She states that grieving is an individual and social process with interaction between an individual's lifestyle (e.g., beliefs, values, and assumptions) and his or her "work-style," which includes the work environment and workplace "rules" (formal and informal, written and unwritten). This interaction affects the normal, healthy fluctuation between avoiding or repressing grief and experiencing grief.

Tasks that must be achieved (Papadatou, 2000) include "making meaning" and "loss transcendence." Making meaning, that is, interpreting events and representing the situation in symbolic terms, allows individuals and teams to gain a sense of mastery and integration and to overcome confusion and doubt. Loss transcendence involves discovering behaviors, thoughts, and emotions that allow reinvestment in life and in oneself.

Tasks for the bereaved professional are further described by Saunders and Valente (1994; Valente & Saunders, 2002). They are

- finding meaning—emotionally and cognitively processing the death
- restoring or maintaining integrity (personal and professional, self-esteem and self-blame)
- responding to and managing feelings
- realigning relationships with family, colleagues, and patients and their families.

References

Kaplan, L.J. (2000). Toward a model of caregiver grief: Nurses' experiences of treating dying children. *Omega, 41,* 187–206.

Papadatou, D. (2000). A proposed model of health professionals' grieving process. *Omega, 41,* 59–77.

Saunders, J.M., & Valente, S.M. (2000). Nurses' grief. *Cancer Nursing, 17,* 318–325.

Valente, S.M., & Saunders, J.M. (2002). Nurses' grief reactions to a patient's suicide. *Perspectives in Psychiatric Care, 39,* 5–14.

Moral Distress

Cynthia A. Stutzer

General Principles

"Moral distress occurs when one knows the right thing to do, but institutional or other constraints make it difficult to pursue the desired course of action" (Raines, 2000, p. 30). Moral distress also can occur in situations of "internal constraints, such as...being socialized to follow orders, the futility of past actions, fear of losing...jobs, self doubts and lack of courage" (Wilkinson, 1987-1988, p. 21). Moral distress results when moral decisions cannot be translated into moral action (Rodney & Starzomski, 1993).

Factors and Situations that Can Produce Moral Distress

The degree of moral distress a healthcare professional experiences depends upon the following areas of potential conflicts and their resolution:

- making the shift from cure to comfort (e.g., when there is no hope for a cure, goals are changed and are redefined to include a peaceful, dignified death)
- decision-making and communication (e.g., having or failing to have input into decisions about patients and their families; implementing decisions with which the healthcare professional might not agree, particularly those related to prolonging life; having to carry on with treatment that is felt to be unwarranted or painful; having a child participate in research when he or she is dying; deciding what or how to tell the child and the family; telling the truth)
- conflicting priorities and determining the "right" thing to do (e.g., the needs of the child, the family, the staff, the clinic, or the inpatient unit, including quality-of-life needs)
- the professional's own values, beliefs, morals, religious beliefs, or spiritual beliefs
- disagreements with physicians and other colleagues on the healthcare team
- recognition that family members may have different opinions about what is happening and may base their decisions relating to terminal care on those opinions
- inability to keep promises made to the child or the family
- the nature, intensity, and assigned meaning of the relationships between the nurse, the child, and the family
- difficult workplace issues (e.g., staffing, work hours, workload, as well as cumulative stressors such as newly diagnosed patients, relapses, deaths, and organizational stresses)
- differing coping styles

Moral distress also can arise in the following situations and conditions:

- caring for patients and families in a research-oriented milieu
- being unable to articulate one's moral stance
- being responsible for the care of a patient but not having the authority to make decisions
- perceiving that a patient's suffering, pain, or symptoms are not being adequately relieved
- perceiving one's lack of influence in the workplace
- perceiving that the institution's ethical decision-making process is unclear or inadequate.

Responses to Moral Distress

Individuals' responses to moral distress include feelings of anger, frustration, resentment, exhaustion, or sorrow; feelings of helplessness or powerlessness; erosion of personal integrity and self-esteem; feelings of passivity, uncertainty, and personal and professional disillusionment; physical or emotional withdrawal; a sense of failure (i.e., feelings of having failed the child or the family); feeling undervalued; and guilt. Some professionals might use sarcasm, cry, or leave their current work assignment, whereas others might manipulate situational constraints to gain control, provide comfort, and advocate for the patient and the family. Others might experience a level of stress that leads to quiet suffering, or diminished self-worth, or burnout. Personal and professional relationships can be affected. Moral outrage can occur when there is a "perceived inability to stop/prevent the immoral actions of others" (Wilkinson, 1987–1988, p. 25).

Strategies for Dealing with Moral Distress

- Increase knowledge regarding their patients' clinical situations.

- Clarify personal beliefs, values, and principles, and determine how these beliefs, values, and principles guide individual nursing practice and influence care decisions.
- Communicate clearly and discuss issues with others.
  - Assess the patient's and the family's understanding of the situation.
  - Clarify the implications of the patient's and the family's decisions.
  - Provide additional information or further education to help the patient and the family make their decisions.
  - Determine how the decisions are communicated because eliciting different points of view can help people clarify their own beliefs and talking with others can help resolve issues, offer explanations, and help them decide on a course of action. Sharing individual concerns with others can provide support.
- Recognize moral dilemmas.
  - Ascertain whether the decisions made by the patient, family, and other members of the team are consistent with the nurse's personal beliefs, values, and principles, and determine the level of comfort. Sometimes the best way for professionals to recognize a moral dilemma is by acknowledging their own discomfort with a situation.
- Identify resources, both personal and professional.
- Identify how an institution can help healthcare professionals resolve their ethical dilemmas (e.g., by instituting ethics rounds or ethics committees, providing education and mentorship about ethical decision-making, and developing policies and procedures for identifying and working through ethical dilemmas).
- Develop a plan of action for dealing with ethical dilemmas. As situations arise, decide on a moral course of action after compiling background information and data pertaining to the situation and identifying all of the people involved in the dilemma that might be affected by the decisions.
- Plan how to advocate for the child and the family. Advocacy "involves assisting an individual in making informed choices and advancing his or her interests and life goals...it is not acting instead of someone else or acting to rescue someone from a...situation" (Rushton, 1992, p. 305).
  - Consider different courses of action.
  - Identify the potential obstacles and the consequences of each alternative.
  - Prepare to defend actions. There may be times when the wishes of a patient or a family cannot be carried out. For example, there would be legal ramifications if a child asked for help in taking his or her own life and the nurse complied with that request; in this instance.
- Consider the consequences of each action on patients, the patients' families, colleagues, the workplace, and on the nurse.
- Develop a self-awareness of the triggers that result in moral distress by identifying which situations conflict with one's own moral principles and which ones can cause moral distress. Individuals who are able to recognize such triggers take action to reduce moral distress.
- Discuss moral and ethical issues with colleagues. Decide how to work together to create an ethical environment.

References

Raines, M.L. (2000). Ethical decision making in nurses: Relationships among moral reasoning, coping style, and ethics stress. *JONA's Healthcare Law, Ethics, and Regulation, 2,* 29–41.

Rodney, P., & Starzomski, R. (1993). Constraints on the moral agency of nurses. *The Canadian Nurse, 89*(9), 23–26.

Rushton, C.H., (1992). Caregiver suffering in critical care nursing. *Heart and Lung, 21,* 303–306.

Wilkinson, J.M. (1987–1988). Moral distress in nursing practice: Experience and effect. *Nursing Forum, 23*(1), 16–29.

Ethical Dilemmas in Terminal Care

Lorraine Cogan

General Principles

Gaining insight into ethical dilemmas can require professionals to review the issues by using an ethical framework. A number of ethics-related concepts should be considered when examining issues related to the care of terminally ill children.

Autonomy: The patient's family has the right to choose medical care for the patient. Adults can exercise their right to refuse medical care. Children should be involved in the decision-making process to the extent that they are developmentally ready.

Justice: Distributive justice means the fair allocation of resources. Healthcare providers should determine whether patients in all situations are being treated equally and fairly.

Beneficence: The principle of beneficence means "doing what is good" and providing selected medical interventions that will benefit patients.

Nonmaleficence: The principle of nonmaleficence means "doing no harm." This principle applies to providing selected medical interventions that will do no harm and determining how some interventions could place a burden on a patient and the family.

Double effect: The concept of double effect applies to the process of producing a desired outcome that may risk a negative effect. It is ethically permissible to proceed if the outcome has been determined to be acceptable, right reasons govern the decision, and an acceptable reason (e.g., administering pain medication to comfort a patient) justifies a bad effect. It is acceptable to risk the possibility of respiratory suppression or even early death if a patient's death is imminent or inevitable because pain relief, not the shortening of the patient's life, is the desired outcome.

Nursing Assessment and Interventions

Assessment:

- Recognize situations that create ethical dilemmas (**Table 9-3**).
- Examine the benefits and risks of a particular intervention.
- Analyze ethical dilemmas by using an ethical framework and concepts.
- Determine the patient's and the family's values and wishes, and facilitate a determination of what is in the child's best interests.

Table 9-3. Common Ethical Dilemmas Encountered when Caring for Terminally Ill Children

Dilemma	Rationale for Providing Life-Prolonging Measures to the Patient	Rationale for Withholding Life-Prolonging Measures or Other Measures from the Patient
Medications for pain control	Comfort is the primary goal. The quality of the child's life will improve. The dying process will be easier if the child is free from pain.	Opioid narcotics may cause a decreased level of cognition. Depending on the child's level of pain and stage of illness, pain medications may shorten life (see the brief discussion of double effect in this section). Taking narcotics can result in addiction (this fear in relation to terminally ill patients is unfounded).
Chemotherapy or experimental therapy	These therapies can prolong the patient's life span. The patient may possibly have an increase in the quality of life. Providing these therapies conveys the message that the family has done everything it could have to save the child.	These therapies decrease the child's blood counts and increase the risk of infection. The side effects of treatment may be painful or uncomfortable.
Supplemental nutrition and hydration (intravenous, nasogastric, g-tube)	The child may be hungry or thirsty. The child cannot and will not eat. These measures alleviate the fear that the child will starve to death. The primary role of parents is to feed and nourish their child. These measures relieve parental guilt feelings.	Supplemental oral feedings beyond what a child can ingest may actually cause nausea and vomiting. These measures can cause an increase in the tumor's growth (i.e., they feed the tumor). An increase in fluid volume can result in congestive heart failure, increased respiratory secretions and/or pulmonary congestion–which leads to the question of whether to administer a diuretic and have the child endure its side effects. Increased urine output can lead to increased risk of skin breakdown if the child is incontinent. There is a risk of ascites. Withholding IV fluids decreases nausea and vomiting, shortness of breath, and incontinence. Death is more comfortable and natural when supplemental nutrition is not provided. Ice chips are effective in managing a dry mouth. Complaints of being thirsty are associated with the dying process, not the patient's level of hydration (Zerwekh, 1997).
Families that resist do-not-resuscitate orders	The family believes they are giving up. This directive conflicts with the family's cultural or religious beliefs. The family is in denial about the fact that the child is actually going to die. The family cannot assume responsibility for stopping interventions that might prolong the child's life.	The directive allows nature to take its course. The family believes the child has suffered enough.
Autopsy	An autopsy will aid in research that may help other children. An autopsy may be able to establish or determine if the disease has a genetic link.	The child and family have endured enough. The autopsy will not provide valuable medical information.

- Recognize that some families will not be able to address some difficult issues that will determine the child's medical treatment later in the child's illness, and plan to readdress them as the situation changes.
- Maintain an expert level of knowledge concerning how to manage patients' end-stage symptoms in the best way possible.

Interventions:

- Consult with other healthcare team members to obtain their advice, expertise, and assistance.
- Discuss current issues related to managing the patient's treatment with the patient and the family.
- Introduce as early as possible potential issues that the patient and the family will have to confront. It may be easier for parents to consider alternatives when they are not in a crisis situation.
- Support the patient and the family in the decisions they make regardless of how those fit with one's personal philosophy.
- Provide options for treatment and explain the sequelae of each option.

Reference

Zerwekh, J.V. (1997). Do dying patients really need I.V. fluids? *American Journal of Nursing, 97*(3), 23–30.

Legal Concerns

Lorraine Cogan

General Principles

Providing care to children who are terminally ill requires careful planning to adhere to state regulations and institutional policies.

Legal Considerations

Individual states have different laws governing do-not-resuscitate orders and time limitations for do-not-resuscitate orders. Other legal issues that may apply include notification of a death that occurs at home (state or county laws governing medical examiners' jurisdiction when a child's death occurs at home must be considered), the process or legality of a nurse's pronouncement of death, autopsy (mandatory in some states), transportation of dead bodies, observance of do-not-resuscitate orders by paramedics or school system authorities, and the control of narcotic substances, such as those that might be used to control pain in terminally ill patients.

Nursing Assessment and Interventions

Assessment:

- Research state and county laws governing medical examiners' jurisdiction regarding home deaths, a nurse's pronouncement of death, autopsy, and transportation of dead bodies.
- Determine the legal criteria for a do-not-resuscitate order.

Interventions:

- Research the institution's policies and state regulations for guidelines on narcotics use. Prescriptions that allow titration to comfort patients may require that specific procedures be followed prior to filling the prescription.
- If appropriate, contact local paramedics, school officials, or both to notify them about a child's do-not-resuscitate status.

Bibliography

Children and Death

Bluebond-Langner, M. (1977). *The private words of dying children.* Princeton, NJ: Princeton University Press.

Brown-Hellsten, M. (2002). Family-centered end-of-life care. In M.J. Hockenberry, *Wong's nursing care of infants and children* (7th ed., pp. 947–1030). St. Louis: Mosby.

Physical Care of the Terminally Ill Child

Brown, M., Hockenberry-Eaton, M., Lamb, D., Chordas, C., Kline, N., & Bottomley, S. (2000). *End of Life Care for Children.* Austin, TX: Texas Cancer Council.

Dougherty, M., & Debaun, M.R. (2003). Rapid increase of morphine and benzodiazepine usage in the last three days of life in children with cancer is related to neuropathic pain. *Journal of Pediatrics, 142*, 373–376.

Hellsten, M.B. (2000). All the king's horses and all the king's men: Pain management from hospital to home. *Journal of Pediatric Oncology Nursing, 17*, 149–159.

Hockenberry-Eaton, M., Barrera, P., Brown, M., Bottomley, S.J., & O'Neill, J. (1999). *Pain management in children with cancer.* Austin, TX: Texas Cancer Council.

Kane, J.R., & Primono, M. (2001). Alleviating the suffering of seriously ill children. *The American Journal of Hospice and Palliative Care, 18*, 161–169.

Mitchell, A.M., Gale, D.D., Matzo, M.L., McDonald, M.C., & Gadmer, N. (2002). Critique of transcultural practices in end-of-life clinical nursing practice. *Nursing Forum, 37*(4), 24–31.

Psychosocial Care of the Terminally Ill Child

Brown, M., Hockenberry-Eaton, M., Lamb, D., Chordas, C., Kline, N., & Bottomley, S. (2000). *End of life care for children.* Austin, TX: Texas Cancer Council.

Contro, N., Larson, J., Scofield, S., Sourkes, B., & Cohen, H. (2002). Family perspectives on the quality of pediatric palliative care. *Archives of Pediatric & Adolescent Medicine, 156*, 14–19.

Hongo, T., Watanabe, C., Okada, S., Inoue, N., Yajima, S., & Fujii, Y., et al. (2003). Analysis of the circumstances at the end of life in children with cancer: Symptoms, suffering, and acceptance. *Pediatrics International, 45*, 60–64.

Zwerdling, T., Davies, S., Lazar, L., Crawford, B., Tucker, L., & Boughner, A., et al. (2000). Unique aspects of caring for dying children and their families. *The American Journal of Hospice and Palliative Care, 17*, 305–311.

Bereavement

Field, M.J., & Behrman, R.E. (Eds.). (2003). *When children die: Improving palliative and end-of-life care for children and their families.* Washington, D.C.: The National Academies Press.

Fochtman, D. (2002). Palliative care. In C.R. Baggott, K.P. Kelly, D. Fochtman, & G.V. Foley (Eds.), *Nursing care of children and adolescents with cancer* (3rd ed., pp. 400–425). Philadelphia: W.B. Saunders.

Hilden, J., & Tobin, D.R. (2003). *Shelter from the storm: Caring for a child with a life-threatening condition.* Cambridge, MA: Perseus Publishing.

Kushner, H.S. (2001). *When bad things happen to good people.* New York: Schocken Books.

Woznick, L.A., & Goodheart, C.D. (Eds.) (2002). *Living with childhood cancer.* Washington, D.C.: American Psychological Association.

Professionals' Grief, Distress, and Bereavement

Papadatou, D., Bellali, T., Papazoglou, I., & Petraki, D. (2002). Greek nurse and physician grief as a result of caring for children dying of cancer. *Pediatric Nursing, 28,* 345–353.

Rich, S. (2002). Caregiver grief: Taking care of ourselves and our patients. *International Journal of Trauma Nursing, 8,* 24–28.

Moral Distress

Corley, M.C., Elswich R.K., Gorman, M., & Clor, T. (2001). Development and evaluation of a moral distress scale. *Journal of Advanced Nursing, 33,* 250–256.

Erlen, J.A. (2001). Moral distress: A pervasive problem. *Orthopaedic Nursing, 20,* 76–80.

Georges, J.J., & Grypdonck, M. (2002). Moral problems experienced by nurses when caring for terminally ill people: A literature review. *Nursing Ethics, 9,* 155–178.

Hamric, A.B. (2000). Moral distress in everyday ethics. *Nursing Outlook, 48,* 199–201.

Rodney, P., Varcoe, C., Storch, J.L., McPherson, G., Mahoney, K., & Brown, H., et al. (2002). Navigating towards a moral horizon: A multisite qualitative study of ethical practice in nursing. *Canadian Journal of Nursing Research, 34,* 75–102.

Ethical Dilemmas in Terminal Care

Beauchamp, T.L, & Childress, J.F. (2001). *Principles of biomedical ethics.* New York: Oxford University Press.

Field, M.J., & Behrman, R.E. (Eds.). (2003). *When children die: Improving palliative and end-of-life care for children and their families.* Washington, D.C.: The National Academies Press.

SECTION X

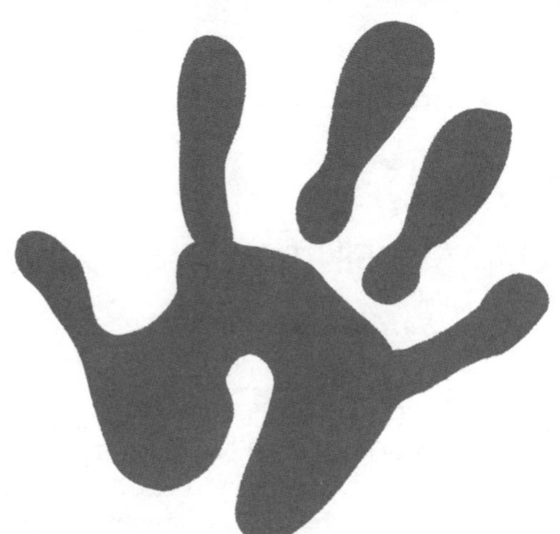

Late Effects of Childhood Cancer

Jill E. Brace O'Neill

Section Outline

Definition and Overview

Sarah J. Bottomley

Definition

The late effects of childhood cancer and its treatment can be defined as a broad range of persistent adverse effects related to the disease process, its therapy, or both. The onset of some late effects can be unpredictable and can occur months or even years after therapy is completed. Early recognition and prompt management of these sequelae can, in some cases, lessen the severity of the residual problems.

Overview

Epidemiology: Approximately 8,600 new cases of cancer occur annually in children younger than 15 years of age. More than 75% of these children can expect to be cured. It is estimated that currently in the United States, 1 in 900 people aged 15–45 years is a survivor of childhood cancer. This number is expected to increase to 1 in 250 people by 2010. Significant disabilities affect the quality of life of almost half of these long-term survivors.

Causes: Late effects can be caused by the cancer itself, by its treatment, or by a combination of both (**Table 10-1**). Treatments that can cause late effects include surgery, radiation therapy, chemotherapy, supportive care (e.g., administration of aminoglycosides, immunosuppressives).

Factors associated with the development of late effects: Late effects can be associated with

- the location and extent of the primary disease.
- the type and intensity of the initial treatment.
- the age as well as the physiological and developmental status of the person at the time of diagnosis and treatment.
- a genetic or familial predisposition that may interact with treatment-related injuries.

Categories of late effects: Late-effects categories include physical, emotional, economic and other effects. With physical late effects, all organ systems can be affected. A second malignant neoplasm also can manifest itself. Emotional late effects can include psychological and social adjustments. Economic late effects include concerns about finances and insurability. Other late effects can include difficulties in academic achievement and employment issues, such as job discrimination.

Central Nervous System

Sarah J. Bottomley

Definition

Neuropsychological deficits and neurological abnormalities are significant late effects of cancer for many long-term survivors. Their incidence is variable and depends upon the type and location of the original disease, the timing and method of central nervous system (CNS) treatment, and the patient's age at diagnosis. CNS changes can occur as a result of irradiation of the whole brain, surgery, or intrathecal chemotherapy. Neuropsychological deficits typically are manifested as a significant decline in a person's intelligence quotient (IQ) (i.e., 10–20 points), in academic achievement scores, and as specific deficits in integration of visual and motor functions, memory, attention, and motor skills. The most common neurological abnormalities include atrophy and decreased subcortical white matter. Calcifications and leukoencephalopathy are less common.

Risk Factors

Radiation therapy: Radiation therapy is the treatment most commonly associated with late CNS toxicities. Irradiation of the whole brain produces structural changes such as dystrophic calcification, mineralizing microangiopathy, and cerebral atrophy. Children treated before the age of 6 years usually have more serious toxicities than do children who were older when they received treatment. Children who are less than 2 years of age when they are treated are particularly vulnerable to CNS radiation-related toxicity.

Leukoencephalopathy is associated with irradiation of the whole brain at a dosage greater than 1,800 centrigrays (cGy). There is a noted synergy between radiation therapy and drugs such as methotrexate (Mexate). Radiation therapy disrupts the blood-brain barrier, which leads to increased levels of methotrexate in the CNS, which in turn, increases the risk of producing leukoencephalopathy. Hyperfractionated radio therapy may be less damaging to a normal CNS.

Neurocognitive deficits. Learning disabilities are dependent upon the cumulative radiation dosage; they occur with irradiation of the whole brain at levels greater than 1,800 cGy. Neurocognitive deficits are more severe and frequent in children who were less than 5 years old when they received cranial radiation therapy. There is no age limit above which the CNS is spared. Neurocognitive deficits are not progressive; however, children may experience difficulty in learning new concepts and with the increased academic challenges experienced during adolescence and adulthood.

Chemotherapy: High doses of methotrexate (Mexate), given intravenously or intrathecally, are associated with neuroanatomic pathology and neurocognitive deficits. Vinca alkaloids (vincristine [Oncovin], vinblastine [Velban], etoposide [VP-16], cisplatin [Platinol]) are associated with peripheral neuropathy. Intrathecal or intravenous methotrexate (Mexate) and intravenous cytarabine (Cytosine Arabinoside) are associated with leukoencephalopathy.

Surgery: Resection of a CNS tumor puts a patient at risk to develop neurocognitive deficits, which are related to the location of, and the extent of the surgery required to remove the tumor.

Clinical Presentation

Neurocognitive deficits: Neurocognitive deficits can present as difficulties with reading, verbal and nonverbal memory, arithmetic, receptive and expressive language, speed of mental processing. Other negative effects include attention deficits, a decreased IQ, behavioral problems, poor school attendance, poor hand-eye coordination, or personality changes.

Table 10-1. Late Effects Associated with Childhood Cancer Treatments

Organ System	Risk Factors	Potential Late Effects	Evaluation/Interventions
Central nervous system–cognitive	Radiation therapy to brain >1,800 cGy Methotrexate (Mexate) (high-dose intravenous or intrathecal) Resection of a CNS tumor ARA = C (interthecal or high dose intervention)	Learning disabilities Leukoencephalopathy Mineralizing microangiopathy Cerebral atrophy	Arrange for the following: – neurocognitive testing – psychoeducational assistance – a CT or an MRI scan (a baseline and when there are symptoms) – an EEG – an audiogram – vision screening – a neurological consultation as indicated – educational or vocational testing – referral to school liaison program
Central nervous system–peripheral neuropathy	Vincristine (Oncovin) Vinblastine (Velban) Etoposide (VP-16) Cisplatin (Platinol)	Generalized weakness Tingling and numbness Foot drop Parasthesias Areflexia	Arrange for a thorough neurological examination on an annual basis. Encourage the patient to protect the affected area from exposure to extreme temperature. Arrange for physical/occupational therapy. Refferal to pain team (for neuropathic pain management).
Endocrine–hypothalamic-pituitary axis	Radiation therapy to HPA >1,800 cGy Resection of tumor in HPA region Radiation therapy to HPA of >3,000 to 4,000 cGy Resection of tumor in HPA region	Growth hormone deficiency TSH deficiency Adrenocorticotropic hormone (ACTH) deficiency Gonadotropin deficiency Hyperprolactinemia Obesity	Obtain the patient's height, weight, and sitting height measurement annually (every 6 months at ages 9–12 years). Chart measurements on a growth curve. Obtain a bone age film as clinically indicated. Assess Tanner stage during a physical exam. Ensure that appropriate hormone testing is done. Consult an endocrinologist if growth hormone therapy is indicated. Delay puberty with GnRH therapy. Ensure that thyroid studies are done at baseline and every 3–5 years or as directed by an endocrinologist. Check cortisol level to assess for ACTH deficiency. Measure LH, FSH, estradiol, or testosterone levels to assess for gonadotropin deficiency. Obtain prolactin levels to assess for hyperprolactinemia. Ensure that the patient is on appropriate hormone replacement for the specific deficiency. Provide anticipatory guidance on symptoms related to the specific deficiency.
	Radiation therapy to the HPA >2,000 cGy, effects may be seen at doses as low as 1,000 cGy Resection of tumor in the HPA region	Precocious puberty	Obtain height and plot it on a growth curve annually. Determine bone age every 2 years until growth is complete. Measure LH, FSH, estradiol, or testosterone levels. Consult an endocrinologist as needed. Obtain a pelvic ultrasound and GnRH stimulation testing, as needed. Ensure that patient is on appropriate hormone therapy as indicated. Delay puberty with GnRH therapy.
Thyroid	Radiation therapy to the neck or cervical spine >2,000 cGy Total body irradiation >750 cGy Partial or complete thyroidectomy Prior lymphangiogram Total body irradiation (>1,000 cGy)	Hypothyroidism Overt (elevated TSH, decreased T4) Compensated (elevated TSH, normal T4) Thyroid nodules Hyperthyroidism (Graves' disease) (decreased TSH, elevated T4) Thyroiditis Benign or malignant tumors	Obtain at least annual thyroid studies, usually thyroxine and TSH (may include free T4). Refer the patient to an endocrinologist. Patient may require thyroxine replacement. Provide anticipatory guidance on symptoms related to hyperthyroidism or hypothyroidism.

(continued on the next page)

Table 10-1. Late Effects Associated with Childhood Cancer Treatments *(continued)*

Organ System	Risk Factor	Potential Late Effects	Evaluation/Interventions
Ophthal-mology	Steroids Radiation > 800 cGy TBI	Cataracts	Recommend an annual ophthalmoscopic exam. Assess for a decreased red reflex. Patient may require cataract extraction.
	Radiation >4,500 cGy	Decreased tear production (lacrimal gland) Fibrosis of the lacrimal duct Ulcerations or telangiectasis of the eyelids Decreased visual acuity/vision loss Conjunctive necrosis or scarring Thinning of the sclera Ulceration of the cornea (Radiation retinopathy, optic atrophy, xeropthalmia)	Recommend an annual ophthalmologic examination and appropriate follow-up for identified problems (Patient may require cataract extraction). Recommend tear replacement, as needed. Provide education regarding proper eye care.
Ears/Hearing	Aminoglycosides Recurrent otitis media Carboplatin Cisplatin (Platinol) –cumulative dose ≥360mg/m2 CNS neoplasm Age <3 years at treatment Loop diuretics Radiation to the head/neck/ cranial radiation	Sensorineural high-frequency hearing loss Tinnitus Vertigo Abnormal speech development Otosclerosis, chronic otitis media Cerumen impaction	Perform baseline audiogram brainstem auditory evoked response (BAER) and then one every 2–3 years and at every 3 and 5 years if abnormal; follow every year until stable, then every 3 years. Examine the canal. Recommend preferential seating in school, amplification, hearing aids, as indicated. May require speech therapy, as indicated. Consult with an ENT, an audiologist, and a neurologist, as indicated.
Head and neck	Radiation >4,000 cGy	Xerostomia Intranasal scarring Epilation, Alopecia Fibrosis Hypoplasia, bony deformity Decreased salivary function Muscle hypoplasia, constricting fibrosis Osteoradionecrosis Chronic sinusitus Dysphagia	Inspect the mucosa. Recommend dental examination every 6 months. Encourage behaviors that promote dental, head, and neck health: meticulous oral hygiene, no tobacco use, stretching exercises, PT as indicated, and a diet low in concentrated sugars. Provide resource information on wigs and alternative hairstyles. Patient may require saliva substitutes. Sinus CT and otolaryngology consult as needed (Refer to gastroenterology with dysphagia and obtain endoscopy).
	Radiation ≥1,000 cGy	Thyroid nodules/cancer Thyroid dysfunction (hypo or hyper) Dysphagia	Annual physical examination Annual thyroid ultrasound Annual TSH for minimum of 7 years post radiation. Obtain endoscopy with dysphagia and refer to gastroenterology
Dental	Radiation >100 cGy given when the patient is <5 years old Chemotherapy: vincristine (Oncovin), dactinomycin (Actinomycin-D), methotrexate (Mexate), mercaptopurine (Purinethol), cyclophospha-mide (Cytoxan), procarbazine (Matulane), mechlorethamine (nitrogen mustard)	Abnormal tooth and root development, thinning or shortening Dental caries Enamel dysplasia Periodontal disease Tooth decay Malocclusion Craniofacial abnormalities	Recommend orthodontic evaluations as indicated. Provide periodontal prophylaxis. Obtain radiographic studies of irradiated bone every 3–5 years. Dental examination and hygiene every 6 months. Regular fluoride applications.

(continued on the next page)

Table 10-1. Late Effects Associated with Childhood Cancer Treatments *(continued)*

Organ System	Risk Factor	Potential Late Effects	Evaluation/Interventions
Cardiovascular	Anthracyclines >300 mg/m^2 >200 mg/m^2 with radiation therapy to the thorax (including chest, mantle, mediastinal, whole lung, spinal) Other chemotherapy, primarily high-dose cyclophosphamide (Cytoxan)	Arrythmias Cardiomyopathy Pericardial damage	Obtain MUGA/echo, EKG, and chest X ray (baseline and then <300 mg/m^2: every 5 years; <300 mg/m^2 and radiation to the heart: every 2 years; ≥300–400 mg/m^2: every 2 years; ≥300 mg/m^2 + radiation to heart; yearly ≥400 mg/m^2: yearly Refer to a cardiologist, as indicated. Use Holter monitor and have exercise testing done as clinically indicated.
	Radiation >3,000 cGy to mediastinum, or whole lung or mantle >2,500 cGy when given with anthracyclines >3,000 cGy to spine Total body irradiation Female gender Black race <5 years old at treatment		Patient may require cardiac medication. Provide anticipatory guidance for symptoms of cardiac dysfunction and the side effects of cardiac medications. End-stage cardiomyopathy may require a heart transplant. Additional evaluation reccommendation for patients who receive >300 mg/m^2 in the following situations: Pregnancy Prior to initiation of exercise (especially isometric programs).
	Radiation >4,000 cGy	Valvular damage	Obtain echocardiogram and chest X ray (baseline, then every 3–5 years if normal or if the patient is symptomatic). Patient will require penicillin prophylaxis when having surgery or dental procedures.
	Radiation >3,000 cGy	Coronary artery disease	Obtain an EKG (baseline, then every 2–3 years if normal, or if the patient is symptomatic). Obtain a stress test (baseline, then every 3–5 years if normal, or if the patient is symptomatic). Arrange for a consultation with a cardiologist, as indicated. Provide education on the importance of a physical conditioning program and a low-sodium, low-fat diet.
Respiratory	Radiation >1,000 cGy to the pulmonary field Chemotherapy: (bleomycin [Blenoxane], Busulfan (myleran), chlorambucil [Leukeran], mitomycin [Mutamycin], methotrexate [Mexate], cytarabine [Cytosine Arabinoside, carmustine [BCNU], lomustine [CCNU], vinca alkaloids, alkylating agents) Increased risk with radiation dose ≥4,000 cGy Large lung volume in radiation field Combination of radiation and radiation-sensitizing chemotherapy	Pneumonitis Fibrosis	Obtain a chest X ray (baseline, then every 2–5 years, if normal). Perform pulmonary function tests, including diffusion capacity (baseline, then every 3–5 years, if normal and prior to anesthesia). Perform a CT, which may help to define lung volumes. Perform a ventilation quotient scan, as indicated. Prescribe pneumococcal (Pneumovax) and influenza virus vaccines (Fluogen) annually. Refer patient to a pulmonologist, as needed. Provide education regarding healthy behaviors, avoidance or cessation of smoking, maintaining physical conditioning. Treat the patient's symptoms with corticosteroids, bronchodilators, expectorants, antibiotics, oxygen, and bed rest, as needed. Provide anticipatory guidance for those who have received bleomycin (Blenoxane) regarding the risk of respiratory failure with high levels of oxygen (avoid scuba diving).

(continued on the next page)

Table 10-1. Late Effects Associated with Childhood Cancer Treatments *(continued)*

Organ System	Risk Factor	Potential Late Effects	Evaluation/Interventions
Gastro-intestinal	Radiation >4,000 cGy Chemotherapy: doxorubicin (Adriamycin) and dactinomycin (Actinomycin-D); radiation therapy enhances methotrexate (Mexate) and 6-mercaptopurine (Purinethol) Surgery, which may enhance radiation therapy and is also associated with obstruction Bone marrow transplant	Fibrosis, strictures, obstruction Enteritis Adhesions Ulcers Malabsorption Splenomegaly and thrombocytopenia, which can occur after radiation therapy Graft-versus-host disease leading to GI tract strictures, fibrosis GI malignancy	Obtain height and weight on an annual basis. Obtain stool guaiac on an annual basis, and annual rectal examination after the age of 40 years. Obtain a CBC with mean corpuscular value on an annual basis. Obtain blood chemistries on an annual basis. Provide anticipatory guidance regarding dietary modification as needed. Refer to or: Consult a gastroenterologist, as needed. Dilate the fibrotic or obstructed area. Obtain radiographic studies, as indicated. Educate the patient regarding medication administration and side effects, as indicated. Educate the patient regarding a high fiber diet.
Hepatic	Radiation >2,600 cGy Chemotherapy: dactinomycin (Actinomycin-D) radiotherapy enhancer, methotrexate (Mexate), 6-mercaptopurine (Purinethol) Surgery (a hepatic resection can enhance the development of sequelae) Blood transfusions (especially prior to 1992)	Fibrosis Cirrhosis Hepatitis –radiation-induced hepatitis –transfusion-mediated viral hepatitis, which may include hepatitis B, C, or cytomegalovirus	Refer to or consult a gastroenterologist, as needed. Obtain the following: –chemistry panel on an annual basis –baseline hepatitis panel –abdominal ultrasound or livel biopsy, as indicated to assess for hepatitis. Patient may require dietary management for fibrosis. Hepatitis may require treatment with interferon. End-stage liver disease may require a liver transplant. Educate patient about healthy behaviors as well as avoiding alcohol or other hepatoxic drugs. Educate the patient regarding medication administration and side effects as indicated.
Genitourinary	Radiation – Kidney > 2,000-2,500 cGy – Bladder >3,000 cGy (before puberty) – Bladder >5,000 cGy (after puberty) – Prostate >4,000-6,000 cGy – Vagina >4,000 cGy – Uterus >2,000 cGy (before puberty) – Uterus > 4,000-5,000 cGy (after puberty) – Ureter/urethra >5,000 cGy – Pelvic >5,000 cGy Chemotherapy – Cisplatin (Platinol) – Ifosfamide (Ifex) – Cyclophosphamide (Cytoxan) Supportive therapies –Aminoglycosides –Cyclosporine [Sandimmune] –Amphotericin Surgery – nephrectomy	Hypoplastic kidney Nephrotic syndrome Bladder fibrosis or hypoplasia Decreased volume of seminal fluid Hypoplastic or atrophied prostate Fibrosis (vaginal, uterine, ureter) Stricture of urethra Glomerular dysfunction (cisplatin [Platinol]) Tubular dysfunction (cisplatin and ifosfamide [Ifex]) Fibrosis, hypoplasia, or secondary malignancy of bladder (cyclophosphamide, (ifosfamide) Hemorrhagic cystitis (cyclophosphamide, ifosfamide) Incontinence	Perform an annual examination with close attention to the patient's blood pressure, height, and weight. Obtain a urinalysis, BUN, creatinine, hemoglobin/hematocrit, creatinine clearance or GFR (yearly). Consult a nephrologist or urologist as indicated, for patients with hypertension, proteinuira, culture-negative hematuria, or progressive renal insufficiency. Patient may require low-protein, low-salt dietary modifications. Serum sodium, potassium chloride, carbon dioxide, calcium, magnesium phosphorus (for those at risk for tubular dysfunction (baseline; if normal repeat every 5 years). Supplement magnesium and phosphorus as indicated. End-stage kidney disease may require dialysis or a kidney transplant. Patient may require medication for hypertension as indicated. Educate the patient regarding kidney health after a nephrectomy, recommend that the patient avoid contact sports and maintain hydration, and encourage the patient to wear a Medic-Alert bracelet.

(continued on the next page)

Table 10-1. Late Effects Associated with Childhood Cancer Treatments *(continued)*

Organ System	Risk Factor	Potential Late Effects	Evaluation/Interventions
Genitourinary *(continued)*	– removal of other genitourinary organs – damage to nerves Age (young children may experience increased effects, which may not become apparent until the child reaches an age when the organ is unable to compensate)	Infertility	Provide anticipatory guidance related to potential problems with incontinence and infertility as it is needed. Counsel/educate patient regarding prompt reporting of dysuria or gross hematuria.
Reproductive–Testes	Radiation > 100 to 600 cGy to testes Radiation to the hypothalamic-pituitary axis Total body radiation	Testicular atrophy Delayed or arrested pubertal development Infertility	Assess pubertal history. Assess Tanner stage annually. Determine testicular size. (volume and turgor). Obtain LH, FSH, and testosterone levels for delayed pubertal development and when it is clinically indicated. Obtain thyroxine and TSH levels. Refer to or consult with an endocrinologist when necessary. Semen analysis, as needed.
	Chemotherapy: alkylating agents (procarbazine [Matulane], cisplatin [Platinol], cyclophosphamide [Cytoxan], ifosfamide [Ifex]), nitrosoureas (carmustine [BCNU], lomustine [CCNU]) Busulfan (myleran) Mechlorethamine (mustargen) Melphalan (Alkeran) Chlorambucil (Leukeran) Surgery (orchiectomy, or peritoneal node dissection) Age (pubertal males have the highest risk for toxicity) Thyroid dysfunction	Oligospermia or azospermia Ejaculatory or other dysfunction Infertility Hypogonadism	Obtain a bone age film, as indicated. Obtain analysis of sperm at maturity and when clinically indicated. Provide anticipatory guidance regarding symptoms of testosterone deficiency or germ cell damage. Consult an endocrinologist when it is indicated. Provide fertility counseling. Educate the patient regarding performing testicular exams on himself. Provide education regarding hormone replacement therapy and side effects if it is indicated. Prevention of osteoporosis and atherosclerosis. Counsel women at risk of early menopause regarding fertility options.
Reproductive–Ovaries	Radiation >400 cGy to ovaries Radiation to the hypothalamic-pituitary axis Total body irradiation Chemotherapy alkylating agents; procarbazine (Matulane), nitrosoureas; carmustine (BCNU), lomustine (CCNU) Busulfan (myleran) Ifosfamide (Ifex) Cyclophosphamide (Cytoxan), Mechlorethamine (mustargen) Melphalan (Alkeran) Chlorambucil (Leukeran) Surgery (oophorectomy, oophoropexy)	Delayed menarche Delayed or arrested pubertal development Oligomenorrhea or amenorrhea after puberty Infertility Early menopause	Assess pubertal history. Assess Tanner stage annually. Obtain LH, FSH, and estradiol levels for delayed pubertal development and when it is clinically indicated. Obtain thyroxine and TSH levels. Menstrual and pregnancy history Obtain a bone age film, as indicated. Obtain an ultrasound of the ovaries, as indicated. Recommend measurement of basal body temperature. Consult with an endocrinologist when indicated. Provide anticipatory guidance regarding the symptoms of estrogen deficiency and early menopause. Provide fertility counseling and education regarding alternate strategies for parenting. Patient may require hormone replacement.

(continued on the next page)

Table 10-1. Late Effects Associated with Childhood Cancer Treatments *(continued)*

Organ System	Risk Factor	Potential Late Effects	Evaluation/Interventions
Reproductive–Ovaries *(continued)*	Age (older females are at greater risk of ovarian failure) Total body irradiation		Provide education regarding hormone replacement therapy and prevention of osteoporosis and atherosclerosis. Counsel women at risk of early menopause regarding fertility options.
Musculoskeletal/ growth	Radiation > 1,000-2,000 cGy Surgery – muscle loss or resection – amputation – limb salvage – laminectomy Younger age at the time of treatment Chemotherapy – steroids – vinca alkaloids –methotrexate Hypogonadism GH deficiency	Partial or complete arrest of the growth of epiphysis Spinal abnormalities Muscle hypoplasia Asymmetry of muscles Decreased range of motion Gait abnormalities Discrepancy in the length of an extremity Osteonecrosis (AVN) Slipped capitofemoral epiphysis Pathological fracture Osteoporosis Osteopenia	Make a careful comparison and measurement of irradiated and unirradiated areas. Obtain a bone age film as indicated. Obtain and plot on growth chart the patient's height, weight, and sitting height measurements annually. Perform radiographic studies of the irradiated area (baseline, yearly during rapid growth, and if normal, then every 5 years). Refer to or consult an orthopedist as clinically indicated. Encourage a routine physical exercise program for both range of motion and strengthening. Educate the patient about the importance of weight control and exercise. Provide anticipatory guidance regarding realistic expectations about potential growth and function of the affected area and educate regarding osteoporosis prevention with calcium and vitamin D. Treat exacerbating or predisposing conditions (i.e., hypogonadism).
Hematopoietic and immunologic	Radiation – marrow-containing bones – total body irradiation –asplenia, if spleen was in radiation field Blood transfusion(s) (prior to 1985) Surgery – splenectomy Chemotherapy – high doses for extended periods –Etoposide (VP–16) Tenopside (VM–26) –Alkylators—melphalan or nitrogen mustard	Hypoplastic or aplastic bone Frequent, recurrent infection Decreased immunoglobulin levels Overwhelming bacterial infection Acute myeloid leukemia Human Immunodeficiency Virus (HIV)	Obtain a CBC with differential. Perform a bone marrow aspiration as clinically indicated. Obtain immunoglobulin levels as indicated. Obtain T-cell studies as indicated. Consult with an immunologist when it is indicated. Encourage annual evaluations. Recommendations for asplenic individuals: – prophylactic penicillin – pneumococcal vaccine, meningococcal, H. influenza – prompt treatment with symptoms of fever, chills, or infection Medic-Alert bracelet noting asplenia Test for HIV
All Systems (including skin/ dermatologic)	Radiation –higher daily fractions or cumulative treatment dose –extended treatment volumes Chemotherapy –alkylators	Secondary benign or malignant neoplasm in radiation field	Perform annual physical exam with inspection of skin and soft tissues in radiation treatment field(s). Refer to oncology, as indicated. Refer to dermatology, as indicated.

Leukoencephalopathy: Leukoencephalopathy can present as dementia, dysarthria, dysphagia, ataxia, spasticity, seizures, or coma. In some cases, blindness also can occur.

Peripheral neuropathy: Peripheral neuropathy can present as foot drop, parasthesias, or numbness of the hands or feet.

Diagnostic Work-up

A diagnostic work-up consists of a comprehensive yearly history and a physical examination. The patient should receive a baseline computed tomography (CT) scan of the head to evaluate for calcifications. Follow-up CT scans of the head should be obtained if clinically indicated. Magnetic resonance imaging (MRI) should be done if clinically indicated to provide greater anatomic detail and better detection of white matter changes and leptomeningeal and spinal disease. Neuropsychological testing should be done when the patient has completed therapy to establish a baseline, then routinely (i.e., every 2–3 years) during the hallmark stages of academic advancement. In addition, a patient's school performance should be monitored.

Medical Treatment

Medical treatment involves neurocognitive and behavioral rehabilitation, including appropriate school placement, provision of community and school resources to meet the patient's special needs, counseling, and training in behavior management. Psychopharmocological intervention can include administration of methylphenidate (Ritalin) or other psychotropic drugs to control behavioral outbursts or seizures.

Nursing Assessment and Interventions

Assessment:

- Review the survivor's academic performance, including parents' and teachers' appraisals of performance, grade level in school, conduct or behavioral problems, attention problems, as well as strengths and weaknesses in school and attendance.
- Make an assessment of additional available resources as well as those already being used by the child.

Interventions:

- Reinforce the importance of having lifelong follow-up assessments annually with a healthcare provider who is familiar with the survivor's cancer history, treatment, and risks for developing late effects.
- Review neuropsychological results with the family and school staff, as necessary.
- Encourage early intervention with specialized educational programs, tutoring, and resource classes.
- Educate teachers about the child's previous cancer history and the potential for long-term side effects.
- Encourage the parents to advocate for their child's educational needs.
- Advocate for occupational and physical therapies when they are needed.
- Educate the child about peripheral neuropathy, and caution that affected areas should be protected from exposure to excessive heat or cold.

Expected Patient Outcomes

- The survivor is knowledgeable about the risks for neuropsychological and neurological toxicities.
- The survivor has annual follow-up visits.
- The survivor has access to and uses resources in the school and the community to help achieve academic goals.
- The survivor's teachers are knowledgeable about his or her previous treatment and late effects and are providing appropriate intervention.
- The survivor or the family can advocate for the child's needs.

Hypothalamic-Pituitary Axis

Barbara Anne Hieb, Susan K. Ogle, and Wendy Hobbie

Definition

The hypothalamus and the pituitary gland work synergistically to maintain homeostasis of the endocrine system and are connected by the pituitary stalk. Abnormalities of the hypothalamic-pituitary axis (HPA) are commonly seen after a patient has received radiation to the head, neck, and face. Surgery near the HPA also may contribute to abnormalities. A hypothalamic-pituitary injury can result in abnormal levels of growth hormone, thyrotropin, gonadotropins, adrenocorticotropin hormone (ACTH), prolactin, antidiuretic hormone (ADH), or vasopressin.

Risk Factors

Radiation therapy: Injuries from radiation therapy can result from dosages ranging from 1,000 to 5,000 centrigrays (cGy) as listed below:

- Growth abnormalities: dosages greater than 1,800–2,000 cGy
- Precocious puberty: dosages greater than 1,000–2,000 cGy
- Gonadotropin deficiency: dosages greater than 3,000–4,000 cGy
- Thyroid-stimulating hormone (TSH) deficiency: dosages greater than 3,000 cGy
- ACTH deficiency: dosages greater than 3,000–4,000 cGy
- Hyperprolactinemia: dosages greater than 4,000–5,000 cGy.

Higher dosages of radiation are associated with greater risk of developing a hormone deficiency. These deficiencies can occur more rapidly after the completion of cancer treatment for people exposed to higher dosages of radiation. Growing children are most profoundly affected.

Surgery: Surgery, including on the HPA, also may be a risk factor in the development of HPA abnormalities.

Tumor location: Children with tumors in the HPA region have a 30% chance of developing an ADH deficiency before surgery and a 16% chance after surgery.

Clinical Presentation

Growth hormone deficiency: Growth hormone (GH) deficiency is the most common, and generally the first, abnormality noted after a patient has had radiation to the HPA. This can result in a reduction in growth velocity that is inappropriate for a child's age and stage of puberty. Postpubertal patients may note a decrease in relative muscle mass and an increase in adipose tissue. Furthermore, there is new evidence of a relation between GH deficiency and a metabolic syndrome, which includes increased amount of adipose tissue, high cholesterol levels, hypertension, and early onset artherosclerosis.

Precocious puberty: Precocious puberty is manifested by breast development before the age of 8 years in females and signs of genital development and testicular enlargement in males who are younger than 9 years old. Additional manifestations include accelerated bone maturation, premature epiphyseal fusion, and reduced final height.

Gonadotropin deficiency: A gonadotropin deficiency is a failure to progress through puberty, arrested puberty, or amenorrhea. The influence of adrenal androgen on the development of pubic and axillary hair without corresponding breast development must be distinguished from true puberty. Breasts that have been irradiated might not grow during puberty. Testicular enlargement may be delayed. Primary gonadal failure occurs in boys who have received testicular irradiation (see the discussion of the reproductive system and testes later in this section).

Adrenocorticotropin (ACTH) deficiency: ACTH presents as decreased stamina, lethargy, fasting hypoglycemia, and dilutional hyponatremia similar to inappropriate vasopressin secretion.

Hyperprolactinemia: Hyperprolactinemia (noted most commonly in females) is a failure to proceed through puberty, arrested puberty, galactorrhea or amenorrhea, decreased libido, and impotence in males.

Antidiuretic hormone (ADH) deficiency: ADH deficiency is referred to as neurogenic diabetes insipidus and is manifested by increased urination and thirst, as well as dilute urine.

Diagnostic Work-up

A diagnostic work-up includes taking an annual comprehensive history and a physical examination. Specific assessments are described below.

Growth hormone deficiency: Assessment includes a determination of the patient's bone age or organ dysfunction, testing of thyroid function, and routine blood studies to exclude other systemic illnesses that can affect growth (e.g., renal dysfunction). Growth hormone stimulation testing also is done because standard testing may not uncover a growth hormone deficiency (GHD). False negatives are common in this test. If testing is normal and growth continues to be abnormal, a physiological assessment with frequent serum sampling of growth hormone over a period of 12–24 hours may be warranted.

Insulinlike growth factor-1 (IGF-1) serum testing may be done by an endocrinologist. IGF-1 is a growth hormone-dependent serum growth factor.

Insulinlike growth factor-binding protein3 (IGF BP3) serum testing also may be done by an endocrinologist. IGF BP3, in conjunction with another protein (acid labile subunit), is primarily responsible for maintaining a reservoir of IGFs in the serum circulation.

Gonadotropin deficiency: Obtain thyroid function tests on patients who have had radiation therapy to the neck. Obtain basal serum concentration of prolactin in patients who have had high-dose radiation therapy to the HPA. Luteinizing hormone (LH) and follicle-stimulating hormone (FSH) are obtained before puberty, and then periodically throughout puberty if there are delays or arrests in pubertal progression. In addition, testosterone levels are obtained in males and estradial levels usually are obtained in females. Gonadotropin-releasing hormone (GnRh) stimulation testing may provide additional clinical information.

Precocious puberty: Diagnostic tests to assess for precocious puberty include determining the patient's bone age and testing for GnRh. A pelvic ultrasound also may be a helpful and noninvasive means of determining precocious puberty in females. Growth hormone testing may be indicated, given that the patients with precocious puberty also may be GH-deficient.

Thyroid-stimulating hormone deficiency: To assess for thyroid-stimulating hormone deficiency, basal plasma concentrations of thyroxine, thyroid hormone-binding capacity (e.g., T3 resin uptake), and TSH level should be obtained. TSH stimulation testing may be helpful in confirming a diagnosis.

Adrenocorticotropin (ACTH) deficiency: To assess for ACTH deficiency, a random serum cortisol level should be obtained. If this level is abnormal, provocative metyrapone testing should be done.

Hyperprolactinemia: To assess for hyperprolactinemia, random samples of serum plasma prolactin should be obtained. This testing should be directed by an endocrinologist.

ADH deficiency: To assess for an ADH deficiency, a urinalysis, with specific gravity, serum and urine electrolytes, and osmolarity, should be obtained.

Medical Treatment

Growth hormone deficiency: It is recommended that growth hormone therapy not be given for at least 1 year after completion of cancer treatment. Ongoing studies are investigating whether a correlation exists between growth hormone replacement and secondary malignancies. However, there is currently no evidence that children treated with growth hormone are at increased risk of experiencing a relapse of their primary tumor.

Gonadotropin deficiency: Gonadotropin deficiency is treated primarily by replacing the appropriate hormones—estrogen for females and testosterone for males. Care for this condition should be directed by an endocrinologist (see the discussion of reproductive systems later in this section).

Precocious puberty: A gonadotropin-releasing hormone analog is used to suppress pubertal development. Preliminary data show that treatment with growth hormone while a patient is being treated with gonadotropin-releasing hormone increases a patient's overall height.

Thyroid-stimulating hormone (TSH) deficiency: Treatment consists of thyroxine replacement therapy with medications such as levothyroxine (Synthroid). Care of survivors with TSH deficiency should be directed by an endocrinologist.

Adrenocorticotropin deficiency: Hydrocortisone is used to treat adrenocorticotropin deficiency. A low dosage, given twice a day, usually is sufficient. During times of stress (e.g., febrile illness), an increased dosage will be required. Mineralocorticoids also may have to be replaced. Care of survivors with adrenocorticotropin deficiency should be directed by an endocrinologist.

Hyperprolactinemia: Hyperprolactinemia is treated with bromocriptine or related dopaminergic agents. Care of survivors with hyperprolactinemia should be directed by an endocrinologist.

ADH deficiency: Desmopressin (DDAVP) is used to treat an antidiuretic hormone deficiency. Care of survivors with ADH deficiency should be directed by an endocrinologist.

Nursing Assessment and Interventions

Assessment:

- Review the patient's history for the following:
  - poor linear growth
  - halted, absent, or early pubertal development
  - symptoms of hypothyroidism
  - symptoms of antidiuretic hormone deficiency
  - symptoms of hyperprolactinemia, including menstrual and/or pregnancy history and history of sexual function.
- Assess the following during a physical examination of the patient:
  - the patient's height and weight plotted on a growth chart that notes the growth velocity over time as well as parental heights
  - the patient's sitting height (if the spine has been irradiated, subtract the standing height from the sitting height to assess the amount of leg growth)
  - Tanner stage of development.

Interventions:

- Reinforce the importance of having lifelong, annual, follow-up assessments with a healthcare provider familiar with the survivor's cancer history and treatment and with the risks of developing late effects.
- Obtain accurate measurements of the patient's height and weight and plot them on a growth curve.
- Educate the survivor about the particular endocrine dysfunction that he or she is at risk for developing and the corresponding signs and symptoms.
- Educate the survivor who is taking replacement hormones regarding proper administration.

Expected Patient Outcomes

- The survivor knows about his or her risks for developing endocrine dysfunction.
- The survivor continues to have annual follow-up visits.
- The survivor complies with the medication regime.
- The survivor is asymptomatic on replacement medication and reports abnormal symptoms if or when they occur.
- The survivor maintains appropriate serum levels and growth indices.

Thyroid Function

Barbara Anne Hieb, Susan K. Ogle, and Wendy Hobbie

Definition

Thyroid abnormalities can occur after radiation therapy in the thyroid gland or the hypothalamic-pituitary axis (see the discussion of the hypothalamic-pituitary axis earlier in this section). The most common effects are either overt or compensatory. Other abnormalities include Graves' disease (hyperthyroidism), thyroiditis, and benign or malignant tumors (see the discussion of second malignant neoplasms later in this section). The peak incidence of thyroid abnormalities occurs 2–5 years after treatment.

Risk Factors

The risk factors for thyroid abnormalities include having had radiation therapy greater than 2,000 centrigrays (cGy) to the head, neck, chest, or spinal axis, or single-dose or total body irradiation equaling 750 cGy. Also, patients who are pubertal while receiving treatment may be at greater risk for thyroid late effects. Lymphangiograms done at the time of diagnosis have been associated with the development of thyroid late effects. In addition, a thyroid malignancy is highly associated with thyroid dysfunction (see the discussion of second malignant neoplasms later in this section).

Clinical Presentation

Hypothyroidism: The symptoms of hypothyroidism are intolerance of cold, constipation, weight gain, dry skin, generalized muscle weakness, fatigue, lethargy, hoarseness, bradycardia, hypotension, puffy round face, brittle hair, alopecia, periorbital edema, poor linear growth, amenorrhea, arrested pubertal development, and an elevated serum TSH level with a corresponding decrease in serum thyroxine (T-4).

Compensatory hypothyroidism: This type of hypothyroidism generally is asymptomatic, but testing reveals an abnormal thyroid profile suggesting impending thyroid failure (i.e., elevated TSH and normal T-4).

Graves' disease (hyperthyroidism): The symptoms of Graves' disease are a rapid pulse, excitability, nervousness, intolerance of heat, weight loss, increased appetite, diarrhea, moist skin, tremors of the hand, and exophthalmos. Serum blood studies will reveal a decrease in TSH and an elevation of T-4.

Thyroiditis: Thyroiditis presents with the signs and symptoms of hypothyroidism and an elevation in serum thyroid antibodies.

Benign or malignant tumor: Presentation may vary. Any palpable nodule or enlargement of the thyroid should be evaluated by an endocrinologist.

Diagnostic Work-up

An annual examination should include careful palpation of the patient's thyroid gland. Serum TSH and thyroxine (usually free T-4, but may vary depending upon the institution) and other thyroid studies are done as directed by an endocrinologist. Survivors who have received cranial or craniospinal radiation and/or women on birth control pills should be evaluated for thyroid function based on free T-4, rather than T-4.

Medical Treatment

Hypothyroidism: Patients are given replacement levothyroxine (Synthroid).

Compensatory hypothyroidism: Most centers treat this condition with levothyroxine, but treatment decisions are based upon the potential increased risk of tumor development.

Graves' disease (hyperthyroidism): Graves' disease is treated with surgical removal of part or all of the thyroid gland, thyroid ablation with radioactive iodine, or antithyroid drugs.

Thyroiditis: Thyroiditis may be self-limiting and may require no intervention except for periodic serum thyroid studies to monitor levels. If treatment is required for persistent or symptomatic thyroiditis, it usually consists of hormone replacement.

Benign or malignant tumor: Tumors are surgically resected. If they are benign, no further treatment is necessary. A differentiated carcinoma may require additional therapy. These conditions should be monitored by an endocrinologist.

Nursing Assessment and Interventions

Assessment:

- Review the patient's history for any signs or symptoms of thyroid abnormalities.
- Perform a physical examination that includes careful palpation of the patient's thyroid gland.

Interventions:

- Reinforce the importance of having lifelong, annual, follow-up assessments with a healthcare provider who is familiar with the survivor's cancer history, treatment, and risk of developing late effects.
- Order appropriate follow-up studies.
- Inform the survivor about the risk of developing thyroid abnormalities and corresponding signs and symptoms.
- Inform the survivor about the importance and benefits of hormone replacement therapy.
- Inform the survivor about the potential side effects of hormone replacement therapy.

Expected Patient Outcomes

- The survivor is knowledgeable about the potential for thyroid dysfunction.
- The survivor complies with recommendations for follow-up evaluations.
- The survivor is asymptomatic on replacement medication and reports to medical providers abnormal symptoms if or when they occur.
- The survivor maintains appropriate serum levels of thyroid hormones.

Vision and Hearing

Debra A. Eshelman

Definition

Visual deficits can result from neoplastic involvement of the optic tracts, high dose steroids, or radiation injury. Hearing deficits can result from neoplastic involvement, but chemotherapy, radiation therapy, or prolonged use of antimicrobials are more common causes.

Risk Factors

Abnormalities of the ear

Radiation: In general, radiation doses greater than 30 to 40 Gy alone or in combination with host factors, such as central nervous system tumors, younger age at treatment, and certain ototoxic agents like cisplatin (Platinol) or aminoglycosides, can result in hearing problems, such as sensorineural hearing loss or tinnitus. High doses of radiation (>50 Gy) alone or in combination with host factors, such as younger age at treament, can result in typanosclerosis, otosclerosis, conductive hearing loss, or eustachian tube dysfunction.

Chemotherapy: Platinum derivatives have known ototoxic effects that may be potentiated by radiation or other chemotherapeutic agents such as ifosfamide (Ifex), or ototoxic drugs (aminoglycosides). Generally, cumulative cisplatin doses greater than or equal to 360 mg/m2 result in hearing problems. Additional studies to determine ototoxic dose/effects relationships for carboplatin are warranted.

Radiation: Radiation is the primary treatment modality known to result in eye problems. Late effects vary, depending upon the radiation dose and the area of the eye that is involved:

- Reduced visual acuity and orbital hypoplasia generally are caused by doses greater than 1.8–2.0 Gy and fraction doses greater than 2 Gy.
- Cataracts generally are caused by doses greater than 10 Gy, single daily fraction; may be exacerbated by steroids and busulfan.
- Lacrimal duct atrophy generally is caused by doses greater than 40 Gy.
- Xerophthalmia (severe) generally is caused by doses greater than 30 Gy.
- Keratitis and keratoconjunctivitis generally are caused by doses greater than 50 Gy.
- Retinopathy generally is caused by doses greater than 45 Gy.
- Optic chiasm neuropathy generally is caused by doses of 50–65 Gy, with exacerbation by other comorbid conditions, such as diabetes mellitus or hypertension.

Chemotherapy: Chemotherapy produces no known late effect. Steroids, however, are a known risk factor for cataracts, glaucoma, and uveitis.

Clinical Presentation

Abnormalities of the ear: The signs and symptoms of ear problems include hearing abnormalities (e.g., high frequency hearing loss or permanent hearing loss) indicated by abnormal speech development. Other hearing problems include tinnitus, vertigo, or symptoms of structural problems caused by (e.g., fibrosis) that lead to an inability to visualize ear landmarks, or abnormal cerumen production.

Abnormalities of the eye: The signs and symptoms include decreased visual acuity, visual loss, blurred vision, or cataract. Additional symptoms may include lacrimal duct atrophy, severe xerophthalmia, keratitis, keratoconjunctivitis, telangiectasias, retinopathy, optic chiasm neuropathy, enophthalmos, and/or painful eye.

Glaucoma presents with eye pain, headache, nausea, vomiting, and decreased peripheral vision.

Diagnostic Work-up

Ears: An otoscopic examination should be done at least annually to visualize the tympanic membranes and ear structures. A baseline audiogram or brainstem auditory evoked response should be performed, and then done periodically as clinically indicated. An evaluation for hearing aids should be done, as appropriate. Referral to an otorhinolaryngologist or neurologist should be made when clinically indicated.

Eyes: Evaluation is dependent upon which structure of the eye is affected. Evaluation may include slit lamp examination, fundoscopic examination, testing for visual acuity, or measurement of ocular pressure. Referral to an ophthalmologist should be made, as appropriate.

Medical Treatment

Ears: Treatment consists of amplification (e.g., an FM system in the patient's school); hearing aids, if they are needed; an audiology consultation when it is clinically indicated; and removal of impacted cerumen.

Eyes: Treatment consists of extraction of an extracapsular cataract if it is interfering with a survivor's activities of daily living; steroid eye drops for iritis; tear replacement, as needed, for abnormalities of the lacrimal gland; photocoagulation to prevent progression of neovascularization and retinopathy; corneal transplants; medications to lower intraocular pressure if the patient has glaucoma; and dilation of the tear duct when a patient has fibrosis.

Nursing Assessment and Interventions

Assessment:

- Review the survivor's history to determine if there were any previous speech, hearing, or visual problems.
- Assess for poor school performance or problems in school.
- Assess for headaches, blurred vision, lazy eye, squinting, pain, double vision, myopia, tinnitus, and current speech problems.
- Assess for speech discernibility during the physical examination.
- Assess for red reflex during the physical examination.

Interventions:

- Reinforce the importance of having lifelong, annual, follow-up assessments with a healthcare provider who is familiar with the survivor's cancer and treatment history, and emphasize the risk for developing late effects.
- Ensure that the survivor obtains appropriate diagnostic tests.
- Educate the survivor about the potential long-term effects of previous therapy on vision and hearing.
- Educate school personnel about the survivor's special needs; ensure that the child has preferential seating in school if he or she has hearing or visual problems.
- Reinforce the need for protective ultraviolet sunglasses and other methods to preserve vision (e.g., tear replacement).
- Reinforce the need for hearing conservation, as appropriate (i.e., avoid environments with very loud noises).

Expected Patient Outcomes

- The survivor is knowledgeable about the risk factors for developing visual or hearing impairments.
- The survivor continues to have annual ophthalmic examinations and audiograms when they are needed.
- The survivor has access to hearing amplification and correction of visual problems when they are needed.

Head and Neck

Sarah J. Bottomley

Definition

The head and neck region may be affected by tumors or by treatments that include surgery, radiation, or chemotherapy. Late effects of treatment can include bone hypoplasia, deformity, dental abnormalities, and changes in mucous membranes.

Risk Factors

Skin and mucous membranes:

Radiation therapy: With a dosage of 4,000 cGy or more, late effects may occur, primarily from vascular injury that can lead to fibrosis in vessel walls and the perivascular interstitial spaces. Eventually, fibrosis and thinning of the vessels can lead to telangiectasia and atrophy of the skin and membranes. Radiation can stimulate the production of melanin, leading to permanent darkening of irradiated areas, and can affect hair follicles.

Chemotherapy: There are limited data available regarding changes of the mucosa in children related to chemotherapeutic late effects.

Bone and connective tissue:

Radiation therapy: Radiation can cause hypoplasia, deformity, fractures, necrosis, and poor healing related to a decreased blood supply to bone. Connective tissue may exhibit fibrosis and hypoplasia.

Chemotherapy: There are no documented late effects.

Salivary glands and taste buds:

Radiation therapy: If the field of radiation has included the major salivary glands (parotid, submandibular, and sublingual), decreased salivation may occur because of atrophy of the secretory cells. This effect usually is seen in patients who have had dosages greater than 5,000 cGy; with dosages less than 4,000 cGy, the salivary glands and taste buds appear to retain their ability to secrete saliva.

Chemotherapy: There is little evidence of long-term effects.

Dental:

Radiation therapy: Children under 6 years of age have the highest rate of dental abnormalities. These include tooth and root agenesis, enamel dysplasias, caries, incomplete calcification, microdontia, arrested and altered root development, abnormal eruption, and periodontal disease.

Chemotherapy: The following agents have demonstrated late effects on dentition: vincristine (Oncovin), dactinomycin (Actinomycin-D), cyclophosphamide (Cytoxan), methotrexate (Mexate), 6-mercaptopurine (Purinethol), prednisone (Deltasone), procarbazine (Matulane), and mechlorethamine (nitrogen mustard). Dental abnormalities occur as a result of the impact of chemotherapy on ameloblasts, odontoblasts, and cementoblasts during development and include malocclusion, enamel hypoplasia and opacities, hypodontia, microdontia, supranumerary teeth, enlarged pulp chambers, altered root development, marked shortening of premolar root, and thinning and constriction of the roots.

Clinical Presentation

Skin and mucous membranes: The skin may be pale, and there may be thinning of the epithelium, loss of pliability, submucosal induration, and chronic ulcerations. Patients also may have intranasal scarring, along with changes in normal production of mucus and sinus drainage. These conditions may lead to chronic sinusitis, chronic nasal discharge, postnasal drip, nasal obstruction, facial pain, and headache. Other late effects include hyperpigmentation or hypopigmentation, telangiectasias, atrophy, dryness, trismus, and xerostomia. Hair color and texture changes may occur at the radiation site. Patients can experience permanent loss of hair with dosages of 4,500–5,000 cGy. Chronic sinusitis has been reported in patients who have either sinus-involved malignancies or who receive radiation involving the sinuses.

Bone and connective tissue: Patients may present with bony deformities, muscle hypoplasia, loss of elasticity, constricting fibrosis, osteoradionecrosis, and necrosis or ulcers of the soft tissue.

Salivary glands and taste buds: The signs and symptoms include xerostomia, dental caries, and decay that can lead to osteoradionecrosis and changes in the ability to taste.

Dental: Patients can have root and crown abnormalities, root agenesis, premature apical closure, enamel hypoplasia, and microdontia, as well as foreshortening or agenesis of their developing teeth, and gingival hyperplasia.

Diagnostic Work-up

A diagnostic work-up includes the following elements:

- inspection of the oral mucosa, nares, and the skin and soft tissue of the neck
- assessment of neck and jaw mobility for trismus, crepitus, limited mandibular movement, and abnormal growth
- radiographic studies of irradiated bone every 3–5 years, and as indicated
- salivary flow rate and appropriate dental prophylaxis for high-risk patients
- periodontal prophylaxis, including a thorough dental and radiological examination
- CT scan of sinus and otolaryngology consult, as needed.

Medical Treatment

Bone and connective tissue: Treatment includes orthopedic and plastic surgery, as well as dental and orthodontic follow-up care, when needed; physical therapy when needed for maintaining the mobility of the oral cavity, head, and neck; and stretching exercises for the oral cavity to minimize microstomia.

Oral cavity: Treatment consists of a periodontal consultation, with a professional cleaning every 6 months and prophylactic fluoride treatment, an orthodontic consultation when it is needed, and a saliva substitute, if it is needed.

Nursing Assessment and Interventions

Assessment:

- Review the survivor's history for dental problems, neck and jaw mobility, and skin problems.
- Inspect the patient's oral mucosa and teeth, neck mobility, skin appearance, and distribution of hair.
- Determine the patient's level of participation in prophylactic measures, such as dental cleaning, daily oral care, skin care, and physical activity.

Interventions:

- Reinforce the importance of having lifelong, annua, follow-up assessments with a healthcare provider who is familiar with the survivor's cancer history, treatment, and risk for developing late effects.
- Educate the survivor about the long-term effects of cancer therapy on the oral cavity, bones, and connective tissues.
- Educate the survivor, especially one who has altered taste ability and who may have a tendency to consume increased amounts of sweets, regarding dietary controls to decrease the potential for developing caries.
- Educate the survivor regarding the importance of maintaining mobility of the jaw and neck.
- Encourage the survivor to follow up with subspecialists, as indicated.
- Educate the survivor on lifestyle behaviors that promote dental health and maintain adequate head and neck mobility.
  - Discourage the survivor from using tobacco products.
  - Encourage daily oral care, including brushing, flossing, and use of a mouth rinse.
  - Encourage the survivor to maintain a diet low in concentrated sugars.

- Encourage the survivor to do stretching and other exercises to maintain head and neck mobility, as needed.

Expected Patient Outcomes

- The survivor is knowledgeable about the potential long-term effects of therapy to the oral cavity, bones, and connective tissues.
- The survivor adopts healthy lifestyle behaviors.
- The survivor complies with recommendations for follow-up care.

Cardiovascular System

Sarah J. Bottomley

Definition

Cardiac toxicity can result from both chemotherapy and radiation therapy. It most commonly takes the form of cardiomyopathy, pericarditis, or coronary artery disease, and can occur within months, or for as many as 20 years, after exposure.

Risk Factors

Females and young children have a higher incidence of late cardiovascular effects.

Anthracyclines: The incidence of cardiomyopathy is related to the total cumulative dosage of anthracycline (doxorubicin [Adriamycin], daunomycin [Cerubidine], idarubicin [Zavedos], mitoxantrone [Novatrone], epirubicin [Pharmorubicin]). With a cumulative dosage of greater than 600 mg/m2, the incidence rate exceeds 30%; with a cumulative dosage of 500 to 600 mg/m2, it is 11%. The schedule under which anthracycline is administered also is a factor; there is less toxicity with continuous infusion or weekly doses, compared with the administration of a bolus on a schedule of every 3 weeks.

Radiation: Mediastinal radiation enhances anthracycline toxicities. A dose of 4,000 cGy is the usual radiation threshold. Total body irradiation—mantle, whole lung, whole abdominal, left flank, and spinal—may enhance anthracycline toxicity, or may be a risk factor alone.

Exposure to other chemotherapeutic agents: Chemotherapeutic agents that pose a risk are cyclophosphamide (Cytoxan), dactinomycin (Actinomycin-D), mitomycin (Mutamycin), dacarbazine (DTIC), vincristine (Oncovin), bleomycin (Blenoxane), and methotrexate (Mexate).

Other factors that enhance the possibility of myocardial toxicity include an underlying cardiac abnormality, a tumor in the chest, pregnancy, recreational drug use, health behaviors (diet, exercise) and uncontrolled hypertension.

Clinical Presentation

Pericarditis: The signs and symptoms of pericarditis include fatigue, cyanosis, ascites, peripheral edema, hypotension, chest pain, dyspnea, fever, venous distention, pulsus paradoxus, muffled heart sounds, effusion, and friction rub.

Cardiomyopathy: The signs and symptoms of cardiomyopathy include tachycardia, tachypnea, shortness of breath, dyspnea, edema, hepatomegaly, fatigue, cough, hypertension, syncope, arrhythmias, cardiomegaly, gallop rhythms, palpitations, congestive heart failure, or pleural effusion.

Valvular damage: The signs and symptoms of valvular damage include weakness, cough, dyspnea, new murmur, and pulsating liver.

Coronary artery disease: The signs and symptoms of coronary artery disease include chest pain on exertion, dyspnea, diaphoresis, pallor, hypotension, or arrhythmias.

Diagnostic Work-up

A diagnostic work-up consists of the following:

- baseline studies at entry to long-term follow-up; then follow-up studies based on age at diagnosis and initiation of treatment, cumulative anthracycline dose, and/or cumulative radiation dosage exposure; and results of all follow-up studies.
- a comprehensive annual history and physical examination
- gated radionuclide angiography wall motion and quantitative angiocardiography (MUGA), or echocardiogram (echo) and electrocardiogram (EKG)
- chest X rays
- stress studies, as indicated
- use of a Holter monitor, as indicated
- a cardiology consultation for a survivor before a pregnancy, before receiving general anesthesia, or if there are signs or symptoms of cardiomyopathy.

Medical Treatment

Pericarditis: If tamponade develops, a patient may require pericardiocentesis. Effusion usually is resolved in 1–10 months, but can persist for years. If effusion becomes chronic, a patient may require a pericardiectomy.

Cardiomyopathy: Treatment can include digoxin, diuretics, and under certain circumstances, afterload-reducing agents. Cardiac transplantation may be a consideration for patients with congestive heart failure that persists or progresses despite medical therapy.

Valvular damage: Penicillin prophylaxis should be given when a patient is scheduled for surgery or dental procedures. A patient may require surgical replacement of the damaged valve.

Coronary artery disease: Treatment includes diuretics and other cardiac medications. Dietary restrictions may include low-sodium, low-fat foods. A patient may require balloon dilatation angioplasty or coronary artery bypass surgery.

Nursing Assessment and Interventions

Assessment:

- Review the survivor's history for exercise tolerance, fatigue, chest pain, dizziness, dyspnea, cough, shortness of breath, palpitations, fever, and lifestyle behaviors (e.g., smoking, drugs, activity level).

- Ensure that a physical examination assesses for
  - abnormalities in vital signs (blood pressure, pulse, respiration)
  - heart-sound abnormalities (murmurs, rubs, thrills, gallops)
  - edema
  - venous distention
  - hepatomegaly
  - perfusion (i.e., capillary refill)

Interventions:

- Reinforce the importance of having lifelong, annual, follow-up assessments with a healthcare provider who is familiar with the survivor's cancer history, treatment, and risk for developing late effects.
- Ensure that appropriate diagnostic tests are obtained.
- Educate the survivor about lifestyle behaviors that limit cardiac compromise.
  - Encourage close supervision of a survivor's cardiac function during pregnancy.
  - Discourage the use of tobacco products and alcohol.
  - Reinforce healthy dietary habits, including a low-fat, low-sodium, high-fiber diet to prevent obesity and hyperlipidemia.
  - Encourage routine aerobic activity; tell the patient to avoid isometric exercise.
- Ensure that adequate information is available to survivors being treated for cardiomyopathy.
  - Encourage the patient to follow up with a cardiologist, as needed.
  - Provide anticipatory guidance regarding symptoms of cardiac dysfunction and the side effects of cardiac medications.
  - Educate a survivor with valvular damage about the need for prophylactic penicillin before having surgery or dental procedures.
  - Provide education on the side effects of specific cardiac medications.
- Educate survivors diagnosed with prolonged QT interval about medications that may exacerbate the problem.

Expected Patient Outcomes

- The survivor is knowledgeable about the risk of cardiac toxicity.
- The survivor has adopted healthy lifestyle behaviors.
- The survivor complies with recommendations for follow-up care.

Respiratory System

Barbara Anne Hieb, Susan K. Ogle, and Wendy Hobbie

Definition

Radiation therapy to the lungs or systemic chemotherapy may result in acute or chronic impairment of respiratory function. Decreases in lung volumes and compliance as well as perfusion of gases can occur. Chronic changes may occur even if the acute course of treatment has proven to be asymptomatic.

Risk Factors

Combinations of therapies (i.e., methotrexate, cyclophosphamide, doxorubicin, thoracic/spin radiation, and/or total body irradiation), higher cumulative dosages, concurrent infection, and baseline dysfunction (asthma or smoking effects) increase the toxic effects of therapy.

Radiation therapy: Dose-related effects are seen with bleomycin (Blenoxane) greater than 600 u/m^2 and with busulfan greater than 500 mg/m^2. Other agents, including alkylating agents and melphalan, also are associated with pulmonary disease. Alkylating agents can also cause pneumonitis and fibrosis.

Age: Young children, especially those younger than 3 years of age at the time of treatment, are at greatest risk because, in addition to the direct effects of treatment on their lungs, radiation also can impair normal growth and development of the thoracic cage, airways, and lung parenchyma.

Clinical Presentation

Pneumonitis: Pneumonitis can occur 1–3 months after radiation therapy or chemotherapy. Symptoms include low-grade fever, congestion, cough, and fullness in the chest. Severe pneumonitis will result in dyspnea, nonproductive cough, pleuritic chest pain, and production of sputum.

Fibrosis: Fibrosis can occur months or even years after treatment; it stabilizes after 1–2 years, so most patients are asymptomatic. There are minimal symptoms if fibrosis occurs in only one lung and less than 50% of that lung is affected. Patients with severe fibrosis may have chronic respiratory failure and dyspnea on exertion, fatigue, cough, decreased exercise tolerance, orthopnea, cyanosis, and chronic cor pulmonale. The symptoms of fibrosis are the same as those of restrictive lung disease.

Diagnostic Work-up

A diagnostic work-up consists of the following:

- A comprehensive annual history and physical exam.
- Baseline radiography (anteroposterior and lateral chest films); if normal, repeat every 2–5 years and before the patient receives general anesthesia.
- Baseline pulmonary function tests (including DLCO and spirometry) repeated every 2–3 years or before general anesthesia; if the patient is symptomatic or has evidence of pulmonary dysfunction or progression, obtain tests, as needed.

Medical Treatment

Prevention: Preventive measures consist of monitoring a patient's pulmonary function and obtaining chest X rays during treatment. Pneumococcal vaccine (Pneumovax) and influenza virus vaccines (Fluogen) should be given to treated patients to prevent infections that can exacerbate symptoms. Corticosteroids, bronchodilators, expectorants, antibiotics, oxygen, and bed rest may be needed to relieve symptoms.

Nursing Assessment and Interventions

Assessment:

- Review the survivor's treatment history to determine his or her risk factors.
- Review the survivor's medical history for symptoms of respiratory compromise, including fatigue, intolerance to or change in tolerance to activity, chronic cough with or without fever, orthopnea, and dyspnea.
- Determine oxygen saturation via pulse oximetry (if patient is symptomatic).
- Ensure that the survivor's physical examination includes assessment for
  - abnormalities in vital signs (heart rate or respiratory rate)
  - color of skin and/or nails for evidence of pallor, jaundice, or cyanosis
  - respiratory effort and use of accessory muscles or nasal flaring
  - abnormal or decreased breath sounds (e.g., rales, crackles).

Interventions:

- Reinforce the importance of having lifelong, annual, follow-up assessments with a healthcare provider who is familiar with the survivor's cancer history, treatment, and risks for developing late effects.
- Ensure that the survivor obtains appropriate diagnostic tests.
- Educate the survivor about behaviors that will limit respiratory compromise:
  - avoidance of smoking, recreational drugs, second-hand smoke, and strong odors and chemicals
  - receiving vaccinations to prevent respiratory infection, including pneumococcal vaccine (Pneumovax) and influenza virus vaccine (Fluogen)
- Educate the survivor who has received bleomycin and other pulmonary-toxic therapy about the need to inform healthcare providers about his or her treatment history before being given anesthesia because of the risk of respiratory failure with high levels of oxygen (i.e., the patient should avoid FiO_2 of more than 30% intraoperatively and postoperatively).
- Avoid scuba diving due to potential barotraumas and exacerbation of pulmonary fibrosis with high oxygen concentration.
- Ensure that the survivor has adequate information regarding the respiratory diagnosis when he or she is being treated for respiratory dysfunction.
- Encourage the survivor to have a follow-up visit with a pulmonologist.
- Review the instructions for administering medications and discuss their potential side effects.

Expected Patient Outcomes

- The survivor is knowledgeable about the risks for pulmonary toxicity.
- The survivor adopts healthy lifestyle behaviors and is knowledgeable about health behaviors that may cause pulmonary injury or increase his or her risk for a second cancer.
- The survivor complies with recommendations for follow-up care.
- The survivor uses medications correctly for symptom relief.

Gastrointestinal and Hepatic Systems

Sarah J. Bottomley

Definition

Fibrosis and enteritis are the most common pathological abnormalities of the gastrointestinal tract in long-term survivors of cancer, and they can arise at any site—from the esophagus to the rectum. Strictures, adhesions, obstruction, ulcers, and malabsorption also can occur. Fibrosis and cirrhosis are the most common pathological abnormalities of the liver in long-term survivors. Hepatitis also can occur and can be symptomatic or subclinical.

Risk Factors

Radiation therapy: Therapy may cause intestinal fibrosis, stricture, and malabsorption. Incidence is related to the total dose, volume, and site of radiation. The stomach and small intestine appear to be more sensitive to radiation than are the colon or rectum. The incidence of intestinal fibrosis is 5% with a cumulative dosage of 4,000–5,000 cGy. The incidence of fibrosis is greater than 36% with a cumulative dosage of 6,000 cGy. Intestinal fibrosis usually occurs within 5 years of treatment, whereas strictures have been reported to develop as long as 20 years after therapy. Radio-enhanced chemotherapy or abdominal surgery may increase the incidence and severity of intestinal fibrosis, stricture, or malabsorption. Chronic diarrhea, malabsorption, or graft-versus-host disease of the GI tract can occur after either abdominal or total body irradiation.

Hepatic fibrosis: Irradiation of the liver can cause varying degrees of hepatic damage. The incidence is difficult to estimate because the damage often is subclinical and unreported. Children's livers are more sensitive than those of adults. Dosages of 1,200–2,500 cGy delivered to the liver have caused abnormal liver functions in 50% of patients.

Dosages of 2,300–3,500 cGy have resulted in abnormal liver studies in 63% of patients. Dactinomycin (Actinomycin-D) given in conjunction with radiation to the liver can increase the risk of toxicity. A hepatic resection in conjunction with radiation therapy also can contribute to the development of sequelae.

Splenomegaly and thrombocytopenia: Splenomegaly and thrombocytopenia may develop as a consequence of portal hypertension and hypersplenism after a patient has had radiation to the abdomen.

Hepatitis: Hepatitis may be a consequence of radiation therapy to the abdomen.

Chemotherapy: Dactinomycin (Actinomycin-D) and doxorubicin (Adriamycin) can enhance hepatic effects. Although the two are normally excreted through the biliary system, their toxicity may be exaggerated when the patient has hepatic fibrosis. Methotrexate (Mexate) is associated with the development of hepatic dysfunction, fibrosis, and cirrhosis. The incidence of these conditions can be as high as 80% for those treated for more than 2½ years with daily administrations of low-dose methotrexate; however, these conditions usually are stabilized or are resolved once therapy has been completed. The agent 6-mercaptopurine (Purinethol) has been associated with liver damage; however, it has not been well studied. Esophageal varices and bleeding as a symptom of chronic liver disease may be related to the use of either methotrexate, 6-mercaptopurine, or other therapy; however, these reactions are rare.

Surgery: Laparotomy has been associated with intestinal obstruction in less than 2% of patients. Bowel obstructions have been associated with previous abdominal surgery.

Bone marrow transplant: Graft-versus-host disease can lead to strictures of the gastrointestinal tract or perimuscular fibrosis. Chronic graft-versus-host disease and chronic active hepatitis are the most common causes of chronic liver disease.

Other: Transfusion-mediated hepatitis B, hepatitis C, or cytomegalovirus may be symptomatic or subclinical and may cause chronic liver damage.

Clinical Presentation

Presenting signs depend upon the degree of injury. If the injury is mild, patients may be asymptomatic, and the abnormalities may be detected incidentally.

Intestinal fibrosis and enteritis: The signs and symptoms of intestinal fibrosis and enteritis are severe, intermittent abdominal pain; dysphagia; vomiting; diarrhea; constipation; bleeding with or without anemia; weight loss; poor linear growth; fatigue; obstruction; or rectal pain. Enteritis, ulceration, and bowel resection can lead to malabsorption, perforation, or fistulization.

Adhesions and strictures: The signs and symptoms of adhesions and strictures are abdominal pain, bilious vomiting, hyperactive bowel sounds, or dysphagia.

Hepatic fibrosis: Transaminase levels may or may not be elevated. Other signs and symptoms can include elevated bilirubin, hepatomegaly, icterus (often not present until fibrosis and cirrhosis develop), itching, jaundice, bruising, portal hypertension, and encephalopathy.

Hepatitis: The signs and symptoms of hepatitis can include elevation of transaminase levels, and bilirubin levels, anorexia, malaise, nausea, vomiting, abdominal pain, arthralgia, jaundice, hepatomegaly, hepatic fibrosis, positive hepatitis screens for hepatitis B surface antigen (HBsAG), antihepatitis B core (anti-HBC), antihepatitis C virus (anti-HCV), or hepatitis C virus by polymerase chain reaction (HCV RNA by PCR).

Diagnostic Work-up

A diagnostic work-up consists of the following:

- A comprehensive annual history and physical that includes an evaluation for hepatomegaly, icterus, and malabsorption.
- Annual measurements of the survivor's height and weight as a screen for malabsorption.
- A chemistry panel that includes alanine aminotransferase (ALT), aspartate aminotransferase (AST), albumin, gamma-glutamyl transferase (GGT), electrolytes, calcium, phosphorus, magnesium, uric acid, amylase, cholesterol, total protein, bilirubin, and alkaline phosphatase obtained every 2–5 years, depending upon risk and findings.
- A complete blood count on an annual basis.
- A stool guaiac every year (for those who have had abdominal irradiation or surgery, or who are more than 50 years old).
- Serum total protein and albumin levels every 3–5 years for patients at risk for enteritis.
- Serology studies for hepatitis A, B, and C if the survivor has had previous blood transfusions or if the survivor's chemistry panel is elevated.
- An abdominal ultrasound and liver biopsy, if the survivor has persistent elevations of transaminase or bilirubin levels, or if hepatitis B or C has been detected.
- A radiograph of any symptomatic area to assess for adhesions or an obstruction.

Medical Treatment

Suspected late GI and hepatic effects should be evaluated in collaboration with a gastroenterologist.

Intestinal fibrosis: Management consists of dilatation of the affected area and dietary management.

Enteritis: Dietary management is the treatment for enteritis.

Bowel obstruction: A bowel obstruction is evaluated with abdominal radiographs, decompression (if needed), and appropriate contrast studies. The survivor may require surgery to alleviate an obstruction.

GI strictures: Assessment includes a barium test followed by an endoscopy. Treatment may include dilatation of the affected area.

Esophagitis: Esophagitis can be managed with pharmacological agents.

Chronic intestinal obstruction: A chronic intestinal obstruction may require surgical resection or balloon dilatation.

Hepatic fibrosis or cirrhosis: Hepatic fibrosis or cirrhosis can be treated by administering diuretics or managing a patient's diet. End-stage hepatic disease may require a liver transplant.

Hepatitis: Viral hepatitis can be treated with interferon; if a patient develops end-stage cirrhosis, a liver transplant may be required.

Nursing Assessment and Interventions

Assessment:

- Review the history of the survivor's GI symptoms: difficulty swallowing, heartburn, loss of appetite, nausea, vomiting, indigestion, constipation, diarrhea, change in bowel habits, rectal bleeding, abdominal pain, food intolerance, hemorrhoids, or jaundice.
- Assess the amount of the survivor's consumption of alcohol and hepatotoxic over-the-counter or prescription medications.
- Ensure that the survivor is carefully assessed for
  - abnormalities in blood pressure
  - hepatomegaly
  - jaundice, or icterus.

Interventions:

- Reinforce the importance of having lifelong, annual, follow-up assessments with a healthcare provider who is familiar with the survivor's cancer history, treatment, and risk for developing late effects.
- Ensure that the survivor obtains appropriate diagnostic tests.
- Educate the survivor about the importance of avoiding alcohol or other hepatotoxic drugs, especially if he or she has a history of liver dysfunction.
- Educate the survivor about dietary management; chronic malabsorption and malnutrition may require strict dietary management. Low-fat, low-residue, gluten-free, and lactose-free diets can aid in controlling the symptoms associated with GI dysfunction. Intestinal fibrosis may require the patient to maintain a high-fiber diet; intestinal enteritis may require a modification in his or her diet to control symptoms.
- Educate the survivor about taking medication when it is necessary.

Expected Patient Outcomes

- The survivor is knowledgeable about the risks for gastrointestinal and hepatic toxicities.
- The survivor adopts healthy lifestyle behaviors.
- The survivor complies with recommendations for follow-up care.
- The survivor complies with dietary and pharmocological recommendations.

Genitourinary System

Debra A. Eshelman

Definition

Late genitourinary complications primarily involve the kidneys and bladder, but they also can include damage to the ureters and organs involved in reproduction (i.e., testes, ovaries, vagina, uterus, and prostate). Damage usually occurs because of treatments that can compromise the growth, development, or integrity of the genitourinary structures. Abnormalities take the form of structural or functional impairment of the involved organ(s).

Risk Factors

Radiation therapy: Whole abdominal, para-aortic/splenic, spinal and total body irradiation (TBI), will include structures of the genitourinary system in the radiation portal and may cause subsequent dysfunction (e.g., fibrosis, difficulty voiding).

Kidney. Renal insufficiency and hypertension is usually associated with doses greater than 20 Gy to the whole kidney.

Bladder. Dysfunctional voiding and fibrosis are associated with doses greater than 50 Gy and may be exacerbated with concomitant use of cyclophosphamide.

Ureter, urethra. Risk of late effects generally is associated with dosages greater than 5,000 cGy.

Radiation therapy and chemotherapy used in combination: Lower doses of radiation (<20 Gy) coupled with certain chemotherapeutic agents, such as cisplatin (Platinol), cyclophosphamide (Cytoxan), methotrexate (Mexate), dactinomycin (Actinomycin D), nitrosoureas, and anthracyclines, have been associated with exacerbation of genitourinary late effects. A mononephric patient may be at additional risk.

Chemotherapy: Cisplatin (Platinol), ifosfamide (Ifex), and cyclophosphamide (Cytoxan) can cause glomerular dysfunction, hemorrhagic cystitis, and atypical bladder epithelium. With methotrexate, acute toxicities predominate; the majority of patients recover from them without late sequelae. Cyclophosphamide effects are generally reported at doses greater than 3 gm/m^2. Ifosfamide generally is associated with late toxicity at doses greater than 60 g/m^2, when used in combination with other nephrotoxic agents (Cisplatin, aminoglycosides, amphotericin B, immunosuppressants) and in younger children (<5 years old at treatment).

Surgery: Removal of a paired organ usually is not associated with increased risk of late effects unless there is underlying damage to the remaining organ, whereas removal of a nonpaired organ (e.g., prostate, uterus, bladder) can lead to infertility and incontinence. Retroperitoneal lymph node dissection may be associated with parasympathetic dysfunction leading to retrograde ejaculation or impotence.

Age: Renal and bladder dysfunction might not become apparent until a survivor grows to a size that exceeds the ability of the affected organ to compensate. Children less than 5 years old may experience greater radiation toxicities at lower dosages.

Supportive therapies: Therapies include antimicrobials and graft-versus-host disease prophylactic medications (e.g., cyclosporine [Sandimmune]), with prolonged use, resulting in kidney damage.

Clinical Presentation

Renal insufficiency: The signs and symptoms can include either tubular dysfunction or nephritis presenting with hematuria, fatigue, hypertension, hypomagnesemia, Fanconi syndrome, proteinuria, anemia, or growth abnormalities.

Bladder dysfunction: The signs and symptoms can include mucosal irritation, microscopic or macroscopic hematuria, urgency, frequency, dysuria, hemorrhagic cystitis, incontinence, and fibrosis.

Prostate: A patient can have diminished ejaculum.

Vagina, uterus: A patient can present with alteration in sexual function, infertility, or miscarriage.

Ureter, urethra: There are limited data on late effects in children.

Diagnostic Work-up

A diagnostic work-up consists of the following:

- an annual comprehensive history and physical examination and a blood pressure reading
- an annual urinalysis and assessment of serum BUN, creatinine, electrolytes, and magnesium levels
- a baseline creatinine clearance test (if any abnormalities are noted in the blood studies listed above), glomerular filtration rate (GFR), and organ-specific tests based on toxicity (e.g., cystoscopy, voiding cystourethogram, intravenous pyelogram, CT or MRI of the affected area, or glomerular filtration rate)
- an infertility evaluation.

Medical Treatment

Cystitis: Treatment can include hydration, instillation of alum solutions, cauterization of bleeding sites, sometimes a partial or total cystectomy, bladder augmentation, and urological follow-up care.

Kidney dysfunction: The survivor should be evaluated by a nephrologist as clinically indicated for treatment of hypertension, progressive proteinuria, progressive renal insufficiency and/or culture negative, and hematuria. Antihypertensives or electrolyte supplementation may be indicated.

Strictures: Treatment involves dilatation or placement of stents; urinary diversion is sometimes necessary.

Damage to reproductive organs: Treatment for damage to the reproductive organs usually involves surgical revisions or corrections.

Nursing Assessment and Interventions

Assessment:

- Review the survivor's history for urinary tract infections, hematuria, polyuria, dysuria, urgency, frequency, enuresis, and alteration in sexual function.
- Ensure that a physical examination includes an assessment of vital signs (especially blood pressure), and appropriate blood work, such as kidney function tests, electrolytes, calcium, phosphorus and magnesium, and urinalysis.
- Assess the skin, organs, and structures that were in the radiation field during the survivor's treatment.

Interventions:

- Educate the survivor about long-term effects of treatment.
- Reinforce the importance of having lifelong, annual, follow-up assessments with a healthcare provider who is familiar with the survivor's cancer history, treatment, and risk for developing late effects.
- Ensure that appropriate diagnostic tests are obtained.
- Caution the survivor against engaging in contact sports and explain the need to protect the remaining kidney if he or she has had a nephrectomy.
- Ensure that appropriate referrals have been made to a nephrologist or urologist.
- Emphasize that the survivor should have prompt treatment when he or she has symptoms related to urinary tract infection.
- If renal late effects are evident, caution against any nonsteroidal anti-inflammatory agents (aspirin, ibuprofen, naproxen). Caution against taking any new medications (prescription or over-the-counter) without checking with a healthcare provider.
- If patients have salt wasting tubular dysfunction, advise them that low magnesium levels may bring on coronary atherosclerosis.

Expected Patient Outcomes

- The survivor is knowledgeable about his or her individual risk factors.
- The survivor seeks prompt attention for urinary tract infections or symptoms or both.
- The survivor complies with recommendations for follow-up care.

Reproductive System: Testes

Barbara Anne Hieb, Susan K. Ogle, and Wendy Hobbie

Definition

Primary testicular failure can occur after chemotherapy; or after radiation to the abdomen, pelvis, or testes; or after surgical removal of the testes. The germinal cells that produce sperm are more sensitive to the toxic effects of therapy than the Leydig's cells that produce testosterone. Therefore, for the majority of males, normal pubertal development and adult sexual function usually will be preserved, but fertility may be affected. It is important to note, however, that recovery of spermatogenesis can occur 3–5 years after the use of some chemotherapeutic agents has ceased.

Risk Factors

Chemotherapy: Males are placed at increased risk of infertility if given more than three cycles of nitrogen mustard, vincristine, procarbazine, and prednisone; combination therapy for Hodgkin's disease; or higher cumulative doses of chemotherapy, including more than 600 mg/m^2 of busulfan or more than 7 Gm/m^2 (or 200 mg/m^2) of cyclophosphamide. In addition, any aklylating agent combined with testicular or pelvic radiation or total body irradiation may increase the risks. Alkylating agents also can affect the function of the Leydig's cells in pubertal or postpubertal males, but the effect usually is compensated by increased stimulation of luteinizing hormone (i.e., normal testosterone).

Radiation therapy: Radiation to the testes, whether direct or scattered, can cause azospermia. Low dosages (10 cGy) can cause temporary azospermia, while dosages of 200 cGy or greater are likely to result in permanent azospermia. Leydig's cells that produce testosterone are damaged by dosages of greater than 2,000 cGy.

Surgery: Retroperitoneal lymph node dissection, which is done for staging of germ cell or testicular tumors, can damage ejaculatory function. Orchiectomy (removal of a testicle) decreases testosterone and sperm production, but normal function may be maintained if the remaining testicle is unaffected.

Age: Pubertal males are at highest risk of toxicity because of the high rate of activity in their developing gonads. Prepubertal males are not as resistant as was once believed. Secondary testicular failure is a result of damage to the hypothalamic-pituitary axis as a result of radiation therapy (see the discussion of the hypothalamic-pituitary axis earlier in this section). Thyroid dysfunction and chronic illness also can affect reproductive function and should be included as a factor during an evaluation.

Clinical Presentation

The signs and symptoms of primary testicular dysfunction can include delayed or arrested pubertal development, testicles that are small for the patient's Tanner stage, oligospermia or azospermia, elevated gonadotropin levels, and Leydig's cells dysfunction. Leydig's cells dysfunction is manifested by decreased testosterone production, increased follicle-stimulating hormone (FSH), and luteinizing hormone levels, as well as by germinal cell dysfunction that is associated with increased FSH and normal LH levels and normal testosterone levels.

Diagnostic Work-up

A diagnostic work-up consists of the following:

- comprehensive annual history and physical examination including height, weight, Tanner staging, including testicular volume measured by Prader orchiometry
- comprehensive annual history, including sexual function, erection, nocturnal emissions, libido, and medicinal or recreational drug usage
- laboratory tests, including serum follicle-stimulating hormone (FSH), luteinizing hormone (LH), and testosterone levels at age 11 years or older, and for children with signs of delayed puberty or testosterone deficiency
- semen analysis, as requested by the patient, if age-appropriate and a sufficient length of time has passed since treatment ended
- laboratory tests, including serum follicle-stimulating hormone, LH, and testosterone levels; thyroxine and TSH levels (other thyroid studies as directed by an endocrinologist); and a semen analysis
- bone age radiological studies.

Medical Treatment

Before receiving treatment that is known to affect fertility, pubertal young men should be offered the option of sperm analysis and banking. Treatment of gonadal failure includes hormone replacement with testosterone supplementation during the patient's pubertal development. Also, testosterone may be given to enhance the patient's well-being and decrease the risk of osteoporosis in postpubertal males who have low levels of testosterone.

Nursing Assessment and Interventions

Assessment:

- Review the survivor's treatment history to determine his risk factors.
- Review the survivor's medical history for symptoms of testosterone deficiency, which can include decreased testicular volume, poor erectile function, and decreased libido.
- Ensure that the survivor receives a complete annual physical examination, that his growth has been charted, and that Tanner staging has been assessed.

Interventions:

- Reinforce the importance of lifelong, annual, follow-up assessments with a healthcare provider who is familiar with the survivor's cancer history, treatment, and risk for developing late effects.
- Educate the survivor about the use of contraceptives to avoid an unwanted pregnancy because testicular dysfunction may not be permanent.
- Ensure that adequate information is made available for survivors being treated for reproductive dysfunction.
  - Follow up with an endocrinologist and/or urologist.
  - Review instructions for the proper administration of medications with the patient.
- Make referrals for survivors who need counseling on fertility or parenting.

Expected Patient Outcomes

- The survivor is knowledgeable about the risk for reproductive failure and available interventions.
- The survivor is knowledgeable about his contraceptive options.
- The survivor complies with recommendations for follow-up care.
- The survivor is knowledgeable about his parenting options.

Reproductive System: Ovaries

Barbara Anne Hieb, Susan K. Ogle, and Wendy Hobbie

Definition

Primary, secondary, or premature ovarian failure is defined as elevated serum gonadotropins, undetectable estrogen levels, and failure to progress pubertally. These effects can occur after chemotherapy, abdominal or pelvic irradiation, or surgical removal of the ovaries. Normal pubertal development, postpubertal production of estrogen, and production of mature ova for fertilization can be affected. Treatment can cause depletion of oocytes, but the results might not be immediately evident.

Risk Factors

Chemotherapy: Higher cumulative doses of alkylating agents, or combinations of alkylating agents with or without radiation below the diaphragm, and total body irradiation all can damage oocytes. In addition, female survivors of Hodgkin's disease are at increased risk of developing early menopause. Total body irradiation also may be associated with ovarian failure, but current studies are inconclusive; premature menopause has been reported.

Radiation: Direct, scattered, or transmitted radiation to the ovaries in dosages of 400–1,200 cGy can result in ovarian failure. In addition, radiation to the head, neck, or central nervous system in doses greater than 4,000 cGy may cause secondary ovarian failure.

Surgery: If one ovary is removed and if the second ovary has been unaffected by treatment, normal function can be maintained.

Age: The number of oocytes in the ovaries is proportional to a female's age; older females are at greater risk of failure. Secondary ovarian failure is a result of damage to the hypothalamic-pituitary axis caused by radiation (see the discussion of the hypothalamic-pituitary axis earlier in this section). Thyroid dysfunction and chronic illness also can affect reproductive function and should be assessed during an evaluation.

Clinical Presentation

A survivor can have delayed or arrested pubertal development (i.e., no breast buds by the age of 12). The female also may not have progressed beyond Tanner Stage II by 14 years of age. Other signs are delayed menarche (i.e., menarche has not been achieved by age 16), oligomenorrhea or amenorrhea in a postpubertal female, and early menopause.

Diagnostic Work-up

A diagnostic work-up consists of the following:

- A comprehensive annual history, including menstrual and pregnancy history (if applicable), and physical exam.
- Laboratory tests to measure follicle-stimulating hormone, luteinizing hormone, and estradiol levels, as well as thyroxine and thyroid-stimulating hormone. Other thyroid studies should be done as directed by an endocrinologist.
- Radiological studies, including a bone age film and an ultrasound of the survivor's ovaries, may be useful.

Medical Treatment

Prevention: Preventive measures include oophoropexy or shielding the ovaries from radiation. Efforts currently are underway to establish procedures for ovarian tissue preservation for newly diagnosed patients whose treatment increases the risk for infertility.

Hormone replacement therapy: In prepubertal females, hormone replacement therapy (HRT) may be given to stimulate development of the gonadal organs if primary ovarian failure has been established. HRT might be given with growth hormone to maximize the survivor's growth potential. Hormone replacements can be given after puberty to decrease menopausal symptoms as well as to prevent osteoporosis and heart disease.

Nursing Assessment and Interventions

Assessment:

- Review the survivor's treatment history to determine her risk factors.
- Review the survivor's history for symptoms of estrogen deficiency, including primary or secondary amenorrhea, menstrual changes, decreasing size of breasts, breast discharge, hot flashes, mood swings, headache, vaginal dryness, dyspareunia, and low libido.
- Ensure that the survivor has a complete physical examination, that her growth has been charted, and that Tanner staging has been done.
- Review and interpret the patient's laboratory results.

Interventions:

- Reinforce the importance of having annual, lifelong, follow-up examinations with a healthcare provider familiar with her cancer history, treatment, and risk for developing late effects.
- Educate the survivor about the use of contraceptive methods to prevent unwanted pregnancy if the status of her fertility is uncertain.
- Ensure that adequate information is given to a survivor being treated for ovarian failure.
- Ensure that the survivor visits an endocrinologist and gynecologist for an annual Papanicolaou test and pelvic examination.
- Ensure that medications are properly administered.
- Encourage the survivor who is at risk for early menopause not to postpone pregnancy if she wants to have children.
- Provide a referral for a survivor who needs counseling on fertility matters or parenting issues.

Expected Patient Outcomes

- The survivor is knowledgeable about her risk for ovarian failure and what interventions are available.
- The survivor complies with recommendations for follow-up care.

- The survivor is knowledgeable about her contraceptive options.
- The survivor is knowledgeable about her parenting options.

Musculoskeletal System

Debra A. Eshelman

Definition

Damage to the musculoskeletal system is caused most often by radiation that disrupts the cytoarchitecture and damages small vessels, thus preventing full muscle development (because of ischemia). Damage also can be the result of surgical removal of a portion of the musculoskeletal system. Surgery, radiation, chemotherapy, and steroids can result in musculoskeletal late effects, including weakness, alteration or loss of function, osteopathy (such as osteopenia and osteoporosis), or fracture. Survivors may experience psychological late effects, including an altered body image and self concept.

Risk Factors

Radiation therapy: In general, the higher the cumulative radiation dose and the younger the age at treatment, the greater the potential deficits. Second neoplasms (malignant or benign) may occur in radiated areas (see second malignant neoplasms Section 10)

Quantity of radiation. Generally a dose of less than 1,000 cGy causes no detectable effect; a dosage of 1,000–2,000 cGy produces partial arrest of the growth of the epiphysis and muscle hypoplasia. Dosages greater than 2,000 cGy usually result in complete arrest of the epiphysis. Fractionated dosages of radiation decrease the risk of late effects, when compared with a single-dose schedule. Orthovoltage radiation (used more commonly before 1970) results in more musculoskeletal damage than does megavoltage because of increased absorption by bone and skin.

Field size and location. Larger fields can produce greater deficits. Modern radiation techniques have made possible better control of field size by permitting more symmetrical delivery of radiation. As an example of field size significance, abdominal radiation (e.g., Wilms' tumor) can result in scoliosis, but its incidence has decreased with the use of modern techniques. As an example of location significance, radiation to soft tissues of the face (such as may be done to treat rhabdomyosarcoma) may result in cosmetic problems, secondary to alteration in the growth of the tissue and structures in the radiation field.

Age at the time of treatment. Radiation therapy produces greater effects on the bones and muscles of younger children. The epiphyseal plate of the bone may be damaged, causing slower or halted growth of bones. Hypoplasia of the irradiated developing muscle tissue also can occur.

Chemotherapy: Prolonged use of steroids can result in avascular necrosis of the femoral heads, osteopenia, or osteoporosis. Corticosteroid-associated bone morbidity has been linked with the treatment of leukemia. Acute vincristine-related neuropathy can predispose a patient to chronic foot drop. Antimetabolite therapy, especially methotrexate, has been implicated in the development of osteopathy.

Surgery: The loss of muscle groups, especially in the lower extremities, can result in gait disturbances and weakness. Effects of limb-sparing procedures include functional deficits, limb length discrepancies, problems with internal hardware, pain, infection and contractures. Amputation of a part of or an entire extremity also may result in muscle imbalance or functional deficits that may require rehabilitation. Laminectomies may contribute to chronic back pain and have the potential to restrict mobility of the spine.

Clinical Presentation

Effects on bone: Patients may experience the following effects on bone as a result of radiation: spinal abnormalities (kyphosis, lordosis, loss of stature), discrepancies in limb length, exostosis, slipped capitofemoral epiphysis, pathologic fracture, osteonecrosis/avascular necrosis of the femoral head, and delayed or arrested tooth development. The effects on bone from surgery may include alterations in gait or functional impairment of the affected part. The effects on bone from chemotherapy (steroids) include increased risk for osteopenia or osteoporosis. Survivors may present with history of a bone fracture.

Effects on muscle: The effects on muscle due to radiation include soft tissue hypoplasia and muscle asymmetry because of reduced or uneven growth.

Diagnostic Work-up

A diagnostic work-up consists of the following:

- a comprehensive annual history and physical exam.
- X rays of the affected or irradiated area (the frequency is determined by the type of deficit or problem)
- serial measurements of the survivor's standing and sitting height and weight
- observation of the survivor's gait, posture, muscle tone, size, and strength
- an orthopedic consultation and follow-up
- measurement of the circumference of the involved part or extremity and comparison with unirradiated areas
- bone age radiograph, as indicated
- careful inspection and palpation of structures in irradiated fields.

Medical Treatment

Limb length discrepancies: Treatment includes using a shoe lift, contralateral epiphysiodesis to arrest growth in the nonaffected limb, and contralateral limb shortening or ipsilateral lengthening procedures.

Slipped capitofemoral epiphysis: This condition is a medical emergency that requires fixation.

Pathological fractures: This type of fracture can require internal fixation, immobilization, and bone grafting; if it recurs, it may require amputation.

Scoliosis: Bracing is indicated in the growing patient with curves greater than 20 degrees that are rapidly progressing, or curves greater than 30 degrees. Curves greater than 45 degrees usually require fusion.

Exostosis: Treatment depends upon the site and the size of the exostosis.

Amputation: Treatment consists of monitoring the functional capability and condition of the stump and the functioning of the adaptive prosthesis.

Osteopenia and osteoporosis: Treatment normally is patient-specific and usually includes calcium supplementation, bisphosphonates, and treatment of exacerbating conditions (e.g., hormone replacement for hypogonadism). Scans to evaluate bone mineral density should be done as clinically indicated.

Avascular necrosis/osteonecrosis: Treatment is patient-dependent, and orthopedic follow-up is indicated.

Psychological/psychosocial concerns: Referrals should be made to appropriate healthcare providers and resources.

Nursing Assessment and Interventions

Assessment:

- Review the patient's history for reports of pain, as well as for alterations in growth, functional status, and activities of daily living.
- Assess the survivor for alterations in self-esteem and body image.
- Ensure that a physical examination assesses for the following:
  - abnormalities in the skin or structures in the irradiated fields, with prompt evaluation of bony growths or suspicious skin lesions
  - gait changes, posture, functional deficits
  - muscle growth, symmetry, tone, size, and strength
  - scoliosis
  - active and passive range of motion of all joints that were in the radiation field
- Assess the fit and function of the prosthesis or orthotic device in collaboration with an orthopedist and a physical therapist

Interventions:

- Reinforce the importance of lifelong, annual, follow-up assessments with a healthcare provider who is familiar with the survivor's cancer history, treatment, and risk for developing late effects.
- Ensure that proper diagnostic tests are obtained.
- Assist with strategies to help the survivor adapt to changes in body image (e.g., support groups, psychological counseling, or therapy) or changes in function (occupational therapy; physical therapy; modifications to automobiles, workspace, etc.)
- Educate the survivor and the family about precautions and potential late effects:
  - preventive measures, such as calcium supplementation and overall good nutrition the risk for potential fracture
  - realistic expectations about growth and function
  - avoidance of excessive weight gain
  - the impact of nutrition on growth
  - necessary restrictions to involvement in contact sports (if clinically indicated)
  - the risk for second malignant neoplasms
- Stress the importance of having ongoing orthopedic, orthotic, and physical therapy evaluations.

Expected Patient Outcomes

- The survivor is knowledgeable about the risk for musculoskeletal late effects and second malignant neoplasms.
- The survivor is functional in activities of daily living.
- The survivor complies with follow-up visits.

Hematopoietic System

Jill E. Brace O'Neill

Definition

Compromised bone marrow function, or myelosuppression, secondary to radiation therapy or chemotherapy is the primary hematopoietic late effect. To date, only limited research exists on the late-developing hematologic effects of cancer treatment. The hematopoietic symptoms of the long-term effects of radiation therapy and chemotherapy can include hypoplastic or aplastic bone marrow aspirates, decreased white blood cell and platelet counts, and increased susceptibility to infections.

Risk Factors

Chemotherapy: The degree of marrow damage depends upon the age of the patient at the time he or she received the chemotherapy (older patients who often experience delayed recovery of T-cell function are at higher risk). Another risk factor is high-dose myelosuppressive chemotherapy. Anemia may be a secondary effect of chemotherapy-related chronic renal failure or hypothyroidism, but this is only a theory at present.

Radiation therapy: The degree of marrow damage depends upon the radiation dosage and volume the patient received. A 4,000 cGy dose of total nodal irradiation impairs bone marrow reserve for up to 7 years after therapy has been completed. Recovery from 4,000–5,000 cGy given over 4–6 weeks can take more than 2 years. Twenty-five percent of patients who have received 850–1,000 cGy (as a single-dose total body irradiation) have platelet counts below 100,000 for more than 4 months.

Chemotherapy used in conjunction with radiation therapy: Chemotherapy used in conjunction with radiation therapy may have a synergistic effect and therefore may increase the overall risk of hematopoietic late effects. Therefore, hematopoietic stem cell transplant places the survivor at the highest risk for hematopoietic disorders.

Clinical Presentation

A survivor can present with hypoplastic or aplastic bone marrow and, less commonly, peripheral cytopenia.

Diagnostic Work-up

A diagnostic work-up consists of the following:
- a detailed history and physical examination
- laboratory studies
- a CBC with a differential
- a bone marrow aspirate, as indicated.

Medical Treatment

Treatment is based upon the survivor's presenting symptoms and clinical findings.

Nursing Assessment and Interventions

Assessment:
- Obtain a detailed medical history, paying particular attention to recurring infections, symptoms of anemia, or a tendency for bleeding.
- Examine the patient for symptoms of anemia or bleeding diathesis.
- Identify the factors and characteristics of the survivor that are associated with specific adverse hematologic sequelae.

Interventions:
- Reinforce the importance of lifelong, annual, follow-up assessments with a healthcare provider who is familiar with the survivor's cancer history, treatment, and risk for developing late effects.
- Encourage ongoing surveillance to identify and treat late hematologic effects resulting from therapy.
- Educate the survivor about the need for regular medical evaluations.

Expected Patient Outcomes

- The survivor and the family will understand any late-developing symptoms of the hematologic system related to cancer treatment.
- The survivor and the family will understand the importance of and maintain long-term follow-up contact with a pediatric oncology center so that potential hematologic late effects of treatment can be evaluated and managed.

IMMUNE SYSTEM

Jill E. Brace O'Neill

Definition

Immune function may be compromised because of surgery, chemotherapy, or radiation therapy, or a combination of these cancer treatments.

Risk Factors

Radiation therapy: Total body irradiation of 1,000 cGy can impair cell-mediated immunity; incomplete T-cell reconstitution has been reported up to 4 years after a bone marrow transplant. The effects of radiation involving smaller nodal or marrow fields on the immune system vary. The function of the spleen may be partially or completely compromised by radiation of the splenic field with doses of 4,000 cGy.

Surgery: Infection is the major risk after a splenectomy, particularly the risk of sudden and overwhelming infection from encapsulated organisms (i.e., pneumococci, *Haemophilus influenzae*, *Neisseria meningococcus*). One function of the spleen is to filter out substances, such as waste and infectious organisms. It also is responsible for early antibody response. Without the spleen, the immune response is decreased.

Chemotherapy: The long-term effects of chemotherapeutic agents on the immune system have not been well documented.

Clinical Presentation

A survivor may have frequent recurring infections and a decrease in immunoglobulin levels.

Diagnostic Work-up

A diagnostic work-up consists of the following:
- a detailed history and physical examination, paying particular attention to infections
- tests to determine immunoglobulin levels (i.e., IgG, IgM, IgA, IgE levels)
- T-cell studies, T-4, T-8 subsets studies
- consultation with an immunologist, as necessary.

Medical Treatment

Treatment depends upon the diagnosis. There should be a follow-up with an immunologist, when warranted.

Nursing Assessment and Interventions

Assessment:
- Obtain a detailed patient history and evaluate for any recurrent infections.
- Assess the results of the survivor's physical examination.

Interventions:
- Reinforce the importance of lifelong, annual, follow-up assessments with a healthcare provider familiar with the survivor's cancer history, treatment, and risk for developing late effects.
- Educate the survivor and the family about potential immunological late effects and their presenting symptoms.
- Educate the survivor and the family about potential complications associated with having had a splenectomy.
  - Splenectomized patients have a 10% risk or less of having an overwhelming bacterial infection (most often pneumococcal).
  - Emphasize the importance of having a pneumococcal vaccination (before a splenectomy is performed and a booster every 5 years), as well as *Haemophilus b* conjugate vaccine, meningococcal vaccine, and annual influenza vaccine.

- A daily prophylactic dose of penicillin (Pen-Vee-K) or erythromycin (EES) is strongly recommended in splenectomized children. Young adult survivors can be given a prescription for penicillin (or erythromycin, if survivor is penicillin allergic) to keep at home to take in case they develop a fever of 101° F. or higher, but also should seek medical attention from a primary care provider.

Expected Patient Outcomes

- The survivor and the family will understand the importance of early intervention in the event of fever or other signs and symptoms of infection if he or she has had a splenectomy.
- The survivor and the family will understand and identify late-developing symptoms of the immunologic system related to cancer treatment.
- The survivor and the family will understand the importance of, and compliance with, long-term follow-up care at a clinic that specializes in treating cancer survivors for evaluation and management of potential late effects of treatment on the immune system.

Second Malignant Neoplasms

Nancy E. Kline

Definition

Second malignant neoplasms can result either from exposure to previous cancer therapy or from genetic determinants that caused the initial childhood cancer. The risk of a second cancer 20 years after a childhood cancer is estimated to be 3%–8%.

Risk Factors

Genetic mutations: Certain familial genetic mutations predispose family members to specific cancers, including Von Recklinghausen's neurofibromatosis or Li-Fraumeni family cancer syndrome.

Chemotherapeutic agents: Exposure to chemotherapeutic agents (e.g., alkylating agents, epipodophyllotoxins) is a risk factor for the subsequent development of acute myelogenous leukemia; peak incidence occurs 4–5 years after initial therapy ceases. Hodgkin's disease and non-Hodgkin's lymphoma also are associated with alkylating agents. Peak incidence occurs 3–10 years after initial therapy ceases (**Table 10-2**).

Exposure to radiation: Exposure to therapeutic radiation causes an increased incidence of chronic myelogenous leukemia, sarcomas, breast cancer, central nervous system tumors, skin and thyroid cancer(s).

Clinical Presentation

Table 10-3 presents the primary cancer diagnoses associated with second malignant neoplasms.

Leukemia: The symptoms include fatigue, anemia, thrombocytopenia, granulocytopenia, bone pain, bleeding, fevers, and frequent infections.

Solid tumors: The symptoms include fatigue, anorexia, palpable mass, bloody stools, anemia, or pain.

Central nervous system: The symptoms include seizures, headaches, altered mental states, change in vision, nausea, and vomiting.

Diagnostic Work-up

A diagnostic work-up consists of the following:

- a comprehensive annual history and detailed physical exam.
- a complete blood count on a yearly basis for patients who received alkylating agents (e.g., mechlorethamine [nitrogen mustard], chlorambucil [Leukeran], cyclo-phosphamide

Table 10-2. Therapeutic Modalities Associated with Second Malignant Neoplasms

Treatment	Associated Secondary Malignant Neoplasm	Latency Period
Epipodophyllotoxins – etoposide (VP-16) – teniposide (VM-26)	Myeloid leukemia	4–5 years
Alkylating agents – mechlorethamine (nitrogen mustard) – chlorambucil (Leukeran) – procarbazine (Matulane) – carmustine (BCNU), lomustine (CCNU) – cyclophosphamide (Cytoxan) – melphalan (Alkeran)	Myeloid leukemia Hodgkin's disease Non-Hodgkin's lymphoma	3–10 years
Radiation		
– children < 6 years: cranial radiation for ALL	Increased risk of brain tumors	Variable
– children < 5 years: cranial radiation including the neck	Increased risk of thyroid cancer	
– adolescents: radiation to the chest	Increased risk of breast cancer	
– field of treatment for a primary malignancy	Increased risk of bone or soft tissue sarcoma	

Table 10-3. Second Malignant Neoplasms: Primary Diagnosis with Associated Second Malignant Neoplasms

Primary Diagnosis	Predisposing Factors in Development of Secondary Malignant Neoplasms	Associated Secondary Malignant Neoplasms	Latency Period	Recommendation for Follow-up
Retinoblastoma	Genetic type (usually bilateral) Family history of retinoblastoma or *p53* mutation Chromosome 13q14 deletion Radiation dosages >3,000 cGy Alkylating agents	Bone or soft tissue sarcoma Osteosarcoma Chondrosarcoma Pineoblastoma (not a true secondary malignant neoplasm; usually occurs within radiation field, may occur outside field)	Can vary; if within the radiation field, may appear earlier	Radiographic studies, other imaging studies (of the irradiated area) (baseline and every 5 years or when a patient is symptomatic)
Hodgkin's disease	Mechlorethamine (nitrogen mustard) Vincristine (Oncovin) Procarbazine (Matulane)	Leukemia (myeloid) Non-Hodgkin's lymphoma	Plateaus at 10 years (mean 5–7 years)	CBC with differential
	Radiation > 2,000 cGy Treatment for recurrent Hodgkin's in adolescents Female predominance	Sarcoma (bone and soft tissue)		Radiograph, other imaging studies (of the irradiated area) (baseline and every 5 years or when a patient is symptomatic)
	Age > 10 years	Thyroid cancer	Long latency period, no plateau	Annual palpation of thyroid
	Adolescents who receive radiation to the chest when mammary tissue is proliferating	Breast cancer		Mammography at age 25 then every 2 years until age 40, then every year
Genetic conditions	Neurofibromatosis (NF1)	Neurofibrosarcoma CNS tumors Juvenile chronic myelocytic leukemia	Can vary	CBC with differential Radiographic studies, other imaging studies (of the irradiated area) (baseline and every 5 years if normal, or when a patient is symptomatic)
	Li-Fraumeni syndrome (a rare familial cancer; syndrome is characterized by a mutation of the *p53* gene)	Breast Childhood sarcoma CNS tumors Leukemia		
Ewing's sarcoma	Radiation	Bone or soft tissue sarcomas Acute nonlymphocytic leukemia	>4 years, can be a long latency of >30 years	Radiographic studies, other imaging studies (of the irradiated area) (baseline and every 5 years if normal, or when a patient is symptomatic)
Acute lymphoblastic leukemia	Radiation (increased risk among children 5 years of age or less at diagnosis) The risk of secondary malignant neoplasms after treatment for ALL is relatively low overall.	CNS tumors Non-Hodgkin's lymphoma Acute nonlymphocytic leukemia Hodgkin's disease Other neoplasms –thyroid cancers –skin cancers	Can vary (ongoing follow-up studies are being done to assess the latency period)	CBC with differential
Wilms' tumor	Bilateral Wilms' tumor Certain congenital anomalies	Thyroid gland tumors Bone and connective tissues CNS Leukemia	Reported highest incidence is 20 years after treatment	CBC with differential

[Cytoxan], or melphalan [Alkeran]) or epipodophyllotoxins (e.g., etoposide [VP-16], teniposide [VM-26]); or radiation therapy
- other diagnostic tests, as warranted by a physical exam.
- genetic counseling (if the family is interested), with a discussion of the risks and benefits of testing.

Medical Treatment

Medical treatment depends upon the diagnosis of the second malignancy, previous treatment for the primary malignancy, and current available therapies.

Nursing Assessment and Interventions

Assessment:

- Review the survivor's interval medical history for reports of recent weight loss, fatigue, malaise, pain, bleeding abnormalities, persistent fevers, recurrent infections, and hematochezia.
- Review the family's medical history for malignancies, hematological disorders, and genetic disorders.
- Perform a physical examination, which should include these assessments:
  - complete vital signs, particularly attention to weight changes
  - a complete blood count (CBC) with a differential and platelet count
  - a skin assessment for evidence of bleeding, change in pigmentation, or change in nevi
  - gastrointestinal assessment for oral ulcers and perirectal abscess, abdominal pain
  - stool guaiac
  - palpation of the abdomen for hepatosplenomegaly.

Interventions:

- Reinforce the importance of lifelong, annual, follow-up assessments with a healthcare provider familiar with the survivor's cancer history, treatment, and risk for developing late effects.
- Educate the survivor and the family about the early warning signs of cancer.
- Educate the survivor about the benefits of having routine cancer screenings and the appropriate time interval for such screenings (e.g., monthly breast examinations, yearly Papanicolaou tests and pelvic examinations, mammograms).
- Ensure that appropriate diagnostic tests are ordered and that the patient receives the results, as appropriate.
- Perform an assessment of the patient that will ensure early identification of second malignant neoplasms.
- Educate the survivor about healthy lifestyle behaviors to reduce his or her risk of second malignant neoplasms (e.g., dietary recommendations; avoidance of tobacco products, tanning beds, and excessive alcohol consumption; use of sunscreen).

Expected Patient Outcomes

- The survivor and the family know the risk factors for developing second malignant neoplasms and can identify their signs and symptoms early enough to seek medical intervention if it is needed.
- The survivor returns for follow-up examinations, as recommended, and obtains yearly evaluations at a clinic for long-term cancer survivors.

Psychosocial Effects: Personal-Emotional

Sarah J. Bottomley

Definition

Living with a diagnosis and history of cancer equates to living with uncertainty and compromise, which are feelings that can persist long after treatment has been completed. Living with uncertainty can lead to increased feelings of vulnerability. Long-term survivors of childhood cancer and their families also have the challenge of compromised living. Together, uncertainty and compromise can affect long-term survivors' self-concept, self-esteem, body image, and other aspects of their personal and emotional lives. Additionally, posttraumatic stress disorder (PTSD) has been identified recently as a significant problem in as many as 20% of the young adult survivor population.

Risk Factors

Age: A cancer diagnosis is traumatic for any child; however, the age of the child and his or her developmental level influence the entire cancer experience.

Family support: The emotional support of and adaptation by the family to the cancer diagnosis contribute to a child's overall adjustment.

Medical problems: The amount and severity of continuing medical problems often affect a survivor's emotional outlook.

Coping abilities: Survivors of cancer and other serious illnesses often report that they have been changed by the experience. The coping style of a survivor and a family will affect their ability to adjust and assimilate the experience into their lives. Coping with their cancer histories and with the reactions of their peers and society in general are major challenges for survivors of childhood cancer.

Education: Educational performance can have a great impact on the development of a child's self-image and self-esteem. Working through their fears, identifying abilities, addressing social issues, and gaining control are paramount to academic success. A child's anxiety and embarrassment with regard to his or her educational abilities, physical limitations, or differences can significantly contribute to the development of a reluctance to attend school.

Communication style of the individual and the family: A family's ways of communicating about cancer and life issues in general influence how a survivor will communicate about the same issues.

Clinical Presentation

When a survivor is having difficulty with personal or emotional adjustments, he or she can have one or more of the following complaints: sleep disturbances, flat or depressed affect, inability to concentrate, weight loss, change in appetite, anxiety related to returning to the clinic or school, fear of recurrence of the disease, mood swings, feelings of helplessness or hopelessness, problems with self-esteem, issues related to body image, school- or work-related problems that include frequent absences, decreased achievement, or reluctance to attend. Specific symptoms associated with PTSD include: reexperiencing the cancer event, feeling psychologically numb, avoidance behavior (not wanting to return to clinic or to address health issues), and a heightened sense of arousal.

Nursing Assessment and Interventions

Assessment:

- Assess the survivor's general mood and note any wide variations in affect.
- Inquire about sleep patterns and note any changes.
- Plot the survivor's height and weight on a growth chart.
- Obtain a dietary history and note any changes in the child's appetite.
- Assess the survivor's anxiety level related to returning to the clinic, a previous diagnosis, or other concerns.
- Assess the survivor's general level of self-esteem:
  - the survivor's ability to interact and maintain eye contact during a visit
  - the survivor's expressed involvement in activities at school or work
  - the survivor's reported ability to relate to peers through the development of friendships outside the family circle
- Evaluate the survivor's comfort level with his or her physical appearance after treatment (body image).
- Assess the survivor's ability to adapt to life with cancer and a life with possible compromise.
- Assess the survivor's ability to adapt emotionally:
  - Have the survivor and the family incorporated the survivor's cancer history into their daily life and history?
  - Have the survivor and the family established a new state of normalcy in adapting to the emotional and physical changes related to the cancer history and survivorship.
- Assess the parents' expectations:
  - Are parents' expectations of the survivor's physical and neurocognitive abilities consistent with the survivor's actual functional abilities?
  - Have the parents been able to maintain discipline and encourage the survivor's independence?
- Assess the survivor's school or work performance, including progress and attendance patterns.
- Assess the survivor's rehabilitation needs.

Interventions:

- Provide anticipatory guidance in relation to the survivor's medical history, including the disease process, its treatment, and its potential late effects.
- Educate the survivor about lifestyle behaviors that promote and encourage good health and viable coping skills.
- Educate the survivor about available resources that can provide information and support regarding survivorship issues (e.g., the Candlelighters Childhood Cancer Foundation, the American Cancer Society, the National Coalition for Cancer Survivorship, the Leukemia Society, and the National Cancer Institute).
- Provide information about counseling services and local support groups when it is needed.
- Provide referrals to a psychologist or a psychiatrist if they become clinically necessary.

Expected Patient Outcomes

- The survivor is able to identify emotional adjustment issues related to survivorship.
- The survivor verbalizes an understanding of available community and counseling resources.
- The survivor is attending school or work and has stated goals for the future.

Psychosocial Effects: Political-Social

Sarah J. Bottomley

Definition

A history of cancer can provide an avenue for discrimination in several aspects of the survivor's life. Discrimination most often occurs in the form of employment problems, difficulty in obtaining health and life insurance, legal issues, and education-related issues.

Risk Factors

Employment problems: The employment problems of cancer survivors can take many forms. Childhood cancer survivors experience discrimination in employment that is based primarily on the survivor's history of cancer. Employers may have misconceptions about cancer ("Cancer is a death sentence," "Cancer is contagious," "Cancer survivors are an unproductive drain on the economy"). Other employment-related problems are the difficulties in getting a job, denial of promotions, denial of insurance or other benefits, lower salaries, the lack of an employment history, and rejection for military service.

Insurance problems: Attempting to secure adequate insurance (health, life, or disability) can create frustration. Policy cancellations, increased premiums, preexisting-condition clauses, extended waiting periods, and denial of benefits exemplify types of discrimination shown toward a survivor.

Education-related issues: (See "Psychosocial Effects: Educational Issues" later in this section.)

Legal issues: Legal issues relate to employment and education-related discrimination (see the discussions of these topics later in this section).

Clinical Presentation

Survivors may report having experienced discrimination at school or at work. They also may state that they are having insurance or legal problems related to denial of insurance coverage, high premiums, or denial of supplemental security income (SSI).

Assessment and Interventions

Assessment:

- Assess the survivor's educational abilities, progress, and goals.
- Assess the survivor's employment status.
- Assess the survivor's insurance status.
- Assess the survivor's understanding of his or her legal rights.

Interventions:

Employment:

- Provide the survivor with information about federal and state laws that protect the survivor from discrimination:
  - The Americans with Disabilities Act (ADA) of 1990 prohibits discrimination in employment on the basis of a disability and provides for equal access to public facilities. The ADA protects survivors from having potential employers inquire about their disability or medical history before making a job offer. This law is enforced by the U.S. Equal Employment Opportunity Commission (EEOC). Anyone who has specific questions regarding the ADA can contact the agency at 800/669-6820, or 202/663-4900, or www.eeoc.gov.
  - The Family and Medical Leave Act (FMLA) of 1993 mandates job security for workers in large companies who must take a leave of absence of up to 12 weeks to care for a seriously ill child, spouse, parent, or themselves. The law requires an employer to continue to provide benefits, including health insurance, during the leave period.
  - Military service applications are considered on a case-by-case basis. The Department of Defense, under Directive No. 6130 (March 31, 1986), provides a means for cancer survivors to be considered for military service. Survivors who have not required any cancer-related surgical or medical treatment for 5 years and who are considered free of cancer can be granted a medical waiver and be considered fit for military service. However, a survivor must meet the physical requirements of the position for which he or she has applied. Military recruiters may be unfamiliar with the directive. Encourage the survivor to read the directive and to self-advocate.
- Educate the survivor about ways to avoid discrimination:
  - The survivor should not volunteer information regarding his or her cancer history unless it might directly affect his or her ability to perform a job or participate in an educational program.
  - The survivor should not lie about his or her medical history on either a job or an insurance application.
  - The survivor should answer questions truthfully when asked about his or her cancer history and should be prepared to explain his or her current health status and prognosis. The survivor also should be prepared to educate the interviewer about cancer.
  - The survivor should apply for positions for which he or she is qualified.
  - The survivor should provide a letter from the treating healthcare facility that addresses his or her current health status, prognosis, and ability to work.
  - The survivor should not ask about health insurance benefits during the interview process. Once a job offer has been made, the survivor should review the benefits package before accepting the position.
  - The survivor should seek employment in larger companies (those with more then 300 employees) because smaller companies may be exempt from meeting certain provisions of the aforementioned laws.
  - The survivor should seek assistance from a job counselor or a school counselor.
- Encourage the survivor to tell appropriate legislative representatives about any discrimination he or she has experienced.

Education: See Section VIII, "Patient and Family Education," for additional information.

- Educate survivors about the importance of advocating for themselves.
- Provide resource information on organizations that can assist with advocacy efforts.
  - Candlelighters Childhood Cancer Foundation is a nonprofit organization that provides information about the legal rights of cancer survivors. This organization provides assistance in resolving problems with health insurance claims, employment discrimination, waivers into military service, and access to equal education. This organization can be contacted at 800/366-2223 or at www.candlelighters.org.
  - The National Coalition for Cancer Survivorship is a nonprofit organization that provides information about legal rights and advocacy services. This group can be contacted at 301/650-9127 or at www.canceradvocacy.org.
  - The American Cancer Society is a nonprofit organization that provides information and publications on cancer

and insurance issues. This organization can be contacted at 800/ACS-2345 or at www.cancer.org.

Legal counsel:

- Provide survivors with information about cancer organizations that can help them obtain appropriate legal counsel: Candlelighters Childhood Cancer Foundation (800/366-2223), the National Coalition for Cancer Survivorship (301/650-9127), and some units of the American Cancer Society.

Health insurance:

- Provide survivors with resource information about their rights in obtaining health insurance. At presstime, no laws guaranteeing a legal right to adequate health insurance existed; however, there are resources that might be able to help survivors obtain coverage.
  - A state-sponsored comprehensive health insurance plan (CHIP) or risk pool are designed to assist people who are considered medically uninsurable to secure health insurance. Survivors should be directed to contact the office of the insurance commissioner of their state for specific information.
  - Some insurance companies and employers offer an open-enrollment period each year. Coverage usually can be obtained regardless of a person's medical history. Survivors should be directed to contact the office of the insurance commissioner of their state.
  - The Comprehensive Omnibus Budget Reconciliation Act (COBRA) requires employers to offer group medical coverage to employees and their dependents who otherwise would lose their group coverage due to individual circumstances.
  - The Medical Information Bureau is a health data bank that provides information for insurance companies. Survivors can contact this organization to find out what information healthcare plans are using for their eligibility criteria.
- Encourage the survivor and the family to be persistent in pursuing coverage.
- Remind the survivor that lobbying also is an essential mechanism for pursuing changes in health insurance laws.

Expected Patient Outcomes

- The survivor understands that resources are available.
- The survivor is knowledgeable about the issues that have been discussed and about recommended interventions.

Psychosocial Effects: Educational Issues

Sarah J. Bottomley

Definition

School attendance, academic performance, and career achievement may be challenged by a diagnosis and treatment of childhood cancer. Survivors can be further challenged by possible late effects of treatment, including cognitive deficits, hearing and visual impairments, physical limitations, and missed educational opportunities (see Section VII, "Psychosocial Issues: School Reentry").

Risk Factors

High rate of absenteeism: Excessive absenteeism from school because of chronic illness can affect educational achievement and expectations as to future school attendance.

Delayed or altered socialization: The need for frequent visits to a clinic or frequent hospitalizations can affect the development of a child's social skills. Children who have not had an opportunity to develop age-appropriate social skills may have difficulty forming friendships, working with others, and advocating for themselves.

School phobia: Anxiety related to school performance, fear of failure, and missed school days can interfere with a child's enjoyment of school and learning opportunities.

Treatment: Cranial irradiation and intrathecal chemotherapy are associated with neurocognitive disabilities. Children who were younger than 5 years of age when they received these treatments may be at higher risk of having educational difficulties.

Clinical Presentation

A survivor can have problems associated with school performance that include poor grades, an inability to achieve an age-appropriate academic level, or school phobia. The child also may have an attention deficit or hyperactivity problem, or both. The child's parents also may have inappropriate expectations. In addition, the child may have medical problems that impede his or her full participation in school.

Assessment and Interventions

Assessment:

- Assess the survivor's school attendance record and academic performance.
- Evaluate the need for neurocognitive testing.
- Evaluate the communication style among the parents, the child, and the school.
- Assess the parents' expectations about the survivor's abilities and his or her progress in school.

Interventions:

- Provide necessary information to the school about the child's cancer history (see Section VII, "Psychosocial Issues: School Reentry").

- Reinforce recommendations for curriculum modifications when they are indicated.
- Refer the survivor for neuropsychological testing, which may provide a beneficial assessment of the child's cognitive strengths and weaknesses.
- Inform the survivor and his or her parents about organizations that provide school resource and advocacy information:
  - Candlelighters Childhood Cancer Foundation (800/366-2223)
  - National Children's Cancer Society (301/650-9127)
- Educate the survivor and his or her family about the three federal laws that ensure equal access to education:
  - The Individuals with Disabilities Education Act (IDEA) requires states to provide free and appropriate education to all children aged 3–21 years.
  - The Americans with Disabilities Act (ADA) prohibits discrimination against people with an actual disability, perceived disability, and history of a disability. This law is enforced by the U.S. Equal Employment Opportunity Commission (800/669-6820; 202/663-4900).
  - The Rehabilitation Act prohibits schools that receive federal funding from discriminating against qualified students because of their cancer history.
- Educate parents about the importance of maintaining normalcy in their child's life and of encouraging they achieve academically.

Expected Patient Outcomes

- The survivor and the family demonstrate their understanding of available resources, including written materials, community organizations, and academic testing opportunities.
- The survivor is knowledgeable about the issues that have been discussed and about recommended interventions.

Promoting Health After Childhood Cancer

Sarah J. Bottomley

- Encourage the survivor to develop an understanding of his or her previous diagnosis, treatment, and risk for health problems related to the treatment, and provide him or her a written summary of the diagnosis and treatment that can be used as a reference.
- Encourage the survivor to have lifelong, annual, follow-up assessments with a healthcare provider who is familiar with the survivor's cancer history, treatment, and risk for developing late effects.
- Encourage a female survivor to perform or have performed these routine screenings for cancer:

Survivorship Resources

American Cancer Society
800/227-2345
www.cancer.org

Association of Online Cancer Resources
www.acor.org

Cancer Care
800/813-4673
www.cancercare.org

Cancer Cured Kids
516/484-8160

Cancervive
800/486-2873
www.cancervive.org

Candlelighters Childhood Cancer Foundation
800/366-2223 or 301/962-3520
www.candlelighters.org

Lance Armstrong Foundation
512/236-8820
www.laf.org

National Cancer Institute
800/422-6237
www.nci.nih.gov

National Children's Cancer Society, Inc.
314/241-1600
www.children-cancer.org

Outlook, Life Beyond Childhood Cancer
www.outlook-life.org

Long Term Effects of Childhood Cancer Treatment
www.cancersurvivorchild.org

Employment

Equal Employment Opportunities Commission
800/669-6820
www.eeoc.gov

Health Care Financing Administration
www.hcfa.gov

- breast self-examinations every month for all females who have begun to have menstrual cycles
- annual clinical breast examinations
- mammography (or other imaging studies, radionuclide scan, or sonography). All females should have a baseline mammogram when they are 20 to 25 years old, or 10 years following irradiation, whichever occurs first, then yearly. Those who have a family history of breast cancer should have an individualized mammogram or imaging schedule. Patients who have had radiation to the chest should follow the aforementioned mammogram schedule.
- a pelvic examination with a Papanicolaousmear every year beginning at age 18 years, or earlier if the patient is sexually active

- Encourage all male survivors 14 years of age or older to perform a testicular self-examination every month.
- Encourage all survivors to have these tests:
  - serum cholesterol starting at age 25, then on a yearly basis
  - a rectal examination starting at age 45, then on a yearly basis
  - stool testing for occult blood starting at age 50 (American Cancer Society recommendation)
  - a sigmoidoscopy starting at age 50 (American Cancer Society recommendation).
- Encourage the survivor to engage in healthy lifestyle behaviors:
  - Use sunscreen with a sun protection factor of 30 or more and avoid tanning beds.
  - Maintain a well-balanced diet that is low in fat and high in fiber (e.g., fruits, vegetables, whole grains), eat foods rich in vitamin C (e.g., dark-green leafy vegetables, citrus fruits, orange or yellow vegetables), and avoid excessive intake of salt.
  - Maintain an ideal body weight.
  - Engage in moderate exercise for 20–30 minutes at least three times a week.
  - Avoid using tobacco products.
  - Avoid excessive intake of alcoholic beverages.
  - Avoid the use of controlled substances.
  - Practice safe sexual behaviors.
  - Allow adequate time for rest.
  - Avoid prolonged stress.
  - Schedule routine annual visits to a healthcare provider knowledgeable about the survivor's cancer history and treatment and remain informed about the late effects and any advances that can reduce or prevent them.

Bibliography

Definition and Overview

American Cancer Society. (2001). Cancer facts & figures 2001 (No. 5008.01, pp.11-12). National Media Office, New York: American Cancer Society.

Bottomley, S.J., & Kassner, E. (2003). Late effects of childhood cancer therapy. *Journal of Pediatric Nursing,18*(2), 126-132.

Dreyer, Z.E., Blatt, J., & Bleyer, A. (2002). Late effects of childhood cancer and its treatment. In P.A. Pizzo & D.G. Poplack (Eds.), *Principles and practice of pediatric oncology* (4th ed., pp.1431–1461). Philadelphia: Lippincott, Williams & Wilkins.

Friedman, D.L., & Meadows, A.T. (2002). Late effects of childhood cancer therapy. *Pediatric Clinics of North America, 49*(5):1083-106.

Ganz, P.A. (2001). Late effects of cancer and its treatment. *Seminars in Oncology Nursing*, 17(4):241-248.

Hobbie, W., Ruccione, K., Harvey, J., & Moore, I.M. (2002). Care of survivors. In C.R. Baggott, K.P. Kelly, D. Fochtman, & G.V. Foley (Eds.), *Nursing care of children and adolescents with cancer,* (3rd ed). (pp. 426–464). Philadelphia: W.B. Saunders.

Keene, N., Hobbie, W., & Ruccione, K. (2000). *Childhood cancer survivors: A practice guide to your future.* Sebastopol, CA: O'Reilly & Associates, Inc.

Parisi, M.T., Fahmy, J.L., Kaminsky, C.K., & Malogolowkin, M.H. (1999). Complications of cancer therapy in children: a radiologist's guide. *Radiographis, 9*(2), 283-297.

Ries, L.A.G., Smith, M.A., Gurney, J.G., Linet, M., Tamra,T., Young, J.L., Bunin, G.R. (Eds.). (1999). *Cancer incidence and survival among children and adolescents: United States SEER Program 1975-1995* (NIH Publication No. 99-4649). Monographs of the *National Cancer Institute, SEER Program.* Bethesda, MD.

Central Nervous System

Challinor, J., Miaskowski, C., Moore, I., Slaughter, R., & Franck, L. (2000). Review of research studies that evaluated the impact of treatment for childhood cancers on neurocognition and behavioral and social competence: Nursing implications. *Journal of the Society of Pediatric Nursing, 5*, 57–74.

Dreyer, Z.E., Blatt, J., & Bleyer, A. (2002). Late effects of childhood cancer and its treatment. In P.A. Pizzo & D.G. Poplack (Eds.), *Principles and practice of pediatric oncology* (4th ed., pp. 1437–1439). Philadelphia: Lippincott Williams & Wilkins.

Moleski, M. (2000). Neuropsychological, neuroanatomical, and neurophysiological consequences of CNS chemotherapy for acute lymphoblastic leukemia. *Archives of Clinical Neuropsychology, 15*, 603–630.

Hypothalamic-Pituitary Axis

Cohen, L.E. (2003). Endocrine late effects of cancer treatment. *Current Opinion in Pediatrics, 15*, 3–9.

Thyroid Function

Cohen, L.E. (2002). Endocrine late effects of cancer treatment. *Current Opinions in Pediatrics, 15*, 3–9.

Lando, A., Holm, K., Nyson, K., Rasmussen, K., Feldt-Rasmussen, U., Petersen, J.H., et. al. (2001). Thyroid function in survivors of childhood acute lymphoblastic leukaemia: The significance of prophylactic cranial radiation. *Clinical Endocrinology, 55*, 21–25.

Rose, S.R., Lustig, R.H., Pitukcheewanont, P., Broome, D.C., Burghen, G.A, Li, H., et al. (1999). Diagnosis of hidden central hypothyroidism in survivors of childhood cancer. *The Journal of Clinical Endocrinology & Metabolism, 84*, 4472–4479.

Vision and Hearing

Holstrom, G., Borgstrom, B., & Callissendorff, B. (2002). Cataract in children after bone marrow transplantation: Relation to conditioning regime. *Acta Ophthalmologica Scandinavica, 80,* 211–215.

Oberlin, O., Rey, A., Anderson, J., Carli, M., Raney, R.B., Treuner, J., et al. (2001). Treatment of orbital rhabdomyoscarcoma: Survival and late effects of treatment. Results of an international workshop. *Journal of Clinical Oncology, 19* (1), 197–204.

Ondrey, F.G., Robert, G. J., & Herscher, L. (2000). Radiation dose to otologic structures during head and neck cancer radiation therapy. *Laryngoscope, 110* (2, Part 1): 217–221.

Paulino, A.C., Simon, J.H., Zhen, W., & Wen, B. (2000). Long term effects in children treated with radiotherapy for head and neck rhabdomyosarcoma. *International Journal of Radiation Oncology Biology Physics, 48,* 1489–1495.

Head and Neck

Dahllof, G., Jonsson, A., Ulmner, M., & Huggare, J. (2001). Orthodontic treatment in long-term survivors after pediatric bone marrow transplantation. *American Journal of Orthodontic Dentofacial Orthop, 120,* 459–465.

Duggal, M.S. (2003). Root surface areas in long-term survivors of childhood cancer. *Oral Oncology, 39,* 178–183.

Handschel, J., Sunderkotter, C., Kruse-Losler, B., & Prott, F.J. (2001). Late effects of radiotherapy on oral mucosa in humans. *European Journal of Oral Science, 109,* 95–102.

Karsila-Tenovuo, S., Jahnukainene, K., Peltomaki, T., Minn, H., & Kulmala, J. (2001). Disturbances in craniofacial morphology in children treated for solid tumors. *Oral Oncology, 37,* 586–592.

Minicucci, E.M., Lopes, L.F., & Crocci, A.J. (2003). Dental abnormalities in children after chemotherapy treatment for acute lymphoid leukemia. *Leukemia Res, 27,* 45–50.

Paulino, A.C., Simon, J.H., Zhen, W., & Wen, B.C. (2000). Long-term effects in children treated with radiotherapy for head and neck rhabdomyosarcoma. *International Journal of Radiation Oncology Biology and Phys, 48,* 1489–1495.

Sims, S.A., Barker, G.J., & Gilman, A. (2002). Oral complications associated with the treatment of pediatric neuroblastoma case study. *Journal of Clinical Dentistry, 26,* 401–404.

Cardiovascular System

Bossi, G., Lanzarini, L., Laudisa, M.L., Klersy, C., Raisaro, A., & Arico, M. (2001). Echocardiographic evaluation of patients cured of childhood cancer: A single center study of 117 subjects who received anthracyclines. *Medical and Pediatric Oncology, 36,* 593–600.

Gupta, M., Steinherz, P.G., Cheung, N.K., & Steinherz, L. (2003). Late cardiotoxicity after bolus versus infusion anthracycline therapy for childhood cancers. *Medical Pediatric Oncology, 40,* 343–347.

Kremer, L.C., van Dalen, E.C., Offringa, M., Ottenkamp, J., & Voute, P.A. (2001). Anthracycline-induced clinical heart failure in a cohort of 607 children: Long-term follow-up study. *Journal of Clinical Oncology, 19,* 191–196.

Postma, A., Elzenga, N.J., Haaksma, J., Schasfoort-Van Leeuwen, M.J.M., Kamps, W.A., & Bink-Boelkens, M.T.E. (2002). Cardiac status in bone tumor survivors up to nearly 19 years after treatment with doxorubicin: A longitudinal study. *Medical Pediatric Oncology, 39,* 86–92.

Respiratory System

Dreyer, Z.E., Blatt, J., & Bleyer, A. (2002). Late effects of childhood cancer and its treatment. In P.A. Pizzo & D.G. Poplack (Eds.), *Principles and practice of pediatric oncology* (4th ed., pp. 1445-1447). Philadelphia: Lippincott Williams & Wilkins.

Gastrointestinal and Hepatic Systems

Bismar, M.M., & Sinicrope, F.A. (2002). Radiation enteritis. *Current Gastroenterology Report, 4,* 361–365.

Dreyer, Z.E., Blatt, J., & Bleyer, A. (2002). Late effects of childhood cancer and its treatment. In P.A.Pizzo & D.G.Poplack (Eds.), *Principles and practice of pediatric oncology,* (4th ed., pp. 1447–1448). Philadelphia: Lippincott Williams & Wilkins.

Halonen, P., Mattila, J., Ruuska, T., Salo, M.K., & Makipernaa, A. (2003). Liver histology after current intensified therapy for childhood acute lymphoblasti leukemia: Microvesicular fatty change and siderosis are the main findings. *Medical Pediatric Oncology, 40,* 148–154.

Nguyen, N.P., Antoine, J.E., Dutta, S., Karlsson, U., & Sallah, S. (2002). Current concepts in radiation enteritis and implications for future clinical trials. *Cancer, 95,* 1151–1163.

Regimbeau, J.M., Panis, Y., Gouzi, J.L., Fagniez, P.L., & French University Association of Surgical Research. (2001). Operative and long term results after surgery for chronic radiation enteritis. *The American Journal of Surgery, 182,* 237–242.

Strickland, D.K., Jenkins, J.J., & Hudson, M.M. (2001). Hepatitis C infection and hepatocellular carcinoma after treatment of childhood cancer. *Journal of Pediatric Hematology & Oncology, 23,* 527–529.

Genitourinary System

Ceremuzynski, L., Gebalska, J., Wolk, R., & Makowska, E. (2000). Hypomagnesmia in heart failure with ventricular arrhythmias. *Journal of Internal Medicine, 247,* 78–86.

Liao, F., Folsom, A.R., & Brancati, F.L. (1998). Is low magnesium concentration a risk factor for coronary heart disease? The Atherosclerosis Risk in Communities (ARIC) Study. *American Heart Journal, 136,* 480–490.

Ritchey, M.L., Green, D.M., Thomas, P.R., et al. (1996). Renal failure in Wilms' tumor patients: A report from the National Wilms' Tumor Study Group. *Medical and Pediatric Oncology, 26,* 75–80.

Reproductive System: Testes

Dreyer, Z.E., Blatt, J., & Bleyer, A. (2002). Late effects of childhood cancer and its treatment. In P.A. Pizzo & D.G. Poplack (Eds.). *Principles and practice of pediatric oncology* (4th ed., pp. 1439–1441), Philadelphia: Lippincott Williams & Wilkins.

Houell, S.J. & Shalet, S.M. (2001). Testicular function following chemotherapy. *Human Reproduction Update, 7,* 363–369.

Kenney, L.B., Laufer, M.R., Grant, F.D., Grier, H., & Diller, L. (2001). High risk of infertility and long-term gonadal damage in males treated with high dose cyclophosphamide for sarcoma during childhood. *Cancer, 91,* 613–620.

Sklar, C. (1999). Reproductive physiology and treatment-related loss of sex hormone production. *Medical and Pediatric Oncology, 33,* 2–8.

Reproductive System: Ovaries

Cohen, L.E. (2003). Endocrine late effects of cancer treatment. *Current Opinions in Pediatrics, 15,* 3–9.

Dreyer, Z.E., Blatt, J., & Bleyer, A. (2002). Late effects of childhood cancer and its treatment. In P.A. Pizzo & D.G. Poplack (Eds.), *Principles and practice of pediatric oncology* (4th ed., pp. 1441–1442). Philadelphia: Lippincott Williams & Wilkins.

Sklar, C. (1999). Reproductive physiology and treatment-related loss of sex hormone production. *Medical and Pediatric Oncology, 33*, 2–8.

Musculoskeletal System

Kaste, S.C., Jones-Wallace, D., Rose, S.R., Boyett, J.M., Lustig, R.H., Rivera, G.K., et al. (2001). Bone mineral decrements in survivors of childhood acute lymphoblastic leukemia: Frequency of occurrence and risk factors for their development. *Leukemia, 15*, 728–734.

Mattano, L.A., Sather, H.N., Trigg, M. E., & Nachman, J.B. (2000). Osteonecrosis as a complication of treating acute lymphoblastic leukemia in children: A report from the Children's Cancer Group. *Journal of Clinical Oncology, 18*, 3262–3272.

Nagarajan, R., Neglia, J.P., Clohisy, D.R., & Robison, L.L. (2002). Limb salvage and amputation in survivors of pediatric lower extremity bone tumors: What are the long-term implications? *Journal of Clinical Oncology, 20*, 4493–4501.

Paulino, A.C., Simon, J.H., Zhen, W., & Wen, B. (2000). Long term effects in children treated with radiotherapy for head and neck rhabdomyosarcoma. *International Journal of Radiation Oncology Biology Physics, 48*, 1489–1495.

Pfeilschifter, J. & Diel, I.J. (2000). Osteoporosis due to cancer treatment: Pathogenesis and management. *Journal of Clinical Oncology, 18*, 1570–1593.

Raney, R.B., Asmar, L., Vassilopoulou-Sellin, R., Klein, M.J., Donaldson, S.S., Green, J., et al. (1999). Late complications of therapy of 213 children with localized nonorbital soft-tissue sarcoma of the head and neck: A descriptive report from the Intergroup Rhabdomyosarcoma Studies (IRS)-II and III. *Medical and Pediatric Oncology, 33*, 362–371.

Hematopoietic System

Dreyer, Z.E., Blatt, J., & Bleyer, A. (2002). Late effects of childhood cancer and its treatment. In P.A. Pizzo & D.G. Poplack (Eds.). *Principles and practice of pediatric oncology* (4th ed., pp. 1449–1450). Philadelphia: Lippincott Williams & Wilkins.

Immune System

Dreyer, Z.E., Blatt, J., & Bleyer, A. (2002). Late effects of childhood cancer and its treatment. In P.A. Pizzo & D.G. Poplack (Eds.). *Principles and practice of pediatric oncology* (4th ed., pp. 1449–1450). Philadelphia: Lippincott Williams & Wilkins.

Second Malignant Neoplasms

Aung, L., Gorlick, R.G., Shi, W., Thaler, H., Shorter, N.A., Healey, J.H., et al. (2002). Second malignant neoplasms in long-term survivors of osteosarcoma: Memorial Sloan-Kettering Cancer Center experience. *Cancer, 95*, 1728–1734.

de Vathaire, F., Hawkins, M., Campbell, S., Oberlin, O., Raquin, M-A., Schlienger, J-Y., et al. (1999). Second malignant neoplasms after a first cancer in childhood: temporal pattern of risk according to type of treatment. *British Journal of Cancer, 79*, 1884–1893.

Dreyer, Z.E., Blatt, J., & Bleyer, A. (2002). Late effects of childhood cancer and its treatment. In P.A. Pizzo & D.G. Poplack (Eds.). *Principles and practice of pediatric oncology* (4th ed., pp. 1450–1452). Philadelphia: Lippincott Williams & Wilkins.

Hobbie, W., Ruccione, K., Harvey, J., & Moore, I.M. (2002). Care of survivors. In C. R. Rasco-Baggott, K.P. Kelly, D. Fochtman & G.V. Foley (Eds.), *Nursing care of children and adolescents with cancer* (3rd ed., pp. 426–464). Philadelphia: W. B. Saunders Company.

Jemal, A., Murray, T., Samuels, A., Ghafoor, A., Ward, E., & Thun, M. (2003). Cancer statistics, 2002. *CA: A Cancer Journal for Clinicians, 53*, 5–26.

Neglia, J.P., Friedman, D.L., Yasui, Y., Mertens, A.C., Hammond, S., Stovall, M., et al. (2001). Second mailignant neoplasms in five-year survivors of childhood cancer: childhood cancer survivor study. *Journal of the National Cancer Institute, 93*, 618–629.

Travis, L.B., Gospodarowicz, M., Curtis, R.E., Clarke, E.A., Anderson, M., Glimelius, B., et al. (2002). Lung cancer following chemotherapy and radiotherapy for Hodgkin's disease. *Journal of the National Cancer Institute, 94*, 182–190.

Psychosocial Effects

Bhatia, S., Jenney, M.E.M., Bogue, M.K., Rockwood, T.H., Feusner, J.H., Friedman, D.L., et al. (2002). The Minneapolis-Manchester quality of life instrument: Reliability and validity of the adolescent form. *Journal of Clinical Oncology, 20*, 2692–2698.

Eiser, C., Hill, J.J., & Blakclay, A. (2000). Surviving cancer: What does it mean for you? An evaluation of a clinic based intervention for survivors of childhood cancer. *PsychoOncology, 9*, 214–220.

Hobbie, W.L., Stuber, M., Meeske, K., Wissler, K., Rourke, M.T., Ruccione, K., et al. (2000). Symptoms of posttraumatic stress in young adult survivors of childhood cancer. *Journal of Clinical Oncology, 18*, 4060–4066.

Hoffman, B. (1999). Cancer survivors' employment and insurance rights: A primer for oncologists. *Oncology, 13*, 841–852.

Keene, N., Hobbie, W., & Ruccione, K. (2000). *Childhood cancer survivors: A practical guide to your future.* Sebatopol, CA: O'Reilly.

Langeveld, N.E., Stam, H., Grootenhuis, M.A., & Last, B.F. (2002). Quality of life in young adult survivors of childhood cancer. *Support Care Cancer, 10*, 579–600.

Langeveld, N.E., Ubbink, M.C., Last, B.F., Grootenhuis, M.A., Voute, P.A., & De Haan, R.J. (2003). Educational achievement, employment, and living situation in long-term young adult survivors of childhood cancer in the Netherlands. *Psycho-Oncology, 12*, 213–225.

Mitby, P.A., Robison, L.L., Whitton, J.A., Zevon, M.A., Gibbs, I.C., Tersak, J.M., et al. (2003). Utilization of special education services and educational attainment among long-term survivors of childhood cancer. A report from the Childhood Cancer Survivor Study. *Cancer, 97*, 1115–1126.

Van Dongen-Melman, J.E.W.M. (2000). Developing psychosocial aftercare for children surviving cancer and their families. *ACTA Oncologica, 39*, 23–31.

Zebrack, B.J., Zeltzer, L.K., Whitton, J., Mertens, A.C., Odom, L., Berkow, R., et al. (2002). Psychological outcomes in long-term survivors of childhood leukemia, Hodgkin's disease, and non-Hodgkin's lymphoma: A report from the Childhood Cancer Survivor Study. *Pediatrics, 110*, 42–52.

INDEX

Note. Page numbers followed by *f* refer to figures; page numbers followed by *t* refer to tables.
The index uses letter-by-letter alphabetization.

A

B

D

E

F

G

H

I

J

K

L

M

N

O

P

Q

R

U

V

W

X

Y

Z